Anemia: Diagnosis and Treatment

Anemia: Diagnosis and Treatment

Edited by **Rudy Willis**

hayle
medical

New York

Published by Hayle Medical,
30 West, 37th Street, Suite 612,
New York, NY 10018, USA
www.haylemedical.com

Anemia: Diagnosis and Treatment
Edited by Rudy Willis

International Standard Book Number: 978-1-63241-420-5 (Hardback)

The publisher's policy is to use permanent paper from mills that operate a sustainable forestry policy. Furthermore, the publisher ensures that the text paper and cover boards used have met acceptable environmental accreditation standards.

Trademark Notice: Registered trademark of products or corporate names are used only for explanation and identification without intent to infringe.

Printed in the United States of America.

Contents

Preface

Anemia is a condition that arises due to the lack of hemoglobin or red blood cells. Hemoglobin is the factor that binds oxygen to blood and supplies it to all the parts of the body. It may be caused due to decreased production of red blood cells, sudden blood loss, and genetic conditions like sickle cell anemia, etc. Slow anemia results in fatigue, problems in breathing, while a quick anemia may result in unconsciousness and increased thirst. The diagnosis and treatment of this disease involves complete blood count, blood smear test, flow cytometry and providing iron supplements. This book explores all the important aspects related to anemia in the present day scenario. It will provide comprehensive knowledge to the readers. This text includes some of the vital pieces of work being conducted across the world, on various aspects related to anemia. It strives to provide a fair idea about this discipline and to help develop a better understanding of this field. It will serve as an essential guide for hematologists, researchers and students alike.

This book unites the global concepts and researches in an organized manner for a comprehensive understanding of the subject. It is a ripe text for all researchers, students, scientists or anyone else who is interested in acquiring a better knowledge of this dynamic field.

I extend my sincere thanks to the contributors for such eloquent research chapters. Finally, I thank my family for being a source of support and help.

Editor

Presence and Characterisation of Anaemia in Diabetic Foot Ulceration

J. A. Wright,[1] M. J. Oddy,[2] and T. Richards[1]

[1] *Department of Vascular Surgery, Royal Free and University College Hospitals, London, UK*
[2] *Department of Orthopaedic Surgery, University College Hospital, London, UK*

Correspondence should be addressed to J. A. Wright; josephine.wright@nhs.net

Academic Editor: Bruno Annibale

Introduction. Diabetic foot ulceration (DFU) is the commonest cause of severe limb ischaemia in the western world. In diabetes mellitus, anaemia is frequently unrecognized, yet studies have shown that it is twice as common in diabetics compared with nondiabetics. We aimed to assess the incidence of anaemia and further classify the iron deficiency seen in a high-risk DFU patient group. *Methods.* An observational study was undertaken in a multidisciplinary diabetic foot clinic setting. All patients with DFU attending over a four-month period were included. Anaemia was defined as haemoglobin (Hb) levels < 12 g/dL. Iron deficiency was classified according to definitions of AID (absolute iron deficiency) and FID (functional iron deficiency). *Results.* 27 patients had DFU; 14 (51.9%) were anaemic; two (7.41%) had severe anaemia (Hb < 10 g/dL). No patient had B12 or Folate deficiency. In patients with anaemia, there was significant spread of indices. Only one patient had "textbook" absolute iron deficiency (AID) defined as low Hb, MCV, MCH, and ferritin. Functional iron deficiency (FID) was seen in a further seven patients (25.5%). *Conclusion.* Anaemia and iron deficiency are a common problem in patients with DFU. With current clinical markers, it is incredibly difficult to determine causal relationships and further in-depth scientific study is required.

1. Introduction

Since the earliest descriptions by Aretaeus of Cappadocia in the 2nd century AD, "*Diabetes is a dreadful affliction, not very frequent among men, being a melting down of the flesh and limgs [sic] into urine. . .life is short, unpleasant and painful*" [1]; diabetes mellitus remains one of the most serious worldwide health challenges.

Diabetic foot ulceration (DFU) continues to be the commonest cause of severe limb ischaemia in vascular surgery. Up to 25% of diabetic patients are at risk of developing DFU during their lifetime and poor wound healing is a principle reason for morbidity and mortality [2]. Diabetes carries an increased risk of a person undergoing lower extremity amputation over twenty times that of age-matched healthy individuals [3].

The pathophysiology of DFU is complex and the reasons for slow and poor healing are incompletely understood. It is known that micro- and macrovascular disease, dysfunctional glycaemic control, polyneuropathy, foot deformity, altered biomechanics, active infection, inflammation and impaired immunity are of key importance and associated with poor outcome [4]. Clinically, crucial aspects of therapy to promote wound healing include prompt revascularisation, offloading, and treatment of infection [5].

As with many chronic diseases, anaemia is found in diabetes but is frequently unrecognized. Studies suggest that anaemia is twice as common in diabetics compared with nondiabetics [6–8]. Development of anaemia is an additional burden to the microvascular complications of diabetes [9]. To date the association between anaemia and DFU has undergone limited study as most literature investigating diabetes and anaemia has been led by nephrologists and diabetes is the leading cause of "renal anaemia" [10].

The overall adult anaemia "cutoffs" or definitions have been unchanged since 1968. By the time anaemia is detected, iron deficiency is usually advanced. Iron deficiency has consequences even when no anaemia is apparent clinically [11].

Traditionally, anaemic patients have been divided into two groups: those with "iron deficiency anaemia" (IDA) and those with "anaemia of chronic disease" (ACD). IDA is classically defined as microcytic hypochromic anaemia, but ACD can be difficult to diagnose, often considered a diagnosis of exclusion. This is because chronic disease and inflammation are associated with elevated ferritin as part of the acute-phase response. The alternative terminology "anaemia of inflammation" is also in use.

More recently, definitions of "absolute" (AID) and "functional iron deficiency" (FID) have been proposed [12]; see Figures 1(a) and 1(b). FID is characterised by an inflammatory state where iron is gathered by macrophages and stored as ferritin with failure of delivery of iron from the reticuloendothelial system to the bone marrow. Although iron stores appear normal, the pathways for delivery to the place of need (bone marrow) are blocked.

The associations between anaemia and DFU are poorly understood. A previous retrospective study by our group has suggested correlation between anaemia and clinical stage of DFU [13]. To date, there have been no studies that have characterized the cause of anaemia seen in DFU.

2. Aims

Our specific aims were to assess the incidence of anaemia in patients presenting with severe (high-risk) DFU. Secondly, in order to optimize diabetic foot-care and develop therapeutic strategies, we wished to characterize the anaemia seen into AID and FID.

3. Research Design and Methods

A prospective observational study of a consecutive cohort of DFU patients receiving outpatient multidisciplinary diabetic-foot care at a university teaching hospital was undertaken. All patients with severe DFU (Texas classification IIc&d/IIIc&d or Wagner grades 2–5) attending over a four-month period (1 September 2010 to 31 December 2010) were included. As part of their routine medical care, these patients attended initial and 3-month follow-up outpatient diabetic-foot care appointments.

At the initial outpatient diabetic-foot care visit, in all severe DFU patients we assessed the following investigations: blood-tests including haemoglobin (Hb), B12, Folate, iron studies, reticulocyte count, C-reactive protein (CRP), erythrocyte sedimentation rate (ESR), full blood count, renal profile, and glycated haemoglobin (HbA1c). These investigations were repeated at three-month follow-up assessment. Additionally, we assessed outcome of wound-healing status (healed or nonhealed) at three months.

Anaemia was defined as haemoglobin (Hb) levels < 12 g/dL; severe anaemia was defined as Hb <10 g/dL. Classification of DFU patients anaemia at both initial and three-month follow-up assessment was undertaken. Iron deficiency

was classified according to definitions of AID (total body iron depletion) and FID (apparently normal iron stores with inability to mobilise iron from reticuloendothelial system), with blood investigations assessed according to Figure 1(b) and our hospital laboratory normal reference ranges.

At our centre, multidisciplinary diabetic foot care is established with overarching clinical governance and care pathways under vascular surgery. Patient referrals were received directly from three principal primary care trusts with some tertiary referrals nationally. In this study, no patient included underwent diabetic foot care at institutions elsewhere. Those patients taking ferrous sulphate or vitamin supplements continued to do so through the study. Patients with other foot deformities, Charcot foot, gout, and ischaemic or venous ulceration were excluded. Patients requiring renal replacement therapy at the time of study were also excluded as this service was not provided on-site. Approval for this study was granted by our hospital clinical audit department.

Statistical analysis was performed using Prism for Windows version 6.0 (GraphPad Software, La Jolla, CA, USA; http://www.graphpad.com/). Continuous data are expressed as median ± range or mean ± standard deviation as appropriate. For comparisons of both initial and three-month nonanaemic and anaemic patients investigations, Mann-Whitney t-tests (for white blood cell count, creatinine, CRP, and ESR) and unpaired t-tests with welsh correction (for eGFR) were applied. All data were subject to normality testing and two-tailed P values were quoted. Spearman rank correlation was performed to assess presence of relationship between patients initial and three-month follow-up CRP and Ferritin levels, with two-tailed P and R values quoted. To assess associations between anaemia and wound healing and endovascular intervention, Fisher's exact test was performed, with P value quoted.

4. Results

4.1. Demographics. Of the 218 vascular outpatient cases seen, 27 patients with severe DFU (Texas classification IIc&d/IIIc&d or Wagner grades 2–5) were identified over a four-month period. Of these patients, 22 (81.5%) were male; median age was 67 years (range 27–86). Median initial HbA1c of all patients was 62.8 mmol/mol (<30–121.9 mmol/mol). Only 3 patients (16.6%) continued ferrous sulphate treatment throughout the study. No patient underwent blood transfusion within the study period. At three-month followup, a further five patients did not undergo further investigations to determine presence or characterization of anaemia; in one case this was due to hospital admission at another institution, one was due to transfer of outpatient care to another institution, and three patients were lost to followup. No patient died during the study period.

4.2. Initial Presence and Characterisation of Anaemia. Half, 14 patients (51.9%), were anaemic (Hb < 12 g/dL) at initial presentation. Two patients (7.4%) had severe anaemia (Hb < 10 g/dL). The median initial Hb of all patients was

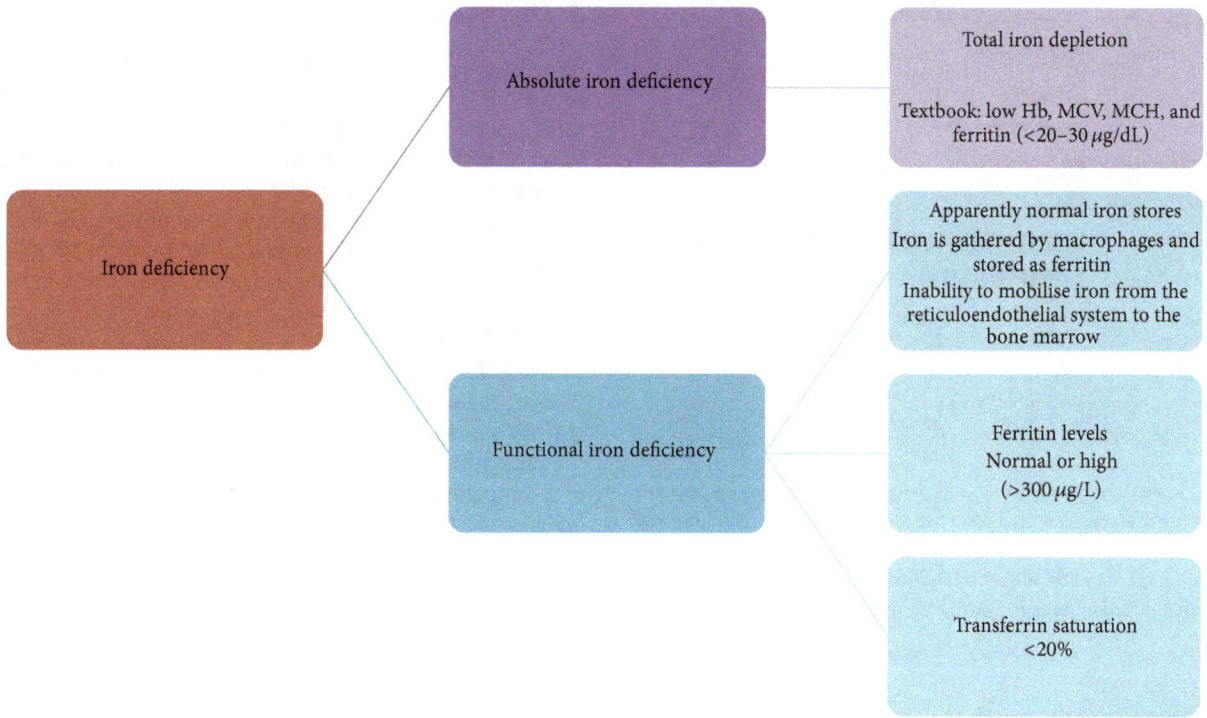

(a)

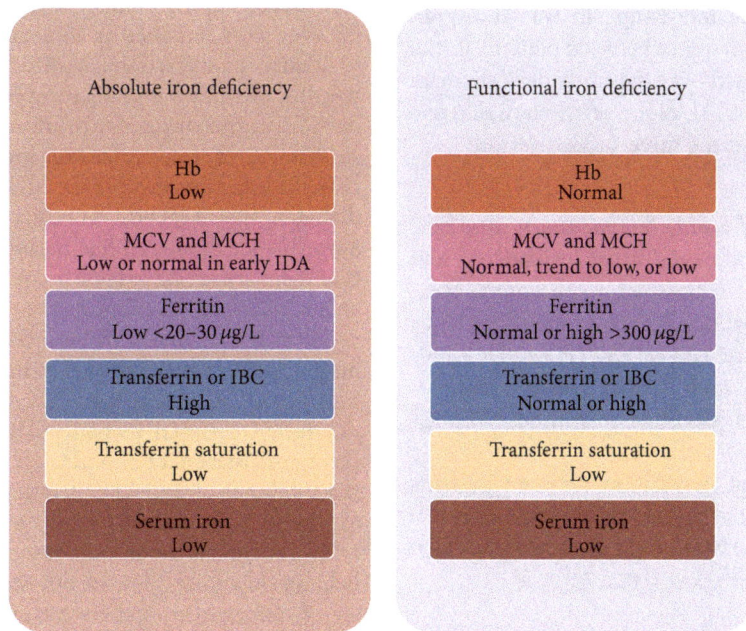

(b)

FIGURE 1: (a) Definitions of iron deficiency. (b) Interpretation of blood investigations in absolute iron deficiency and functional iron deficiency.

11.60 g/dL (range 7.90–16.50 g/dL). Median initial HbA1c of anaemic patients was 67.2 mmol·mol (44.3–102.2 mmol/mol). No patient had B12 or Folate deficiency. In patients with anaemia, there was significant spread of iron studies (see Figure 2 and Table 1). Only one patient had AID. FID was seen in seven "nonanaemic" patients. *Thus for definitions of anaemia and iron deficiency combined, twenty-one (77.8%) severe DFU patients could be classified in this abnormal group.*

4.3. Persistence of Anaemia at Three-Month Followup. At three-month followup, half (50.0%) of the patients were anaemic. In all patients who were initially anaemic

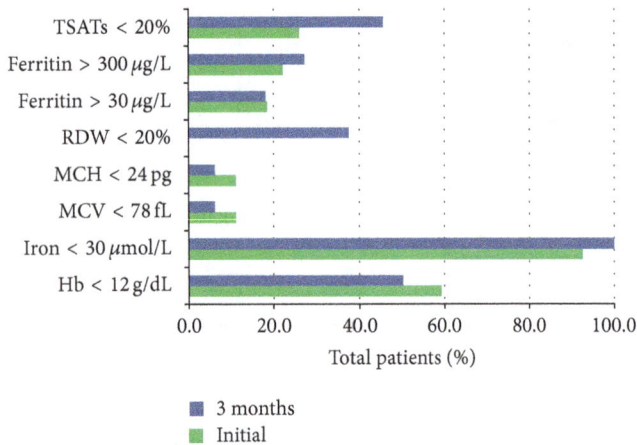

FIGURE 2: Percentage of initial and three-month follow-up patients with abnormal indices and iron studies. *Definitions of abnormal indices listed are indicated on the y-axis. Key: percentage of initial follow-up patients with abnormal indices is indicated in green; three-month follow-up patients are indicated in blue.*

(by definition: Hb < 12 g/dL), their anaemia persisted and did not resolve. The median follow-up Hb was 11.65 g/dL (range 10.0–14.1 g/dL). The difference between patients initial and three-month Hb decreased over the study period; mean decrease was 0.21 g/dL (SD 1.34). None of the nonanaemic patients became anaemic over the three-month period.

4.4. Haematological, Renal, and Inflammatory Markers. There was no significant difference between anaemic and nonanaemic patients' initial white blood cell count, creatinine, eGFR, and C-reactive protein. In anaemic patients, there was a significantly elevated initial ESR ($P = 0.0065$); see Table 2. There was no significant difference between anaemic and nonanaemic white blood cell count, creatinine, eGFR, C-reactive protein, and ESR.

There was no significant correlation between patients CRP or Ferritin levels at initial presentation (*two-tailed P = 0.2149, Spearman rank R = 0.2466*) or at three months (*two-tailed P = 0.5307, Spearman rank R = 0.2270*).

4.5. Relationship between Anaemia, Wound Healing, and Endovascular Intervention. Five patients had healed during the three-month follow-up period. Initial presence or absence of anaemia (Hb < 12 g/dL) was not associated with healing status at three months (*two-tailed P = 0.3705, Fisher's exact test*).

Interestingly, five separate patients required admission for endovascular interventions (including crural angioplasty or stenting), all of whom were anaemic with Hb <12 g/dL (two of these had severe anaemia Hb < 10 g/dL). This association between anaemia and endovascular intervention approached statistical significance, $P = 0.0598$, Fisher's exact test.

5. Discussion

This prospective study showed a high incidence of anaemia in patients with severe DFU. It demonstrates the significant difficulties encountered in the interpretation of iron indices to provide clear classification of anaemia seen in severe DFU.

We found that at initial assessment, sixteen patients (59.3%) were classified as anaemic by definition Hb < 12 g/dL. Only one of these patients had absolute or textbook IDA. This finding is comparable to earlier studies undertaken in developing countries where percentages of DFU patients with IDA range from 49% to 62%. In a cross-sectional study of fifty DFU patients attending a Nigerian hospital, 49% of patients had IDA at the time of their presentation [14]. In a similar prospective case series of forty-seven DFU patients (this patient cohort included Wagner grades 2-3) 57% of patients were classified as "anaemic" [15]. Further cross sectional study of forty-two Nigerian patients with all grades of DFU (Wagner grade 1–5) showed that 61.8% of patients had "anaemia," which was found to be a significant risk factor for in-hospital mortality [16]. Our study in the UK provides some evidence to suggest that the anaemia observed in severe DFU patients may be more than nutritional in its nature.

Additionally, we found that for definitions of anaemia and iron deficiency combined, twenty-one (77.8%) severe DFU patients were classified as abnormal. There was a high initial incidence of altered haematinics and FID. Although the handful of studies investigating anaemia in DFU mentioned above document presence of anaemia, they do not include full assessment of iron indices or attempt classification of DFU patients into those with FID. In a study of UK patients with diabetes, the "Teesside Anaemia in Diabetes Study" found a prevalence of altered haematinics of 40% [17]. We suggest that there are multiple factors contributing to the presence of anaemia in DFU; see Figure 3.

Studies of anaemic diabetic patients have found that they have a higher rate of stroke, ischaemic heart disease, hypertension, and CKD, as mentioned above [18]. In an analysis of seven UK based diabetic patient cohorts, Kengne et al. [19] found that anaemia and CVD conferred similar mortality risks. Studies of patient outcomes in anaemic DFU patients are limited. In a single study of one hundred and eighty DFU patients, anaemia was associated with adverse wound-healing outcomes [20]. In our study, we did not detect any significant association between anaemia and major or minor amputation or mortality. This is likely due to the low numbers of patients included and positive outcomes experienced at our centre which has a proactive multidisciplinary approach to diabetic foot care. Currently, retrospective analysis of existing hospital-based and research databases is virtually impossible owing to lack of haematinic investigations being undertaken and recorded in this severe DFU patient group and hospital coding systems which do not permit identification of those patients suffering from diabetic foot disease.

The impact of anaemia on cardiovascular function in DFU patients has undergone limited investigation. The ACORD trial (Anaemia CORrection in Diabetes) investigated the effects of anaemia correction with epoetin beta

TABLE 1: Initial DFU patients indices and iron studies: functional and absolute iron deficiency.

Indices and iron studies	Nonanaemic patients with functional iron deficiency		Anaemic patients with absolute iron deficiency*		Anaemic patients with abnormal indices and iron studies**	
	Median values	Range	Value	Range	Median values	Range
Haemoglobin g/dL	12.2	12.0–16.5	11.2	—	11.1	7. 0–11.5
MCV fL	91.6	87.1–95.2	72.4	—	93.0	61.6–122.5
MCH pg	29.3	27.0–32.9	21.1	—	29.6	18.6–37.8
RDW %	13.7	12.3–14.5	15.9	—	14.6	13.6–18.7
Ferritin ug/L	131.0	70.0–983.0	13.0	—	125.0	24.0–744.0
Transferrin saturation %	24.0	22.0–49.0	15.1	—	19.0	13.0–45.0
Iron umol/L	12.5	9.0–24.0	8.0	—	12.0	5.0–45.0
Reticulocytes %	1.6	0.5–1.5	0.6	—	1.20	0.6–10.0

Anaemia defined as Hb < 12.0 g/dL. Initial visit patient values presented only. *Only one anaemic patient initially had a text book absolute iron deficiency; hence these data are presented without range. **The remaining thirteen anaemic patients had abnormal iron indices and studies (iron < 30 umol/L, MCH < 24 pg, MCV < 78 fL, RDW < 12%, TSATS < 20%, ferritin < 30 ug/L or >300 ug/L). Normal hospital laboratory reference ranges: MCV fL 80–99; MCH 27.0–33.5; RDW 11.5–15.0; ferritin 300–400 ug/L; transferrin saturation 20–50%; iron 10.6–28.3 umol/L; reticulocytes 0.38–2.64%.

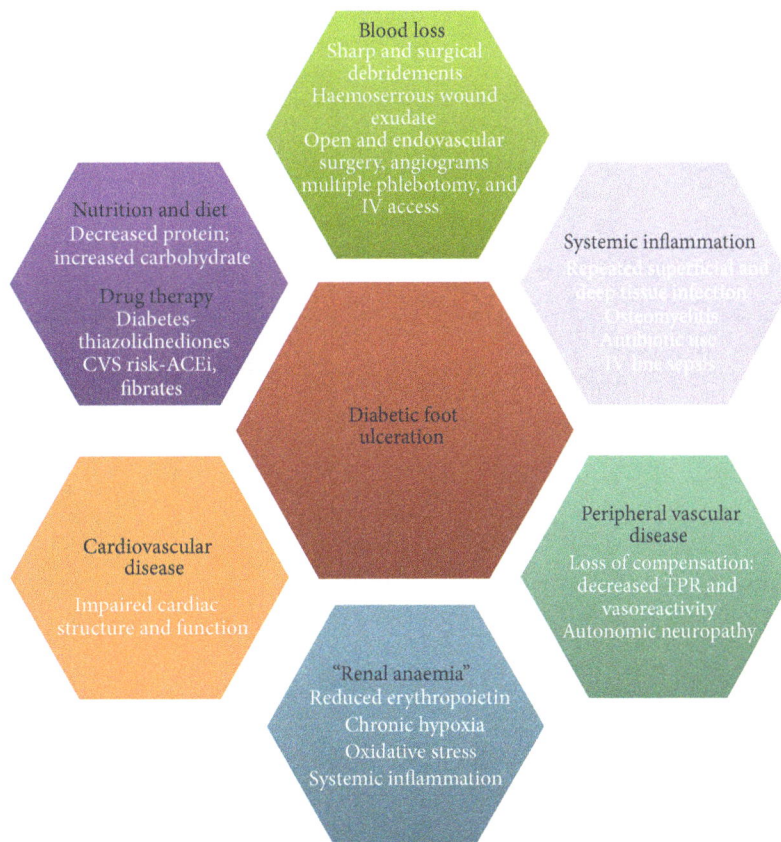

FIGURE 3: Mechanisms contributing to anaemia in poorly healing diabetic foot ulceration.

on cardiac structure and function in patients with early diabetic nephropathy and moderate LVH. Normalisation of Hb level (to target 13–15 g/dL) did not decrease LVMI but did prevent additional increase in LVH and improved quality of life [21]. Further studies in diabetic patients undertaken by Srivastava et al. [22] found that anaemia was associated with cardiac dysfunction and a correlation with plasma markers of cardiac risk, including BNP, CRP, and AVP. Whilst these studies suggest that diabetes-related anaemia is associated with cardiovascular dysfunction, only one study has addressed such cardiovascular dysfunction specifically in a DFU patient cohort [23]. Furthermore, there are no studies that have investigated the effect of iron correction treatment (erythropoietin or IV iron) on DFU healing rates.

TABLE 2: Nonanaemic and anaemic patients initial and three-month follow-up haematological, renal, and inflammatory markers.

| Markers | Initial | | | | | | Three-month followup | | | | | |
| | Nonanaemic patients | | Anaemic patients | | Two-tailed P value | | Nonanaemic patients | | Anaemic patients | | Two-tailed P Value |
	Median values	Range	Median values	Range			Median values	Range	Median values	Range	
White blood cell count ×10^9/L	8.19	6.28–12.78	7.85	4.74–17.05	ns 0.6448		8.70	7.67–18.42	6.87	5.51–12.78	ns 0.2743
Creatinine umol/L	83.0	61.0–234.0	94.0	46.0–364.0	ns 0.6041		86.5	70.0–288.0	109.0	48.0–472.0	ns 0.7618
eGFR mL/min/1.73 sqm	84.0	57.0–90.0	64.5	15.0–90.0	ns 0.1572		78.5	54.0–90.0	59.0	12.0–90.0	ns 0.3536
C-reactive protein (CRP) mg/L	1.70	1.2–49.0	4.50	0.6–84.6	ns 0.4734		8.65	0.6–144.0	3.70	0.6–59.4	ns 0.5596
Erythrocyte sedimentation rate (ESR) mm/hr	5.5	4.0–28.0	14.0	8.0–119.0	** 0.0065		20.0	16.0–20.0	24.0	13.0–86.0	ns 0.5000

Definition of anaemia: Hb < 12 g/dL. Normal hospital laboratory reference ranges: white blood cell count 3–10 × 10^9/L; creatinine 66–112 umol/L; CRP 0–50 mg/L; ESR 1–20 mm/hr. Mann-Whitney t-test applied for comparisons of white blood cell count, creatinine, CRP, and ESR. Unpaired t-test with Welsh correction applied for comparisons of eGFR. **Two-tailed $P < 0.05$.

Patients with severe DFU require multiple endovascular intervention. We found that all severe DFU patients requiring endovascular intervention were classified as anaemic. This finding is consistent with recent literature that has shown that, in diabetic patients with PVD, Hb decline correlates with both clinical symptom deterioration and disease progression [24]. Furthermore, in diabetic patients undergoing open-bypass surgery for PVD, preoperative low Hb is associated with major cardiac events and death [25]. Further study is required to establish causal relationships. The impact of anaemia on both the macrovascular and microvascular diseases seen in DFU requires more specific study.

CKD is an independent risk factor for the development of foot lesions in the diabetic population [26]. We found that there was no significant difference between anaemic and nonanaemic patients' initial and three-month follow-up creatinine and eGFR. This is due to the fact that we did not include DFU patients undergoing renal replacement therapy, as this service is provided at a different hospital site. More recent studies have suggested that screening for anaemia in current diabetes management should be extended. New et al. [27] found that, below an eGFR of $83 \, \text{mL/min/1.73 m}^2$, for every $1 \, \text{mL/min/1.73 m}^2$ fall in eGFR, there was an associated 0.4 (0.3–0.5) g/L fall in haemoglobin. The contribution of "renal-anaemia" to poor wound healing seen in DFU requires further investigation.

We also found that anaemic patients had a significantly elevated initial ESR, although no significant difference was found between anaemic and nonanaemic patients' initial and three-month follow-up white blood cell count and C-reactive protein. In the study by Ekpebegh et al. [16], leucocytosis was shown to be a significant risk factor for inpatient mortality, although association between Hb decline and other inflammatory markers was not described. Our finding of ESR being elevated at initial visit is most likely related to the inflammatory and infective processes occurring in DFU. Although further experimental study of hepcidin levels would be of interest, in order to fully characterize the anaemia seen in severe DFU. Hepcidin binds to ferroportin (iron export protein) present on macrophages leading to iron trapping and further FID [28].

The relationships between anaemia and wound-healing outcomes (wound-healing rates, healing following amputation) are difficult to comment on based on the findings of this study. Only five patients had healed during the three-month follow-up period and presence or absence of anaemia was not associated with healing status at three months. Furthermore, the impact of AID and FID on wound healing could not be determined owing to the current significant difficulties encountered in the interpretation of iron indices; the underlying pathophysiological mechanisms require detailed scientific study.

6. Conclusion

Anaemia and iron deficiency are a common problem in patients with DFU. Identification of both the presence of anaemia and FID in DFU patients is necessary to assess the role of iron replacement and therapeutic strategies. With current clinical markers, it is incredibly difficult to determine causal relationships. In-depth scientific study of the mechanisms underlying poorly healing DFU in the presence of AID and FID is required.

Abbreviations

ACD: Anaemia of chronic disease
IDA: Iron deficiency anaemia
AID: Absolute iron deficiency
FID: Functional iron deficiency
eGFR: Estimated glomerular filtration rate
CRP: C-reactive protein
ESR: Erythrocyte sedimentation rate
ACEi: Ace inhibitor
TSATs: Transferrin saturation.

Conflict of Interests

The authors declare that there is no conflict of interests associated with this paper.

References

[1] J. A. H. Wass, P. M. Stewart, S. A. Amiel, and M. J. Davies, Eds., *Oxford Text Book of Endocrinology & Diabetes*, Oxford University Press, Oxford, UK, 2nd edition, 2002.

[2] N. Singh, D. G. Armstrong, and B. A. Lipsky, "Preventing foot ulcers in patients with diabetes," *The Journal of the American Medical Association*, vol. 293, no. 2, pp. 217–228, 2005.

[3] A. D. McInnes, "Diabetic foot disease in the United Kingdom: about time to put feet first," *Journal of Foot and Ankle Research*, vol. 5, no. 1, article 26, 2012.

[4] J. R. W. Brownrigg, J. Apelqvist, K. Bakker, N. C. Schaper, and R. J. Hinchliffe, "Evidence-based management of PAD & the diabetic foot," *European Journal of Vascular and Endovascular Surgery*, vol. 45, no. 6, pp. 673–681, 2013.

[5] M. Edmonds, "Body of knowledge around the diabetic foot and limb salvage," *Journal of Cardiovascular Surgery*, vol. 53, no. 5, pp. 605–616, 2012.

[6] M. C. Thomas, R. J. MacIsaac, C. Tsalamandris, D. Power, and G. Jerums, "Unrecognized anemia in patients with diabetes: a cross-sectional survey," *Diabetes Care*, vol. 26, no. 4, pp. 1164–1169, 2003.

[7] T. J. Cawood, U. Buckley, A. Murray et al., "Prevalence of anaemia in patients with diabetes mellitus," *Irish Journal of Medical Science*, vol. 175, no. 2, pp. 25–27, 2006.

[8] P. E. Stevens, D. J. O'Donoghue, and N. R. Lameire, "Anaemia in patients with diabetes: unrecognised, undetected and untreated?" *Current Medical Research and Opinion*, vol. 19, no. 5, pp. 395–401, 2003.

[9] M. Thomas, C. Tsalamandris, R. MacIsaac, and G. Jerums, "Anaemia in diabetes: an emerging complication of microvascular disease," *Current Diabetes Reviews*, vol. 1, no. 1, pp. 107–126, 2005.

[10] S. Al-Khoury, B. Afzali, N. Shah et al., "Diabetes, kidney disease and anaemia: time to tackle a troublesome triad?" *International Journal of Clinical Practice*, vol. 61, no. 2, pp. 281–289, 2007.

[11] WHO, *Haemoglobin Concentrations for the Diagnosis of Anaemia and Assessment of Severity*, 2011, http://www.who.int/indicators/haemoglobin.pdf.

[12] T. Richards, "Anaemia in hospital practice," *The British Journal of Hospital Medicine*, vol. 73, no. 10, pp. 571–575, 2012.

[13] M. L. S. Khanbhai, J. A. Wright, S. Hurel, and T. Richards, "Anaemia, inflammation, renal function, and the diabetic foot: what are the relationships?" *The Diabetic Foot Journal*, vol. 15, no. 4, pp. 150–158, 2012.

[14] A. O. Akanji, O. O. Famuyiwa, and A. Adetuyibi, "Factors influencing the outcome of treatment of foot lesions in Nigerian patients with diabetes mellitus," *Quarterly Journal of Medicine*, vol. 73, no. 271, pp. 1005–1014, 1989.

[15] O. A. Ogbera, E. Osa, A. Edo, and E. Chukwum, "Common clinical features of diabetic foot ulcers: perspectives from a developing nation," *International Journal of Lower Extremity Wounds*, vol. 7, no. 2, pp. 93–98, 2008.

[16] C. O. Ekpebegh, S. O. Iwuala, O. A. Fasanmade, A. O. Ogbera, E. Igumbor, and A. E. Ohwovoriole, "Diabetes foot ulceration in a Nigerian hospital: in-hospital mortality in relation to the presenting demographic, clinical and laboratory features," *International Wound Journal*, vol. 6, no. 5, pp. 381–385, 2009.

[17] S. C. Jones, D. Smith, S. Nag et al., "Prevalence and nature of anaemia in a prospective, population-based sample of people with diabetes: teesside anaemia in diabetes (TAD) study," *Diabetic Medicine*, vol. 27, no. 6, pp. 655–659, 2010.

[18] C. X. R. Chen, Y. C. Li, S. L. Chan, and K. H. Chan, "Anaemia and type 2 diabetes: implications from a retrospectively studied primary care case series," *Hong Kong Medical Journal*, vol. 19, no. 3, pp. 214–221, 2013.

[19] A. P. Kengne, S. Czernichow, M. Hamer, G. D. Batty, and E. Stamatakis, "Anaemia, haemoglobin level and cause-specific mortality in people with and without diabetes," *PLoS ONE*, vol. 7, no. 8, Article ID e41875, 2012.

[20] E. N. Hokkam, "Assessment of risk factors in diabetic foot ulceration and their impact on the outcome of the disease," *Primary Care Diabetes*, vol. 3, no. 4, pp. 219–224, 2009.

[21] M. Laville, "New strategies in anaemia management: ACORD (Anaemia CORrection in Diabetes) trial," *Acta Diabetologica*, vol. 41, no. 1, pp. S18–S22, 2004.

[22] P. M. Srivastava, M. C. Thomas, P. Calafiore, R. J. MacIsaac, G. Jerums, and L. M. Burrell, "Diastolic dysfunction is associated with anaemia in patients with type II diabetes," *Clinical Science*, vol. 110, no. 1, pp. 109–116, 2006.

[23] M. Löndahl, P. Katzman, O. Fredholm, A. Nilsson, and J. Apelqvist, "Is chronic diabetic foot ulcer an indicator of cardiac disease?" *Journal of Wound Care*, vol. 17, no. 1, pp. 12–16, 2008.

[24] Y. Dang, Y. Xia, Y. Li, and D. C. W. Yu, "Anemia and type 2 diabetes mellitus associated with peripheral arterial disease progression in Chinese male patients," *Clinical Biochemistry*, vol. 46, no. 16-17, pp. 1673–1677, 2013.

[25] O. A. Oshin and F. Torella, "Low hemoglobin concentration is associated with poor outcome after peripheral arterial surgery," *Vascular and Endovascular Surgery*, vol. 47, no. 6, pp. 449–453, 2013.

[26] S. Lewis, D. Raj, and N. J. Guzman, "Renal failure: Implications of chronic kidney disease in the management of the diabetic foot," *Seminars in Vascular Surgery*, vol. 25, no. 2, pp. 82–88, 2012.

[27] J. P. New, T. Aung, P. G. Baker et al., "The high prevalence of unrecognized anaemia in patients with diabetes and chronic kidney disease: a population-based study," *Diabetic Medicine*, vol. 25, no. 5, pp. 564–569, 2008.

[28] T. Ganz and E. Nemeth, "Hepcidin and iron homeostasis," *Biochimica et Biophysica Acta*, vol. 1823, no. 9, pp. 1434–1443, 2012.

2

Prevalence and Severity of Anaemia Stratified by Age and Gender in Rural India

Gerardo Alvarez-Uria, Praveen K. Naik, Manoranjan Midde, Pradeep S. Yalla, and Raghavakalyan Pakam

Department of Infectious Diseases, Bathalapalli Rural Development Trust Hospital, Kadiri Road, Bathalapalli, Anantapur District, Andhra Pradesh 515661, India

Correspondence should be addressed to Gerardo Alvarez-Uria; gerardouria@gmail.com

Academic Editor: Aurelio Maggio

Anaemia is a major public health problem in India. Although nearly three quarters of the Indian population live in rural areas, the epidemiology of anaemia in rural settings is not well known. We performed a retrospective observational study using routine clinical data from patients attending the out-patient clinics of a rural hospital in India from June 2011 to August 2014. The study included 73,795 determinations of haemoglobin. 49.5% of patients were female. The median haemoglobin concentration was 11.3 g/dL (interquartile range (IQR), 9.8–12.4) in females and 12.5 g/dL (IQR, 10.6–14.2) in males. Anaemia was present in the majority of children <10 years, women after puberty, and older adults. Children <5 years had the highest prevalence of anaemia, especially children aged 1-2 years. The high proportion of microcytic anaemia and the fact that gender differences were only seen after the menarche period in women suggest that iron deficiency was the main cause of anaemia. However, the prevalence of normocytic anaemia increased with age. The results of this study can be used by public health programmes to design target interventions aimed at reducing the huge burden of anaemia in India. Further studies are needed to clarify the aetiology of anaemia among older adults.

1. Introduction

According to the World Health Organization (WHO), there are two billion people with anaemia in the world and half of the anaemia is due to iron deficiency [1]. Anaemia is a late indicator of iron deficiency, so it is estimated that the prevalence of iron deficiency is 2.5 times that of anaemia [1, 2]. The estimated prevalence of anaemia in developing countries is 39% in children <5 years, 48% in children 5–14 years, 42% in women 15–59 years, 30% in men 15–59 years, and 45% in adults >60 years [1]. These staggering figures have important economic and health consequences for low- and middle-income countries. Anaemia and iron deficiency lead to substantial physical productivity losses in adults [2]. Iron deficiency during pregnancy is associated with maternal mortality, preterm labour, low birth-weight, and infant mortality [2]. In children, iron deficiency affects cognitive and motor development and increases susceptibility to infections [3].

Anaemia is a major health problem in India. In the 2005-2006 National Family Health Survey (NFHS-3), a household survey aimed at having national and state representative data on population health and nutrition; the prevalence of anaemia was 70% in children aged 6–59 months, 55% in females aged 15–49 years, and 24% in males aged 15–49 years [4]. Although the NFHS-3 showed that the prevalence of anaemia was higher in rural areas, there is a paucity of data about the epidemiology of anaemia in rural settings [5]. The aim of this study is to describe the prevalence of anaemia among patients who attended the outpatient clinics of a rural hospital in Andhra Pradesh, India.

2. Methods

2.1. Setting. The study was performed in Anantapur, a district situated in the South border of Andhra Pradesh, India. Anantapur has a population of approximately four million

TABLE 1: Haemoglobin concentrations (g/dL) for the diagnosis of anaemia and assessment of severity according to the World Health Organization.

Age	Mild	Moderate	Severe
6–59 months	10–10.9	7–9.9	<7
5–11 years	11–11.4	8–10.9	<8
12–14 years	11–11.9	8–10.9	<8
Female >14 years	11–11.9	8–10.9	<8
Male >14 years	11–12.9	8–10.9	<8

people. In Anantapur, 72% of the population live in rural areas and 36% are illiterate [5]. Rural Development Trust General Hospital is a nonprofit 220-bed hospital in Bathalapalli, a rural village in Anantapur. The hospital belongs to a nongovernmental organization called Rural Development Trust.

2.2. Study Design. We collected epidemiological data (age and sex) and laboratory data from the hospital database of patients who attended outpatient clinics from June 1, 2011, to August 31, 2014. HIV infected patients were excluded. In patients who had more than one determination of haemoglobin during the study period, only one determination per year of age was allowed in order to avoid repeated measurements in the same patient. We used definitions of anaemia according to recommendation from the WHO (Table 1) [6]. Microcytic anaemia was defined according to cut-offs proposed by the US Centers for Disease Control and Prevention (CDC) (1-2 years: <77 fL; 3–5 years: <79 fL; 6–11 years: <80 fL; 12–15 years: <82 fL; >15 years: <85 fL) [7].

The study was approved by the Hospital Ethical Committee. Statistical analysis was performed using Stata Statistical Software (Stata Corporation. Release 12.1 College Station, Texas, USA).

3. Results

The study included 73,795 determinations of haemoglobin from 69,440 patients, of which 34,399 (49.45%) were female. The median haemoglobin concentration was 11.8 g/dL (interquartile range (IQR), 10.2–13.3) and the median age was 25 years (IQR, 12–42). The median haemoglobin concentration was 11.3 g/dL (IQR, 9.8–12.4) in females and 12.5 g/dL (IQR, 10.6–14.2) in males. Haemoglobin concentrations did not change significantly during the duration of the study (Figure 1).

In Figure 2, we present the median concentration of haemoglobin and interquartile range stratified by age and gender. Children aged 6–30 months had the lowest haemoglobin concentrations. Females and males had similar haemoglobin concentrations until the onset of puberty (around age 13 years). After puberty, females had median concentrations of haemoglobin around 11.5 g/dL, whereas males had a rapid increase in haemoglobin concentrations reaching a plateau of about 14 g/dL at age 20 years and experienced a progressive decline after age 40 years.

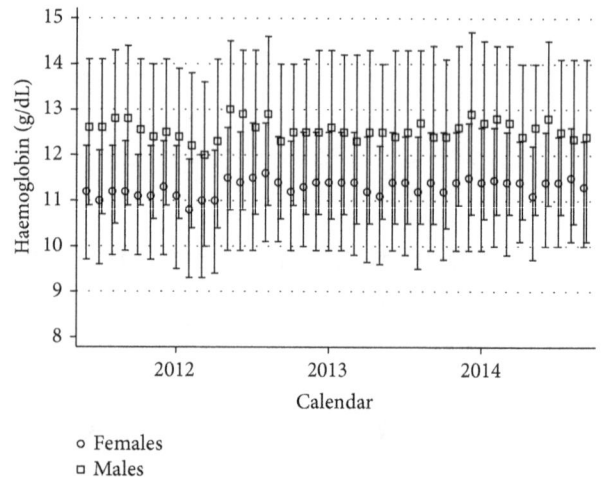

FIGURE 1: Median and interquartile range of haemoglobin concentration stratified by gender and calendar month.

The prevalence of mild, moderate, and severe anaemia is presented in Figure 3. The highest prevalence of mild and moderate anaemia was seen in children <10 years. The highest prevalence of moderate anaemia was seen in children aged 1-2 years. Both female and male children experienced a rapid improvement in the prepuberty period. After puberty, the prevalence of anaemia was constantly over 50% in females, having older women higher prevalence of moderate and severe anaemia than younger women. Males had a peak of anaemia during puberty and a progressive increase of mild, moderate, and severe anaemia with age.

The median and interquartile range of the mean corpuscular volume (MCV) in patients with anaemia is presented in Figure 4. The vast majority of children with anaemia had low MCV and there were no gender differences. In adults with anaemia, males tended to have a higher MCV than women, but differences reduced with age.

The prevalence of macrocytic, normocytic, and microcytic anaemia is presented in Figure 5. In general, macrocytic anaemia was rare. While microcytic anaemia was more prevalent in children and women, the proportion of normocytic anaemia increased progressively with age in male adults and women after menopause age.

4. Discussion

In this retrospective observational study using routine clinical data from a large number of patients attending the outpatient clinics of a rural hospital in India, anaemia was present in the majority of children <10 years, women after the onset of puberty, and older adults.

The high proportion of microcytic anaemia and the fact that gender differences were only seen after the menarche period in women indicate that iron deficiency was the main cause of anaemia. In a study of children aged 12–23 months in two rural districts in India, 72% of children with anaemia had low ferritin levels [8]. Other Indian studies have also shown high prevalence of iron deficiency anaemia among

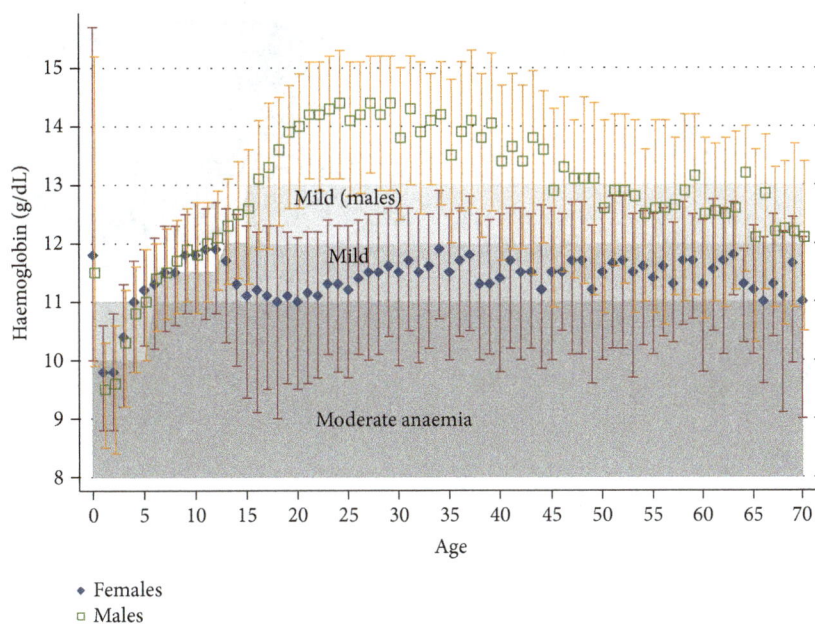

FIGURE 2: Median and interquartile range of haemoglobin concentration stratified by gender and age.

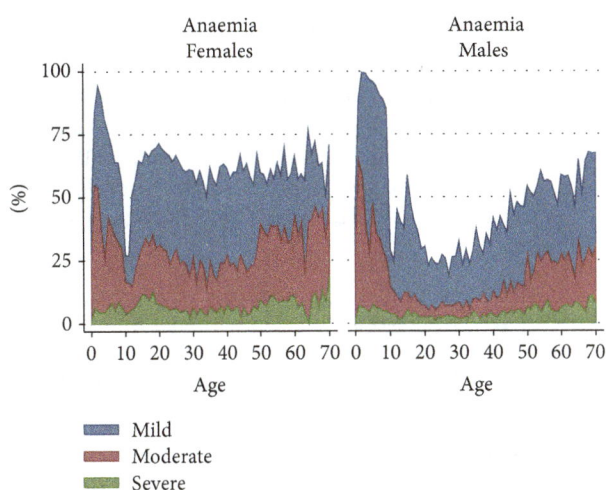

FIGURE 3: Prevalence of mild, moderate, and severe anaemia by age in males and females.

young women [9, 10]. The high prevalence of iron deficiency anaemia among women in childbearing age has important public health implications. It is estimated that anaemia accounts for 12.8% of maternal mortality in Asia [11]. Iron requirements are greater in pregnancy, and iron deficiency is associated with maternal death, preterm delivery, and low birth-weight [12, 13]. In India, only 28% of women consume meat, fish, or eggs on a weekly basis [4], and the iron bioavailability of the vegetarian diet is poor [10, 14]. Effective public health programmes aimed at reducing iron deficiency among young women could have a major impact in reducing maternal and infant mortality [15].

The highest prevalence of anaemia was seen in children <10 years, especially in those <5 years. In India, over

95% of children are breastfed [4]. The WHO organization recommends introducing solid and semisolid food at the age of six months because breastfeeding does not suffice to maintain optimal growth after this age. However, at age 6–8 months only 45% of children receiving breastfeeding are given solid or semisolid food [4, 16]. Moreover, only 10% of breastfeeding children and 20% of nonbreastfeeding children aged 6–35 months eat meat, fish, or eggs [4], which are rich in haem iron with high bioavailability [17, 18]. In the NFHS-3, only 14.6% of children aged 6–35 months consumed food rich in iron in the previous 24 hours of the survey [4]. At this age, the effect of iron deficiency on the neurological development can be not totally reversible [3, 19]. Consequently, the Indian Government recommends iron and folic acid supplementations to younger children [20]. However, the programme implementation has been poor due to lack of logistic planning and accountability [20]. In our study, we did not observe an increase in haemoglobin concentrations during the study period suggesting that the programme has not achieved a reduction in the prevalence of anaemia in our setting. Our results are in agreement with other studies in India [21] and indicate that the iron supplementation programme for children aged <24 months should be better monitored.

In this study, we observed an increased prevalence of anaemia with age. Interestingly, the proportion of normocytic anaemia was highest in older adults, suggesting that other causes than iron deficiency might have contributed to the high prevalence of anaemia in this group. Recent studies have shown the poor bioavailability of vitamin B12 in the typical Indian vegetarian diet [14] and substantial prevalence of vitamin B12 deficiency in Indian patients with anaemia [9, 10, 22]. However, new studies investigating the aetiology of anaemia among older adults are needed.

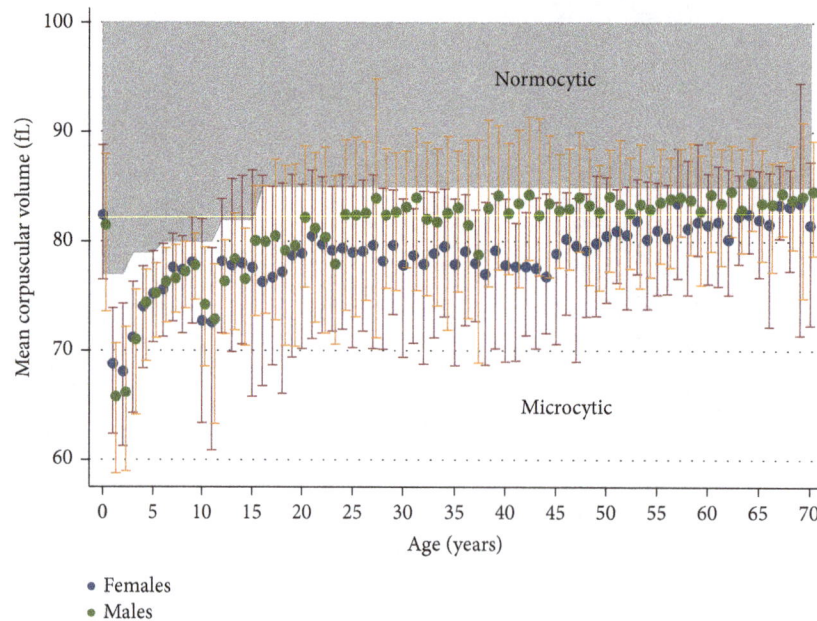

FIGURE 4: Median and interquartile range of the mean corpuscular volume in patients with anaemia stratified by gender and age.

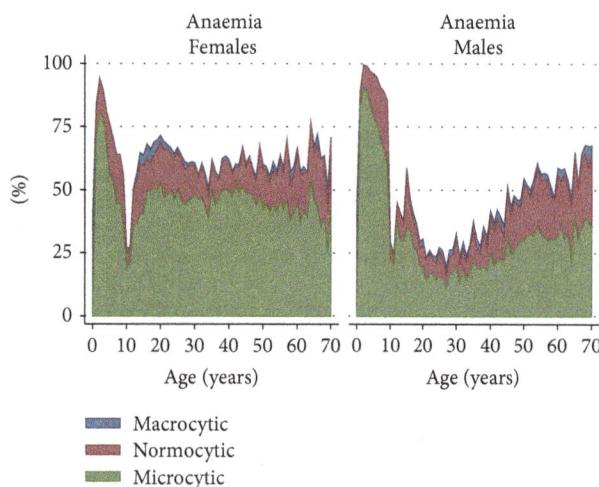

FIGURE 5: Prevalence of macrocytic, normocytic, and microcytic anaemia by age in males and females.

seen in children <10 years followed by women and older adults. The vast majority of anaemia cases were microcytic, suggesting that iron deficiency was the main cause of anaemia. However, the prevalence of normocytic anaemia increased with age, so further studies are needed to clarify the cause of anaemia among older adults. The results of this study can be used by public health programmes to design target interventions aimed at reducing the huge burden of anaemia in India.

Conflict of Interests

The authors declare that they have no competing interests.

References

[1] WHO, UNICEF, and UNU, *Iron Deficiency Anaemia: Assessment, Prevention and Control, A Guide for Programme Managers*, WHO, UNICEF, UNU, Geneva, Switzerland, 2001, http://www.who.int/nutrition/publications/micronutrients/anaemia_iron_deficiency/WHO_NHD_01.3/en/index.html.

[2] M. B. Zimmermann and R. F. Hurrell, "Nutritional iron deficiency," *The Lancet*, vol. 370, pp. 511–520, 2007.

[3] R. D. Baker, F. R. Greer, and Committee on Nutrition American Academy of Pediatrics, "Diagnosis and prevention of iron deficiency and iron-deficiency anemia in infants and young children (0–3 years of age)," *Pediatrics*, vol. 126, pp. 1040–1050, 2010.

[4] F. Arnold, S. Parasuraman, P. Arokiasamy, and M. Kothari, "Nutrition in India," in *National Family Health Survey (NFHS-3) India 2005-06*, 2009, http://www.rchiips.org/nfhs/nutrition_report_for_website_18sep09.pdf.

[5] Office of The Registrar General & Census Commissioner, Census of India, 2011.

The study has some limitations. We used data from patients coming to the hospital to assess the prevalence of anaemia in the population. This might have led to an overestimation of anaemia in our setting. However, we excluded patients admitted to the hospital, and the prevalence of anaemia was similar to the ones reported in Andhra Pradesh in the NFHS-3 (70.8% in children 6–59 months; 62.9% in females 15–49 years; 23.3% in males 15–49 years) [4].

5. Conclusions

In our rural setting, most patients attending out-patient clinics had anaemia. The highest prevalence of anaemia was

[6] WHO, *Haemoglobin Concentrations for the Diagnosis of Anaemia and Assessment of Severity*, WHO, Geneva, Switzerland, 2011, http://www.who.int/vmnis/indicators/haemoglobin/en/.

[7] "Recommendations to prevent and control iron deficiency in the United States. Centers for Disease Control and Prevention," *MMWR Recommendations and Reports*, vol. 47, pp. 1–29, 1998.

[8] S.-R. Pasricha, J. Black, S. Muthayya et al., "Determinants of anemia among young children in rural India," *Pediatrics*, vol. 126, no. 1, pp. e140–e149, 2010.

[9] K. C. Menon, S. A. Skeaff, C. D. Thomson et al., "Concurrent micronutrient deficiencies are prevalent in nonpregnant rural and tribal women from central India," *Nutrition*, vol. 27, no. 4, pp. 496–502, 2011.

[10] P. Thankachan, S. Muthayya, T. Walczyk, A. V. Kurpad, and R. F. Hurrell, "An analysis of the etiology of anemia and iron deficiency in young women of low socioeconomic status in Bangalore, India," *Food and Nutrition Bulletin*, vol. 28, no. 3, pp. 328–336, 2007.

[11] K. S. Khan, D. Wojdyla, L. Say, A. M. Gülmezoglu, and P. F. van Look, "WHO analysis of causes of maternal death: a systematic review," *The Lancet*, vol. 367, no. 9516, pp. 1066–1074, 2006.

[12] K. Kalaivani, "Prevalence & consequences of anaemia in pregnancy," *Indian Journal of Medical Research*, vol. 130, no. 5, pp. 627–633, 2009.

[13] L. H. Allen, "Anemia and iron deficiency: effects on pregnancy outcome," *The American Journal of Clinical Nutrition*, vol. 71, no. 5, pp. 1280s–1284s, 2000.

[14] K. Shridhar, P. K. Dhillon, L. Bowen et al., "Nutritional profile of Indian vegetarian diets—the Indian Migration Study (IMS)," *Nutrition Journal*, vol. 13, article 55, 2014.

[15] Z. A. Bhutta, J. K. Das, R. Bahl et al., "Can available interventions end preventable deaths in mothers, newborn babies, and stillbirths, and at what cost?" *The Lancet*, vol. 384, no. 9940, pp. 347–370, 2014.

[16] C. J. Chantry, C. R. Howard, and P. Auinger, "Full breastfeeding duration and risk for iron deficiency in U.S. infants," *Breastfeeding Medicine*, vol. 2, no. 2, pp. 63–73, 2007.

[17] M. B. Zimmermann, N. Chaouki, and R. F. Hurrell, "Iron deficiency due to consumption of a habitual diet low in bioavailable iron: a longitudinal cohort study in Moroccan children," *The American Journal of Clinical Nutrition*, vol. 81, no. 1, pp. 115–121, 2005.

[18] R. Hurrell, "How to ensure adequate iron absorption from iron-fortified food," *Nutrition Reviews*, vol. 60, supplement 7, pp. S7–S15, 2002.

[19] S. More, V. B. Shivkumar, N. Gangane, and S. Shende, "Effects of iron deficiency on cognitive function in school going adolescent females in rural area of central India," *Anemia*, vol. 2013, Article ID 819136, 5 pages, 2013.

[20] P. V. Kotecha, "Nutritional anemia in young children with focus on Asia and India," *Indian Journal of Community Medicine*, vol. 36, no. 1, pp. 8–16, 2011.

[21] R. K. Singh and S. Patra, "Extent of anaemia among preschool children in EAG States, India: a challenge to policy makers," *Anemia*, vol. 2014, Article ID 868752, 9 pages, 2014.

[22] A. Bhardwaj, D. Kumar, S. K. Raina, P. Bansal, S. Bhushan, and V. Chander, "Rapid assessment for coexistence of vitamin B12 and iron deficiency anemia among adolescent males and females in northern himalayan state of India," *Anemia*, vol. 2013, Article ID 959605, 5 pages, 2013.

3

Hospitalization Events among Children and Adolescents with Sickle Cell Disease in Basra, Iraq

Zeina A. Salman[1] and Meaad K. Hassan[1,2]

[1]*Center for Hereditary Blood Diseases, Basra Maternity and Children Hospital, Basra, Iraq*
[2]*Department of Pediatrics, College of Medicine, University of Basra, Basra, Iraq*

Correspondence should be addressed to Meaad K. Hassan; alasfoor_mk@yahoo.com

Academic Editor: Maria Stella Figueiredo

Objectives. Despite improvements in the management of sickle cell disease (SCD), many patients still experience disease-related complications requiring hospitalizations. The objectives of this study were to identify causes of hospitalization among these patients and factors associated with the length of hospital stay (LOS) and readmission. *Methods.* Data from 160 patients (<14 years old) with SCD who were admitted to the Basra Maternity and Children's Hospital from the first of January 2012 through July 2012 were analyzed. *Results.* The main causes of hospitalization were acute painful crises (73.84%), infections (9.28%), acute chest syndrome (8.02%), and acute splenic sequestration crisis (6.32%). The mean LOS was 4.34 ± 2.85 days. The LOS for patients on hydroxyurea (3.41 ± 2.64 days) was shorter than that for patients who were not (4.59 ± 2.86 days), $P < 0.05$. The readmission rate (23.1%) was significantly higher among patients with frequent hospitalizations in the previous year (OR 9.352, 95% CI 2.011–43.49), asthma symptoms (OR 4.225, 95% CI 1.125–15.862), and opioid use (OR 6.588, 95% CI 1.104–30.336). Patients on hydroxyurea were less likely to be readmitted (OR 0.082, 95% CI 0.10–0.663). *Conclusions.* There is a relatively high readmission rate among patients with SCD in Basra. The use of hydroxyurea significantly decreases the LOS and readmission rate.

1. Introduction

Sickle cell disease (SCD) is a multisystem disease associated with episodes of acute illness and progressive organ damage, and it represents a major public health problem because of its associated morbidity and mortality [1]. The prevalence of sickle hemoglobin (Hb S) in Basra is 6.48%, with a gene frequency of 0.0324% [2].

Patients with SCD have a chronic hemolytic anemia and can suffer from sudden, severe, and life-threatening complications caused by the acute sickling of red blood cells, with resultant pain or organ dysfunction. Repetitive sickling events can result in irreversible organ damage [3]. Children with SCD should be treated by experts, most often pediatric hematologists, for the management of this disease [4].

Comprehensive care and advances in clinical investigations have reduced the morbidity and mortality associated with SCD, especially in young children, and more patients are now surviving into adulthood. Most children with sickle cell anemia (93.9%) and nearly all children with milder forms of SCD (98.4%) now live to become adults [5, 6].

Severe complications of SCD often require hospitalization. The hospitalization of children with SCD constitutes a significant burden on their caregivers. The hospital admission pattern of children with SCD varies in different parts of the world.

Although acute, painful crises account for the majority of admissions in many countries. Infections are still the main cause of admissions in other areas, particularly in developing countries [7–10].

The average rate of painful crises prompting medical evaluation in sickle cell anemia (SCA) is 0.8 crises per year, although it is often treated inadequately in the emergency department [11, 12].

Approximately 40% of patients never seek medical attention for pain, while approximately 5% of patients account for one-third of all painful crises events requiring medical attention [11].

Acute chest syndrome (ACS), another important cause of morbidity and mortality among patients with SCD, refers to a constellation of findings that include a new radiodensity on chest radiograph, fever, respiratory distress, and pain that occurs often in the chest. Because of the clinical overlap between pneumonia and ACS, all episodes should be treated promptly with antimicrobial therapy including at least a macrolide and a 3rd-generation cephalosporin to treat the most common pathogens associated with ACS [4].

Many patients with SCD experience inpatient hospitalization for complications of the disease, with many who are also readmitted. Inpatient hospitalization for all children younger than 5 years was recommended by many centers because of the high risk of infection. In addition, all children, regardless of age, with the following high-risk features should be admitted: temperature above 38.5°C, marked lethargy, chest pain and/or shortness of breath, sudden onset of severe headache or seizures, sudden onset of pallor, abdominal distension, priapism, ill or toxic appearance, pain refractory to home treatment and joint pain, swelling, and redness [4, 11].

Identifying factors that can predict risk of readmission in SCD patients allows for the early diagnosis and treatment of groups particularly at risk, thus decreasing morbidity, improving quality of life, and reducing the SCD-related burden on health services [8].

The current study was conducted to identify the main causes of hospitalization among patients with SCD in Basra and to determine the factors associated with the length of hospitalization and with readmission of children and adolescents with SCD.

2. Patients and Methods

This descriptive study investigated children and adolescents with SCD who were admitted to the hereditary blood disease ward at the Basra Maternity and Children's Hospital for various reasons between the first of January 2012 and the end of July 2012. A total of 160 patients were recruited; their ages ranged from 9 months to 14 years.

The hospitalization event includes one or more than one admission during a period of more than 30 days from the primary admission [13]. According to this definition the total number of hospitalization events was 237.

Clinical data included age at presentation, sex, history of previous hospitalizations, the number of hospitalizations in the previous year, the number of blood transfusions in the previous year, and asthma symptoms. Disease severity was defined as ≥3 admissions and/or ≥3 blood transfusions in the previous year [13, 14].

The residence and educational level of the mother, the father, and the child (if of school age) were also reported. School attendance was assessed in school age children and was divided into regular, irregular, and left school [15].

Patient's medications like hydroxyurea (HU) and opioid, type of SCD according to the results of High Performance Liquid Chromatography (HPLC), diagnosis, and date of discharge were recorded.

Full clinical examinations were conducted for each patient, including a general examination, vital signs measurements, and a systemic examination.

Treatment, length of hospitalization, complications, outcome, and readmissions (if present) for the patient were recorded. Readmission was defined as a hospital admission occurring within 30 days of the primary admission [13].

In the Center for Hereditary Blood Diseases in Basra, we follow many strategies to reduce infections including penicillin prophylaxis for children ≤5 years old and vaccination (*Haemophilus influenzae* type b, meningococcus group C, and pneumococcal polysaccharide vaccine). It is worthy to mention that all aspects of management of these patients are free of charge. However, unfortunately we do not have neonatal screening program in Basra which enables early detection and when possible prevention of complications.

Informed consent was obtained from one or both parents for enrollment in the study. The study was approved by the Ethical Committee of the Basra Medical College.

2.1. Statistical Analysis. Statistical analysis was performed using SPSS program version (20) software. Data were expressed as the mean ± standard deviation (SD). Proportions were compared using cross-tabulations with chi-square tests. t-tests were used for quantitative comparisons and to compare the difference between two means. Comparisons between groups were made by using one-way analysis of variance (ANOVA) tests. A logistic regression analysis (Multinomial Logistic) was also performed using odds ratios (OR) with a 95% confidence interval (CI). For all tests, a P value of <0.05 was considered to be statistically significant.

3. Results

The total number of patients admitted to the general pediatric wards and the hereditary blood diseases ward at the Basra Maternity and Children's Hospital during the study period was 4140. Of these patients, 160 had SCD, with a total of 237 hospitalization events (excluding patients who were readmitted within one month), which constituted 5.75% of the total admissions during the study period.

Of the 160 admitted patients with SCD during the study period, 91 (56.88%) were male, and 69 (43.12%) were female, Table 1. Their ages ranged from 9 months to 14 years, with a mean age (±SD) of 7.97 ± 3.65 years. The majority of admitted patients with SCD had S/β-Thalassemia (81.9%), and 41.25% were between 5 and 10 years old.

The majority of the mothers (68.75%) and 45.61% of the fathers either were illiterate or had received primary school education. One hundred (62.5%) hospitalized patients were of school age; however, only 13% of them regularly attended school.

Acute painful crisis was the most common cause of hospitalization events (73.84%), followed by infection (9.28%), ACS (8.02%), and acute splenic sequestration crisis (ASSC) in 6.32%, Table 2. However, when considering the causes of admission in relation to number of patients both infections and ACS were found to be the second cause of admission (11.8%).

TABLE 1: Selected sociodemographic characteristics of patients.

Variable	SCA		S/β-Thalassemia		Total	
	Number	%	Number	%	Number	%
Age (years)						
≤5	10	6.24	34	21.26	44	27.5
>5–10	14	8.74	52	32.51	66	41.25
>10–14	5	3.12	45	28.13	50	31.25
Sex						
Male	14	8.74	77	48.14	91	56.88
Female	15	9.36	54	33.76	69	43.12
Residence						
Urban	13	8.11	70	43.76	83	51.87
Rural	16	9.99	61	38.14	77	48.13
Educational level of father						
Illiterate	1	0.62	10	6.25	11	6.87
Primary	15	9.36	47	29.38	62	38.74
Secondary	6	3.75	54	33.75	60	37.5
High education	7	5.45	20	12.5	27	16.95
Educational level of mother						
Illiterate	2	1.25	17	10.63	19	11.88
Primary	18	11.23	73	45.64	91	56.87
Secondary	7	4.37	30	18.75	37	23.12
High education	2	1.25	11	6.88	13	8.13
Total	29	18.1	131	81.9	160	100
School attendance for children (number, 100)						
Regular	2	2	11	11	13	13
Irregular	15	15	49	49	64	64
Left	1	1	22	22	23	23

The extremities were the most common site of pain in both sexes (33.4% overall; 10.5% of female patients and 22.9% of male patients), followed by pain in more than one site (30.7%). The least common site of pain was joint pain (0.7%), Figure 1. There were no significant differences between the sexes concerning the site of pain, $P = 0.178$.

The presence of infections was also recorded. Urine cultures for patients with urinary tract infections (UTI) revealed *E. coli* in 5 cases, *Klebsiella* spp. in 2 cases, and *Proteus* spp. in 1 case. Two patients presented with fever, and all available investigations were negative, including a blood culture.

The pattern of admissions in relation to the type of SCD was studied and it was found that there is no significant difference except for ACS which was significantly higher among patients with Hb SS disease compared to those with S/β-Thalassemia, Table 3.

Forty-two (26.25%) patients had no history of blood transfusion. The mean frequency of blood transfusion was 4.43 ± 0.54/year; this frequency was significantly higher among patients with S/β-Thalassemia (5.19 ± 0.64/year) compared to those with SCA (1.00 ± 0.21/year), $P = 0.020$.

Compared to those patients with ASSC, patients with ACS stayed for a significantly longer time at the hospital, $P = 0.030$. The mean LOS for patients on HU was significantly shorter than the LOS for patients who did not receive this drug, $P = 0.032$. However, there was no statistically

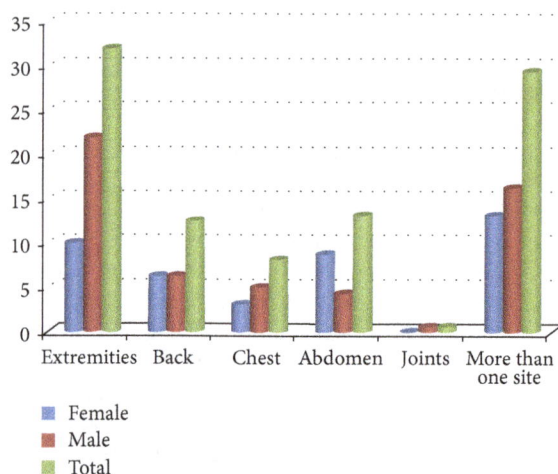

FIGURE 1: Frequency of sickle cell pain by body region and sex. P value $= 0.178$ (chi-square test).

significant difference in LOS in relation to age, sex, or SCD type, Table 4.

Age, sex, type of SCD, LOS, clinical events, and main treatment modalities (blood transfusion, opioid, and HU) provided to children and adolescents with SCD who were

TABLE 2: Causes of hospital admission.

Cause	Admitted patients		Hospitalization events	
	Number	%	Number	%
Acute painful crisis	104	65	175	73.84
ACS/pneumonia	19	11.88	19	8.02
ASSC	13	8.13	15	6.32
Infection				
Urinary tract infection	8	5	10	4.23
Hepatitis A	4	2.5	4	1.69
Gastroenteritis	3	1.88	4	1.69
Fever	2	1.25	2	0.84
Cervical lymphadenitis	2	1.25	2	0.84
Bleeding due to hypersplenism	2	1.25	3	1.27
AVN	1	0.63	1	0.42
Stroke	1	0.63	1	0.42
Neuroblastoma	1	0.63	1	0.42
Total	160	100	237	100

ACS: acute chest syndrome, ASSC: acute splenic sequestration crises, and AVN: avascular necrosis.

readmitted compared to those not readmitted were evaluated. The rate of readmissions among hospitalized patients was 23.1%. The mean LOS for readmitted patients was significantly longer than for patients who were not readmitted, $P = 0.022$, Table 5. A history of ≥ 3 hospitalization in the previous year, asthma symptoms, and opioid use were significant risk factors for readmission, $P < 0.05$. Patients on HU were less likely to be readmitted, $P = 0.006$, Table 6.

4. Discussion

There is still a high utilization of medical resources by patients with SCD despite the reductions in morbidity and mortality associated with early screening and the use of prophylactic antibiotics. Interventions directed at the prevention of SCD complications and hospitalizations may reduce the significant economic burden of the disease [16].

In this study, the hospitalization of patients with SCD constituted about 6% of the total number of hospitalizations in the pediatric wards, excluding patients who were admitted to the Emergency Unit and discharged.

The current study showed that approximately two-thirds of school-aged, hospitalized patients have irregular school attendance and approximately one-fourth of hospitalized patients have left school, most likely because of their illness. Shapiro et al. found that, in the USA, approximately half of school absences of SD patients are associated with SCD-related pain. Other causes of school absences include minor infections, clinic visits, and other medical problems associated with SCD. In addition, families may perceive their

children as vulnerable and keep them out of school for problems that would not interfere with school attendance for most children. SCD-related pain and illness also have been shown to affect the psychosocial function and thus the school attendance of these patients [17].

Acute painful crisis was the most common cause of in-patient hospitalizations of SCD patients in this study. This finding supports results reported by Akar and Adekile in Kuwait (63.2%) [18], Jaiyesimi et al. in Oman (83%) [19], and Brown et al. in Nigeria (61.5%) [7].

Frequent acute painful crises requiring hospitalization are one of the characteristic features of SCD [20]. Individualized pain management in the emergency department is effective in improving the management quality of these crises and is associated with a high level of patient satisfaction and decreases in preventable hospitalizations [12, 20, 21].

In this study, the most common site of pain for both sexes was in the extremities. Similarly, Jaiyesimi et al. in Oman reported that 45% of hospitalized patients with SCD had pain in their extremities [19], and Fosdal and Wojner-Alexandrov in the USA found that the extremities were the most common site of pain. However, Fosdal and Wojner-Alexandrov also found that female patients were the most affected, in contrast with our findings [22].

Infections were found to be the second-leading cause of hospitalization among children and adolescents in Basra, followed by ACS then ASSC. Although infections contributed to a considerable percentage of in-patient hospitalizations, an earlier study in Basra reported a higher rate of infections (21%) among hospitalized children with SCD [23] compared to this study.

Despite the wide use of penicillin prophylaxis, the combination of suboptimal compliance and resistance to penicillin prophylaxis, nonvaccine serotypes of *S. pneumoniae*, and hyposplenism can all explain why children with SCD are still at an increased risk of bacterial infections [24].

ACS was an important cause of hospitalization among both types of SCD in this study. However, it was more common among patients with SCA compared to those with S/β-Thalassemia. This is consistent with research conducted by Hawasawi et al. in Saudi Arabia, who found that ACS was the third-leading cause of hospitalization events among patients with SCD [25], and by Tarer et al. in Guadeloupe, who found it to be the second-leading cause of hospitalization [26].

The LOS among hospitalized patients with SCD in relation to age and sex was not significantly different in Basra. Raphael et al. in the USA found that, after controlling for other factors, older age was the only sociodemographic variable associated with longer LOS [27]. In addition, there was no significant difference in the LOS for patients with both types of SCD, which is consistent with findings by Fosdal and Wojner-Alexandrov in the USA [22].

The mean LOS was longer for patients with ACS than for patients with ASSC. A similar finding was reported by Akar and Adekile in Kuwait, where the LOS for patients with ACS was 5.6 ± 3.3 days, and it was 3.2 ± 2.4 days for ASSC [18].

In this study, the LOS at the hospital was significantly shorter for SCD patients who were on HU compared with those who were not. Patients on HU were also less likely to be

TABLE 3: Causes of admission in relation to type of SCD.

Causes of admission	SCA		S/β-Thalassemia		Total	
	Number	%	Number	%	Number	%
Acute painful crisis	16	55.17	88	67.18	104	65
ACS*	8	27.59	11	8.4	19	11.88
ASSC	2	6.89	11	8.4	13	8.13
Infection						
UTI			8	6.11	8	5
Hepatitis A	1	3.45	3	2.29	4	2.5
Gastroenteritis	1	3.45	2	1.53	3	1.88
Fever			2	1.53	2	1.25
Cervical lymphadenitis	1	3.45	1	0.76	2	1.25
Bleeding due to hypersplenism			2	1.53	2	1.25
AVN			1	0.76	1	0.63
Stroke			1	0.76	1	0.63
Neuroblastoma			1	0.76	1	0.63
Total	29	100	131	100	160	100

*P value = 0.007 (chi-square).
ACS: acute chest syndrome, ASSC: acute splenic sequestration crises, AVN: avascular necrosis, and UTI: urinary tract infection.

TABLE 4: Length of hospital stay in relation to selected variables among patients with SCD.

Variable	LOS (mean ± SD)	P value
Age (year)		
≤5	3.81 ± 2.44	
>5–10	4.63 ± 3.44	0.350
>10	4.42 ± 2.25	
Sex		
Male	4.18 ± 2.62	0.421
Female	4.55 ± 3.14	
Type of SCD		
SCA	4.48 ± 2.16	0.881
S/β-Thalassemia	4.31 ± 2.98	
HU		
Not received	4.59 ± 2.86	0.032
Received	3.41 ± 2.64	
Final diagnosis		
Acute painful crisis	4.10 ± 2.75	
ACS/pneumonia	5.10 ± 2.44	0.030*
ASSC	2.61 ± 0.96	

P value calculated by ANOVA test for age and final diagnosis and by t-test for other variables.
*Significantly different between ACS and splenic sequestration in relation to length of stay.
ACS: acute chest syndrome, ASSC: acute splenic sequestration crises, HU: hydroxyurea, LOS: length of stay, SCD: sickle cell disease, and SCA: sickle cell anemia.

readmitted within 30 days. This can be attributed to the fact that HU improves hematological parameters and decreases the SCD-related complications (mainly acute painful crises), the required hospitalizations, and the LOS [28, 29].

Of all the patients with SCD admitted to the hospital, 23.1% were readmitted within 30 days. This result is higher than that reported by Sobota et al. in the USA (17%) [30].

The readmission rate was significantly higher among patients with ≥3 hospitalizations in the previous year and among patients with asthma symptoms. These results are similar to those reported by Frei-Jones et al. in the USA [13] but in contrast to those reported by Sobota et al. in the USA, who found that asthma was not a risk factor for readmission [30].

Asthma is associated with an increase in SCD-related morbidity. Children with SCA and a clinical diagnosis of asthma had nearly twice as many episodes of ACS and more frequent painful episodes, which are 2 leading causes of hospitalization. Based on the pathogenesis of asthma and the prevalence of airway obstruction and airway liability, ventilation-perfusion mismatching may cause local tissue hypoxia, promote increased sickling of red blood cells, and initiate an ACS or a vasoocclusive pain episode [31].

The current study reported that patients with SCD who received opioids during their hospitalization were more likely to be readmitted, while patients who were on HU were less likely to be readmitted. This result could be because an increase in the levels of acute phase reactants that bind to opioids makes them unavailable to induce pain relief, the development of tolerance to opioids, or changes at the opioid receptor sites [21]. However, Loureiro et al. in Brazil did not find such an association; the only risk factors for readmission found in that study were previous vasoocclusive crises and renal failure [32].

TABLE 5: Readmission among hospitalized patients with SCD.

Variable	Readmission	No readmission	P value
	Number (37)	Number (123)	
Mean age (year) ± SD[*]	8.55 ± 3.53	7.80 ± 3.68	0.272
Mean LOS ± SD[*]	5.45 ± 3.45	4.01 ± 2.56	0.022
	Number (%)	Number (%)	
Sex			
Male	19 (51.35)	72 (58.54)	0.431
Female	18 (48.65)	51 (41.46)	
Type of SCD			
SCA	6 (16.22)	23 (18.70)	0.732
S/β-Thalassemia	31 (83.78)	100 (81.30)	
Final diagnosis			
Acute painful crisis	21 (56.76)	83 (67.48)	
ACS	2 (5.40)	17 (13.82)	0.572
ASSC	3 (8.11)	10 (8.13)	
Hospitalization in previous year			
No	2 (5.41)	42 (34.15)	
<3	9 (24.32)	41 (33.33)	0.000
≥3	26 (70.27)	40 (32.52)	
Blood transfusion in previous year			
No	5 (13.51)	37 (30.10)	
<3	13 (35.14)	50 (40.70)	0.027
≥3	19 (51.35)	36 (29.30)	
Blood transfusion during admission			
Not received	19 (51.35)	64 (52.03)	0.942
Received	18 (48.65)	59 (47.97)	
Asthma symptom			
No	16 (43.24)	88 (71.54)	0.002
Yes	21 (56.75)	35 (28.46)	
Opioid received			
No	19 (51.35)	113 (91.87)	0.000
Yes	18 (48.65)	10 (8.13)	
HU received			
No	33 (89.19)	93 (75.61)	0.077
Yes	4 (10.81)	30 (24.39)	

[*]P values for age and LOS were assessed by t-test and for other variables by chi-square.
ACS: acute chest syndrome, ASSC: acute splenic sequestration crises, HU: hydroxyurea, LOS: length of stay, SCD: sickle cell disease, and SCA: sickle cell anemia.

Most patients were discharged in good health, and no deaths were reported in this study. This result could be related to the severity of the disease or to the short study period.

The main limitation of this study is its short duration. A longer duration may have revealed other causes of morbidity, and it would have enabled the assessment of mortality among these patients.

It can be concluded from this study that although acute painful crises were the most common cause of hospitalization and readmission among patients with SCD, infections were still reported in a significant proportion of patients with SCD. In addition, there was a relatively high rate of readmission, and the use of HU was associated with shorter LOS and fewer hospital readmissions.

Disclaimer

The findings of this study are those of the authors and do not necessarily represent the official position of the Center for Hereditary Blood Diseases.

TABLE 6: Logistic regression analysis of different variables with readmission.

| Variable | OR | 95% (CI) | | P value |
		Lower	Upper	
Age (years)	0.674	0.105	4.327	0.911
LOS	1.073	0.048	24.032	0.688
Sex	0.352	0.087	1.444	0.141
Type of SCD	0.431	0.076	2.445	0.350
Acute painful crisis	1.608	0.150	17.209	0.221
Hospitalization in previous year ≥ 3	9.352	2.011	43.490	0.001
Blood transfusion in previous year ≥ 3	3.325	0.477	23.163	0.393
Asthma symptoms	4.225	1.125	15.862	0.028
Opioid received	6.588	1.104	30.336	0.000
HU received	0.082	0.010	0.663	0.006

HU: hydroxyurea, LOS: length of stay, and SCD: sickle cell disease.

Conflict of Interests

The authors declare no conflict of interests.

Acknowledgments

The authors would like to thank Dr. Assad Yehia, Professor of Animal Production, College of Agriculture, and Dr. Narjis Abd-AL Hasan Ajeel, Professor of Community Medicine, College of Medicine, University of Basra, for their great help in the statistical analysis of the data.

References

[1] R. D. Cançado, "Sickle cell disease: looking back but towards the future," *Revista Brasileira de Hematologia e Hemoterapia*, vol. 34, no. 3, pp. 175–177, 2012.

[2] M. K. Hassan, J. Y. Taha, L. M. Al-Naama, N. M. Widad, and S. N. Jasim, "Frequency of haemoglobinopathies and glucose-6-phosphate dehydrogenase deficiency in Basra," *Eastern Mediterranean Health Journal*, vol. 9, no. 1-2, pp. 45–54, 2003.

[3] A. M. Brandow and R. I. Liem, "Sickle cell disease in the emergency department: atypical complications and management," *Clinical Pediatric Emergency Medicine*, vol. 12, no. 3, pp. 202–212, 2011.

[4] M. R. De Baun, M. Frei-Jones, and E. Vichinsky, "Hemglobinobathies," in *Nelson TextBook of Pediatrics*, E. R. Behrman, R. M. Kliegman, and H. B. Jenson, Eds., pp. 1663–1670, Elsevier Saunders, Philadelphia, Pa, USA, 19th edition, 2011.

[5] R. Colombatti, M. Montanaro, F. Guasti et al., "Comprehensive care for sickle cell disease immigrant patients: a reproducible model achieving high adherence to minimum standards of care," *Pediatric Blood and Cancer*, vol. 59, no. 7, pp. 1275–1279, 2012.

[6] C. T. Quinn, Z. R. Rogers, T. L. McCavit, and G. R. Buchanan, "Improved survival of children and adolescents with sickle cell disease," *Blood*, vol. 115, no. 17, pp. 3447–3452, 2010.

[7] B. J. Brown, N. E. Jacob, I. A. Lagunju, and O. O. Jarrett, "Morbidity and mortality pattern in hospitalized children with sickle cell disorders at the University College Hospital, Ibadan, Nigeria," *Nigerian Journal of Paediatrics*, vol. 40, no. 1, pp. 34–39, 2013.

[8] G. Aljuburi, A. A. Laverty, S. A. Green, K. J. Phekoo, D. Bell, and A. Majeed, "Socio-economic deprivation and risk of emergency readmission and inpatient mortality in people with sickle cell disease in England: observational study," *Journal of Public Health*, vol. 35, no. 4, pp. 510–517, 2013.

[9] C. Booth, B. Inusa, and S. K. Obaro, "Infection in sickle cell disease: a review," *International Journal of Infectious Diseases*, vol. 14, no. 1, pp. e2–e12, 2010.

[10] A. N. Ikefuna and I. J. Emodi, "Hospital admission of patients with sickle cell anaemia pattern and outcome in Enugu area of Nigeria," *Nigerian Journal of Clinical Practice*, vol. 10, no. 1, pp. 24–29, 2007.

[11] P. Lanskowsky, S. Arkin, M. Atlas, B. Aygun, and D. Friedman, "Hemoglobin defects, sickle cell disease," in *Manual of Pediatric Hematology and Oncology*, P. Lanzkowsky, Ed., pp. 200–224, Academic Press, 5th edition, 2011.

[12] L. Krishnamurti, B. Smith-Packard, A. Gupta, M. Campbell, S. Gunawardena, and R. Saladino, "Impact of individualized pain plan on the emergency management of children with sickle cell disease," *Pediatric Blood and Cancer*, vol. 61, no. 10, pp. 1747–1753, 2014.

[13] M. J. Frei-Jones, J. J. Field, and M. R. DeBaun, "Risk factors for hospital readmission within 30 days: a new quality measure for children with sickle cell disease," *Pediatric Blood and Cancer*, vol. 52, no. 4, pp. 481–485, 2009.

[14] D. Jain, K. Italia, V. Sarathi, K. Ghoshand, and R. Colah, "Sickle cell anemia from central India: a retrospective analysis," *Indian Pediatrics*, vol. 49, no. 11, pp. 911–913, 2012.

[15] S. S. Al Arrayed and N. Haites, "Features of sickle cell disease in Bahrain," *Eastern Mediterranean Health Journal*, vol. 1, no. 1, pp. 112–119, 1995.

[16] T. L. Kauf, T. D. Coates, L. Huazhi, N. Mody-Patel, and A. G. Hartzema, "The cost of health care for children and adults with sickle cell disease," *American Journal of Hematology*, vol. 84, no. 6, pp. 323–327, 2009.

[17] B. S. Shapiro, D. F. Dinges, E. C. Orne et al., "Home management of sickle cell-related pain in children and adolescents: natural history and impact on school attendance," *Pain*, vol. 61, no. 1, pp. 139–144, 1995.

[18] N. A. Akar and A. Adekile, "Ten-year review of hospital admissions among children with sickle cell disease in Kuwait," *Medical Principles and Practice*, vol. 17, no. 5, pp. 404–408, 2008.

[19] F. Jaiyesimi, R. Pandey, D. Bux, Y. Sreekrishna, F. Zaki, and N. Krishnamoorthy, "Sickle cell morbidity profile in Omani children," *Annals of Tropical Paediatrics*, vol. 22, no. 1, pp. 45–52, 2002.

[20] Y. Lamarre, M. Romana, X. Waltz et al., "Hemorheological risk factors of acute chest syndrome and painful vaso-occlusive crisis in children with sickle cell disease," *Haematologica*, vol. 97, no. 11, pp. 1641–1647, 2012.

[21] S. K. Ballas, "Current issues in sickle cell pain and its management," *Hematology/the Education Program of the American Society of Hematology*, vol. 2007, no. 1, pp. 97–105, 2007.

[22] M. B. Fosdal and A. W. Wojner-Alexandrov, "Events of hospitalization among children with sickle cell disease," *Journal of Pediatric Nursing*, vol. 22, no. 4, pp. 342–346, 2007.

[23] I. A. Ali and M. K. Hassan, "Sickle cell syndrome in children in Basrah," *Medical Journal of Tikrit*, vol. 5, pp. 10–15, 1999.

[24] S. Chakravorty and T. N. Williams, "Sickle cell disease: a neglected chronic disease of increasing global health importance," *Archives of Disease in Childhood*, vol. 100, no. 1, pp. 48–53, 2015.

[25] Z. M. Hawasawi, G. Nabi, M. S. F. Al Magamci, and K. S. Awad, "Sickle cell disease in childhood in Madina," *Annals of Saudi Medicine*, vol. 18, no. 4, pp. 293–295, 1998.

[26] V. Tarer, M. Etienne-Julan, J.-P. Diara et al., "Sickle cell anemia in Guadeloupean children: pattern and prevalence of acute clinical events," *European Journal of Haematology*, vol. 76, no. 3, pp. 193–199, 2006.

[27] J. L. Raphael, B. U. Mueller, M. A. Kowalkowski, and S. O. Oyeku, "Shorter hospitalization trends among children with sickle cell disease," *Pediatric Blood and Cancer*, vol. 59, no. 4, pp. 679–684, 2012.

[28] S. K. Ballas, R. L. Bauserman, W. F. McCarthy, O. L. Castro, W. R. Smith, and M. A. Waclawiw, "Hydroxyurea and acute painful crises in sickle cell anemia: effects on hospital length of stay and opioid utilization during hospitalization, outpatient acute care contacts, and at home," *Journal of Pain and Symptom Management*, vol. 40, no. 6, pp. 870–882, 2010.

[29] M. Mulaku, N. Opiyo, J. Karumbi, G. Kitonyi, G. Thoithi, and M. English, "Evidence review of hydroxyurea for the prevention of sickle cell complications in low-income countries," *Archives of Disease in Childhood*, vol. 98, no. 11, pp. 908–914, 2013.

[30] A. Sobota, D. A. Graham, E. J. Neufeld, and M. M. Heeney, "Thirty-day readmission rates following hospitalization for pediatric sickle cell crisis at freestanding children's hospitals: risk factors and hospital variation," *Pediatric Blood & Cancer*, vol. 58, no. 1, pp. 61–65, 2012.

[31] J. H. Boyd, E. A. Macklin, R. C. Strunk, and M. R. DeBaun, "Asthma is associated with acute chest syndrome and pain in children with sickle cell anemia," *Blood*, vol. 108, no. 9, pp. 2923–2927, 2006.

[32] M. M. Loureiro, S. Rozenfeld, M. S. Carvalho, and R. D. Portugal, "Factors associated with hospital readmission in sickle cell disease," *BMC Blood Disorders*, vol. 9, article 2, 2009.

4

Assessment of Serum Zinc Levels of Patients with Thalassemia Compared to Their Siblings

Mohamed El Missiry,[1] Mohamed Hamed Hussein,[1] Sadaf Khalid,[1] Naila Yaqub,[2] Sarah Khan,[2] Fatima Itrat,[2] Cornelio Uderzo,[1] and Lawrence Faulkner[1]

[1] *Cure2Children Foundation, Via Marconi 30, 50131 Florence, Italy*
[2] *Children's Hospital Pakistan Institute of Medical Sciences, Islamabad, Pakistan*

Correspondence should be addressed to Mohamed El Missiry; mohamed.elmissiry@cure2children.org

Academic Editor: Aurelio Maggio

Zinc (Zn) is essential for appropriate growth and proper immune function, both of which may be impaired in thalassemia children. Factors that can affect serum Zn levels in these patients may be related to their disease or treatment or nutritional causes. We assessed the serum Zn levels of children with thalassemia paired with a sibling. Zn levels were obtained from 30 children in Islamabad, Pakistan. Serum Zn levels and anthropometric data measures were compared among siblings. Thalassemia patients' median age was 4.5 years (range 1–10.6 years) and siblings was 7.8 years (range 1.1–17 years). The median serum Zn levels for both groups were within normal range: 100 μg/dL (10 μg/dL–297 μg/dL) for patients and 92 μg/dL (13 μg/dL–212 μg/dL) for siblings. There was no significant difference between the two groups. Patients' serum Zn values correlated positively with their corresponding siblings ($r = 0.635$, $P < 0.001$). There were no correlations between patients' Zn levels, height for age Z-scores, serum ferritin levels, chelation, or blood counts (including both total leukocyte and absolute lymphocyte counts). Patients' serum Zn values correlated with their siblings' values. In this study, patients with thalassemia do not seem to have disease-related Zn deficiency.

1. Introduction

Zinc (Zn) is an essential element for cell growth, differentiation, and survival. It is a structural element of many proteins [1]. Zinc affects growth in children. It is known that adequate zinc levels in the body are essential for maintaining suitable levels of growth hormone and insulin-like growth factor in the body [2]. Impairment of zinc levels will consequently lead to growth hormone decrease. Zinc supplement is given to children on growth hormone replacement therapy. In addition, zinc is important for nucleic acid synthesis, cell division, and metabolism of lipids, proteins and carbohydrates. It is also essential in bone homeostasis and bone growth as well as in the maintenance of connective tissues. Decreased Zn may compromise growth and immune functions [2, 3].

Zn is known to be important for the integrity of the immune system, although its role and mechanism of action are not fully understood [1, 4–6]. Zn deficiency affects the adaptive immune system and results in thymus atrophy, lymphopenia, and impaired lymphocyte function [4, 7, 8].

Zinc deficiency is prevalent in children of developing countries where food is often vegetable-based and rarely includes animal products. Zinc is easily absorbed with animal proteins, while excess plant meals lead to decreased zinc absorption due to its binding to phytates [9, 10]. In such countries, Zn deficiency results in growth retardation, hypogonadism, and increased mortality and morbidly from infection-related diarrhea and pneumonia due to compromised immune function [4, 9].

Despite deficits of several specific micronutrients reported in children with thalassemia major, Zn studies yielded conflicting results [7, 11, 12]. Several factors contribute to zinc deficiency in thalassemia. One of these most important factors is chelation therapy. Chelators, namely, deferoxamine and deferiprone, may contribute to Zn deficiency in thalassemia as they tend to eliminate positive divalent ions, like iron and Zn, into urine [7, 13, 14]. On the other side, some studies showed no significant correlation between zinc level and short stature, serum ferritin level, desferrioxamine dose, age at first blood transfusion, and chelation therapy [7]. Zinc can be normal in some patients especially those who are on regular blood transfusions [7, 11, 12]. What is notable that these studies were performed on adequately treated patients subjects which is not the case in many thalassemia affected areas where access to treatment is not always possible.

In the present study, we aimed to assess serum Zn levels in patients with thalassemia and their siblings in a lower middle income country, namely, Pakistan (http://data.worldbank.org/country/pakistan), to determine whether Zn deficiency is present and, if so, if it is related to the disease per se, the use of chelation or to nutritional factors.

2. Patients and Methods

The present study was performed at the Children's Hospital of the Pakistan Institute of Medical Sciences (PIMS), Islamabad, Pakistan, between June 2009 and February 2012. A total of 30 patients with β-thalassemia major and 30 siblings were included. Parental informed consent was obtained. The following data were obtained from the patients' clinical file records: blood transfusion history, last ferritin measurement, onset of chelation therapy and type of chelation used, and infection profile. In addition to serum Zn levels, anthropometric measures such as height, weight, and body mass index (BMI) (BMI = weight (kg)/height^2 (m^2) were obtained).

Sampling and processing: Three mL of peripheral venous blood was withdrawn from each patient and sibling in the early morning, three hours before having breakfast. The samples were left for 20 minutes to clot at room temperature and then centrifuged at 2000 ×g for 10 minutes, and sera were separated and put into aliquots which were stored at −70°C till they were analyzed by atomic absorption spectrometer (AAS; AA300). Zn normal values were estimated to lie between 65 and 120 μg/dL [15].

Statistical analyses were performed by parametric single and paired t-test (after the run of normality test to check that data is normally distributed) and Pearson's correlation coefficient test. A P value ≤ 0.05 was considered to be statistically significant.

3. Results

Median patient age was 4.5 years (ranging from 1 to 10.6 years) and median sibling age was 7.3 years (ranging from 1.1 to 17 years). Patients' serum Zn ranged from 10 μg/dL to 297 μg/dL (median 100 μg/dL), while siblings' serum Zn ranged from 13 μg/dL to 212 μg/dL (median 92 μg/dL) (Figure 1). There were no significant differences in Zn levels between the patients and their corresponding siblings (P = 0.19) on matched pair analysis (Table 1). However, it was found that Zn levels were significantly correlated between patients with their corresponding siblings (r correlation coefficient = 0.63, $P < 0.0001$) (Figure 2).

After measuring the height for age Z-scores for the 30 patients with thalassemia, it was found that heights ranged between −4.2 at minimum and 1.09 at maximum (median = −1.5). Height for age Z-scores and Zn levels did not correlate (r = 0.05).

For siblings, the median height for age Z-scores was −1.2 and ranged from −3.78 to 2.6 (median = −1.2). A comparison of patient height for age Z-scores with corresponding values for siblings revealed that patients' Z-scores levels were significantly lower than corresponding siblings (P = 0.02). Correlation between the two groups was weakly positive (r = 0.4), and pairing between the two groups was statistically significant (P = 0.01).

The median patient serum ferritin level was 2065 ng/mL (range: 5475 ng/mL–81.15 ng/mL) and showed no correlation with patients' Zn level (P = 0.7).

Regular chelation therapy was used by 14 patients: 7 cases were on deferasirox and 7 cases on desferrioxamine, while 16 cases received no chelation therapy. No significant difference in Zn levels was found between chelated and nonchelated groups (median zinc levels were 103.5 μg/dL and 96 μg/dL for chelated and nonchelated patients, respectively, P = 0.63). There was also no significant difference in zinc values between patients on desferrioxamine and those on deferasirox (median zinc levels were 96 μg/dL and 102 μg/dL for patients with desferrioxamine and deferasirox, respectively, P = 0.37).

Absolute lymphocytic count (ALC) ranged between 817 and 9040 microL, with a median of 3882 microL. No correlation was found between patients' Zn values and ALC (r = 0.36).

4. Discussion

Zinc is an essential element for growth and immunity. In this study we aimed to compare serum Zn levels between thalassemia patients and their healthy siblings as to assess whether a possible deficiency is influenced by the disease itself or by nutritional and familial/environmental causes.

Patients' and siblings' Zn median values were within the normal range (median values were 100 μg/dL and 92 μg/dL for patients and siblings, resp.) with no significant difference (patients' serum Zn median value was 100 μg/dL versus 92 μg/dL for siblings) (Figure 1). This finding is in agreement with studies by Rea et al. (1984) [12] and Donma et al. (1990) [11] who noted that the serum Zn levels of patients with thalassemia can be higher than normal [11, 12]. Among the 30 siblings in this study, 18 were carriers for beta thalassemia and 12 were not with no significant differences between the two groups, suggesting that Zn status is not related to thalassemia—the disease itself or trait. The patients' Zn values in this study correlated significantly with corresponding siblings (r correlation coefficient − 0.63, $P < 0.0001$) (Figure 2) suggesting that Zn level was not influenced by thalassemia or its treatment [7], but rather seems more likely related to familial factors either genetic or nutritional/environmental [7].

No correlation between Zn values and growth (height for age Z-scores) was observed in our patients. Similar results

TABLE 1: (a) A collective table for the data of the patients: zinc level in μg/dL, sex (m: male, f: female), age (in years), height (in cm), height-age z-score, ferritin level (in ng/mL), chelation type, and ALC (in microL). (b) A collective table for the data of the patients: zinc level in μg/dL, sex (m: male, f: female), age (in years), height (in cm), and height-age z-score.

(a)

Patient number	Zinc level (μg/dL)	Sex	Age (years)	Height (cm)	Height-age z-score	Ferritin (ng/mL)	Chelation	ALC (microL)
1	94	m	2.6	84	−1.33	694	None	6325
2	58	m	2.9	92	−0.97	2527	None	6200
3	68	f	5.3	100	−2.29	3004	Deferasirox	3903
4	297	m	2.5	92	−0.04	785	None	3891
5	130	m	1	72	−2	641	None	7956
6	66	m	5.5	106	−1.51	2129	Deferoxamine	2156
7	102	f	2.5	91	−1	2000	Deferasirox	8024
8	80	f	8.8	122	−1.57	3513	Deferoxamine	2340
9	109	m	3.8	88	−4	1551	None	7526
10	157	m	4.4	106	−1	2425	Deferoxamine	3872
11	120	m	8.2	115	−2.31	1502	Deferoxamine	3008
12	74	m	2.5	89	−1.17	616	None	4884
13	127	m	5.4	105	−1.48	3810	None	3570
14	75	f	4	95	−1.79	1150	None	1700
15	117	f	4.6	111	0.92	1804	Deferasirox	1218
16	295	m	1.9	81	−1.6	850	None	9040
17	88	m	10.6	131	−1.5	5475	Deferasirox	1160
18	116	f	4	95	−2	2836	None	2813
19	17	m	4.7	113	1.09	658	None	2592
20	111	m	5.6	109	−1.18	2411	Deferoxamine	5002
21	112	m	7.1	114	−1.53	1951	None	1353
22	10	m	1.6	72	−4.2	81.15	None	817
23	79	m	2.2	83	−1.9	2621	None	5490
24	15	f	5	110	0.14	5036	Deferoxamine	1980
25	97	f	10	124	−2.32	706	Deferasirox	4312
26	96	f	10.4	139	−0.32	4487	Deferoxamine	3062
27	120	m	4.5	106	−0.33	5054	None	3180
28	105	f	7.4	117	−1.41	1760	Deferasirox	4260
29	98	m	1.3	75	−1.9	3812	None	5535
30	260	m	4.4	98	−2.01	4100	Deferasirox	3944

(b)

Sibling number	Zinc level (μg/dL)	Sex	Age (years)	Height (cm)	Height-age z-score	Sibling carrier status
Sibling of 1	25	f	12.0	143	−1.23	Not a carrier
Sibling of 2	75	m	5.9	128	2.62	Carrier
Sibling of 3	28	f	9.4	127	−1.31	Not a carrier
Sibling of 4	203	m	6.2	108	−1.85	Not a carrier
Sibling of 5	68	f	11.5	136	−1.8	Carrier
Sibling of 6	35	m	2.4	89	−0.48	Carrier
Sibling of 7	151	f	1.1	77	0.74	Not a carrier
Sibling of 8	89	m	4.1	108	0.95	Carrier
Sibling of 9	212	f	8.7	117	−2.24	Carrier
Sibling of 10	194	f	12.4	150	−0.53	Carrier

(b) Continued.

Sibling number	Zinc level (μg/dL)	Sex	Age (years)	Height (cm)	Height-age z-score	Sibling carrier status
Sibling of 11	138	m	6.9	110	−2.16	Not a carrier
Sibling of 12	72	m	6.9	119	−0.41	Carrier
Sibling of 13	81	m	1.5	75	−2.5	Not a carrier
Sibling of 14	82	m	12.0	140	−1.26	Carrier
Sibling of 15	98	f	2.6	144	−1.51	Not a carrier
Sibling of 16	90	f	5.3	104	−1.39	Carrier
Sibling of 17	79	f	17.0	149	−2.07	Carrier
Sibling of 18	98	m	14.1	150	−1.8	Not a carrier
Sibling of 19	42	f	9.0	137	0.74	Not a carrier
Sibling of 20	94	f	7.5	118	−1.03	Not a carrier
Sibling of 21	107	f	11.9	132	−2.7	Carrier
Sibling of 22	13	m	3.2	89	−2.18	Carrier
Sibling of 23	96	m	11.2	134	1.5	Carrier
Sibling of 24	13	f	7.2	124	0.39	Carrier
Sibling of 25	113	m	8.0	106	−3.78	Carrier
Sibling of 26	87	f	2.4	90	−0.01	Carrier
Sibling of 27	123	f	7.2	130	1.45	Carrier
Sibling of 28	114	f	1.2	73	−1.1	Carrier
Sibling of 29	103	f	9.2	140	0.98	Not a carrier
Sibling of 30	180	f	12.0	138	−1.94	Not a carrier

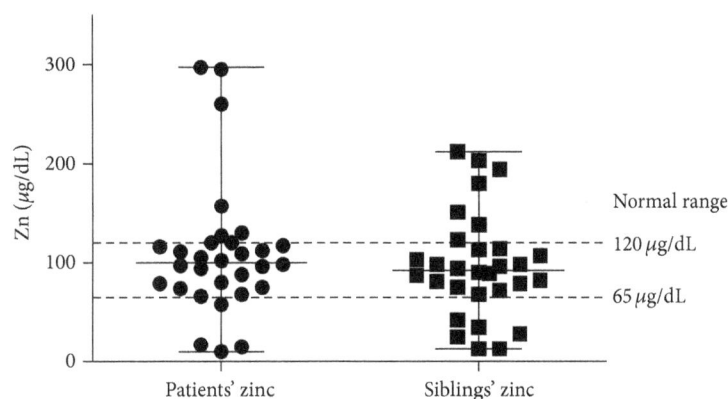

FIGURE 1: Comparison between serum Zn levels for patients and their corresponding siblings. Median levels were within normal range: 100 μg/dL (10 μg/dL–297 μg/dL) for patients and 92 μg/dL (13 μg/dL–212 μg/dL) for siblings.

have been found in several other studies; thus, it is assumed that a Zn deficiency is not related to short stature [7, 16]. However, in a study by Kyriakou and Skordis (2009) [17], the authors proposed that Zn deficiency could be a concomitant factor for growth failure among patients with thalassemia [17]. As patients were found to have significant lower height-for-age compared to their siblings, however there are other concomitant variables such as chronic anemia, iron overload-related endocrine problems, and impaired bone growth which play an important role [18–20]. In our study zinc levels did not seem to differ among siblings suggesting that Zn deficiency may not play a significant role in growth

differences often observed between thalassemic children and their brothers or sisters.

It appears that elevated ferritin levels are inversely related to Zn levels so that as ferritin increases, Zn decreases. However, in this study, the correlation was not statically significant. Decreased zinc levels or increased ferritin values have been previously reported [7, 21] and might be explained by inadequacy of clinical care and proper management affecting independently both ferritin and nutritional Zn levels.

With the limitation of a small sample size, in our study chelation therapy did not seem to affect zinc levels. Deferox-amine and deferiprone have been reported to also chelate and

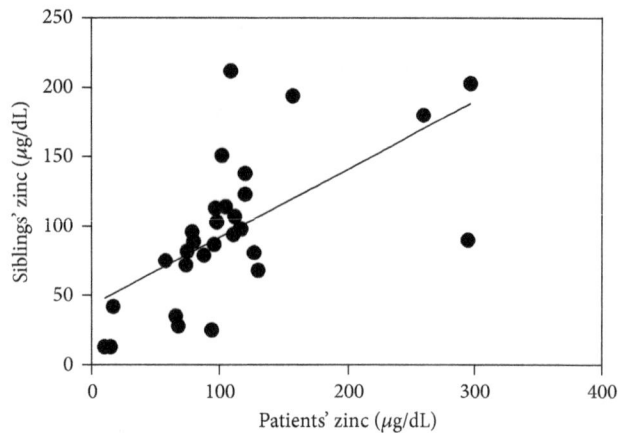

FIGURE 2: Correlation between patients' serum Zn values. Levels correlated positively with corresponding ($r = 0.635$, $P < 0.001$).

eliminate zinc into urine, while for deferasirox, which has a lower affinity for divalent zinc, this seems not to be the case [7, 13, 14].

Several studies have assumed that Zn is important to maintain intact lymphocytic function and counts [4, 7]. Fraker and King (2004) [8] found that a Zn deficiency led to lymphopenia [8]. In conclusion, this study showed that patients with thalassemia do not seem to be prone to Zn deficiency. Patients' serum Zn values correlated with their sibling suggesting that serum Zn levels are possibly more influenced by familial and environmental factors rather than by thalassemia per se or its treatment.

Abbreviations

ALC: Absolute lymphocytic count
BMI: Body mass index
CMV: Cytomegalovirus
IL-2: Interleukin 2
IL-10: Interleukin 10
Treg: T regulatory cells
Zn: Zinc.

Conflict of Interests

The authors declare that there is no conflict of interests regarding the publication of this paper.

Acknowledgments

The authors would like to thank the patients and their families for showing cooperativeness and they acknowledge the support of Cure2Children foundation (C2C), Florence, Italy, and Pakistani-Italian Debt-for-Development Swap Agreement (PIDSA), Islamabad, Pakistan, for the support of the study. Special thanks are due to Assistant Adjunct Professor of Nursing, Julia Challinor, RN, Ph.D., University of California, San Francisco, USA, for revising this paper.

References

[1] T. Hirano, M. Murakami, T. Fukada, K. Nishida, S. Yamasaki, and T. Suzuki, "Roles of zinc and zinc signaling in immunity: zinc as an intracellular signaling molecule," *Advances in Immunology*, vol. 97, pp. 149–176, 2008.

[2] R. S. MacDonald, "The role of zinc in growth and cell proliferation," *Journal of Nutrition*, vol. 130, pp. 1500S–1508S, 2000.

[3] J. Brandão-Neto, V. Stefan, B. B. Mendonça, W. Bloise, and A. V. B. Castro, "The essential role of zinc in growth," *Nutrition Research*, vol. 15, pp. 335–358, 1995.

[4] M. Yu, W.-W. Lee, D. Tomar et al., "Regulation of T cell receptor signaling by activation-induced zinc influx," *The Journal of Experimental Medicine*, vol. 208, no. 4, pp. 775–785, 2011.

[5] J. L. Kadrmas and M. C. Beckerle, "The LIM domain: from the cytoskeleton to the nucleus," *Nature Reviews Molecular Cell Biology*, vol. 5, no. 11, pp. 920–931, 2004.

[6] G. Moshtaghi-Kashanian, A. Gholamhoseinian, A. Hoseinimoghadam, and S. Rajabalian, "Splenectomy changes the pattern of cytokine production in β-thalassemic patients," *Cytokine*, vol. 35, no. 5-6, pp. 253–257, 2006.

[7] M. Mehdizadeh, G. Zamani, and S. Tabatabaee, "Zinc status in patients with major β-thalassemia," *Pediatric Hematology and Oncology*, vol. 25, no. 1, pp. 49–54, 2008.

[8] P. J. Fraker and L. E. King, "Reprogramming of the immune system during zinc deficiency," *Annual Review of Nutrition*, vol. 24, pp. 277–298, 2004.

[9] M. Y. Yakoob, E. Theodoratou, A. Jabeen et al., "Preventive zinc supplementation in developing countries: impact on mortality and morbidity due to diarrhea, pneumonia and malaria," *BMC Public Health*, vol. 11, no. 3, article S23, 2011.

[10] R. S. Gibson and E. L. Ferguson, "Nutrition intervention strategies to combat zinc deficiency in developing countries," *Nutrition Research Reviews*, vol. 11, no. 1, pp. 115–131, 1998.

[11] O. Donma, S. Gunbey, and M. A. M. M. tas Donma, "Zinc, copper, and magnesium concentrations in hair of children from southeastern Turkey," *Biological Trace Element Research*, vol. 24, no. 1, pp. 39–47, 1990.

[12] F. Rea, L. Perrone, A. Mastrobuono, G. Toscano, and M. D'Amico, "Zinc levels of serum, hair and urine in homozygous beta-thalassemic subjects under hypertransfusional treatment," *Acta Haematologica*, vol. 71, no. 2, pp. 139–142, 1984.

[13] R. Galanello, "Deferiprone in the treatment of transfusion-dependent thalassemia: a review and perspective," *Therapeutics and Clinical Risk Management*, vol. 3, no. 5, pp. 795–805, 2007.

[14] M. D. Cappellini, "Exjade (deferasirox, ICL670) in the treatment of chronic iron overload associated with blood transfusion," *Therapeutics and Clinical Risk Management*, vol. 3, no. 2, pp. 291–299, 2007.

[15] M. Hambidge, "Human zinc deficiency," *Journal of Nutrition*, vol. 130, no. 5, pp. 1344S–1349S, 2000.

[16] G. J. Fuchs, P. Tienboon, S. Linpisarn et al., "Nutritional factors and thalassaemia major," *Archives of Disease in Childhood*, vol. 74, no. 3, pp. 224–227, 1996.

[17] A. Kyriakou and N. Skordis, "Thalassaemia and aberrations of growth and puberty," *Mediterranean Journal of Hematology and Infectious Diseases*, vol. 1, no. 1, 2009.

[18] V. de Sanctis, A. Eleftheriou, and C. Malaventura, "Prevalence of endocrine complications and short stature in patients with thalassaemia major: a multicenter study by the Thalassaemia International Federation (TIF)," *Pediatric Endocrinology Reviews*, vol. 2, supplement 2, pp. 249–255, 2004.

[19] C. Theodoridis, V. Ladis, A. Papatheodorou et al., "Growth and management of short stature in thalassaemia major," *Journal of Pediatric Endocrinology and Metabolism*, vol. 11, no. 3, pp. 835–844, 1998.

[20] Guidelines for the clinical management of thalassemia, 2008.

[21] A. Mahyar, P. Ayazi, A. A. Pahlevan, H. Mojabi, M. R. Sehhat, and A. Javadi, "Zinc & copper status in children with Beta-thalassemia major," *Iranian Journal of Pediatrics*, vol. 20, pp. 297–302, 2010.

5

Study of Hematological Parameters in Children Suffering from Iron Deficiency Anaemia in Chattagram Maa-o-Shishu General Hospital, Chittagong, Bangladesh

Abu Syed Mohammed Mujib,[1] Abu Sayeed Mohammad Mahmud,[1] Milton Halder,[1] and Chowdhury Mohammad Monirul Hasan[2]

[1] *Industrial Microbiology Research Division, Bangladesh Council of Scientific and Industrial Research, Chittagong 4220, Bangladesh*
[2] *Department of Biochemistry and Molecular Biology, University of Chittagong, Chittagong 4331, Bangladesh*

Correspondence should be addressed to Abu Sayeed Mohammad Mahmud; sayedrism@gmail.com

Academic Editor: Aurelio Maggio

A total of 150 (30.61%) anemic patients out of 490 patients diagnosed to have iron deficiency anemia (IDA) have been selected for the first time in Bangladesh. For detailed study, blood samples from 150 anemic patients along with 25 controls were analyzed. Analysis of variance showed significant P value between mean platelet volume (MPV) in females (8.08 μm^3) and males (7.59 μm^3) ($P < 0.05$) in iron deficiency anemia patients. Besides, the value of white blood cells (WBC) in males (10946.08/cmm) was significantly higher than in females (9470.833/cmm) ($P < 0.05$). The significant correlation was observed among hemoglobin levels with hematocrits, hemoglobin with RBC, RBC with hematocrits, and MCV with MCH as well as MCH with MCHC. However, the negative correlation was observed between the hematological variables neutrophils and lymphocytes ($r = -0.989$). The common complaints we have found in the survey were weight loss 73.33%, attention problem 68%, dyspepsia 65%, decrease of appetite 72%, weakness 68%, diarrhea 65%, and headache 55% among IDA patients. ANOVA showed significant statistical difference in all the hematological and biochemical parameters. Analysis of variance test between anemias with only one of three biochemical parameters decreased and control showed that this group does not have iron deficiency.

1. Introduction

As the name implies, iron deficiency anemia is due to insufficient iron. Without enough iron, human body cannot produce enough hemoglobin; as a result, iron deficiency anemia causes tired and short breath. Worldwide, the most important cause of iron deficiency anemia is parasitic infection caused by hookworms, whipworms, and roundworms, in which intestinal bleeding caused by the worms may lead to undetected blood loss in the stool. These are especially important problems in growing children [1]. Malaria infections that destroy red blood cells (although the iron is recycled) and chronic blood loss caused by hookworms (where the iron is lost) contribute to anemia during pregnancy in most developing countries [2]. The principal cause of iron deficiency anemia in the developed countries is blood lost during menses in premenopausal women, which is not compensated by intake from food and supplements. Iron deficiency anaemia still remains the most common cause of anaemia not only in Bangladesh but also all over the world. According to the World Health Report, there are 1,788,600 people in this world suffering from iron deficiency anaemia. And iron deficiency anaemia is the foremost prevalent disease causing morbidity in the world [3]. Many surveys had been conducted in Bangladesh to know the prevalence of iron deficiency. A study of 114 healthy, socioeconomically privileged girls demonstrated that 24% of this group had no storage iron of and 42% of girls had suboptimal iron stores [4].

In a study of 85 men and 54 women in Finland, only traces of marrow iron were found in 4 to 7% of men, in 70% of women of 15 to 49 years of age, and in 23% of women of 50 years of age or older [5]. In a survey of 1105 Canadians, iron stores, judged by serum ferritin values, were greatly reduced in about 25% of children, 30% of pregnant women, and 3% of men [6]. In a study conducted by Looker AC. [7], it was found that 9% of toddlers aged up to 2 years, 9% to 11% of adolescent girls, and women of child bearing age were found to be iron deficient. Of these, iron deficiency anaemia was found in 3% and 2% to 5%, respectively. Also 7% of men over 50 years of age and 1% of young men and teenage boys had iron deficiency [8]. In Pakistan, anaemia was present in 47% of children and 30% of the adult females [9]. Iron deficiency is particularly common in infants and pregnant women. The iron deficiency in women occurs most often during the reproductive years, whereas in men the incidence is relatively high in adolescent and low during young adulthood; it increases thereafter with advancing age. In infancy, the occurrence of iron deficiency is equal in both sexes. It is usually detected between the ages of 6 and 20 months; the peak incidence is at a younger age in infants born prematurely than in those born at term.

2. Methods

2.1. Study Design. A cross-sectional study was conducted from November 2010 to June 2011. The subjects were selected depending on the availability in the hospital ward. The hospital has facilities for iron deficiency anaemia diagnoses, treatment, and monitoring.

2.2. Study Subjects. A total of 150 subjects were included in this study. There was no specific predilection for race, religion, and socioeconomic status. The study subjects comprised the following two groups:

group 1:

(a) IDA male: 102 (subjects),
(b) IDA female: 48 (subjects);

group 2:

(a) control male: 17,
(b) control female: 8.

2.3. Ethical Consideration. Informed parental consent was taken before enrolling the children into the study. The procedure was fully explained to the parents and they were informed that if they wish they will be able to withdraw them from the study and it would not in any way hamper the treatment. Permission was also taken from the hospital authority, departmental head of the haematology laboratory, and biochemistry lab in order to undertake the study.

2.4. Inclusion Criteria and Exclusion Criteria

2.4.1. Inclusion Criteria. Inclusion criteria are as follows:

(1) all cases of suspected iron deficiency anaemia belonging the age group of 18 yrs,
(2) all the patients having haemoglobin less than 11 gm/dL.

2.4.2. Exclusion Criteria. Exclusion criteria are as follows:

(1) patients previously transfused with blood within 120 days,
(2) patients already on iron therapy.

2.5. Control and Development of Questionnaire

2.5.1. Control. 25 patients having haemoglobin within normal range were taken as control.

2.5.2. Development of Questionnaire. A questionnaire was developed to obtain relevant information of demographic and socioeconomic data. The questionnaire also included anthropometric data, birth date, immunization history, past medical history, and clinical information. The questionnaire was coded and pretested before finalization. The questionnaire was both closed and open ended.

2.6. Blood Samples. Blood samples were collected by venepuncture using either the antecubital vein or the dorsal vein and dispensed into dipotassium EDTA anticoagulant bottles. Thereafter, informed consents were obtained from their parents/guardians and teachers. All haematological parameters were carried out by automatic methods. Adequate quality control measures were taken on each test procedure to ensure the reliability of the results. Haematological and biochemical investigations were done in haematology laboratory and biochemistry laboratory, respectively.

2.7. Serum Sample. Collect whole blood in a covered test tube. If commercially available tubes are to be used and should use the red toped tubes. These are available from Becton Dickinson (BD). BD's trade name for the blood handling tubes is Vacutainer. After collection of the whole blood, allow the blood to clot by leaving it undisturbed at room temperature. This usually takes 15–30 minutes. Remove the clot by centrifuging at 1,000–2,000 ×g for 10 minutes in a refrigerated centrifuge.

2.8. Biochemical Examination

2.8.1. Serum Iron Estimation. Serum iron estimation was done with the help of the automated Dimension IRON method by Dade Behring Dimension Biochemistry Analyser.

2.8.2. Total Iron Binding Capacity. TIBC estimation was done with the help of kit manufactured by Randox Laboratories LTD, UK.

2.8.3. Serum Ferritin Assay. Serum ferritin assay was done with the help of ferritin serozyme kit manufactured by Biochem Immunosystems, Italy.

2.9. Hematological Examination

2.9.1. Automated Blood Count (Complete Blood Count). A complete blood count (CBC), also known as full blood count

Age distribution of IDA and control patients

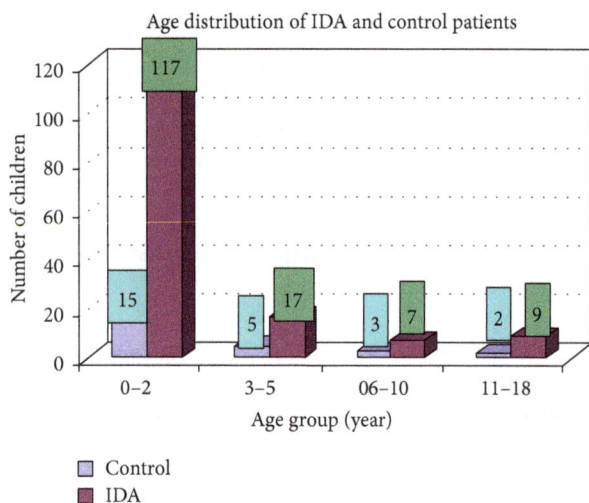

FIGURE 1: Showing age distribution of control and iron deficiency anaemia.

Sex distribution of IDA and control patients

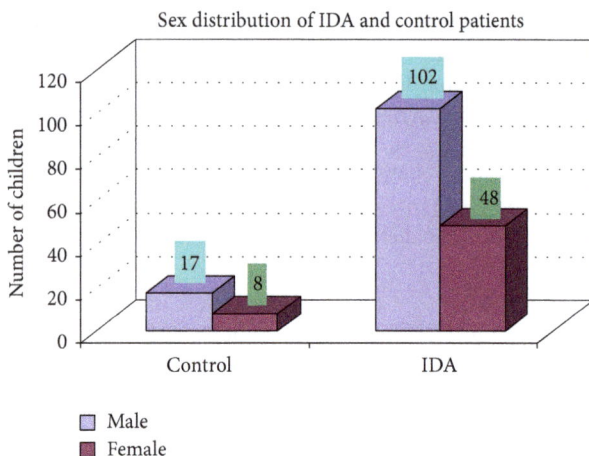

FIGURE 2: Showing sex distribution of IDA and control patients.

Biochemical parameters

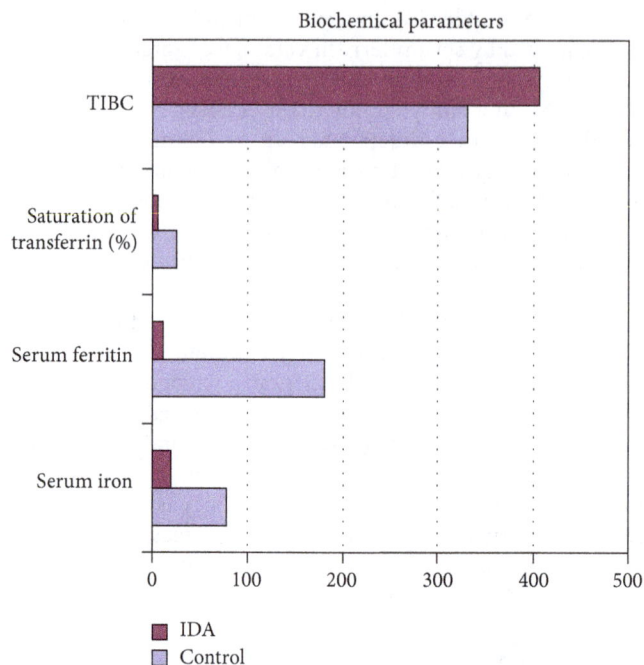

FIGURE 3: Showing biochemical parameters in control and IDA.

The mean value of hemoglobin of IDA and control patients

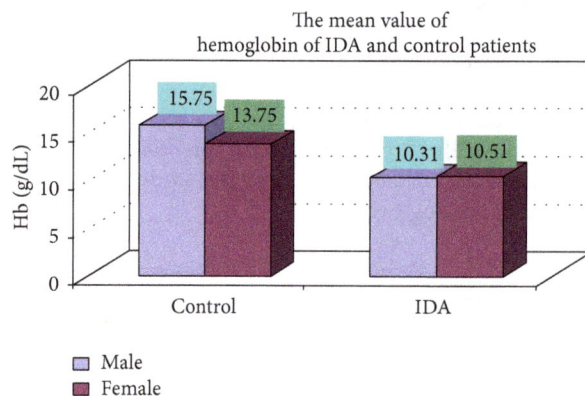

FIGURE 4: Showing the mean value of hemoglobin of control and iron deficiency anaemia.

(FBC), was analyzed by the ABX PENTRA 60 which is a fully automated (Microprocessor controlled) haematology analyser used for the in vitro diagnostic testing of whole blood specimens. The ABX PENTRA 60 is able to operate either in CBC mode (12 parameters) or in CBC + 5DIFF mode (26 parameters). A scientist or lab technician performs the requested testing and provides the requested medical professional with the results of the CBC. The blood is well mixed (though not shaken) and placed on a rack in the analyzer. This instrument has many different components to analyze different elements in the blood. The cell counting component counts the numbers and types of different cells within the blood. The results are printed out or sent to a computer for review.

2.9.2. HCT Measurement. The height of the impulse generated by the passage of a cell through the microaperture is directly proportional to the volume of the analyzed RBC.

The haematocrit is measured as a function of the numeric integration of the MCV.

2.10. MPV Measurement. The MPV (mean platelet volume) is directly derived from the analysis of the platelet distribution curve.

2.11. Erythrocyte Sedimentation Rate (ESR) Measurement. We have followed Westergren method, collecting 2 mL of venous blood into a tube containing 0.5 mL of sodium citrate. It should be stored no longer than 2 hours at room temperature or 6 hours at 4°C. The blood is drawn into a Westergren-Katz tube to the 200 mm mark. The tube is placed in a rack in a strictly vertical position for 1 hour at room temperature, at which time the distance from the lowest point of

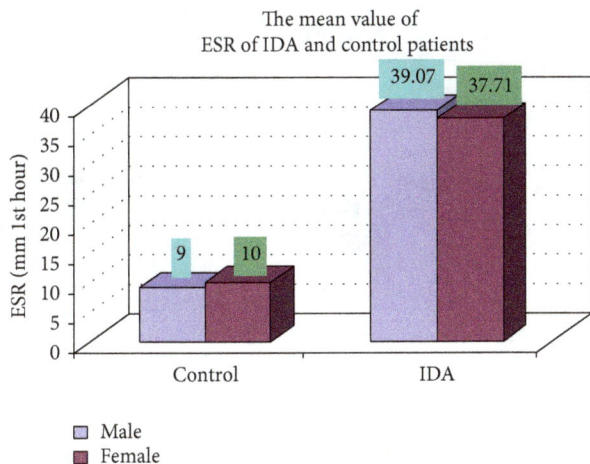

FIGURE 5: Showing the mean value of ESR of control and iron deficiency anaemia.

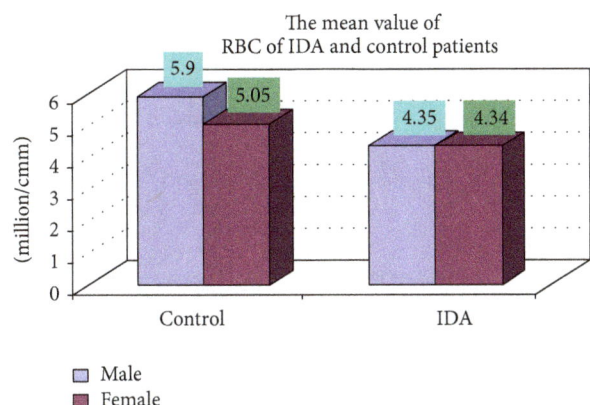

FIGURE 6: Showing the mean value RBC of control and iron deficiency anaemia.

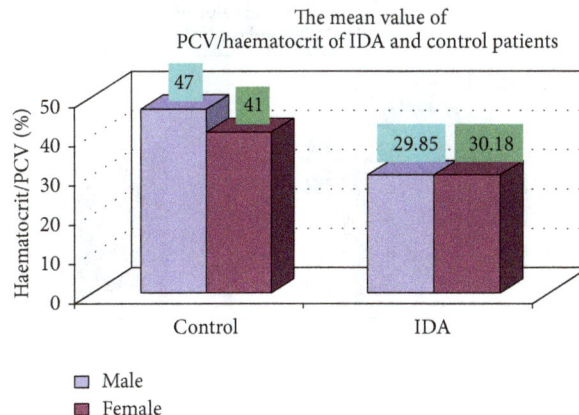

FIGURE 7: Showing PCV/hematocrit of control and iron deficiency anaemia.

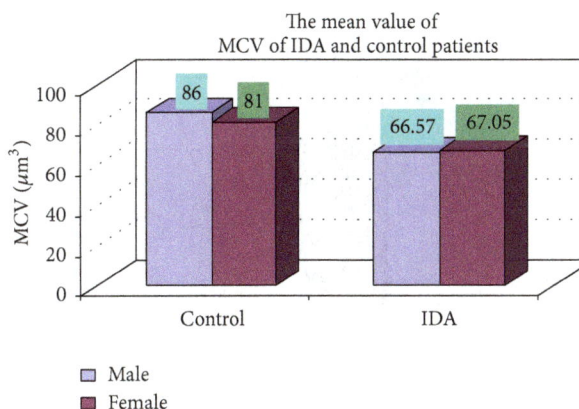

FIGURE 8: Showing the mean value MCV of control and iron deficiency anaemia.

TABLE 1: Mean biochemical parameters of IDA and control.

Biochemical parameters	Control	IDA
Serum iron (g/dL)	78.25	20.85
Serum ferritin (ng/mL)	180.33	9.94
% saturation of transferrin	25.51	5.73
TIBC (g/dL)	329.42	404.47

the surface meniscus to the upper limit of the red cell sediment is measured. The distance of fall of erythrocytes, expressed as millimeters in 1 hour, is the ESR.

3. Results

The diagnosis of iron deficiency anaemia was made only if all the three biochemical parameters like serum iron, serum ferritin, and percentage saturation of transferrin were below normal for the sex. By these criteria 150 (30.61%) out of 490 patients were diagnosed to have iron deficiency anaemia.

3.1. Age Distribution of IDA.
Out of 150 patients of IDA, 117 patients were in the age group of 0–2 years, 17 in the age group of 3–5 years, 7 in the age group of 6–10 years, and 9 in the age group of 11–18 years. The age distribution of iron deficiency anaemia and controls is shown in Figure 1.

3.2. Sex Distribution of IDA.
Of 150 patients with IDA patients, 102 were male and 48 were female and M : F ratio

is 2.1 : 1. Of 25 controls, 17 were male and 8 were female and M : F ratio is 2.12 : 1 (Figure 2).

3.3. Biochemical Parameters.
The mean value of serum iron in IDA was 20.85 g/dL, which is markedly less than that in control. The mean total iron binding capacity was greater in IDA (404.47 g/dL) than in control (Table 1). The mean percentage saturation of transferrin in IDA was found to be 5.73% that is markedly less than control. The mean serum ferritin in IDA was 9.94 ng/mL, which is less than control (Figure 3).

3.4. Complete Blood Count.
The blood samples were collected from suspected anemic patient and control group,

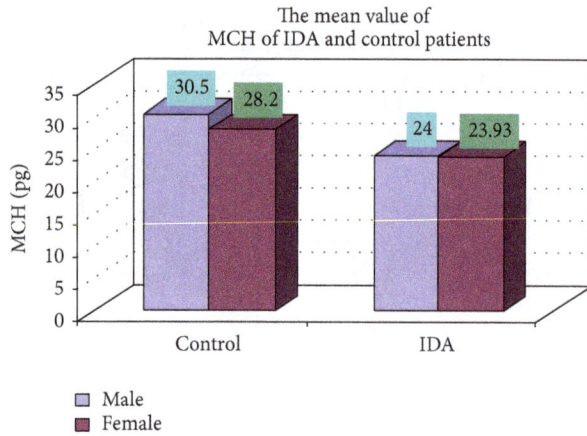

FIGURE 9: Showing mean value MCH of control and iron deficiency anaemia.

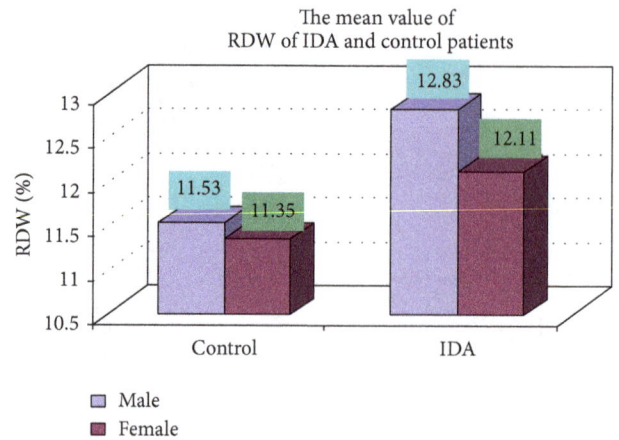

FIGURE 11: Showing the mean value RDW of control and iron deficiency anemia.

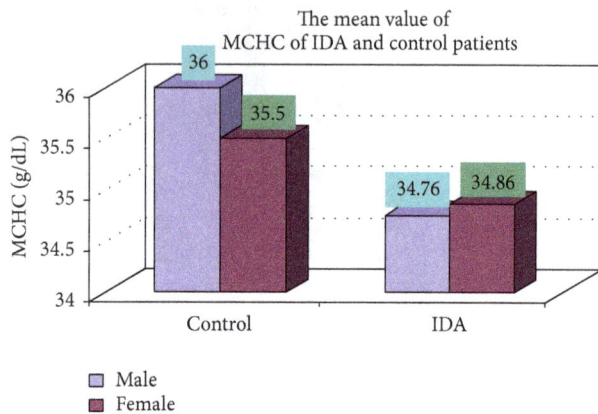

FIGURE 10: Showing the mean value MCHC of control and iron deficiency anemia.

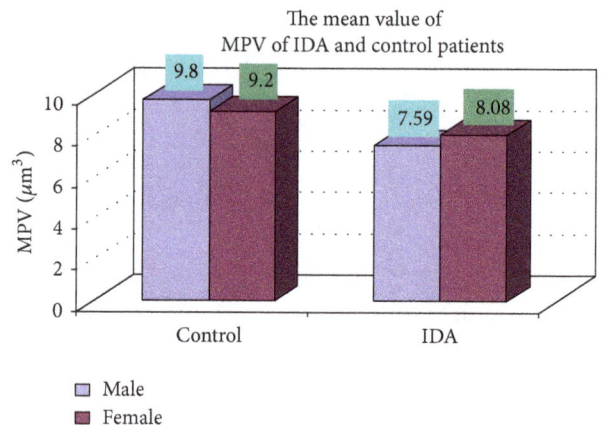

FIGURE 12: Showing the mean value of MPV of control and iron deficiency anaemia.

then complete blood count was conducted for the following hematological values like hemoglobin (Hgb), erythrocyte sedimentation rate (ESR), red blood cell (RBC), hematocrit (HCT), packed cell volume (MCV), mean corpuscular hemoglobin (MCH), mean corpuscular hemoglobin concentration (MCHC), red cell distribution width (RDW), mean platelet volume (MPV), platelet, white blood cell (WBC), neutrophil, lymphocyte, eosinophil, and monocytes. The results are represented graphically (Figures 4, 5, 6, 7, 8, 9, 10, 11, 12, 13, 14, 15, 16, 17, and 18).

3.5. Comparison of Hematological Parameters in Anemic Males and Females.

We conducted complete blood count for various hematological values like hemoglobin (Hgb), erythrocyte sedimentation rate (ESR), red blood cell (RBC), hematocrit (HCT), packed cell volume (MCV), mean corpuscular hemoglobin (MCH), mean corpuscular hemoglobin concentration (MCHC), red cell distribution width (RDW), mean platelet volume (MPV), platelet, white blood cell (WBC), neutrophil, lymphocyte, eosinophil, and monocytes. The following (Table 2) is the comparative study of hematological values for IDA in males and females. Statistical

analysis was carried out using Statistical Package for Social Sciences (SPSS) version 11.5, and an independent-sample t-test ($P < 0.05$) and one-way ANOVA test were used for comparison of hematological parameters. Results were considered to be statistically significant when the two-sided P value was less than 0.05 or ($P < 0.05$). ANOVA (analysis of variance) showed significant P value between mean platelet volume (MPV) in females (8.08 μm^3) and males (7.59 μm^3) ($P < 0.05$) in iron deficiency anemia patients (Tables 2, 3, 4, and 5). On the other hand, the value of white blood cells (WBC) in males (10946.08/cmm) was significantly higher than in females (9470.833/cmm), ($P < 0.05$).

The positive correlation among hematologic and biochemical variables was between hemoglobin and hematocrit ($r = 0.851$), hemoglobin and RBC ($r = 0.659$), RBC and hematocrit ($r = 0.736$), MCV and MCH ($r = 0.806$), and MCH and MCHC ($r = 0.620$), but not with other parameters.

The best negative correlation among hematologic variables was between neutrophils and lymphocytes ($r = -0.989$) but not with other parameters.

TABLE 2: Showing comparative hematological values for iron deficiency anemic males and females.

Parameters	Male mean ± SD	Female mean ± SD	P value
Hb (g/dL)	10.31 ± 1.46	10.51 ± 1.07	0.339
ESR (mm 1st hour)	39.07 ± 27.40	37.71 ± 25.68	0.768
RBC (million/cmm)	4.35 ± 0.59	4.34 ± 0.52	0.918
PCV/haematocrit	29.85 ± 3.75	30.18 ± 3.23	0.589
MCV (fl)	66.57 ± 5.32	67.05 ± 4.86	0.584
MCH (pg)	24.00 ± 2.93	23.93 ± 2.59	0.87
MCHC (g/dL)	34.76 ± 1.43	34.86 ± 0.98	0.626
RDW (%)	12.83 ± 2.08	13.11 ± 2.28	0.485
MPV (μm^3)	7.59 ± 0.85	8.08 ± 0.82	0.001
Platelet (×1000/cmm)	340.49 ± 82.57	332.29 ± 80.99	0.567
WBC (/cmm)	10946.08 ± 3786.32	9470.833 ± 2969.49	0.011
Neutrophil (%)	49.32 ± 16.27	49.43 ± 17.50	0.97
Lymphocytes (%)	45.66 ± 15.98	45.85 ± 17.21	0.947
Eosinophil (%)	2.95 ± 2.95	2.48 ± 1.60	0.208
Monocytes (%)	2.13 ± 1.05	2.25 ± 1.05	0.052

TABLE 3: Showing comparative hematological values between control and iron deficiency anemia (IDA) males and females.

Parameters	Control Male Number (mean)	Control Female Number (mean)	IDA Male Number (mean)	IDA Female Number (mean)
Hb (g/dL)	17 (15.75)	8 (13.75)	102 (10.31)	48 (10.51)
ESR (mm 1st hour)	17 (9)	8 (10)	102 (39.07)	48 (37.71)
RBC (million/cmm)	17 (5.9)	8 (5.05)	102 (4.35)	48 (4.34)
PCV/haematocrit	17 (47)	8 (41)	102 (29.85)	48 (30.18)
MCV (μm^3)	17 (86)	8 (81)	102 (66.57)	48 (67.05)
MCH (pg)	17 (30.5)	8 (28.2)	102 (24.00)	48 (23.93)
MCHC (g/dL)	17 (con)	8 (28.2)	102 (34.76)	48 (34.86)
RDW (%)	17 (11.53)	8 (11.35)	102 (12.83)	48 (13.11)
MPV (μm^3)	17 (9.8)	8 (9.2)	102 (7.59)	48 (8.08)
Platelet (×1000/cmm)	17 (325.25)	8 (315.00)	102 (340.49)	48 (332.29)
WBC (/cmm)	17 (12500.3)	8 (12300.2)	102 (10946.08)	48 (9470.833)
Neutrophil (%)	17 (48.3)	8 (47.2)	102 (49.32)	48 (49.43)
Lymphocytes (%)	17 (29.22)	8 (28.2)	102 (45.66)	48 (45.85)
Eosinophil (%)	17 (2.4)	8 (2.2)	102 (2.95)	48 (2.48)
Monocytes (%)	17 (3)	8 (3.2)	102 (2.13)	48 (2.25)

TABLE 4: Showing correlation among hematologic and biochemical variables in iron deficiency anemia patients.

	Hb	ESR (west)	RBC	PCV/Hct	MCV	MCH	MCHC	RDW	MPV
Hb	1	−0.281**	0.659**	0.851**	0.441**	0.329**	0.159	−0.302**	−0.020
ESR (west)		1	−0.252**	−0.241**	0.016	0.008	−0.064	0.032	−0.138
RBC			1	0.736**	0.070	−0.118	−0.183*	0.040	−0.090
PCV/hct.				1	0.448**	0.289**	0.125	−0.289**	−0.121
MCV					1	0.806**	0.410**	−0.492**	−0.085
MCH						1	0.620**	−0.399**	−0.017
MCHC							1	−0.366**	0.084
RDW								1	0.004
MPV									1

** Correlation is significant at the 0.01 level (2-tailed). * Correlation is significant at the 0.05 level (2-tailed).

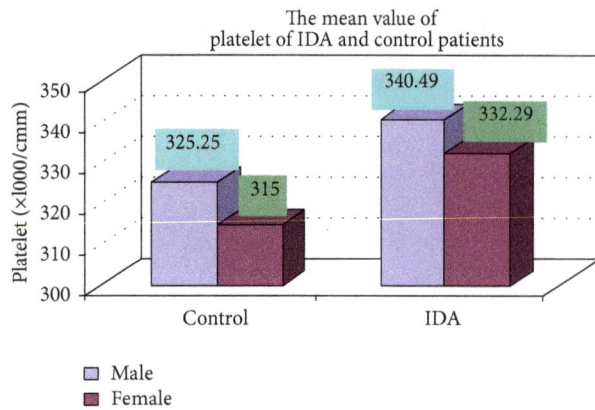

The mean value of platelet of IDA and control patients

FIGURE 13: Showing mean value platelets of control and iron deficiency anemia.

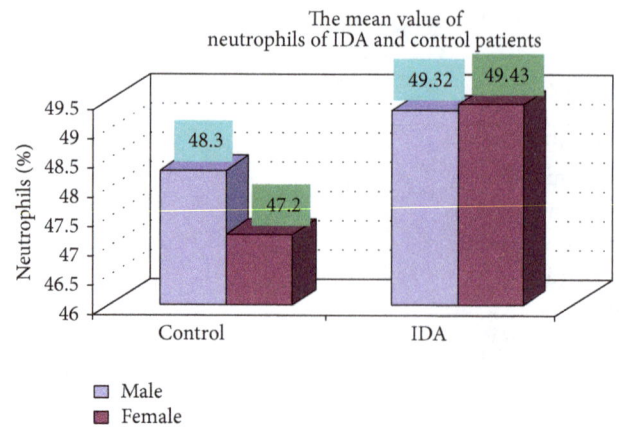

The mean value of WBC of IDA and control patients

FIGURE 14: Showing mean value WBC of control and iron deficiency anaemia.

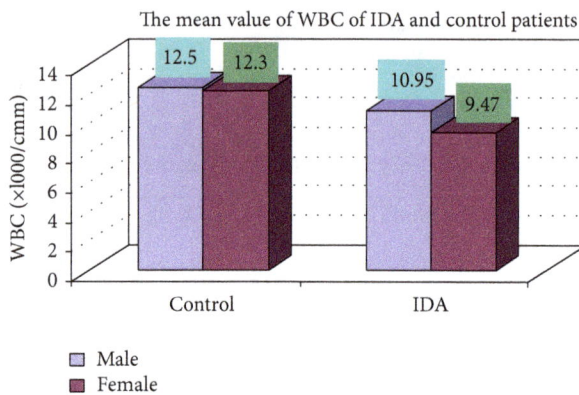

The mean value of neutrophils of IDA and control patients

FIGURE 15: Showing mean value of neutrophils of control and iron deficiency anemia.

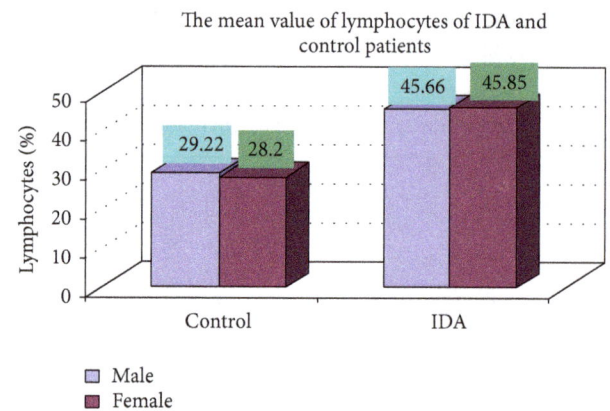

The mean value of lymphocytes of IDA and control patients

FIGURE 16: Showing means value of lymphocytes of control and iron deficiency anemia.

TABLE 5: Showing correlation among hematologic variables in Iron deficiency anemia patients.

	Neutrophils	Lymphocytes	Eosinophils	Monocytes
Neutrophils	1	−0.989**	−0.141	−0.035
Lymphocytes		1	0.035	−0.024
Eosinophils			1	−0.047
Monocytes				1

** Correlation is significant at the 0.01 level (2-tailed).

3.6. Clinical Features of IDA. Regarding the clinical presentation the most common complaints were weight loss 73.33%, attention problem 68%, dyspepsia 65%, decrease appetite 72%, weakness 68%, diarrhea 65%, and headache 55% (Table 6). Pale skin color and premature baby were the least common clinical presentation. The results regarding clinical complaints of iron deficiency have been shown graphically (Figures 19, 20, 21, 22, 23, and 24).

4. Discussion

In our study out of 150 IDA patients (102 males and 48 females) 78% were in age group between 0 and 2 years, 11.3% in age group between 3 and 5 years, 4.7% in age group

TABLE 6: Showing the frequency of clinical features of IDA and control patients.

Clinical features	Control Number (%)	IDA Number (%)
Weight loss	8 (32%)	110 (73.33%)
Attention problem	4 (16%)	102 (68%)
Pale skin colour	3 (12%)	51 (34%)
Dyspepsia	5 (20%)	97 (65%)
Diarrhoea	6 (24%)	98 (65%)
Premature baby	2 (8%)	52 (35%)
Weakness	4 (16%)	102 (68%)
Decrease appetite	5 (20%)	108 (72%)
Headache	7 (28%)	83 (55%)

between 6 and 10 years, and 6% in age group between 11 and 18 years. It should be noted that iron supplements and increased iron stores have recently been linked to maternal complications [10]. In contrast, our study showed that IDA is most commonly prevalent in the 0–2-year age group which includes 78% (male and female) and the sex ratio is

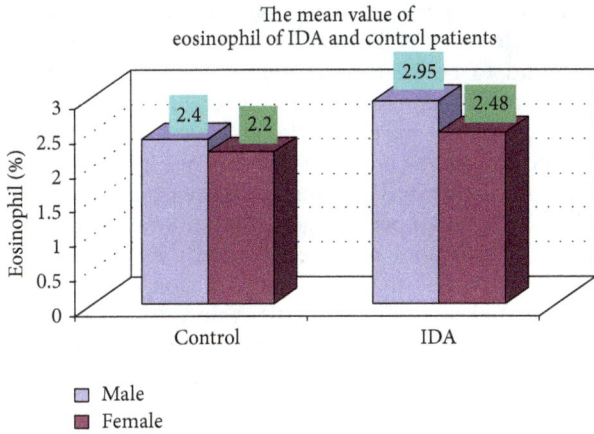

FIGURE 17: Showing mean value of eosinophil of control and iron deficiency anaemia.

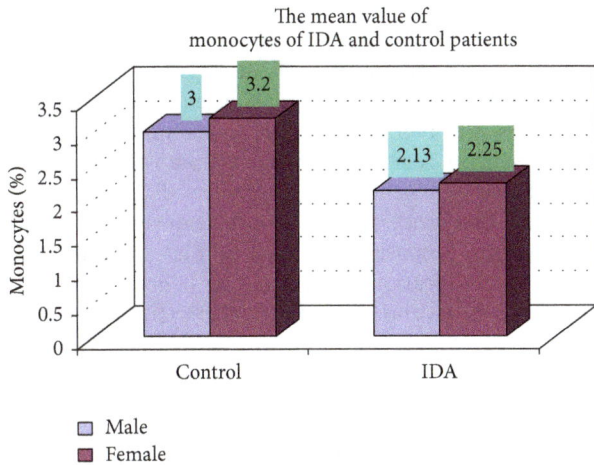

FIGURE 18: Showing the mean value of monocytes of control and iron deficiency anaemia.

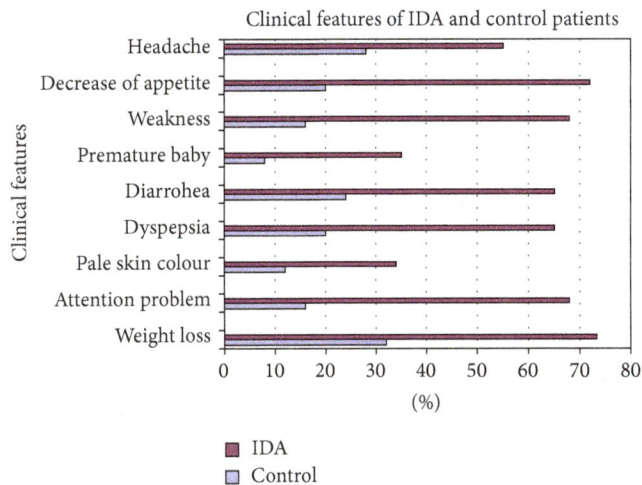

FIGURE 19: Showing clinical features of IDA and control patients.

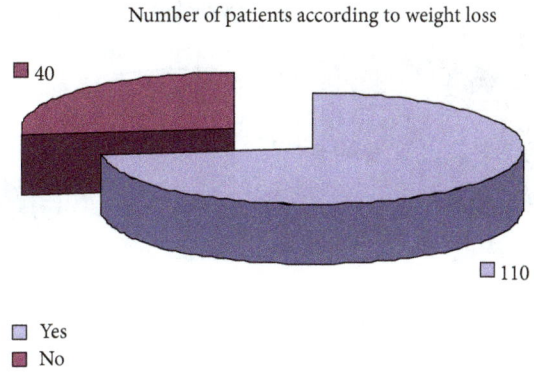

FIGURE 20: Showing the distribution of patients according to complaints of weight loss.

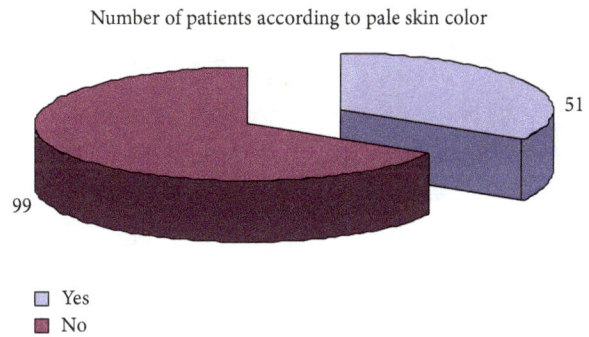

FIGURE 21: Showing the distribution of patients according to complaints of pale skin colour.

also 2.12 : 1. These observations were taken from patients of medical OPD and ward. Moreover, hookworm infestation is more common in our context. Various researches have shown that hookworm is second most prevalent parasitosis in Nepal, incidence of which varies from 11% to 100% [11–13]. This could be the probable factor for the difference in the observations as stated before. Lower class (54%), middle class (31%), and upper class (15%) were mostly affected. These observations show that economically deprived and ignorant people are mostly affected. In clinical manifestations, weight loss, decrease of appetite, diarrhea, attention problems, and weakness were the most common complaints of the patients with IDA. Also, it is equally common among the anaemic individuals who were not iron deficient. Moreover, premature baby, pale skin color, dyspepsia, and headache were other complaints almost equally common among IDA and controls. These are symptoms of anaemia but not specifically concerned with IDA. These observations are in accordance with the previous reports of Elwood [12]. In our observation, the average MCV in IDA was 66.81 fl. Similarly the mean value of MCH was 23.97 pg, mean value of MCHC was 34.81%, and mean hemoglobin was 10.41 gm/dL in IDA. These observations are similar to the report by Bainton [14] and Finch C. A., which showed mean MCV to be 74 fl, mean MCH to be 20 pg, mean MCHC to be 28%, and mean hemoglobin to be 7.6 gm/dL in patients with IDA [15].

Number of patients according to dyspepsia

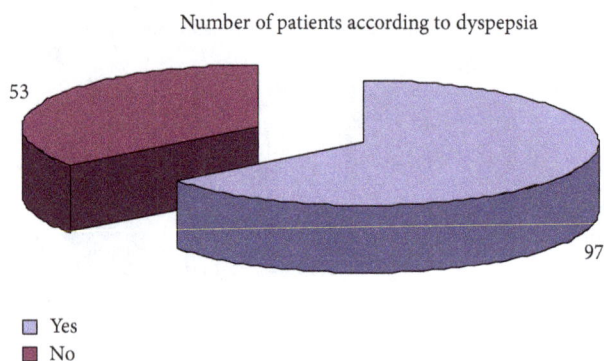

- □ Yes
- ■ No

FIGURE 22: Showing the distribution of patients in accordance with complaints of dyspepsia.

Number of patients according to decrease of appetite

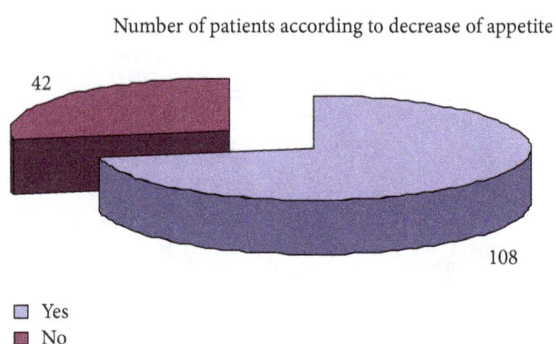

- □ Yes
- ■ No

FIGURE 23: Showing the distribution of patients in accordance with complaints of decrease in appetite.

Number of patients according to headache

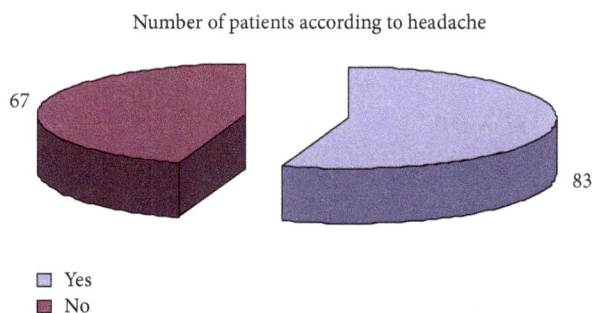

- □ Yes
- ■ No

FIGURE 24: Showing the distribution of patients in accordance with complaints of headache.

In the present study, the mean value of serum iron in IDA was 20.85 g/dL, which was significantly lower than control group (78.25 g/dL). In a study conducted in geriatric patients the mean was found to be 22.7 g/dL [16] which is almost similar to our result. The principal limitation of the serum iron determination is variability in the values [17], which may be due to both technical and physiologic factors [18] such as contamination of glassware and reagents with iron although the use of disposable, plastic equipment has reduced such contamination considerably. Among the biochemical tests, total iron binding capacity (TIBC) was increased in 42% out of the IDA patients (102 male and 48 female). The mean value of TIBC in IDA was 404.47 μg/dL, which

was significantly higher than control group (329.42 μg/dL). A study done in children IDA patients the mean TIBC was found to be 413.6 μg/dL, which is also closer to our observation. Though increased value of TIBC indicates iron deficiency, the normal or even lower value may occur in iron deficiency anaemia [19]. So, TIBC was not included among the three biochemical parameters. Instead, in the present study, we have used percentage saturation of transferrin, the value of which does not overlap with the normal values and the values less than 16% occur in iron deficiency and anaemia of chronic diseases [20]. Values less than 5% are found only in iron deficiency. Statistical analysis was carried out using ($P < 0.05$); one-way ANOVA test was used for comparison of hematological parameters. ANOVA (analysis of variance) showed significant P value between mean platelet volume (MPV) in females (8.08 μm^3) and males (7.59 μm^3), ($P < 0.05$) in iron deficiency anemia patients. Besides, the value of white blood cells (WBC) in males (10946.08/cmm) was significantly higher than that in females (9470.833/cmm) ($P < 0.05$). ANOVA showed statistical significance in hematological and biochemical parameters between IDA and the control group and anaemia due to other diseases. It has also showed that the role of TIBC in diagnosing IDA cannot be overemphasized. ANOVA also showed that anaemia with decrease in any two of the three biochemical parameters might have iron deficiency while anaemia with decrease in one of the three biochemical parameters did not have iron deficiency. This problem must be overemphasized by public health system, because of too easy and available treatment and nutrition education for people. Our people do not know which foods to eat and which foods help their health.

5. Conclusion

Iron deficiency anaemia in children is still considered a major health problem all over the world. This is because of long term effects on mental and cognitive skills and on immunity and general physical wellbeing. More recently, iron deficiency is suggested to be related to DNA damage. This prospective study conducted in Chattagram Maa-O-Shishu General Hospital and Medical College, Agrabad, Chittagong, from November 2010 to June 2011 showed that iron deficiency anaemia is one of the most common anemias and in 30.61% of anaemic patients the diagnosis was confirmed by decrease in three biochemical parameters.

Conflict of Interests

The authors hereby declare that they have no conflict of interests regarding this paper.

Acknowledgment

The authors thank Chattagram Maa-o-Shishu General Hospital, Chittagong, Bangladesh, and department of biochemistry and molecular biology for their logistic support and collaboration.

References

[1] W. Fowler, "Chlorosis-an obituary," *Annals of Medical History*, vol. 8, pp. 168–177, 1936.

[2] S. Ashwell, "Observations on chlorosis, and its complications," *Guy's Hospital Reports*, vol. 1, pp. 529–579, 1836.

[3] World Health Organization, *The World Health Report 1998-Life in the 21st Century: A Vision for All*, The World Health Report 1998: Life in the 21st Century a Vision for All; The World Health Report 1998: Life In The 21st Century a Vision for All, World Health Organization, Geneva, Switzerland, 1998.

[4] D. E. Scott and J. A. Pritchard, "Iron deficiency in healthy young college women," *The Journal of the American Medical Association*, vol. 199, no. 12, pp. 897–900, 1967.

[5] H. Takkunen, *Iron Deficiency in the Finnish Adult Population: An Epidemiological Survey from 1967 to 1972 Inclusive*, Munksgaard, 1976.

[6] L. Valberg, J. Sorbie, J. Ludwig, and O. Pelletier, "Serum ferritin and the iron status of *Canadians*," *Canadian Medical Association Journal*, vol. 114, no. 5, pp. 417–421, 1976.

[7] A. C. Looker, C. C. Johnston Jr., H. W. Wahner et al., "Prevalence of low femoral bone density in older U.S. women from NHANES III," *Journal of Bone and Mineral Research*, vol. 10, no. 5, pp. 796–802, 1995.

[8] A. C. Looker, P. R. Dallman, M. D. Carroll, E. W. Gunter, and C. L. Johnson, "Prevalence of iron deficiency in the United States," *The Journal of the American Medical Association*, vol. 277, no. 12, pp. 973–976, 1997.

[9] P. Hamedani, K. Z. Hashmi, and M. Manji, "Iron depletion and anaemia: prevalence, consequences, diagnostic and therapeutic implications in a developing Pakistani population," *Current Medical Research and Opinion*, vol. 10, no. 7, pp. 480–485, 1987.

[10] T. O. Scholl, "Iron status during pregnancy: setting the stage for mother and infant," *The American Journal of Clinical Nutrition*, vol. 81, no. 5, pp. 1218s–1222s, 2005.

[11] M. Vernet, "The transferrin receptor: its role in iron metabolism and its diagnosis utility," *Annales de Biologie Clinique*, vol. 57, no. 1, pp. 9–18, 1999.

[12] P. C. Elwood, W. E. Waters, W. J. W. Greene, P. Sweetnam, and M. M. Wood, "Symptoms and circulating haemoglobin level," *Journal of Chronic Diseases*, vol. 21, no. 9-10, pp. 615–628, 1969.

[13] L. D. Hamilton, C. J. Gubler, G. E. Cartwright, and M. M. Wintrobe, "Diurnal variation in the plasma iron level of man," *Experimental Biology and Medicine*, vol. 75, no. 1, pp. 65–68, 1950.

[14] D. F. Bainton, J. L. Ullyot, and M. G. Farquhar, "The development of neutrophilic polymorphonuclear leukocytes in human bone marrow," *The Journal of Experimental Medicine*, vol. 134, no. 4, pp. 907–934, 1971.

[15] L. H. Allen, "Pregnancy and iron deficiency: unresolved issues," *Nutrition Reviews*, vol. 55, no. 4, pp. 91–101, 1997.

[16] G. M. Brittenham, "Disorders of iron metabolism: iron deficiency and overload," *Hematology: Basic Principles And Practice*, vol. 3, pp. 397–428, 2000.

[17] B. E. Statland and P. Winkel, "Relationship of day to day variation of serum iron concentrations to iron binding capacity in healthy young women," *American Journal of Clinical Pathology*, vol. 67, no. 1, pp. 84–90, 1977.

[18] P. R. Dallman, "Diagnosis of anemia and iron deficiency: analytic and biological variations of laboratory tests," *The American Journal of Clinical Nutrition*, vol. 39, no. 6, pp. 937–941, 1984.

[19] J. H. Lee, J. S. Hahn, S. M. Lee, J. H. Kim, and Y. W. Ko, "Iron related indices in iron deficiency anemia of geriatric Korean patients," *Yonsei Medical Journal*, vol. 37, no. 2, pp. 104–111, 1996.

[20] S. K. Rai, T. Kubo, M. Nakanishi et al., "Status of soil-transmitted helminthic infection in Nepal," *The Journal of the Japanese Association for Infectious Diseases*, vol. 68, no. 5, pp. 625–630, 1994.

6

Anemia in Patients with Type 2 Diabetes Mellitus

Jéssica Barbieri,[1] **Paula Caitano Fontela,**[2] **Eliane Roseli Winkelmann,**[3,4]
Carine Eloise Prestes Zimmermann,[5,6] **Yana Picinin Sandri,**[4,6]
Emanelle Kerber Viera Mallet,[6] **and Matias Nunes Frizzo**[3,6]

[1]*Regional University of Northwestern Rio Grande do Sul (UNIJUÍ), Ijuí, RS, Brazil*
[2]*Program in Respiratory Sciences, the Federal University of Rio Grande do Sul (UFRGS), Porto Alegre, RS, Brazil*
[3]*Department of Life Sciences, the Regional University of Northwestern Rio Grande do Sul (UNIJUÍ),*
 Rua do Comércio No. 3000, Bairro Universitário, 98700 000 Ijuí, RS, Brazil
[4]*Program in Integral Attention to Health (PPGAIS-UNIJUI/UNICRUZ), Ijuí, RS, Brazil*
[5]*Program in Pharmacology of the Health Sciences Center, The Federal University of Santa Maria (UFSM), RS, Brazil*
[6]*Cenecista Institute for Higher Education, Rua Dr. João Augusto Rodrigues 471, 98801 015 Santo Ângelo, RS, Brazil*

Correspondence should be addressed to Carine Eloise Prestes Zimmermann; carine_zimmermann@yahoo.com.br
and Matias Nunes Frizzo; matias.frizzo@gmail.com

Academic Editor: Eitan Fibach

The objective of this study was to evaluate the prevalence of anemia in DM2 patients and its correlation with demographic and lifestyle and laboratory variables. This is a descriptive and analytical study of the type of case studies in the urban area of the Ijuí city, registered in programs of the Family Health Strategy, with a total sample of 146 patients with DM2. A semistructured questionnaire with sociodemographic and clinical variables and performed biochemical test was applied. Of the DM2 patients studied, 50 patients had anemia, and it was found that the body mass items and hypertension and hematological variables are significantly associated with anemia of chronic disease. So, the prevalence of anemia is high in patients with DM2. The set of observed changes characterizes the anemia of chronic disease, which affects quality of life of diabetic patients and is associated with disease progression, development, and comorbidities that contribute significantly to increasing the risk of cardiovascular diseases.

1. Introduction

Diabetes mellitus (DM) is a metabolic disorder of great impact worldwide. Epidemiological data showed that in 2010 there were 285 million people affected with the disease in the world, and it is estimated that in the year of 2030 we will have about 440 million diabetics [1]. Its worldwide prevalence is increasing fast among developing countries. The type 2 diabetes affects about 7% of the population [2].

The increasing prevalence of type 2 diabetes mellitus (DM2) has become a major public health concern. The diabetic patients' number has been increasing due to population and urbanization growth, increase in the prevalence of obesity and sedentary lifestyle, and the longer survival of patients with DM [3]. Diabetes is a highly disabling disease, which can cause blindness, amputations, kidney disease, anemia, and cardiovascular and brain complications, among others, impairing the functional capacity and autonomy and individual quality of life [4].

The disease can be classified into two predominant types, as type 1 DM (DM1), defined by the destruction of pancreatic β-cells and the absence of endogenous insulin, and as DM2, insulin resistance characterized by a frame, generally associated with obesity. Both types are featured by hyperglycemia above. Insulin resistance reduces glucose tolerance especially in muscle cells and adipocytes, where glucose uptake is insulin dependent. This causes glucose accumulation in the circulation and consequently a hyperglycemic state, generating homeostatic and systemic imbalance [5].

Diabetes is considered a major cause of premature death, because of the increased risk for developing cardiovascular diseases, which contribute to 50% to 80% of patients deaths due to increased levels of serum cholesterol and triglycerides. Cardiovascular diseases include diseases of the circulatory system, comprising a wide range of clinical syndromes, the main cause of atherosclerosis, which also increases the risk of acute coronary syndromes. The incidence of cardiovascular diseases reaches 20% in diabetics after a period of about 7 years [6].

Hyperglycemia has a direct relationship with the development of an inflammatory condition showed by the increased expression of proinflammatory cytokines such as IL-6, TNF-α, and NFκB. Thus, diabetes, as well as hyperglycemia due to its nature, is also an inflammatory disease character. Studies show that the longer the duration of the disease and/or loss of glycemic control, the higher the inflammatory process [7, 8].

The elevation of proinflammatory cytokines plays an essential role in insulin resistance and induces the appearance of cardiovascular complications diabetic micro- and macrovascular, kidney disease and anemia. By increasing especially IL-6, antierythropoietic effect occurs, since this cytokine changes the sensitivity of progenitors to erythropoietin (erythroid growth factor) and also promotes apoptosis of immature erythrocytes causing a decrease, further, in the number of circulating erythrocytes and consequently causing a reduction of circulating hemoglobin [7, 9].

It should also be noted that, due to the development of diabetes mellitus, the nephropathy may arise, which further undermines the renal production of erythropoietin, positively contributing to an increased anemic framework [9, 10]. According to Escorcio et al. [11] approximately 40% of diabetic patients are affected by kidney diseases. The decreased renal function and proinflammatory cytokines are the most important factors in determining reduction of hemoglobin levels in those patients. The inflammatory situation created by kidney disease also interferes with intestinal iron absorption and mobilization of inventories [12]. Therefore, diabetic patients with kidney disease have the highest risk for developing anemia [11].

The National Kidney Foundation defines anemia in chronic kidney disease as Hb level < 13,5 g/dL in men and 12,0 g/dL in women [13]. Anemia represents an emerging global health problem that negatively impacts quality of life and requires an ever-greater allocation of healthcare resources [14]. The anemic framework promotes reduced exercise capacity, fatigue, anorexia, depression, cognitive dysfunction, decreased libido, and other factors, which increase cardiac risk patients and depress the quality and life expectancy of the same [15]. Under these circumstances, anemia in patients with diabetes must be treated once diagnosed, since it may contribute to the pathogenesis and progression of cardiovascular disease and serious diabetic nephropathy and retinopathy. The regular screening for anemia, along with other complications associated with diabetes, can help slow the progression of vascular complications in these patients [16].

Anemia in diabetic person has a significant adverse effect on quality of life and is associated with disease progression and the development of comorbidities [7], as obesity and dyslipidemia that are strongly associated with diabetic framework and significantly contribute to increasing the

risk of cardiovascular diseases [8]. Thus, the present study is to evaluate the prevalence of anemia in a sample of patients with type 2 diabetes who are living in a city in the northwest of the Rio Grande do Sul state, registered in the Family Health Strategies, and check its correlation with demographic, lifestyle, and laboratory variables of patients.

2. Methods

This is a descriptive and analytical study of the type of case studies in patients with DM2 and ages less than 75 years living in the urban area in the city of Ijuí RS, registered in programs of the Family Health Strategy (FHS) in this city. The study was conducted from January 2010 to January 2013, after agreement by the Research Ethics Committee of the Regional University of Rio Grande do Sul State Northwest (UNIJUÍ) (Opinion number 091/2010). All participants signed the informed consent in this research.

The sample size was calculated by StatCalc application EpiInfo 3.5.3, considering the prevalence of nonspecific outcome of 50%, 5% error, and 95% level of reliability, which resulted in a sample of 269 patients. Foreseeing possible losings a percentage of 5% of this number was added, a total sample of 283 patients with DM2.

The study excluded those patients who had difficulties to understand the proposed procedures, those who were bedridden, and those who had difficulty walking.

The invitation to participate in the study was made to patients during home visits, with the monitoring of community health workers when possible. At the moment of visit, the research objectives were explained for the patient and the dates of the interviews were fixed with those who agreed to participate, in addition to scheduling the clinical and laboratory reviews, held, respectively, in Physiotherapy Clinic and the Laboratory of Clinical Analysis of UNIJUÍ (UNILAB).

The interviews and tests were conducted by trained health professionals. Data collection was performed by applying a semistructured instrument. The presence of anemia was considered as the dependent variable; the patient was considered anemic, according to the World Health Organization reference values [17]. Thus, the patient was considered anemic patient when the blood count hemoglobin < 12 g/dL and <14 g/dL for females and males, respectively. The independent variables analyzed were as follows:

(a) Sociodemographic characteristics:

   (i) age (in years);
   (ii) sex (female/male).

(b) Health condition:

   (i) time of diagnosis of type 2 diabetes (in years);
   (ii) advanced age (over 60 years).

(c) Comorbidities:

   (i) presence of hypertension (yes/no);

(ii) cardiac and/or respiratory (yes or no), analyzed according to the patient's report when asked about the presence of these diseases;

(iii) dyslipidemia (yes/no), diagnosed by biochemical tests;

(iv) obesity (yes/no), when the value of body mass index was $\geq 30,0\,kg/m^2$ for patients up to 59 years old and $\geq 27,0\,kg/m^2$ for patients aged 60–75 [18].

(d) Lifestyle:

(i) smoking (yes/no);

(ii) alcohol consumption (yes/no);

(iii) physical inactivity (yes/no);

(iv) stress (yes/no).

(e) Eating habits, investigated through questioning a high salt diet (yes/no).

Every patient who declared himself a smoker at the moment of evaluation is considered smoker, regardless of the amount of cigarettes consumed; and alcoholic is the person who reported excessive consumption of alcohol during the study period, at any frequency. Excessive salt intake was measured by the question: Do you put much salt in your food? Stress was assessed by the question: Do you consider yourself a stressed person? There were classified physically inactive patients who reported not performing any type of regular exercise with the lowest frequency of three times a week.

The evaluation of anthropometric data, including the measurement of body weight (in kilograms) on digital scale, was performed (Toledo); height (in meters) in stadiometer (Toledo) and waist circumference (WC) were measured at the midpoint between the last rib and the iliac crest using flexible standard tape and nonextensible, defining measure of 0,1 cm, according to techniques recommended [19]. The body mass index (BMI) was calculated by dividing body weight and the square of height: kg/m^2.

At the end of the clinical evaluation, an appointment was made with the date and the time of collection of blood from each patient. Patients personally received clarification on the procedures of collection and were instructed to fast for at least eight hours prior to the blood collection, in addition to writing instructions and containers for the collection of the first urine in the morning. Among the laboratory tests that were performed are the creatinine dosage and blood glucose by enzymatic Trinder method [20]. In addition, the collection and enforcement of the blood count were performed to evaluate the presence of hematological disorders in patients with DM2. The blood sample, was also used the serum of patients after venipuncture and centrifugation of whole blood for biochemical measurements, as well as whole blood anticoagulant containing standard for hematologic examinations.

The patient who presented two or more of the following criteria proposed by the National Cholesterol Education Program was classified as having metabolic syndrome: [21] increased waist circumference (>88 cm women and >102 cm men); elevated serum triglycerides (≥150 mg/dL) or

decreased HDL cholesterol (<40 mg/dL men and <50 mg/dL women); and hypertension (diagnosed or identified through the use of antihypertensive medication).

Renal function was assessed by the value of serum creatinine, obtained by biochemical tests. The glomerular filtration rate is estimated by the Cockcroft-Gault calculated using the formula available on the websites of the Brazilian Society of Nephrology (SBN) of the National Kidney Foundation [22]. We considered impaired renal function the values above 1,2 mg/dL in the serum creatinine [23] and the GFR less than $60\,mL/min/1,73\,m^2$ estimated by the Cockroft-Gault equation [24] representing a decrease of about 50% of normal renal function and, below this level, increasing the prevalence of complications of chronic kidney disease [25]. For the use of the Cockcroft-Gault equation, the ideal weight of the patient was computed using the Lorenz formula, which puts the ideal body weight for the subjects height in cm function [26].

For processing the data, we used the Statistical Package for Social Science (SPSS) (version 18.0, one Chicago, IL, USA). In the statistical analysis, all variables were tested for normality using the Kolmogorov-Smirnov (KS) test. The qualitative variables are presented as frequencies and percentages and quantitative variables as average and standard deviation (average ± SD) ormedian (minimumand maximum). Mann-Whitney tests were used to compare two independent groups with abnormal distribution, Student's t-test was used for normally distributed variables, and the Chi-square test and Fisher's exact Pearson were used to compare categorical variables in order to verify differences of variables between patients with and without anemia. The Spearman correlation coefficient was used to evaluate the correlation between clinical and biochemical parameters with the hemoglobin level. $p < 0,05$ was considered statistically significant. All tests were applied with a Confidence Interval (CI) of 95%.

3. Results

283 patients with DM2 were suitable to the study inclusion criteria and were selected for home visits and invitation to participate in the study, according to data collected from health professionals in FHS or the medical records of the patients belonging to nine FHS in the city of Ijuí, RS. Of these, 64 patients were not included in the study for the following reasons: contact absence; refusal to participate; and not identifying the address informed and 73 individuals were not included due to insufficient data to evaluate the hematologic changes, since they did not undergo blood tests for hemoglobin count, a total sample of 146 type 2 diabetic patients in this study, of which 50 had anemia, corresponding to 34,2%.

The study population had an average age of 60,9 ± 8,9 years, body mass index of 31,2 ± 5,8 kg/m^2, and a median of disease diagnosis time of 5,0 years (0,5–40,0 years).

We analyzed the dependent variable "anemia" according to some characteristics of patients with DM2. For time of diagnosis of the disease, old age, metabolic syndrome, renal dysfunction by creatinine, and the Cockcroft-Gault equation, there was no difference between the presence and absence

TABLE 1: Characteristics of patients with diabetes mellitus type 2 according to the presence of anemia.

| Variables | Anemia | | p value |
	Yes (n = 50)	No (n = 96)	
Gender			$0,059^{£}$
Male	23 (46,0)	29 (30,2)	
Female	27 (54,0)	67 (69,8)	
Age (in years)	61,8 ± 9,5	60,5 ± 8,7	$0,274^{\mu}$
Body mass (kg)	83,6 ± 16,8	77,5 ± 13,5	$0,019^{¥*}$
Height (m)	1,61 ± 0,08	1,59 ± 0,09	$0,287^{¥}$
BMI (kg/m²)	32,2 ± 6,0	30,6 ± 5,7	$0,126^{¥}$
Waist circumference (cm)	105,9 ± 15,9	104,7 ± 11,5	$0,626^{¥}$
Time of diagnosis of DM2 (in years)	6 (0,5–40,0)	5 (0,6–40,0)	$0,148^{\mu}$
Advanced age	30 (60,0)	55 (57,3)	$0,753^{£}$
Hypertension	42 (84,0)	65 (67,7)	$0,035^{£*}$
Dyslipidemia	23 (46,0)	48 (50,0)	$0,646^{£}$
Obesity	38 (76,0)	65 (67,7)	$0,297^{£}$
Metabolic syndrome	35 (70,0)	56 (58,3)	$0,167^{£}$
Heart disease	10 (20,0)	18 (18,8)	$0,856^{£}$
Respiratory disease	6 (12,0)	15 (15,6)	$0,627^{€}$
Smoking	8 (18,0)	14 (14,6)	$0,179^{£}$
Alcoholism	4 (8,0)	6 (6,3)	$0,924^{€}$
Physical inactivity	23 (46,0)	50 (52,1)	$0,485^{£}$
Stress	23 (46,0)	53 (55,2)	$0,291^{£}$
Hypersodic diet	6 (12,0)	19 (19,8)	$0,259^{€}$
Alteration of renal function by creatinine	9 (18,0)	18 (18,8)	$0,912^{£}$
Alteration of renal function by Cockcroft-Gault equation	12 (24,0)	25 (26,0)	$0,788^{£}$

DM2: diabetes mellitus type 2; ¥ indicates p value according to Student's t-test; μ indicates p value according to test of Mann-Whitney; £ indicates p value according to test of Chi-square of Pearson; € indicates p value according to the exact test of Fischer; results presented on average ± standard deviation or median (minimal and maximal value) and number (percentage); ∗ was considered statistically significant.

TABLE 2: Biochemical and hematological variables in patients with DM2 according to the presence of anemia.

| Variables | Anemia | | p value |
	Yes (n = 50)	No (n = 96)	
Hemoglobin (g/dL)	11,68 ± 0,81	13,32 ± 0,85	$<0,0001^{¥*}$
Hematocrit (%)	35,08 ± 5,23	40,45 ± 2,88	$<0,0001^{\mu*}$
Red cells (millions/mm³)	4,23 ± 0,37	4,68 ± 0,34	$<0,0001^{¥*}$
Glycemia (mg/dL)	109,4 ± 40,5	133,6 ± 55,2	$0,005^{\mu*}$
Creatinine (mg/dL)	1,05 ± 0,39	1,03 ± 0,27	$0,944^{\mu}$
Glomerular filtration rate (mL/min)	91,7 ± 41,9	79,9 ± 27,2	$0,277^{**}$

¥ indicates p value according to Student's t-test; μ indicates p value according to test of Mann-Whitney; ∗ was considered statistically significant; results presented in average ± standard deviation or median (minimal and maximal value). ∗∗ indicates mean glomerular filtration rate by Cockcroft-Gault equation.

TABLE 3: Coefficients of correlation between clinical and biochemical parameters with the hemoglobin in patients with diabetes mellitus type 2.

| Variables | Hemoglobin | |
	p	R
Age (in years)	0,492	−0,057
BMI (kg/m²)	0,051	−0,155
Time of diagnosis of DM2	0,466	−0,061
Glycemia (mg/dL)	$0,004^{*}$	0,235
Creatinine (mg/dL)	0,209	0,105
Glomerular filtration rate by the Cockcroft-Gault equation (mL/min./1,73 m²)	0,526	0,053

Spearman rank correlation test; ∗ was considered statistically significant.

of anemia ($p > 0,05$). However, variables, body mass, and hypertension showed significance to the outcome studied ($p < 0,05$). These data are presented in Table 1.

We observed statistically significant difference in hematological variables between groups with and without anemia ($p < 0,05$). The same is observed with respect to glucose,

however, with higher values in the group without anemia. There was no statistically significant difference in creatinine variable ($p > 0,05$). These data are presented in Table 2.

Table 3 shows the correlations between the clinical and biochemical parameters with hemoglobin. It is observed that there are positive and weak correlation between glucose and hemoglobin and negative and weak correlation between BMI and hemoglobin.

4. Discussion

Often, chronic diseases, such as DM, are accompanied by mild-to-moderate anemia, often called anemia of inflammation or infection or anemia of chronic disease [27]. Andrews and Arredondo [28] determined the presence of anemia in type 2 diabetic patients as well as evaluating the expression of genes related to inflammation and immune response. The results found by the authors demonstrate that diabetic patients with anemia exhibit increased expression of proinflammatory cytokines as compared to diabetic patients only. In anemic patient increase in IL-6 production, as well as B cell activity, was confirmed which reinforces the association between IL-6 and antierythropoietic action. Moreover, the diabetic and anemic patients had high levels of C-reactive protein and ferritin ultrasensible; however, these diabetic and anemic patients had low iron contents, showing that ferritin increases were associated with chronic inflammatory process present in diabetes [28].

In this study, there was a higher prevalence of obesity and higher mean BMI and waist circumference in anemic patients when compared to nonanemic ones; however, there was a statistically significant difference between the groups only for body mass variable. Anemia in diabetic patients is also related to obesity, BMI, and high waist circumference. The obesity or accumulation of circulating fatty acids is associated with the development of an inflammatory state that predisposes the development of insulin resistance. Insulin resistance reduces glucose tolerance especially in adipocytes and muscle cells, in which glucose uptake is insulin. This causes glucose accumulation in the circulation and consequently a hyperglycemic state [29].

Adipose tissue has more recently been recognized as a metabolically active organ system linking the endocrine and immune systems; furthermore it is the source of a variety of cytokines. Higher baseline BMI remained a predictor of additional adjustments for blood pressure level and the presence or absence of diabetes mellitus. Similar to TNF-alpha, IL-6 is a proinflammatory adipokine that correlates with body weight and insulin resistance [30].

The increased inflammatory activity in adipose tissue of obese patients favors the production of hepcidin that in anemia of chronic disease is increased during infection and inflammation, causing a decrease in serum iron level through a mechanism that limits the availability of iron. The association of higher iron stores with diabetes and insulin resistance has been repeatedly confirmed by many investigators. Ferritin levels were found to predict a higher rate of diabetes in prospective studies and case-control cohorts. Furthermore, serum ferritin was positively associated with body mass index (BMI), visceral fat mass, serum glucose levels, insulin sensitivity, and cholesterol levels [31–33].

In addition, it was found in this study that the prevalence of hypertension in diabetic patients that were anemic was significantly higher when compared to nonanemic ones. This association is of concern considering that hypertension in diabetic increases the risk of cardiovascular complications such as heart failure, stroke, tissue inflammation, and atherosclerosis [4].

According to Ximenes et al. [34] anemia is a prevalent comorbidity in patients with hypertension and when present, patients have more severe symptoms and worse functional capacity as well as increased mortality. The knowledge that anemia worsens the symptoms of hypertension is not new, but, in recent years, the magnitude of the anemia associated with this disease has become more evident. The main causes that contribute to anemia in patients with hypertension are nutritional deficiencies especially iron deficiency and chronic inflammation [34].

It was observed in the present study that there are decreased values of hemoglobin, hematocrit, and red blood cells in anemic patients, which can be associated with a normocytic normochromic anemia, characteristic of an anemia of chronic disease (ACD). ACD is a light-to-moderate anemia shortening the survival of red blood cells (about 80 days instead of 120 days normal). This phenomenon is attributed to hyperactivity state mononuclear phagocyte system, triggered by infectious, inflammatory, or neoplastic process, leading to early removal of circulating red blood cells. Inadequate bone marrow response observed is due basically to inappropriately low Secretion of Erythropoietin (EPO), decreased bone marrow response to EPO, and decreased erythropoiesis consequent to lower supply of iron to the bone marrow [35].

One explanation for this bone marrow response is directly related to the activation of macrophages and the release of inflammatory cytokines, particularly IL-1, IL-6, tumor necrosis factor (TNF a), and interferon gamma (INF g) which act by inhibiting the proliferation of erythroid precursors and therefore inhibit erythropoiesis. Furthermore, the suppressive action of these cytokines on erythropoiesis stimulating overcomes the action of EPO resulting in decreased bone marrow response to EPO and erythropoiesis [36].

Also it should be noted that there was no hemoglobin correlation with creatinine or statistical differences in creatinine values and glomerular filtration rate estimated between groups, indicating once again that anemia by chronic disease was inflammation triggered and the reduction renal function affects the production of EPO.

The limitations in this study refer to the fact that the assessment of glycemic control in diabetic patients was performed by means of fasting glucose that is a momentary biochemical analysis, does not represent the average glucose of patients, and may also occur interfering in the examination, as the effect of hypoglycemic agents, promoting a reduction in glucose levels. In this sense, the gold standard for assessing glycemic control would be the achievement of HbA1c (glycated hemoglobin), which is one of the most important tools to assess glycemic control of patients with diabetes, as they express the average amount of glucose in the last three months, and this can infer the diabetes control efficiency and suggest the need for adjustments.

Therefore, it is suggested that further studies should be conducted using test glycated hemoglobin, which currently is already considered an essential parameter in the DM control evaluation, in order to relate hyperglycemia, inflammation, and anemia.

5. Conclusion

Patients with DM2 and anemia were those with high body mass, hypertension, increased waist circumference, and longer time of the disease. This set of changes characterizes the anemia as chronic disease, which has a significant adverse effect on quality of life of diabetic patients and is associated with the progression of the disease; the development of comorbidities significantly contributes to the increased risk of cardiovascular disease. However, against what was expected, the results of blood glucose were higher in nonanemic patients, which is contradictory due to the anemia of these patients being associated with an inflammatory condition, for being characterized as normocytic normochromic anemia. Deepening the study of the issues raised throughout this work provides knowledge for the establishment of new strategies for glycemic control, which can increase the research and correlate some analytical parameters, such as HbA1c, Il-6, VHS, and PCR.

Conflict of Interests

The authors declare that there is no conflict of interests.

References

[1] J. E. Shaw, R. A. Sicree, and P. Z. Zimmet, "Global estimates of the prevalence of diabetes for 2010 and 2030," *Diabetes Research and Clinical Practice*, vol. 87, no. 1, pp. 4–14, 2010.

[2] P. F. Pereira, R. D. C. G. Alfenas, and R. M. A. Araújo, "Does breastfeeding influence the risk of developing diabetes mellitus in children? A review of current evidence," *Jornal de Pediatria*, vol. 90, no. 1, pp. 7–15, 2014.

[3] Brasil Ministério da Saúde, *Diretrizes da Sociedade Brasileira de Diabetes 2013-2014*, AC Farmacêutica, 2014.

[4] P. M. S. B. Francisco, A. P. Belon, M. B. A. Barros, L. Carandina, M. C. G. P. Alves, and C. L. G. Cesar, "Self-reported diabetes in the elderly: prevalence, associated factors, and control practices," *Cadernos de Saúde Pública*, vol. 26, no. 1, pp. 175–184, 2010.

[5] X. Zhang, X. Cui, F. Li et al., "Association between diabetes mellitus with metabolic syndrome and diabetic microangiopathy," *Experimental and Therapeutic Medicine*, vol. 8, no. 6, pp. 1867–1873, 2014.

[6] T. R. Silva, J. Zanuzzi, C. D. M. Silva, X. S. Passos, and B. M. F. Costa, "Prevalence of cardiovascular diseases in diabetic and nutritional status of patientes," *Journal of the Health Sciences Institute*, vol. 30, no. 3, pp. 266–270, 2012.

[7] A. Angelousi and E. Larger, "Anaemia, a common but often unrecognized risk in diabetic patients: a review," *Diabetes & Metabolism*, vol. 41, no. 1, pp. 18–27, 2015.

[8] B. Martínez-Pérez, I. De La Torre-Díez, and M. López-Coronado, "Mobile health applications for the most prevalent conditions by the World Health Organization: review and analysis," *Journal of Medical Internet Research*, vol. 15, no. 6, article e120, 2013.

[9] S. Fava, J. Azzopardi, S. Ellard, and A. T. Hattersley, "ACE gene polymorphism as a prognostic indicator in patients with type 2 diabetes and established renal disease," *Diabetes Care*, vol. 24, no. 12, pp. 2115–2120, 2001.

[10] V. Jha, G. Garcia-Garcia, K. Iseki et al., "Chronic kidney disease: global dimension and perspectives," *The Lancet*, vol. 382, no. 9888, pp. 260–272, 2013.

[11] C. S. M. Escorcio, H. F. Silva, G. B. S. Junior, M. P. Monteiro, and R. P. Gonçalves, "Evaluation of anemia treatment with EPO and oral and iv iron in patients with chronic kidney disease under hemodialysis," *RBSA*, vol. 42, no. 2, pp. 87–90, 2010.

[12] G. Weiss and L. T. Goodnough, "Anemia of chronic disease," *The New England Journal of Medicine*, vol. 352, no. 10, pp. 1011–1059, 2005.

[13] I. C. Macdougall, K.-U. Eckardt, and F. Locatelli, "Latest US KDOQI Anaemia Guidelines update—what are the implications for Europe?" *Nephrology Dialysis Transplantation*, vol. 22, no. 10, pp. 2738–2742, 2007.

[14] A. MacCiò and C. Madeddu, "Management of anemia of inflammation in the elderly," *Anemia*, vol. 2012, Article ID 563251, 20 pages, 2012.

[15] T. D. Moreira and M. A. Mascarenhas, *Avaliação da prevalência de anemia em grupos diabéticos e não diabéticos e sua relação com insuficiência renal crônica*, 62nd edition, 2004.

[16] D. K. Singh, P. Winocour, and K. Farrington, "Erythropoietic stress and anemia in diabetes mellitus," *Nature Reviews Endocrinology*, vol. 5, no. 4, pp. 204–210, 2009.

[17] WHO, *Anaemia*, World Health Organization, 2012.

[18] D. A. Lipschitz, "Screening for nutritional status in the elderly," *Primary Care*, vol. 21, no. 1, pp. 55–67, 1994.

[19] V. H. Hevward and L. M. Stolarczyc, *Avaliação da composição corporal aplicada*, Manole, São Paulo, Brazil, 2000.

[20] J. B. Henry, *Diagnósticos Clínicos e Tratamento por Métodos Laboratoriais*, São Paulo, Brazil, Manole, 2008.

[21] Expert Panel on Detection, Evaluation, and Treatment of High Blood Cholesterol in Adults, "Executive summary of the third report of the National Cholesterol Education Program (NCEP) Expert Panel on Detection, Evaluation, and Treatment of High Blood Cholesterol in Adults (Adult Treatment Panel III)," *Journal of the American Medical Association*, vol. 285, no. 19, pp. 2486–2497, 2001.

[22] National Kidney Foundation, "K/DOQI clinical practice guidelines for chronic kidney disease: evaluation, classification and stratification," *American Journal of Kidney Diseases*, vol. 39, no. 2, supplement 1, pp. S1–S266, 2002.

[23] F. M. Di Napoli, J. E. Burmeister, D. R. Miltersteiner, B. M. Campos, and M. G. Costa, "Estimation of renal function by the cockcroft and gault formula in overweighted or obese patients," *Jornal Brasileiro de Nefrologia*, vol. 30, pp. 185–191, 2008.

[24] E. J. C. Magacho, A. C. Pereira, H. N. Mansur, and M. G. Bastos, "Nomogram for estimation of glomerular filtration rate based on the CKD-EPI formula," *Jornal Brasileiro de Nefrologia*, vol. 34, no. 3, pp. 313–315, 2012.

[25] M. G. Bastos, R. Bregman, and G. M. Kirsztajn, "Chronic kidney diseases: common and harmful, but also preventable and treatable," *Revista da Associacao Medica Brasileira*, vol. 56, no. 2, pp. 248–253, 2010.

[26] T. P. Sanso, "Neurofisiologia dela alimentación: su incidencia em la obesidad común," *Estudios de Psicologia*, vol. 14, pp. 126–138, 1983.

[27] M. C. Carvalho, E. C. E. Baracat, and V. C. Sgarbieri, "Anemia ferropriva e anemia de doença crônica: distúrbios do metabolismo de ferro," *Revista Segurança Alimentar e Nutricional*, vol. 13, no. 2, pp. 54–63, 2006.

[28] M. Andrews and M. Arredondo, "Ferritin levels and hepcidin mRNA expression in peripheral mononuclear cells from anemic type 2 diabetic patients," *Biological Trace Element Research*, vol. 149, no. 1, pp. 1–4, 2012.

[29] P. L. Hooper and P. L. Hooper, "Inflammation, heat shock proteins, and type 2 diabetes," *Cell Stress and Chaperones*, vol. 14, no. 2, pp. 113–115, 2009.

[30] C. Rüster and G. Wolf, "Adipokines promote chronic kidney disease," *Nephrology Dialysis Transplantation*, vol. 28, supplement 4, pp. iv8–iv14, 2013.

[31] T. Iwasaki, A. Nakajima, M. Yoneda et al., "Serum ferritin is associated with visceral fat area and subcutaneous fat area," *Diabetes Care*, vol. 28, no. 10, pp. 2486–2491, 2005.

[32] C. E. Wrede, R. Buettner, L. C. Bollheimer, J. Schölmerich, K.-D. Palitzsch, and C. Hellerbrand, "Association between serum ferritin and the insulin resistance syndrome in a representative population," *European Journal of Endocrinology*, vol. 154, no. 2, pp. 333–340, 2006.

[33] P. Galan, N. Noisette, C. Estaquio et al., "Serum ferritin, cardiovascular risk factors and ischaemic heart diseases: a prospective analysis in the SU.VI.MAX (SUpplementation en VItamines et Minéraux AntioXydants) cohort," *Public Health Nutrition*, vol. 9, no. 1, pp. 70–74, 2006.

[34] R. M. O. Ximenes, A. C. P. Barretto, and E. P. Silva, "Anemia in heart failure patients: development risk factors," *Revista Brasileira de Cardiologia*, vol. 27, no. 3, pp. 189–194, 2014.

[35] R. D. Cançado, "Multiple myeloma and anemias," *Revista Brasileira de Hematologia e Hemoterapia*, vol. 29, no. 1, pp. 67–76, 2007.

[36] L. F. Amador-Medina, "Anemia in chronic kidney disease," *Revista Médica del Instituto Mexicano del Seguro Social*, vol. 52, no. 6, pp. 660–665, 2014.

7

Cormic Index Profile of Children with Sickle Cell Anaemia in Lagos, Nigeria

Samuel Olufemi Akodu, Olisamedua Fidelis Njokanma, and Omolara Adeolu Kehinde

Department of Paediatrics, Lagos State University Teaching Hospital, P.O. Box 11950, Ikeja, Lagos 100001, Nigeria

Correspondence should be addressed to Samuel Olufemi Akodu; femiakodu@hotmail.com

Academic Editor: Aurelio Maggio

Background. Sickle cell disorders are known to have a negative effect on linear growth. This could potentially affect proportional growth and, hence, Cormic Index. *Objective*. To determine the Cormic Index in the sickle cell anaemia population in Lagos. *Methodology*. A consecutive sample of 100 children with haemoglobin genotype SS, aged eight months to 15 years, and 100 age and sex matched controls (haemoglobin genotype AA) was studied. Sitting height (upper segment) and full length or height were measured. Sitting height was then expressed as a percentage of full length/height (Cormic Index). *Results*. The mean Cormic Index decreased with age among primary subjects (SS) and AA controls. The overall mean Cormic Index among primary subjects was comparable to that of controls (55.0 ± 4.6% versus 54.5 ± 5.2%; 54.8 ± 4.5% versus 53.6 ± 4.9%) in boys and girls, respectively. In comparison with AA controls, female children with sickle cell anaemia who were older than 10 years had a significantly lower mean Cormic Index. *Conclusion*. There was a significant negative relationship between Cormic Index and height in subjects and controls irrespective of gender. Similarly, a significant negative correlation existed between age, sitting height, subischial leg length, weight, and Cormic Index in both subjects and controls.

1. Introduction

Sickle cell anaemia is a group of genetic disorders most commonly seen in man and it is found in people of African descent but it is also seen in people of other ethnic groups [1]. It has been shown that, as a group, children with sickle cell anaemia have poor growth [2, 3]. Anthropometry is the principal method of assessing growth and height/length-for-age is the most useful linear measurement that gives an indication of past nutrition [4].

The Cormic Index expresses sitting height as a proportion of full height. It is a measure of the relative length of trunk and lower limb and it varies between individuals and groups [5]. It is the most common bivariate index of shape [5]. The Cormic Index is most often used to correct for variability in body shape when Body Mass Index (BMI) is used to compare the nutritional status in or between different populations [6]. For example, individuals who are very tall may be wrongly classified as being underweight despite having normal body weight for their culture. Similarly, in muscular people BMI may be more likely to indicate overweight, as lean body mass

tissue is denser than fat tissue. The BMI can be modified using Cormic Index to help correct for this variability in body shape. Used as such, it adjusts for population differences in phenotype that may impact BMI. It is important to recognize that this type of adjustment mainly has been applied to adults and not to children or adolescents [7].

It has been evident that there is variability in the growth of spinal length compared with limb length during the prepubertal period and during adolescence. Previous studies have shown that increase in sitting height is relatively faster than leg length in later childhood [8, 9]. The negative effect of sickle cell anaemia on spinal growth and, hence, Cormic Index would therefore be expected to be more obvious in older children during the period of expected rapid growth. Shorter spinal length relative to the height increases the Cormic Index.

To the best of the authors' knowledge, there is no prior report of the Cormic Index among children with sickle cell anaemia in Nigeria or elsewhere. Studies have been conducted among African [10], Australian aborigines [11], and Asian [12] population without specific reference to haemoglobin genotype. However, the direct effect of sickle cell anaemia on linear growth may limit the application of findings in the general population to affected children.

The appraisal of the Cormic Index among children with sickle cell anaemia is therefore of clinical and scientific interest. Therefore, the main objective of the present report was to determine the Cormic Index among children with sickle cell anaemia.

2. Materials and Methods

The cross-sectional study was conducted between October and December 2009 among children with sickle cell anaemia attending the sickle cell disease clinic of the Department of Paediatrics of Lagos State University Teaching Hospital, Ikeja, in Southwest Nigeria. The hospital is an urban tertiary health centre in Lagos State, Western Nigeria. It is a major referral center serving the whole state, which is a major point of entry into Nigeria from different parts of the world and is the economic nerve centre of Nigeria.

Approval for the study was obtained from the Ethics Committee of Lagos State University Teaching Hospital and written informed consent was obtained from each parent. Consecutive patients with sickle cell anaemia who came for routine follow-up clinic that gave consent and met the study criteria were eligible for enrollment in the study. Healthy controls were children with haemoglobin genotype "AA" from the general outpatient and follow-up clinics and healthy children attending other specialist clinics like the Paediatric Dermatology Clinic. Controls were matched with primary subjects for age and sex. Two hundred children were studied—one hundred each with haemoglobin genotypes SS and AA. In order to have fairly equal representation of ages, the subjects stratified as follows: <2 years, >2 to 5 years, >5 to 10 years, and >10 to 15 years.

2.1. Inclusion Criteria

(1) Age six months to fifteen years.

(2) Confirmed HbSS by electrophoresis.

(3) Signed, informed consent of the caregiver.

(4) Subjects who were in steady state, that is, absence of any crisis in the preceding four weeks, no recent drop in the haemoglobin level, and absence of any symptoms or signs attributable to acute illness [13].

(5) Children who were not taking medications known to affect growth, for example, steroids.

2.2. Exclusion Criteria

(1) Children with congenital cardiac abnormality, chronic renal disease, or abnormal chest wall deformity or chronic respiratory disorder.

(2) Refusal of consent.

(3) Children with history of cerebrovascular accident.

(4) Sickle cell anaemia patients with history of long-term transfusion therapy.

The inclusion and exclusion criteria for the controls were the same as for subjects except that the haemoglobin genotype was AA.

2.3. Measurement of Height. Children two years of age and older had their heights measured using a stadiometer while the length of those below two years was measured using an infantometer.

2.4. Measurement of Weight. Subjects' weights were measured barefooted and wearing light clothing. Weight measurements were taken on a Seca 761 series mechanical floor scale to the nearest 0.1 Kg.

2.5. Measurement of Sitting Height. Sitting height was measured using a sitting height table. Sitting height was measured from the vertex of the head to the seated buttocks. The subject's head was positioned in the Frankfort horizontal plane, the shoulders relaxed, the back straight, and the head plate was brought into firm contact with the vertex [14].

The various linear measurements were taken three times and the mean was recorded. Subjects were measured wearing light clothing and shoes were removed. The measurements were taken following the standard techniques. The measurements were carried out by the researchers.

2.6. Derivation of Subischial Leg Length. It is expressed as the difference between height/length and sitting height.

2.7. Derivation of Body Mass Index. The body mass index was expressed as weight in Kg/height in metre^2 (Kg/m^2).

2.8. Derivation of Cormic Index. It is expressed as

$$\left(\frac{\text{Sitting height}}{\text{height}} \right) \times 100. \qquad (1)$$

Social classification was done using the scheme proposed by Oyedeji [15] in which subjects are grouped into five classes (I–V) based on the occupation and educational attainments of both parents. Analysis was done using Statistical Package for Social Science (SPSS) version 17.0. Comparison of mean values was done using Student's t-test and $P < 0.05$ is considered significant. The Pearson correlation coefficient (r) was attempted for understanding the overall relationship of anthropometric variables and age with Cormic Index.

In order to standardize the calculated BMI, the model developed by Norgan [16] was modified and applied. In the original model, standardized BMI was obtained using the formula $\text{BMI}_{\text{std}} = \text{BMI}_{52.0} + (\text{BMI}_0 - \text{BMI}_1)$, where

BMI_{std} is standardized BMI,

$\text{BMI}_{52.0}$ is estimated BMI at Cormic Index of 54.9% (the mean Cormic Index for the European population),

TABLE 1: Mean Cormic Index distribution of study subjects according to age and gender.

Variable	SS Mean (SD)	AA Mean (SD)	t-value	P value
Age group				
≤2 yrs				
Males	60.3 (2.6)	60.1 (1.8)	−0.228	0.822
Females	59.5 (2.8)	60.8 (2.6)	1.192	0.245
Males and females	59.9 (2.7)	60.5 (2.2)	0.783	0.437
>2 yrs–5 yrs				
Males	54.5 (2.3)	56.6 (3.3)	1.914	0.068
Females	55.0 (2.3)	54.8 (1.5)	−0.267	0.792
Males and females	54.7 (2.2)	55.7 (2.7)	1.408	0.165
>5 yrs–10 yrs				
Males	52.1 (5.6)	51.5 (1.2)	−0.385	0.704
Females	51.4 (1.6)	51.6 (2.2)	0.337	0.739
Males and females	51.8 (4.0)	51.6 (1.7)	−0.208	0.836
>10 yrs–15 yrs				
Males	50.4 (3.6)	51.1 (3.5)	0.475	0.640
Females	48.1 (2.2)	51.5 (2.9)	3.181	0.004
Males and females	49.3 (3.1)	51.3 (3.2)	2.213	0.032
Socioeconomic strata				
Upper	55.15 (5.15)	55.02 (4.89)	0.128	0.899
Other	53.10 (4.70)	54.57 (4.18)	1.612	0.110

SD: standard deviation.

BMI$_0$ is actual (observed) BMI,

BMI$_1$ is estimated BMI at actual (observed) Cormic Index.

Note: Cormic Index should be expressed as a percentage.

Modification to the Norgan model was done by substituting the mean Cormic Index of the European population with that for the haemoglobin AA population in the current study.

3. Results

3.1. Cormic Index of Study Subjects. The Cormic Index of the SS subjects ranged from 44.5% to 68.2% while that for AA controls ranged from 45.9% to 65.0%. The mean Cormic Index of the SS group of 54.1 (±5.1)% was not statistically different from 54.9 (±4.5)% in the AA-control group (t-value = 1.240, P = 0.216). The overall mean Cormic Index was 54.5 (±4.8)%. The mean Cormic Index of the study subjects according to age, gender, and socioeconomic strata was shown in Table 1. Mean Cormic Index decreased with age irrespective of gender or haemoglobin genotype. In each age group, the value observed in males with genotype SS was comparable to that of their AA counterparts. This was also the pattern in females except in the oldest age group in which AA controls had a significantly higher index. Within the haemoglobin "SS" group, the mean Cormic Index values of males were comparable to those of females across all age groups. The same was true of "AA" subjects across all age groups.

The mean Cormic Index was significantly higher in sickle cell anaemia subjects of the upper socioeconomic class than in those of the other classes (P = 0.047). On the other hand, the difference between mean values for upper class and lower class controls was not significant (P = 0.63).

3.2. Correlation between Cormic Index and Height. Table 2 shows the results of correlation analysis between Cormic Index and height of study subjects with and without sickle cell anaemia. Overall, the Cormic Index had strong negative correlations with height (r = −0.850, −0.860, in subjects and controls, resp.). The pattern of negative correlation was observed in both sexes and in all age groups but the coefficients were not consistently significant. Significant positive correlations were detected between sitting height and subischial leg length (r = 0.895, 0.925: P = 0.000 each) in subjects and controls, respectively.

3.3. Correlation between Cormic Index and Other Anthropometrics and Age. Anthropometric variables tested were weight, BMI, sitting height, and subischial leg length. The Pearson correlation coefficient (r) for understanding the overall relationship of anthropometric variables and age with Cormic Index is shown in Table 3. Examination on the Pearson correlation coefficient revealed a significant ($P < 0.05$) negative correlation between age, sitting height, subischial leg length, weight, and Cormic Index in both subjects and controls. Also, a weak correlation was observed between BMI and Cormic Index among subjects with HbSS and controls. However, it was in subjects with sickle cell anaemia that the

TABLE 2: Correlation analysis between height and Cormic Index in study subjects.

Age group	Correlation coefficient (r)		P value	
	AA	SS	AA	SS
≤2 yrs				
Males	−0.679	−0.411	0.011	0.164
Females	−0.786	−0.604	0.001	0.029
Males and females	−0.708	−0.465	0.000	0.017
>2 yrs–5 yrs				
Males	−0.887	−0.680	0.000	0.011
Females	−0.571	−0.861	0.042	0.000
Males and females	−0.827	−0.769	0.000	0.000
>5 yrs–10 yrs				
Males	−0.460	−0.641	0.133	0.025
Females	−0.594	−0.235	0.042	0.462
Males and females	−0.552	−0.569	0.005	0.004
>10 yrs–15 yrs				
Males	−0.453	−0.644	0.139	0.024
Females	−0.299	−0.047	0.345	0.885
Males and females	−0.381	−0.495	0.066	0.014

TABLE 3: The Pearson correlation of Cormic Index with other anthropometrics and age.

Characteristics	Correlation coefficient (r)		P value	
	AA	SS	AA	SS
Age	−0.752	−0.744	0.000	0.000
BMI	0.120	0.386	0.241	0.000
Subischial leg length	−0.922	−0.919	0.000	0.000
Sitting height	−0.728	−0.670	0.000	0.000
Weight	−0.565	−0.700	0.000	0.000

TABLE 4: Regression of BMI on Cormic Index of subjects and controls.

Independent variables	Equation	R^2	SEE (cm)
Sickle cell anaemia subjects			
Males	3.73 + 0.21 CI	0.162	2.448
Females	6.10 + 0.15 CI	0.126	1.951
Males and females	4.60 + 0.18 CI	0.149	2.215
Controls			
Males	6.52 + 0.16 CI	0.063	2.901
Females	15.26 + 0.02 CI	0.000	3.961
Males and females	10.84 + 0.09 CI	0.014	3.459

CI: Cormic Index.

Note: Cormic Index should be expressed as a percentage.

correlation coefficient was significant ($P = 0.000$). Table 3 also shows that the correlation between Cormic Indices and subischial leg length is higher in both subjects with sickle cell anaemia and controls.

3.4. Regression of BMI and Cormic Index. A simple regression equation was derived from the relationship between BMI as dependent variable and Cormic Index as independent variable (Table 4). Separate regression equations for the sexes were derived for BMI on the Cormic Index. Testing by covariance analysis showed that the slopes and intercepts were not significantly different. Therefore, the sexes were combined and a single equation was used to calculate expected BMI values.

Standardized BMI using the modified Norgan model was obtained as follows:

$$BMI_{std} = BMI_{54.9} + (BMI_0 - BMI_1). \quad (2)$$

Using 54.9 (the mean Cormic Index of haemoglobin AA controls) in the regression equation for estimating BMI yielded a value of 14.5.

Thus, the final model is

$$BMI_{std} = 14.5 + (BMI_0 - BMI_1). \quad (3)$$

z-scores were generated for observed BMI as well as the standardized BMI. On the basis of the z-scores, study subjects were then categorized into "thin," "normal," or "overweight." Table 5 shows the prevalence of thinness and overweight using both the actual (observed) and the standardized BMI values. Table 5 shows that, altogether, sixty subjects were classified as thin on the basis of z-scores of observed BMI. Of these 60, six were identified as thin using z-scores of standardized BMI. Also, five subjects were adjudged overweight using observed BMI: four of these five subjects were identified as overweight using standardized BMI.

4. Discussion

Cormic Indices were comparable between male and female children with sickle cell anaemia. Unfortunately, there are no local or international figures for comparison. However, mean Cormic Index decreased progressively with age both in primary subjects and in controls. This is consistent with the expected physiologic trend in which the lower limbs grow relatively faster than the trunk in early childhood.

Specifically, comparison of mean Cormic Index between HbSS subjects and controls older than 10 years showed that controls have significantly higher mean Cormic Index values than sickle cell anaemia subjects irrespective of gender. Interestingly, the significant difference was not recorded in males following gender stratification. The explanation for the different pattern in males and females is not clear. This significantly lower mean value among females with sickle cell anaemia older than 10 years translates to relatively shorter trunks which may be explained by narrowing of intervertebral discs as a result of repeated vasoocclusion [17, 18]. Added to this explanation is the fact that increase in sitting height is relatively faster than leg length in later childhood [8, 19]. The negative effect of sickle cell anaemia on spinal growth would therefore be expected to be more obvious in older children during the period of expected rapid growth.

Thus, the finding of lower Cormic Index in older subjects might be expected but the limitation of the observation to girls is not readily explained. It is plausible that the observation represents a relatively minor trend that has

TABLE 5: The effect of adjusting the BMI of subjects with sickle cell anaemia for a mean Cormic Index of 54.9%.

Age group	Thinness		Overweight	
	Actual	Adjusted	Actual	Adjusted
≤2 yrs				
Males	8 (61.5)	4 (30.8)	1 (7.7)	0 (0.0)
Females	4 (30.8)	1 (7.7)	1 (7.7)	1 (7.7)
Males and females	12 (46.2)	5 (19.2)	2 (7.7)	1 (7.7)
>2 yrs–5 yrs				
Males	7 (53.8)	0 (0.0)	1 (7.7)	0 (0.0)
Females	7 (53.8)	0 (0.0)	0 (0.0)	0 (0.0)
Males and females	14 (53.8)	0 (0.0)	1 (3.9)	0 (0.0)
>5 yrs–10 yrs				
Males	5 (41.7)	0 (0.0)	1 (8.3)	1 (8.3)
Females	8 (66.7)	1 (8.3)	0 (0.0)	0 (0.0)
Males and females	13 (54.2)	1 (4.2)	1 (8.3)	1 (8.3)
>10 yrs–15 yrs				
Males	9 (75.0)	0 (0.0)	1 (8.3)	2 (16.7)
Females	12 (100)	0 (0.0)	0 (0.0)	0 (0.0)
Males and females	21 (87.5)	0 (0.0)	1 (4.2)	1 (4.2)
All				
Males	29 (58.0)	4 (8.0)	4 (8.0)	3 (6.0)
Females	31 (82.0)	2 (4.0)	1 (2.0)	1 (2.0)
Males and females	60 (60.0)	6 (6.0)	5 (5.0)	4 (4.0)

been exaggerated by peculiar circumstances of the female subjects in the current study. Only further studies, possibly with much larger subgroups, can elucidate the situation. A plausible explanation could be that there was a fortuitous concentration of female sickle cell anaemia with relatively less severe affection of height.

Significant negative correlations were detected between Cormic Index and height ($r = -0.868, -0.855$) in boys and girls, respectively. This is purely an arithmetical relationship: height is the denominator in the Cormic Index. Therefore, the ratio should increase as the denominator reduces and vice versa.

It was also observed that strong negative correlations existed between Cormic Index and age (0.752, 0.744). Similar observations have been reported in a study of healthy Bengalee children aged six years to 12 years [5]. Both the sitting height and height are linear measurements which increase physiologically in the same direction with age. Arithmetically, this ratio could be reduced if the sitting height is relatively short. Several previous studies have shown that increase in sitting height is faster than leg length in later childhood [20, 21]. A disease like sickle cell anaemia that affects growth is therefore more likely to adversely affect sitting height in later childhood.

From the result of this study there is significant positive correlation when sitting height was compared to subischial height. This study has also demonstrated that Cormic Index has a direct relationship with sitting height and subischial leg length. That is to say, it is the size of the trunk that mainly determines the body Cormic Index and not subischial leg length.

A positive correlation exists between Cormic Index and BMI in subjects with sickle cell anaemia and controls, although this correlation is relatively weak (<0.4). The low r-values indicate that the Cormic Index is a minor determinant of BMI. This corroborates a study of Nigerians aged between 15 and 56 years in whom weak positive correlation between Cormic Index and BMI was observed [22].

BMI is known to vary with age and body shape. The cutoff used for BMI classification is the same in both children with and children without sickle cell anaemia. There is a marked difference between body shape of children with sickle cell anaemia and that without sickle cell anaemia. In order to account for changes in this documented body shape, the Cormic Index was standardized to compare the BMI of different haemoglobin genotype populations to prevent or reduce the overestimation of prevalence of BMI abnormalities. Upon standardization, the current study showed a 90% reduction in the proportion of subjects otherwise classified as thin. The effect of the standardization was far less felt at the upper end of the BMI spectrum. Indeed, there was only a 17% reduction in the number of subjects classified as overweight. It is thus attractive to argue that the standardization will be more relevant when the objective was to determine proportion of thinness among subjects with sickle cell anaemia.

The extent to which the standardization in the current study applies across races or ethnic groups can only be confirmed by further study. Also, it is plausible that severity of illness may influence the interrelationships between Cormic Index and BMI measurements. Thus, it may be argued that regions with milder or more severe disease expressions may require developing their own standardization models.

In conclusion, the mean Cormic Index decreased with age in both subjects and controls. The mean Cormic Index for children with sickle cell anaemia is comparable with that of HbAA controls except in females older than 10 years that the mean Cormic Index was significantly higher among AA controls than their SS counterparts. The correlation analysis between Cormic Index and height is strongly negative. This may be of great importance for the field of anthropology and forensic medicine. Adjusting for body proportions in classifying BMI drastically reduced the number of sickle cell anaemia subjects who would have been categorized as thin.

Conflict of Interests

The authors declare that there is no conflict of interests regarding the publication of this paper.

Authors' Contribution

The study was conceived by all the authors. Data was collected by all authors except Omolara Adeolu Kehinde. Samuel Olufemi Akodu and Olisamedua Fidelis Njokanma analyzed the data, while Samuel Olufemi Akodu wrote the initial draft of the paper. All authors reviewed and approved the final paper for submission.

References

[1] G. R. Serjeant and B. E. Serjeant, *Sickle Cell Disease*, Oxford University Press, New York, NY, USA, 3rd edition, 2001.

[2] E. M. Barden, D. A. Kawchak, K. Ohene-Frempong, V. A. Stallings, and B. S. Zemel, "Body composition in children with sickle cell disease," *The American Journal of Clinical Nutrition*, vol. 76, no. 1, pp. 218–225, 2002.

[3] A.-W. Al-Saqladi, R. Cipolotti, K. Fijnvandraat, and B. J. Brabin, "Growth and nutritional status of children with homozygous sickle cell disease," *Annals of Tropical Paediatrics*, vol. 28, no. 3, pp. 165–189, 2008.

[4] L. Beker and T. L. Cheng, "Principles of growth assessment," *Pediatrics in Review*, vol. 27, no. 5, pp. 196–198, 2006.

[5] M. C. Ukwuma, "A study of the cormic index in a Southeastern Nigerian population," *The Internet Journal of Biological Anthropology*, vol. 4, no. 1, 2009.

[6] M. Siahkouhian and M. Hedayatneja, "Correlations of anthropometric and body composition variables with the performance of young elite weightlifters," *Journal of Human Kinetics*, vol. 25, no. 1, pp. 125–131, 2010.

[7] N. G. Norgan, "Relative sitting height and the interpretation of the body mass index," *Annals of Human Biology*, vol. 21, no. 1, pp. 79–82, 1994.

[8] B. S. Zemel, D. A. Kawchak, K. Ohene-Frempong, J. I. Schall, and V. A. Stallings, "Effects of delayed pubertal development, nutritional status, and disease severity on longitudinal patterns of growth failure in children with sickle cell disease," *Pediatric Research*, vol. 61, no. 5, pp. 607–613, 2007.

[9] M. T. Ashcroft, G. R. Serjeant, and P. Desai, "Heights, weights, and skeletal age of Jamaican adolescents with sickle cell anaemia," *Archives of Disease in Childhood*, vol. 47, no. 254, pp. 519–524, 1972.

[10] B. A. Woodruff and A. Duffield, "Anthropometric assessment of nutritional status in adolescent populations in humanitarian emergencies," *European Journal of Clinical Nutrition*, vol. 56, no. 11, pp. 1108–1118, 2002.

[11] N. G. Norgan, "Interpretation of low body mass indices: Australian aborigines," *American Journal of Physical Anthropology*, vol. 94, no. 2, pp. 229–237, 1994.

[12] S. Pheasant, "Body space: anthropometry, ergonomics and design," *American Journal of Physical Anthropology*, vol. 4, pp. 331–334, 1986.

[13] O. Awotua-Efebo, E. A. O. Alikor, and K. E. O. Nkanginieme, "Malaria parasite density and splenic status by ultrasonography in stable sickle-cell anaemia (HbSS) children," *Nigerian Journal of Medicine*, vol. 13, no. 1, pp. 40–44, 2004.

[14] M. A. Carpenter, M. S. Tockman, R. G. Hutchinson, C. E. Davis, and G. Heiss, "Demographic and anthropometric correlates of maximum inspiratory pressure: the Atherosclerosis Risk in Communities Study," *American Journal of Respiratory and Critical Care Medicine*, vol. 159, no. 2, pp. 415–422, 1999.

[15] G. A. Oyedeji, "Socio-economic and cultural background of hospitalized children in Ilesha," *Nigerian Journal of Paediatrics*, vol. 12, no. 4, pp. 111–117, 1985.

[16] N. G. Norgan, "Body mass index and nutritional status: the effect of adjusting body mass index for the relative sitting height on estimates of the prevalence of chronic energy deficiency, overweight and obesity," *Asia Pacific Journal of Clinical Nutrition*, vol. 4, no. 1, pp. 137–139, 1995.

[17] M. Sadat-Ali, A. Ammar, J. R. Corea, and A. W. Ibrahim, "The spine in sickle cell disease," *International Orthopaedics*, vol. 18, no. 3, pp. 154–156, 1994.

[18] J. O. Ozoh, M. A. C. Onuigbo, N. Nwankwo, S. O. Ukabam, B. C. Umerah, and C. C. Emeruwa, "'Vanishing' of vertebra in a patient with sickle cell haemoglobinopathy," *British Medical Journal*, vol. 301, no. 6765, pp. 1368–1369, 1990.

[19] M. T. Ashcroft, G. R. Serjeant, and P. Desai, "Heights, weights, and skeletal age of Jamaican adolescents with sickle cell anaemia," *Archives of Disease in Childhood*, vol. 47, no. 254, pp. 519–524, 1972.

[20] P. Dasgupta and S. R. Das, "A cross-sectional growth study of trunk and limb segments of the Bengali boys of Calcutta," *Annals of Human Biology*, vol. 24, no. 4, pp. 363–369, 1997.

[21] J. M. Tanner, R. H. Whitehouse, E. Marubini, and L. F. Resele, "The adolescent growth spurt of boys and girls of the Harpenden growth study," *Annals of Human Biology*, vol. 3, no. 2, pp. 109–126, 1976.

[22] D. O. Adeyemi, O. A. Komolafe, and A. I. Abioye, "Variations in body mass indices among post-pubertal Nigerian subjects with correlation to cormic indices, mid-arm circumferences and waist circumferences," *The Internet Journal of Biological Anthropology*, vol. 2, no. 2, 2009.

8

Determinants of Anemia among Children Aged 6–59 Months Living in Kilte Awulaelo Woreda, Northern Ethiopia

Gebremedhin Gebreegziabiher,[1] Belachew Etana,[2] and Daniel Niggusie[2]

[1] Department of Public Health, College of Health Science, Adigrat University, P.O. Box 50, Adigrat, Ethiopia
[2] School of Public Health, College of Health Science, Mekelle University, P.O. Box 1871, Mekelle, Ethiopia

Correspondence should be addressed to Belachew Etana; belachewetana@yahoo.com

Academic Editor: Edward J. Benz

Introduction. The aim of this study was to determine the prevalence of anemia and determinant factors among children aged 6–59 months living in Kilte Awulaelo Woreda, eastern zone. *Method.* A community based cross-sectional study was conducted during February 2013 among 6 tabias of Kilte Awulaelo Woreda, northern Ethiopia. A total of 568 children were selected by systematic random sampling method. Anthropometric data and blood sample were collected. Bivariate and multivariate logistic regression analyses were performed to identify factors related to anemia. *Result.* The mean hemoglobin level was 11.48 g/dl and about 37.3% of children were anemic. Children who were aged 6–23 months [AOR = 1.89: 95% CI (1.3, 2.8)], underweight [AOR = 2.05: 95% CI (1.3, 3.3)], having MUAC less than 12 cm [AOR = 3.35: 95% CI (2.1, 5.3)], and from households with annual income below 10,000 Ethiopian birr [AOR = 4.86: 95% CI (3.2, 7.3)] were more likely to become anemic. *Conclusion.* The prevalence of anemia among the children is found to be high. It was associated with annual household income, age, and nutritional status of the child. So, improving family income and increasing awareness of the mother/caregiver were important intervention.

1. Introduction

Anemia can be defined as a reduction in the hemoglobin, hematocrit, or red cells number. In physiologic terms, anemia is any disorder in which the patient suffers from tissue hypoxia due to decreased oxygen carrying capacity of the blood [1]. It is mainly caused by iron deficiency in all developing countries, including Africa, where consumption of iron is limited. This is because iron-rich or animal based foods are not affordable by most families. Children <2 years and pregnant women are most at risk for anemia because their requirements for iron are higher than any other group [2].

Anemia is said to be a severe public health problem when its prevalence is 40% or more in any group (all types of anemia). Severe anemia (hemoglobin < 7 g/dL) is a public health problem if prevalence exceeds 2% [2]. According the 2004 World Health Organization (WHO) report, more than 2 billion people worldwide are anemic and about 47.4% of preschool children are affected by the problem. It affects most of countries in Africa and South Asia and some countries in East Asia and the Pacific. The highest prevalence of anemia is in Africa, but the greatest numbers of children affected are found in Asia [3].

Furthermore, according to 2008 WHO report, more than half of the world's preschool-age children (56.3%) reside in countries where anemia is a severe public health problem [3]. In sub-Saharan Africa, it is a sever public health problem among preschool-age children. In this region, much of the national prevalence is estimated to be above 40% among this group [4].

In Ethiopia, more than four out of ten under-five children (44%) were anemic. From these, about 21% of children were mildly anemic, 20% were moderately anemic, and 3% were severely anemic. In Tigray region, the reported prevalence (37.5%) was lower than the national prevalence [5].

Factors associated with anemia among children are complex and multidimensional. These involves socioeconomic, nutritional, biological, environmental, and cultural characteristics [6]. Because of this, understanding these factors in a given population is important for evidence based interventions and policies towards anemia. Many researches have been conducted to show its associated factors. But it remains the main public health problem, especially in developing countries. So, identifying factors associated with anemia is needed to develop appropriate interventions.

Therefore, the study was designed to assess the prevalence of anemia and its associated factors among children aged 6–59 months living in Kilte Awulaelo Woreda, eastern zone, northern Ethiopia. So it provides evidences for policy makers and program managers for policy formulation, problem prioritization, and resource allocation.

2. Methods

2.1. Study Area and Population. The study was conducted during February 2013 in Kilte Awulaelo Woreda which is located in eastern zone of Tigray regional state. It is found 828 km north of the capital city, Addis Ababa. There are 115,762 people within 25,047 households in the Woreda (source: Woreda Kilte Awulaelo Plan and Finance Office, 2012). It is divided into 18 tabias (the smallest administration unit in Tigray) and the main source of income is agriculture. The Woreda has 5 health centers and 16 health posts that provide health services. The main causes of morbidity among children in the Woreda were pneumonia, other respiratory infections, and malnutrition.

2.2. Study Design and Sample. Community based cross-sectional study was conducted among 568 children and their mothers/caregivers. The sample size was calculated using single population proportion formula assuming the prevalence of all types of anemia among children 6–59 months of age in Tigray regional state is 37.5% [7], confidence interval 95%, margin of error 5%, and design effect 1.5. Finally, 5% of the calculated sample size added for any non response to the actual sample size.

Multistage sampling was used to select study participants. For this, first, 6 tabias were selected using lottery method from 18 tabias in the Woreda. Within these tabias, households with children aged 6–59 months were identified after census was conducted and the number of households was allocated by proportional allocation to size method. Finally, individual households were selected by systematic random sampling technique after sampling fraction was prepared for each tabia separately. In case of more than one child within the specified age group within the household, one child was selected by lottery method.

2.3. Data Collection. Data were collected by interviewing mother/caregivers of the child during house to house survey using pretested and interview administered questionnaire which was prepared in English language which was later translated into Tigrigna. Three types of data from respondents were children and their caretaker/mother characteristics, anthropometric data, and blood sample from

children. Diploma graduate clinical nurse interviewed mothers/caregivers and anthropometric data were taken by the three health extension workers. In addition, three laboratory technicians collected blood sample.

One-day training was given for data collectors and supervisors before data collection which was followed by pretesting of the tool. The pretesting was done in one tabia which was not included in the study. The data collection team completed a total of 30 questionnaires during pretest and necessary changes were made accordingly.

Height and length board was used to take height/length of children and mothers. Recumbent length was taken for children aged 6–23 months and standing height was taken from children aged 24–59 months. In addition to this, mid-upper arm circumference was taken by MUAC tape. Furthermore, weighing scale was used to take weight measurements for all children and mothers. Known weight (premeasured) was used daily in the morning and afternoon to check the quality of the weighing scale. To maintain accuracy of anthropometric measurements, anthropometric data was collected twice from children and mothers and the average of the two measurements was taken.

Blood sample was collected using diamine tetraacetic acid (EDTA) test tube and transported to Wukro Hospital every day to measure the hemoglobin level. Laboratory technician did the hemoglobin test using complete blood count (CBC) machine in Wukro Hospital Laboratory Department. To protect the quality of collected blood sample, it was transported using icebox to nearby hospital (Wukro Hospital) within eight hours after collection.

The quality of hemoglobin test was further insured by continuously washing the machine by cleaning solution (cell clean) and measuring blank solution/air/background until it is near to zero (<0.1 g/dL) reading. The machine washing was done every day by cleaning solution until the background/air reading reaches near to zero. In addition to this, the quality of test was also checked by using standard eight checks which are commercially prepared and have known hemoglobin value. After analysis, the samples were discarded to the sink in the laboratory and the test tubes were incinerated in incinerator.

2.4. Measurement. Anemia was defined as presence of hemoglobin level of less than 11 g/dL. It was further categorized into mild, moderate, and severe anemia. Mild anemia was for child with hemoglobin level of 10–<11 g/dL, while moderate anemia was for children with Hb level of 7–<10 g/dL and severe anemia was for hemoglobin level below 7 g/dL.

Besides this, the children national status was assessed and classified into underweight, stunting, and wasted. Children are said to be underweight if they had weight-for-age z-score below −2 standard deviation; stunting was for children with height-for-age z-score below −2 SD while wasted was for those with weight-for-height z-score below −2 SD according to WHO Child Growth Standards median.

2.5. Data Analysis. Data was entered and cleaned using Epi-Info 3.5.1 and analyzed using SPSS 16. The data was cleaned and preliminary analysis was done by the researchers. Descriptive statistics was done to describe the data. Then, binary logistic regression was made to see the crude associations between independent variables and dependent variable. Variables found to have statistically significant association, P value < 0.05, during bivariate analysis were entered to multiple logistic regressions to identify independent predictors of anemia after controlling for confounder. Odds ratios (OR) with their 95% confidence level (CI) were calculated. Anthropometric data was analyzed using ENA software using 2006 WHO standards [8]. All statistical tests are considered significant at $P < 0.05$ level.

Hemoglobin level less than 11 mg/dL was taken as dependent variable while household income, mothers' characteristics, child characteristic, source of water and availability of toilet facility, antenatal care (ANC) visit, child feeding, and child nutritional status were taken as independent variables.

2.6. Ethical Statement. An ethical approval was obtained from the Ethical Review Committee of Mekelle University, College of Health Sciences, Research and Community Service Office. Official support letter was obtained from Mekelle University, Tigray Regional Health Bureau, and Kilte Awulaelo Health Office for conducting the study. Information about objective of the study, procedures, potential risks, and benefits was given to mothers before they were enrolled to the study.

All participants were informed about the purpose and significance of the study before their consent was taken. Their full right to refuse participation was explained. Written informed consent was obtained from each mother/caregiver of children selected for the study. Children found with severe anemia (Hb value of 7–<11 g/dL) got free treatment from the health post and were counselled to visit nearby health facility for further investigation and treatment. In addition to this, referral paper was provided to take the child to the nearby health facility. There is no potential risk occurring to participants except minimal discomfort while blood was drawn from the children. So, the right of participants to anonymity and confidentiality will be ensured by making the questionnaire anonymous.

3. Results

3.1. Characteristics of Study Participants. Total of 568 households participated in the study with the 100% response rate. The mean age of mothers was 28.34 (±6.46) years which ranged from 19 to 51 years. Majority (95%) of the respondents were Orthodox followers while 13 (2.3%) were Muslims. In addition, the majority, 510 (89.8%), of the respondents were married and 264 (46.5%) of the mothers had formal education (they can read and write). Majority of the mothers, 485 (85.4%), were housewives and 83 (14.6%) of them had their own income with mean annual income of 13195 (Table 1).

Agriculture was the main source of income for majority of the respondents (510 (89.8%)) and the remaining 23 (4%) were employed. More than half of the households, 337 (59.3%), use pipe water (hand pipe) and the remaining 329 (40.7%) use water from other sources like river water

TABLE 1: Sociodemographic and other characteristics of the mother in Kilte Awulaelo Woreda, eastern zone, northern Ethiopia, 2013 ($n = 568$).

Variables	Frequency	Percent
Marital status		
Married	510	89.8
Single	24	4.2
Divorced	29	5.1
Widowed	5	0.9
Religion		
Orthodox	553	97.4
Muslim	13	2.2
Catholic	2	0.4
Educational status		
No formal education	305	53.7
1–6	162	28.5
7-8	46	8.1
9–12	46	8.1
Above 12	9	1.6
Earned annual income		
Yes	83	14.6
No	485	85.4
ANC visit		
None	38	6.7
1 time	59	10.4
2 times	175	30.8
3 times	216	38
4 times and more	80	14.1
Annual income of the HH		
≤5000	3	0.5
5001–10000	189	33.3
10001–15000	218	38.3
15001–20000	134	23.6
20001–25000	18	3.2
>25001	6	1.1
Availability of latrine/toilet		
Yes	456	80.3
No	112	19.7
Source of income for the HH		
Agriculture	510	89.8
Employed	23	4
Merchant	27	4.8
Daily laborer	8	1.8

and well. Majority of the households, 456 (80.3%), owned latrine/toilet and the remaining 112 (19.7%) have no latrine (Table 1).

3.2. Child Characteristics. From total of 568 selected children, 282 (49.6%) of them were males and 286 (50.4%) were females. The mean age of the children was 30.18 (15.85) months. Beside this, about 52.4% were stunted and 6.5% were

TABLE 2: Characteristics of child and dietary factors in Kilte Awulaelo Woreda, eastern zone, northern Ethiopia, 2013 ($n = 568$).

Variable	Frequency	Percentage
Age of the child in months		
6–23	231	40.7
24–35	116	20.4
36–47	103	18.1
48–59	118	20.8
Mean age (±SD)	**30.18 (15.85)**	
Sex of the child		
Male	282	49.6
Female	286	50.4
MUAC in cm		
<12	37	6.5
≥12	531	93.5
Stunted		
Yes	298	52.4
No	270	47.6
Underweight		
Yes	117	20.6
No	451	79.4
Wasted		
Yes	37	6.5
No	531	93.5
Number of food groups eaten by the child per day		
≤3	465	81.8
≥4	103	18.2
Mean food groups (±SD)	**2.87 (0.79)**	

TABLE 3: The degree of anemia among children aged 6–59 months in relation to their sex in Kilte Awulaelo Woreda, northern Ethiopia, 2013 ($n = 568$).

Hemoglobin value	Male (%)	Female (%)	Total N (%)
<7 g/dl (severely anemic)	0 (0)	2 (0.7)	2 (0.4)
7–9.9 g/dl (moderately anemic)	33 (11.2)	32 (11.2)	65 (11.4)
10–11.9 g/dl (mildly anemic)	64 (22.7)	81 (28.3)	145 (25.5)
≥11 g/dl (normal)	185 (65.5)	171 (59.8)	356 (62.7)

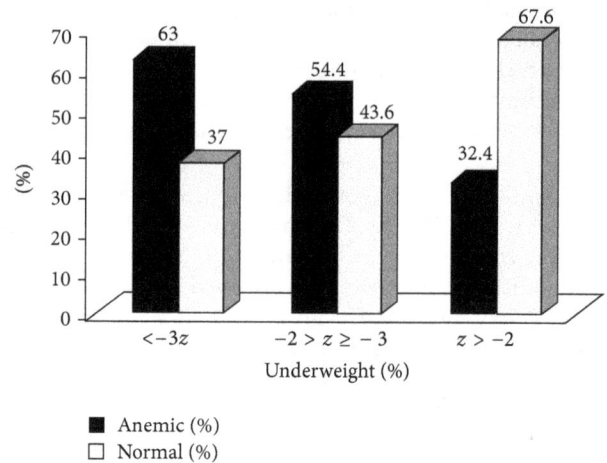

FIGURE 1: Anemia among children aged 6–59 months by their nutritional status in Kilte Awulaelo Woreda, northern Ethiopia, during February 2013.

wasted, while 20.6% were underweight. On average (±SD), the child ate 2.87 (0.79) food groups per day (Table 2).

On average, there are about 3.46 siblings per household and the mean birth interval between the selected child and his/her elder was 32.8 months.

3.3. Magnitude of Anemia among Children. Anemia was measured using the hemoglobin level of the child. So, accordingly, the mean hemoglobin level was about 11.48 (±1.53) g/dL which ranged from 5.5 g/dL to 14.5 g/dL. Accordingly, more than one-third of the children, 212 (37.3%), were anemic and only 2 (0.4%) of them were found to be severely anemic, whereas 65 (11.4%) were moderately anemic and 145 (25.5%) were mildly anemic. The prevalence of anemia was 40.2% among females and 34.5% among males (Table 3).

Figure 1 shows anemia by weight-for-age (underweight) z-score. Anemia was higher among children who are severely underweight and it is lower among children with normal weight-to-age z-score.

Furthermore, it also differs by child age category. Younger children were more anemic than older children and it gradually decreases as the child gets older. Children aged 6–23 months were the most at-risk group in which the risk is

almost 3 times when compared with those of 48–59 months (Figures 2 and 3).

3.4. Factors Associated with Anemia. Bivariate logistic regression analysis was done to assess association of sociodemographic and other maternal factors with child anemia (Table 4). Accordingly, children of mothers with weight of less than 50 kg were 1.77 (1.2, 2.6) times more likely to be anemic than those of mothers greater than 50 kg. But it did not show statistically significant association in multivariate logistic regression. The remaining maternal factors did not show statistically significant association with child anemia even in the bivariate logistic regression (Table 5).

Table 6 shows the association of household factor with anemia among children. Multivariate logistic regression analysis showed that children from household with annual income of less than 10,000 birr were 4.86 [COR, 4.86; 95% CI: (3.2, 7.3)] times more likely to be anemic than their counterparts. The remaining household factors did not show statistically significant association with child anemia in both bivariate and multivariate logistic regression.

Other factors assessed to be associated with child anemia were child age and dietary factors. Multivariate analysis showed that children aged 6–23 months were 1.89 (1.2, 2.8) times more likely to be anemic than those of 24–59 months

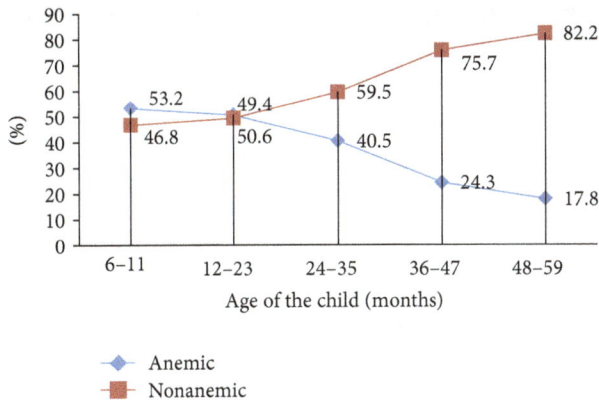

FIGURE 2: Anemia among children aged 6–59 months by their age distribution in Kilte Awulaelo Woreda.

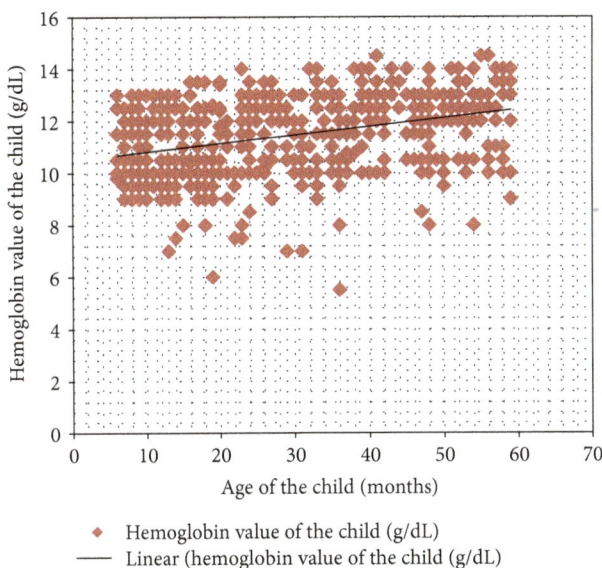

FIGURE 3: Hemoglobin value of the children aged 6–59 months in relation to their age, Kilte Awulaelo Woreda, eastern zone, northern Ethiopia, 2013 ($n = 568$).

of age. Furthermore, anemia also related to nutritional status of the children. Being underweight, that is, with weight-for-age less than −2 z-score, 2.05 (1.3, 3.3), and having mid-upper arm circumference (MUAC) less than 12 cm [3.35 (2.1, 5.3)] were significantly associated with anemia (Table 6).

4. Discussion

This study assessed the prevalence of anemia and factors associated with it among children aged 6–59 months. The prevalence of anemia was found to be 37.3% which is relatively lower than the national prevalence (44%) of the EDHS 2011 findings, but it is similar to the prevalence of Tigray region (37.5%) [9]. Prevalence of anemia reported from several developing countries varied. It is about 16.1% in the Philippines during the year 2008 [10] and 87% in Tanzania [11]. This level of prevalence is considered moderate public

health problem according to WHO classification [2], but it is lower than the estimated global anemia prevalence (47.4%) [3].

We found that the prevalence decreased with age. It is dramatically decreased among children aged above 23 months. This finding is similar to study conducted in Nigeria in 2011 [12]. This may be attributable to lower iron requirements per kg body weight associated with decreasing growth rate and the shift in diet from complementary foods to table foods. This is supported with studies that have found that children under two years of age groups were more anemic than children aged 2–5 years [10, 12–16]. The first 2 years of life carry the highest risk for developing anemia [17, 18]. Iron requirements are related to growth velocity and so requirement per kg of body weight decreases with age. The prevalence of the problem in under-24-month-old children is likely to be a combined result of the increased iron requirements due to rapid growth, low availability of foods rich in iron, and lack of diet variety. Iron intake is also likely to improve with age as a result of a more varied diet, including the introduction of meat and other iron containing foods [13].

In addition to this, age of the child had statistically significant association with anemia using multivariate logistic regression. Children aged 6–11 months were the most affected age groups with anemia prevalence of 53.2% which is almost three times higher than those aged 48–59 months (17.8%). This finding is similar to study findings done in Brazil (2010), Bangladesh (2010), and northern Ethiopia (2007) [8, 16, 19].

In this study, anemia among children was also associated with household income. Children living in household with lower monthly income were more likely to have anemia compared to those with higher income. Similar finding was from study conducted in Brazil (2011 and 2010) and in northern Ethiopia in 2007 [8, 16, 19]. This is due to the reason that children from poor households are less likely to get iron-rich foods like animal foods and vitamin-rich foods especially vitamins A and C which are very important for iron absorption. In addition to these, households were less likely to afford health service during illness. But, study conducted in the state of Pernambuco, Brazil, in 2007 shows no association between household income and child anemia [15].

Nutritional status of the children also related to anemia among children aged 6–59 months. In this study, mal-nourished children were more likely to be anemic than well-nourished children. Children who were underweight and have MUAC less than 12 cm were more likely to be anemic than their counterparts. This finding is supported by findings from Brazil and Tanzania [11, 20]. Since anemia and malnutrition often share common causes, it is expected that multiple nutrition problems would cooccur in the same individuals [8]. These factors are aggravated by poverty and food insecurity [19]. Low intake of iron-rich foods and diminished nutrient absorption caused by changes in the gastrointestinal epithelium in malnourished individuals contribute towards development of anemia [16].

However, mother and child sociodemographic character-istics are not shown to be associated with anemia among children under five. The influence of child sex on anemia shows no association in this study. This finding was also

TABLE 4: Association of sociodemographic and other maternal factors with anemia in children aged 6–59 months in Kilte Awulaelo Woreda, eastern zone, northern Ethiopia, 2013 ($n = 568$).

Variable	Anemic		Odds ratio (95% CI)	
	Yes (%)	No (%)	COR (95% CI)	OR (95% CI)
Maternal factors				
Age of mother				
<30 years	126 (36.3)	217 (63.3)	0.94 (0.6, 1.3)	
≥30 years	86 (38.2)	139 (61.8)	1	
Maternal weight				
<50 kg	133 (44.3)	167 (55.7)	**1.77 (1.2, 2.6)***	2.27 (0.4, 13.7)
≥50 kg	55 (31.1)	122 (68.9)	1	
Religion of the mother				
Orthodox	207 (37.4)	346 (62.6)	1	
Others	5 (33.3)	10 (67)	0.84 (0.28, 2.48)	
Marital status				
Married	185 (36.2)	326 (63.8)	0.79 (0.35, 1.77)	
Divorced	9 (31)	20 (69)	0.28 (0.09, 0.82)	
Others	18 (62)	11 (38)	1	
Employment status of the mother				
Employed	34 (41)	49 (59)	1.20 (0.7, 1.9)	
Not employed	178 (36.7)	307 (63.3)	1	
Mother's ability to read and write				
Yes	99 (37.6)	164 (62.4)	1.03 (0.7, 1.4)	
No	113 (37)	192 (63)	1	
ANC visit				
Yes	13 (34.2)	25 (65.8)	0.86 (0.4, 1.7)	
No	199 (37.5)	331 (62.5)	1	
Maternal BMI				
Underweight	39 (41.5)	55 (58.5)	0.53 (0.1, 2.5)	
Normal	145 (38.6)	231 (61.4)	0.47 (0.1, 2.1)	
Overweight	4 (57.1)	3 (42.9)	1	

*Variables show statistically significant association at P value < 0.05. OR: odds ratio.

TABLE 5: Association of household factors with anemia in children aged 6–59 months in Kilte Awulaelo Woreda, eastern zone, northern Ethiopia, 2013 ($n = 568$).

Variables	Anemic		Odds ratio (95% CI)	
	Yes (%)	No (%)	COR (95% CI)	AOR (95% CI)
Household factors				
Annual income				
<10000	87 (68.5)	40 (31.5)	**5.50 (3.6, 8.4)***	**4.86 (3.2, 7.3)***
≥10000	125 (28.3)	316 (71.7)	1	
Availability of latrine/toilet				
Yes	162 (35.5)	294 (64.5)	0.68 (0.4, 1.0)	
No	50 (44.5)	62 (55.4)	1	
Availability of pipe water (hand)				
Yes	120 (35.6)	217 (64.4)	0.84 (0.6, 1.2)	
No	92 (39.8)	139 (60.2)	1	
Source of income for the household				
Agriculture	188 (36.9)	322 (63.1)	0.97 (0.2, 4.1)	
Employed	5 (21.7)	18 (78.3)	0.46 (0.1, 2.6)	
Merchant	16 (59.3)	11 (40.7)	2.42 (0.5, 12.3)	
Daily laborer	3 (37.5)	5 (62.5)	1	

*Variables show statistically significant association at P value < 0.05. OR: odds ratio.

TABLE 6: Association of child factors with anemia in children aged 6–59 months in Kilte Awulaelo Woreda, eastern zone, northern Ethiopia, 2013 ($n = 568$).

Variable	Anemic		OR (95% CI)	
	Yes	No	Crude OR (95% CI)	Adjusted OR (95% CI)
	Number (%)	Number (%)		
Child factors				
Age				
<24 months	119 (51.5)	112 (48.5)	**2.79 (1.9, 3.9)**[*]	**1.89 (1.2, 2.8)**[*]
≥24 months	93 (27.6)	244 (72.4)	1	
Sex of the child				
Male	97 (34.4)	185 (65.6)	0.78 (0.5, 1.1)	
Female	114 (40.0)	171 (60)	1	
MUAC of the child				
<12 cm	30 (81.1)	7 (18.9)	**8.22 (3.5, 19.1)**[*]	**3.35 (2.1, 5.3)**[*]
≥12 cm	182 (34)	349 (65.7)	1	
Birth order of the child				
≤3	133 (37.3)	224 (62.7)	0.99 (0.7, 1.4)	
≥4	79 (37.4)	132 (62.6)	1	
Birth interval of the child				
≤33 months	16 (32.7)	33 (67.3)	1	
>33 months	11 (15.1)	62 (84.9)	**0.41 (0.1, 0.9)**[*]	0.42 (0.1, 1.3)
Number of children in household				
≤3 children	128 (37.5)	213 (62.5)	1.02 (0.7, 1.4)	
≥4 children	84 (37)	143 (63)	1	
Child wears shoe				
Yes	184 (36.2)	324 (63.8)	0.65 (0.4, 1.1)	
No	28 (46.7)	32 (53.3)	1	
Number of food groups eaten by the child				
≤3 food group	81 (45)	99 (55)	1	
≥4 food group	131 (33.8)	257 (66.2)	**0.32 (0.2, 0.5)**[*]	0.26 (0.04, 1.5)
Stunting				
Yes	129 (43.3)	169 (56.7)	**1.72 (1.2, 2.4)**[*]	2.85 (0.8, 10.3)
No	83 (30.7)	187 (69.3)	1	
Underweight				
Yes	66 (56.4)	51 (43.6)	**2.70 (1.8, 4.1)**[*]	**2.05 (1.3, 3.3)**[*]
No	146 (32.4)	305 (67.6)	1	
Wasting				
Yes	23 (60.5)	15 (39.5)	**2.76 (1.410, 5.430)**[*]	3.06 (0.8, 10.5)
No	189 (35.7)	341 (64.3)	1	

[*]Variables show statistically significant association at P value < 0.05. OR: odds ratio.

supported with studies conducted in Lao People's Democratic Republic in 2011 and Morocco in 2010 [18, 21]. But this is contrary to study done in the Philippines which reported that anemia is more common in male children [10]. Besides this, maternal education and employment status were also not associated with anemia among children aged 6–59 months old. This finding is supported by study conducted in Brazil in 2011 [16]. This may be due to the reason that most of the mothers that were included in the study were illiterate and most of those that attend formal school were at elementary school level. Because of this, our sample is not sufficient to ascertain statistical association.

In this study, numbers of children in the household, birth interval, water supply, and availability of latrine were not associated with presence of anemia among children aged 6–59 months. This result was supported with reports of two studies conducted in Brazil (2011 and 2010) for number of children in the household, water source, and presence of latrine [13, 20]. But study conducted in the Philippines shows an association between anemia and water supply [19]. Availability of latrine was also not associated with anemia in this study. Besides this, our result showed that maternal BMI was not associated with anemia among children aged 6–59 months. Contradictory result was found from study conducted by WHO in Brazil and India [16, 22].

This study has used the best available technology (Cysmex machine) to determine hemoglobin level which has more accuracy and this makes it strong. But it has certain limitations. Most of the questions asked like dietary recall, ANC visit, and age of the child and the mother may be subject to recall bias. Besides this, this study can only show the local prevalence of anemia and cannot show temporal relationship between anemia and other factors considered. Given these limitations, our finding has a great contribution to improving the health of children aged 6–59 months.

5. Conclusion

The prevalence of anemia among children aged 6–59 months was a moderate public health problem with 37.3% according to WHO classification. Annual income below 10,000 Ethiopian birr, age of the child between 6 and 23 months of age, and being underweight (children with WAZ less than -2 z-score and MUAC of children less than 12 cm) were predictors of anemia among children aged 6–59 months.

So, policy makers should focus on activities that can improve household income to ensure sufficient food production. Moreover, interventions like iron supplementation and nutritional education activities are important to decrease the prevalence of anemia. Finally, controlling multiple nutritional deficiencies among children by expanding targeted supplementary feeding programs, at health post level, which targets malnourished children, is mandatory to avert other nutritional problems including anemia.

Conflict of Interests

The authors declare that there is no conflict of interests regarding the publication of this paper.

Authors' Contribution

Gebremedhin Gebreeziabiher and Belachew Etana designed the study, analyzed the data, drafted the paper, and critically reviewed it. All authors read and approved the final paper.

Acknowledgments

The authors would like to thank the Department of Public health, Mekelle University, for giving them a chance to conduct this study and Kilte Awulaelo Woreda Health Office for their unreserved support for this study. In addition, they would like to thank their data collector and participants of this study.

References

[1] WHO, "Overview of the Problem of Diving with Anemi," 2002, http://www.gulftel.com/~scubadoc/anem.html.

[2] World Bank, *Poverty and Income*, The Poverty Group, 2004, http://devdata.worldbank.org/hnpstats/pvd.asp.

[3] E. McLean, M. Cogswell, I. Egli, D. Wojdyla, and B. De Benoist, "Worldwide prevalence of anaemia, WHO Vitamin and Mineral Nutrition Information System, 1993–2005," *Public Health Nutrition*, vol. 12, no. 4, pp. 444–454, 2009.

[4] R. J. S. Magalhaes, "Archie CA Clements: spatial variation in childhood anaemia in Africa," *Bulletin of the World Health Organization*, vol. 89, pp. 459–468, 2011.

[5] Central Statistical Agency [Ethiopia] and ORC Macro, *Ethiopia Demographic and Health Survey 2011*, Central Statistical Agency, Addis Ababa, Ethiopia; ORC Macro, Calverton, Md, USA, 2011.

[6] R. J. Stoltzfus, "Iron-defi ciency anemia: reexamining the nature and magnitude of the public health problem. Summary: implications for research and programs," *Journal of Nutrition*, vol. 131, no. 2S-2, pp. 697S–700S, 2001.

[7] Sysmex Corporation, *Automated Hematology Analyzer, Operator's Manual*, Sysmex Corporation, Kobe, Japan, 2006.

[8] D. N. Oliveira, R. Martorell, and P. Nguyen, "Risk factors associated with hemoglobin levels and nutritional status among Brazilian children attending daycare centers in Sao Paulo city, Brazil," *Archivos Latinoamericanos de Nutrición*, vol. 60, no. 1, pp. 23–29, 2010.

[9] USAID, *Anemia: Beyond Being Tired. Definitions, Prevention and Control*, USAID, Washington, DC, USA, 2011.

[10] L. W. Tengco, P. Rayco-Solon, J. A. Solon, J. N. Sarol Jr., and F. S. Solon, "Determinants of anemia among preschool children in the Philippines," *Journal of the American College of Nutrition*, vol. 27, no. 2, pp. 229–243, 2008.

[11] *Anaemia in Tanzanian Children*, vol. 81, Bulletin of the World Health Organization, 2003.

[12] G. A. Onyemaobi and A. Ikoku, "Anaemia prevalence among under-five children in Imo State, Nigeria," *Australian Journal of Basic and Applied Sciences*, vol. 5, no. 2, pp. 122–126, 2011.

[13] M. K. Uddin, M. H. Sardar, M. Z. Hossain et al., "Prevalence of anaemia in children of 6 months to 59 months in Narayanganj, Bangladesh," *Journal of Dhaka Medical College*, vol. 19, no. 2, pp. 126–130, 2010.

[14] P. H. Nguyen, K. G. Nguyen, M. B. Le et al., "Risk factors for anemia in Vietnam," *Southeast Asian Journal of Tropical Medicine and Public Health*, vol. 37, no. 6, pp. 1213–1223, 2006.

[15] M. A. A. Oliveira, M. M. Osório, and M. C. F. Raposo, "Socioeconomic and dietary risk factors for anemia in children aged 6 to 59 months," *Jornal de Pediatria*, vol. 83, no. 1, pp. 39–46, 2007.

[16] L. P. Leal, M. B. Filho, P. I. C. de Lira, J. N. Figueiroa, and M. M. Osório, "Prevalence of anemia and associated factors in children aged 6–59 months in Pernambuco, Northeastern Brazil," *Revista de Saúde Pública*, vol. 45, no. 3, pp. 457–466, 2011.

[17] D. G. Silva, S. E. Priore, and S. D. C. C. Franceschini, "Risk factors for anemia in infants assisted by public health services: The importance of feeding practices and iron supplementation," *Jornal de Pediatria*, vol. 83, no. 2, pp. 149–156, 2007.

[18] S. Kounnavong, T. Sunahara, M. Hashizume et al., "Anemia and related factors in preschool children in the southern rural Lao People's Democratic Republic," *Tropical Medicine and Health*, vol. 39, no. 4, pp. 95–103, 2011.

[19] A. A. Adish, S. A. Esrey, T. W. Gyorkos, and T. Johns, "Risk factors for iron deficiency anaemia in preschool children in northern Ethiopia," *Public Health Nutrition*, vol. 2, pp. 243–252, 2007.

[20] R. F. dos Santos, E. S. C. Gonzalez, E. C. de Albuquerque et al., "Prevalence of anemia in under five-year-old children in a children's hospital in Recife, Brazil," *Revista Brasileira de Hematologia e Hemoterapia*, vol. 33, no. 2, pp. 100–104, 2011.

[21] M. El Hioui, M. Farsi, Y. Aboussaleh, A. O. T. Ahami, and A. Achicha, "Prevalence of malnutrition and anemia among preschool children in Kenitra, Morocco," *Nutritional Therapy & Metabolism*, vol. 28, no. 2, pp. 73–76, 2010.

[22] World Health Organization, *Worldwide Prevalence of Anemia 1993–2005*, WHO Global Database on Anemia, Geneva, Switzerland, 2008.

9

Anaemia among Female Undergraduates Residing in the Hostels of University of Sri Jayewardenepura, Sri Lanka

Gayashan Chathuranga,[1] Thushara Balasuriya,[1] and Rasika Perera[2]

[1] Medical Laboratory Sciences Unit, Department of Allied Health Sciences, Faculty of Medical Sciences,
University of Sri Jayewardenepura, Gangodawila, 10250 Nugegoda, Sri Lanka
[2] Department of Biochemistry, Faculty of Medical Sciences, University of Sri Jayewardenepura, Gangodawila,
10250 Nugegoda, Sri Lanka

Correspondence should be addressed to Gayashan Chathuranga; gayashanchathu@yahoo.com

Academic Editor: Bruno Annibale

Anaemia is a major public health problem that has affected around 25% of the world's population. An analytical cross-sectional study was performed on 313 female undergraduates residing in hostels of University of Sri Jayewardenepura, Sri Lanka, during year 2011. Objective of this study was to determine prevalence and contributing factors to anaemia among the study population. Haemoglobin concentration was assayed using cyanomethaemoglobin method. A pretested self-administered questionnaire was used to retrieve information regarding dietary habits and personal factors of participants. Descriptive statistical methods, chi-square test, and independent sample t-test were used to analyze data. Of the 302 females, 17.5% ($n = 53$) had mild anaemia and 7.9% ($n = 24$) had moderate anaemia. Severely anaemic individuals were not observed. Participants' dietary habits and personal factors were not significantly associated with prevalence of anaemia (whether a participant is a vegetarian or not ($P = 0.525$), drinking tea within one hour of a meal ($P = 0.775$), frequency of consumption of red meat, fish, and eggs ($P = 0.499$), antihelminthic treatment within past year ($P = 0.792$), and menorrhagia ($P = 0.560$)). Anaemia in the study population is below the average for Sri Lankan data. Diet and selected medical conditions were not a causative factor for anaemia in this population.

1. Introduction

Anaemia is a global public health problem. It causes human death as well as social and economic problems in both developing and developed countries. According to the World Health Organization (WHO), it has affected 24.8% of the world's population [1]. In neighboring India, one in every two women suffers from anaemia [2]. When anaemia prevalence is 20–39.9% of the general population, it is considered as a moderate public health problem by WHO [1]. In Sri Lanka, anaemia has become a moderate public health problem among preschool, nonpregnant, and pregnant populations as the prevalence is 33%, 39%, and 34%, respectively [3]. According to the WHO, the highest number of individuals affected by anaemia is observed in nonpregnant women aged 15–49.99 years [4]. In Sri Lanka, 39% of females in this category are affected by anaemia [3]. Most of the anaemic cases are due to nutritional deficiencies [4].

Women of childbearing age are having an additional risk of developing anaemia because of their monthly menstrual blood loss and nearly 50 percent of females in this age group are anaemic [5]. On average a healthy woman loses about 25–30 mL of blood monthly. Therefore, the body needs to produce blood in order to compensate for this loss and if the essential nutrients required for haemopoiesis are not supplied in their diet, anaemia will develop. Prevalence of anaemia among nonpregnant women is 30.2% worldwide and in Asia it is 33% accounting to about 318.5 million individuals. Out of the total nonpregnant anaemic individuals of the world, nearly 3/4 reside in Asia. Anaemia among nonpregnant women has become a public health problem in 191 countries out of the 192 member countries of WHO [4].

The objective of this study was to determine the prevalence and contributing factors to anaemia among female undergraduates residing in the hostels of University of Sri Jayewardenepura, Sri Lanka. We assumed that the nutrient intake of female undergraduates who reside in the hostels of University of Sri Jayewardenepura is lower than that of the general population because they buy their meals from the canteens in the university premises or from the nearby food stalls. These places sell food for a considerably lower price and therefore quantity and the quality of this food items are very poor. Thus, these female undergraduates may not obtain nutrients to meet the requirement of the body and were likely to have a higher risk of developing anaemia. In turn, nutrient deficiency anemia may reduce these undergraduates' work capacities and that will adversely affect their academic performances [6].

2. Materials and Methods

An analytical cross-sectional study was performed to determine the proportion and contributing factors to anaemia among female undergraduates residing in hostels situated inside the premises of University of Sri Jayewardenepura, Gangodawila, Nugegoda, Sri Lanka.

2.1. Ethics Statement. Ethical clearance for the study was obtained from Ethical Review Committee, Faculty of Medical Sciences, University of Sri Jayewardenepura, and the study protocol was conducted according to the guidelines of the declaration of Helsinki.

A consent form along with an information sheet giving details of the study (nature of the study, what will be expected from the participants, and expected risks and benefits) were provided to all female undergraduates who were randomly selected to the sample. The details were also explained verbally to the potential participants. Afterwards, female undergraduates who provided written consent were included in the study.

2.2. Sample Size. A simple random sample of 332 girls was drawn from the population of female undergraduates residing in the hostels situated inside the university premises. Random numbers were generated by using blind draw method.

2.2.1. Exclusion Criteria. Female undergraduates with the presence of a past history of haematological disorders (i.e., thalassaemia trait, sickle cell trait, and malignant conditions) or HIV status were excluded from the study.

2.3. Methods

2.3.1. Variables. The study used several variables to determine the proportion and contributing factors to anaemia among female undergraduates residing in hostels situated inside the premises of University of Sri Jayewardenepura.

The variables of the study and the methods of analysis are briefly described in the following section.

2.4. Dependent Variables

2.4.1. Severity of Anemia. The subjects who have a blood haemoglobin concentration of 11 g/dL or above were categorized as nonanaemic and subjects who have less than 11 g/dL of blood haemoglobin concentration were categorized as anaemic [3]. The anaemic individuals were further classified as mildly anaemic (haemoglobin concentration between 10.0 and 10.9 g/dL), moderately anaemic (haemoglobin concentration between 8.0 and 9.9 g/dL), and severely anaemic (haemoglobin concentration below 7.9 g/dL) [3].

A total volume of 2 mL of venous blood was obtained from each participant into EDTA (ethylenediaminetetraacetic acid) containers for haemoglobin measurement. Blood was drawn by skilled personal. Universal precautions were followed during blood collection, transportation, storage, and disposal to protect the participants as well as the researchers.

Blood haemoglobin concentrations of the participants were measured using DiaSys (diagnostic reagent for quantitative in vitro determination of haemoglobin in whole blood on photometric systems—cyanomethaemoglobin method). 20 μL of blood was mixed with 5.0 mL of DiaSys solution and was kept at room temperature for 5 minutes. Then the absorbance of this mixture was measured by using a spectrophotometer at 540 nm wavelength. This absorbance value was multiplied by the calibration factor to find the haemoglobin concentration of a particular subject.

Standard haemoglobin reagent Labtest (reagent for standardization of haemoglobin) was used to calculate the calibration factor in order to convert the absorbance values into concentration values.

2.5. Independent Variables. A self-administered questionnaire was provided to the participants to obtain data regarding their dietary habits and personal factors as independent variables.

Dietary habits of the female undergraduates include whether subject is a vegetarian or not (no, yes), consumption of extra meals (no, yes), consumption of tea within one hour of a meal (no, yes), and number of meals supplemented with meat, fish, or egg per day (zero, one, two, and three).

Personal factors of the female undergraduates include taking antihelminthic treatment within the past year (no, yes), subject's awareness of anaemia (no, yes), and passage of clots in menstrual blood (no, yes).

Both questionnaire and blood sample of a particular individual were labeled with same reference number, so that participants could be traced at the end of the data analysis.

2.6. Statistical Analysis. Data were double entered and analyzed using statistical package for social sciences (SPSS) version 15. Descriptive statistical methods were used to calculate the mean values of menstrual period, age, haemoglobin concentration of anemic subjects, and haemoglobin concentration of nonanaemic subjects. Chi-square test was used to determine the difference between anaemic and nonanaemic groups in dietary habits and other personal factors of the study sample.

TABLE 1: Proportion of participants with the four sets of classification of anaemia.

	Number	Percentage
Nonanaemic (haemoglobin 11 g/dL and above)	225	74.5%
Mild anaemic (haemoglobin level between 10 and 10.99 g/dL)	53	17.5%
Moderately anaemic (haemoglobin level between 8.0 and 9.9 g/dL)	24	7.9%
Severely anaemic (haemoglobin level below 7.99 g/dL)	0	0
Total	302	100%

3. Results

313 female undergraduates from five hostels situated inside the university premises participated in this study. Nine incomplete questionnaires and two clotted blood samples were rejected and therefore data from 302 individuals were used in the analysis. Participants' age ranged from 20 years to 27 years and the mean age was 22.16 ($\pm$1.65) years.

3.1. The Proportion of Anaemic Subjects. According to this study, 17.5% ($n = 53$) had mild anaemia (haemoglobin concentration between 10.0 and 10.9 g/dL) and 7.9% ($n = 24$) had moderate anaemia (haemoglobin concentration between 8.0 and 9.9 g/dL). Severely anaemic individuals (haemoglobin concentration below 7.9 g/dL) were not observed during the study (Table 1). Blood haemoglobin levels of the study group ranged from 8.45 to 15.73 g/dL. Mean haemoglobin level of the anaemic individuals was 10.22 g/dL and the mean haemoglobin level of the nonanaemic individuals was 12.23 g/dL. There was a statistically significant difference between these two means according to the independent sample t-test.

3.2. Dietary Habits of the Study Sample. A questionnaire was used to gather information regarding the dietary habits of the female undergraduates. There were 16 (5.3%) vegetarians among the participants. Majority of the sample consume fish, meat, or egg twice a day. 83.4% of the participants take extra meals between their three main meals. There were 30 (9.9%) individuals who drink tea within one hour of a meal as a habit.

3.3. Personal Factors of the Study Sample. Participants' awareness about anaemia showed a statistically significant ($P < 0.05$) association with the faculty in which they are studying (Table 2). However, the proportion of anaemia was not significantly associated with the awareness of the participants.

Mean number of days that the nonanaemic subjects had their menstrual blood flow was 4.18 days and for anaemic subjects this was 4.32 days. There was no statistically significant difference between the two groups when independent sample t-test was performed. According to data gathered, menstrual blood of 47% of subjects ($n = 142$) contained clots. 79.5% of the subjects ($n = 240$) have taken antihelminthic treatment within past year.

Proportion of anaemia in the study group did not show a statistically significant association ($P > 0.05$) with these dietary habits and selected personal factors (Table 3).

4. Discussion

According to WHO data, the prevalence of anaemia in this age group in Asia and in Sri Lanka is 33% and 31.6%, respectively. But according to a survey done in Sri Lanka, the prevalence of anaemia among nonpregnant females is 39%, whereas the prevalence is 32% among 20–29-year-old nonpregnant females [3]. When we consider the above statistics, the importance of screening for anaemia among the above population is clearly evident, especially because included in the above age group are the female university undergraduates whose academic performance may be adversely affected due to anaemia. According to WHO, global anaemia prevalence among nonpregnant females is 30.2% and the proportion that we found does not significantly differ from this value ($P = 0.075$). When compared with the WHO data available on anaemia for Sri Lanka for nonpregnant females, the proportion of anaemia found in this research is at a lower value (WHO prevalence 31.6%) and our value significantly differs from WHO prevalence ($P = 0.022$) [4]. This prevalence is also lower than the prevalence among nonpregnant females of 20–29 years of age (32%) as found in an island wide research conducted by the Department of Census and Statistics in year 2007 yet the difference is not statistically significant ($P = 0.12$) [3].

The mean haemoglobin value of the study sample was 11.71 g/dL ($\pm$1.19). It was 10.22 g/dL among the anaemic participants and 12.23 g/dL among nonanaemic participants. These two figures are statistically significant according to the independent sample t-test. However, a research done at the University of Sharjah reported a mean Hb of 12.5 g/dL, which exceeded the mean which we acquired [7]. Also a research done in Dubai, UAE, among Medical College girls, reported a higher mean Hb value of 12.83 g/dL [8]. However, our mean Hb value is comparatively higher than that of Indian nursing students (10 g/dL $\pm$ 1.47) [9].

According to this research, over two-thirds of the anaemic students (68.83%) ($n = 53$) suffer from mild anaemia. A research conducted at the Vadodara nursing school in India, among female students within the age limit of 17–21 years, it was revealed that the prevalence of mild and moderate anaemia was almost equal (mild = 42.5%, moderate = 43.11%). Also it revealed that a higher percentage of female students were anaemic (86.6%) [9].

Food habits, which were considered in this study, including drinking tea after main meals and the frequency in which fish and meat products were consumed, did not show a statistically significant association with anaemia.

A research has been carried out in a Bangladesh university in year 2011, based on a similar hypothesis as our research, has found a higher anaemia prevalence of 55.3% and majority of them are girls (63.3%). They have also observed a significant higher proportion of male students who were unaware of anaemia [10]. In our research, there was no

TABLE 2: Subjects' awareness on anaemia according to the faculty in which they are studying.

Name of the faculty	Subject's awareness of anaemia		P value
	Yes	No	
Faculty of Medical Sciences	55 (100%)	0	
Faculty of Humanities and Social Sciences	34 (29.3%)	82 (70.7%)	0.000
Faculty of Management Studies and Commerce	34 (30.9%)	76 (69.1%)	
Faculty of Applied Sciences	17 (81.0%)	4 (19.0%)	

TABLE 3: Distribution of nonanaemic and anaemic subjects according to dietary habits and selected medical conditions.

	Nonanaemic ($n = 225$)		Anaemic ($n = 77$)		P value
	n	%	n	%	
Consumption extra meals					
Yes	193	85.8	59	76.6	0.062
No	32	14.2	18	23.4	
Vegetarian or not					
Yes	13	5.8	3	3.9	0.525
No	212	94.2	74	96.1	
Number of meals supplemented with meat, fish, or egg per day					
Zero	14	6.2	2	2.6	
One	57	25.3	24	31.2	0.499
Two	129	57.3	44	57.1	
Three	25	11.1	72	9.1	
Drinking tea within one hour of a main meal					
Yes	23	10.2	7	9.1	0.775
No	202	89.8	70	90.9	
Subject's awareness about anaemia					
Yes	101	44.9	39	50.6	0.382
No	124	55.1	38	49.4	
Passage of clots in menstrual blood					
Yes	108	48.0	34	44.2	0.560
No	117	52.0	43	55.8	
Antihelminthic treatment within the past year					
Yes	178	79.1	62	80.5	0.792
No	47	20.9	15	19.5	

significant relationship between the awareness on anaemia and anaemic proportion.

A similar research carried out in the Kingdom of Saudi Arabia in King Abdulaziz University has revealed the prevalence of anaemia to be 26% among female university students [11]. Also 26.7% of anaemia prevalence was found among female students in a research carried out in the University of Sharjah [7]. In a research carried out on nonpregnant women in University of Peshawar in Pakistan, the anaemia prevalence was found to be 23.9%. [12]. Thus, the inference is that the anaemic proportion found in our research does not have a statistically significant difference from data obtained in King Abdulaziz University, University of Sharjah, and University of Peshawar (respective P values = 0.84, 0.63, and 0.51).

Anaemia can be caused by drinking tea after main meals. This is caused by the chemical "tanin" in tea, which reduces the absorption of iron from food [13]. However, the finding of this study as well as a study conducted in the Abdulaziz

University did not show a statistically significant association between drinking tea and anaemia.

In our study the mean number of days that the nonanaemic subjects had their menstruation was 4.18 days and for nonanaemic it was 4.32 days. There was no statistically significant difference between these two values. Heavy menstrual blood loss is an important risk factor to develop iron deficiency anaemia but in our study there was no statistically significant relationship between anaemia and the number of days participants have menstruated. In this study, the number of anaemic subjects ($n = 34$) who had clots in menstrual blood was lower than the number of anaemic subjects who did not have clots in menstrual blood ($n = 43$). The research at the king Abdulaziz University too revealed that there was no significant relationship between anaemia and clots in the menstrual blood [11]. The study at University of Hail revealed that there was no relation between duration of menstruation cycle and anaemic and nonanaemic groups [14]. However, another research done among females of childbearing age in King Khalid University Hospital in Riyadh had identified menstrual blood loss lasting for more than eight days or a heavy menstrual cycle as risk factors for iron deficiency anaemia [15].

5. Conclusions

Anaemia in the study population is below the average for Sri Lankan data. Yet nearly one in every four female undergraduates was found to be anaemic and these results warrant serious attention to be paid regarding anemia among this population because, among other things, their academic performance may be adversely affected due to anaemia.

Conflict of Interests

The authors declare that there is no conflict of interests regarding the publication of this paper.

References

[1] The World Bank, *Malnutrition in Sri Lanka. Scale, Scope, Causes and Potential Response. Health Nutrition and Population, Human Development Network*, Human Development Unit, South Asia Region, Washington, DC, USA, 2007, http://un.lk/un_team_in_SL/pdf.

[2] National Family Health Survey (NFHS-III), 2005-2006, http://www.nfhsindia.org/pdf/India.pdf.

[3] Department of Census and Statistics, Ministry of Healthcare and Nutrition, Sri Lanka. Prevalence of anaemia among children and women. Demographic and Health Survey 2006/7, 2011, http://www.statistics.gov.lk.

[4] WHO Report, *World Prevalence of Anemia 1993–2005. WHO Global Database on Anemia*, World Health Organization, Geneva, Switzerland, 2008, http://www.WHO.Int/hinari/en/.

[5] I. P. Kaur and S. Kaur, "A comparison of nutritional profile and prevalence of anemia among rural girls and boys," *Journal of Exercise Science and Physiotherapy*, vol. 7, no. 1, pp. 11–18, 2011.

[6] J. D. Haas and T. Brownlie IV, "Iron deficiency and reduced work capacity: a critical review of the research to determine a causal relationship," *Journal of Nutrition*, vol. 131, no. 2, supplement 2, pp. 676S–688S, 2001.

[7] A. H. Sultan, "Anemia among female college students attending the University of Sharjah, UAE: prevalence and classification," *The Journal of the Egyptian Public Health Association*, vol. 82, no. 3-4, pp. 261–271, 2007.

[8] A. I. Ayoub, "Iron deficiency anemia in Dubai Medical College for Girls: a preliminary study," *The Journal of the Egyptian Public Health Association*, vol. 70, no. 1-2, pp. 213–228, 1995.

[9] P. D. Karkar and P. V. Kotecha, "Prevalence of anemia among students of Nursing School of Vadodara," *The Nursing Journal of India*, vol. 95, no. 11, pp. 257–258, 2004.

[10] K. B. Shill, P. Karmakar, M. G. Kibria et al., "Prevalence of iron-deficiency anaemia among university students in Noakhali region, Bangladesh," *Journal of Health, Population and Nutrition*, vol. 32, no. 1, pp. 103–110, 2014.

[11] F. Al-Sayes, M. Gari, S. Qusti, N. Bagatian, and A. Abuzenadah, "Prevalence of iron deficiency anaemia among females at university stage," *Journal of Medical Laboratory and Diagnosis*, vol. 2, no. 1, pp. 5–11, 2011.

[12] M. T. Khan, T. Akhtar, and M. Niazi, "Prevalence of anemia among university of Peshawar students," *Journal of Postgraduate Medical Institute*, vol. 24, no. 4, pp. 265–269, 2010.

[13] A. V. Hoffbrand, J. E. Pettit, and P. A. H. Moss, Eds., *Essential Haematology*, Blackwell Science, Malden, Mass, USA, 4th edition, 2001.

[14] S. Mohamed and S. Sweilem, "Prevalence of anemia levels in a sample of university female students," *International Journal of Science and Research*, vol. 3, no. 6, pp. 805–809, 2014.

[15] J. M. Al-Quaiz, "Iron deficiency anemia: a study of risk factors," *Saudi Medical Journal*, vol. 22, no. 6, pp. 490–496, 2001.

10

Magnitude of Anemia and Associated Factors among Pediatric HIV/AIDS Patients Attending Zewditu Memorial Hospital ART Clinic, Addis Ababa, Ethiopia

Hylemariam Mihiretie,[1,2] Bineyam Taye,[2] and Aster Tsegaye[2]

[1]*Department of Medical Laboratory Sciences, Faculty of Medical and Health Sciences, Wollega University,*
P.O. Box 395, Nekemte, Ethiopia
[2]*Department of Medical Laboratory Sciences, School of Allied Health Sciences, College of Health Science, Addis Ababa University,*
P.O. Box 1176, Addis Ababa, Ethiopia

Correspondence should be addressed to Hylemariam Mihiretie; hylemariam@gmail.com

Academic Editor: Duran Canatan

Background. Anemia is one of the most commonly observed hematological abnormalities and an independent prognostic marker of HIV disease. The aim of this study was to determine the magnitude of anemia and associated factors among pediatric HIV/AIDS patients attending Zewditu Memorial Hospital (ZMH) ART Clinic in Addis Ababa, Ethiopia. *Methods.* A cross-sectional study was conducted among pediatric HIV/AIDS patients of Zewditu Memorial Hospital (ZMH) between August 05, 2013, and November 25, 2013. A total of 180 children were selected consecutively. Stool specimen was collected and processed. A structured questionnaire was used to collect data on sociodemographic characteristics and associated risk factors. Data were entered into EpiData 3.1.1. and were analyzed using SPSS version 16 software. Logistic regressions were applied to assess any association between explanatory factors and outcome variables. *Results.* The total prevalence of anemia was 22.2% where 21 (52.5%), 17 (42.5%), and 2 (5.0%) patients had mild, moderate, and severe anemia. There was a significant increase in severity and prevalence of anemia in those with CD4+ T cell counts below 350 cells/μL ($P < 0.05$). Having intestinal parasitic infections (AOR = 2.7, 95% CI, 1.1–7.2), having lower CD4+ T cell count (AOR = 3.8, 95% CI, 1.6–9.4), and being HAART naïve (AOR = 2.3, 95% CI, 1.6–9.4) were identified as significant predictors of anemia. *Conclusion.* Anemia was more prevalent and severe in patients with low CD4+ T cell counts, patients infected with intestinal parasites/helminthes, and HAART naïve patients. Therefore, public health measures and regular follow-up are necessary to prevent anemia.

1. Background

Hematological complications have been documented to be the second most common cause of morbidity and mortality in HIV positive persons [1]. Anemia, one of the commonest hematological complications with HIV infection, refers to a condition in which the hemoglobin content of the blood is lower than normal for a person's age, gender, and environment, resulting in the oxygen carrying capacity of the blood being reduced [2]. Anemia is a common feature of HIV infection, occurring in approximately 35% of patients who initiate antiretroviral treatment (ART) in Europe and North America [3].

In HIV-infected patients, anemia may be caused by nutrient deficiencies (iron, folic acid, and vitamin B12), sickle cell disease, HIV/AIDS itself, malaria, hookworm, and other infections. Other mechanisms for HIV-associated anemia, although uncommon, include autoimmune destruction of erythrocytes [4]. Direct infection of marrow precursor cells [5] has been hypothesized but not proven. The incidence of anemia ranges from 10% in people who have no HIV symptoms to 92% in individuals who have advanced AIDS [6]. Anemia has been reported as a very common complication of pediatric HIV infection, associated with a poor prognosis [7]. It has been identified as one of the predictors of early mortality in a cohort of HIV-infected children receiving HAART [8].

In established HIV infection, lower hemoglobin levels have been shown to correlate with decreasing CD4+ T cell counts which is supported by many studies demonstrating an association between anemia during established infection and a faster progression of AIDS as well as death. Therefore, interventions (like HAART administration) to prevent anemia may lead to improved health and survival potential of HIV-infected persons [9]. Anemia in children can be caused by iron deficiency and by health factors such as parasite infections or other causes. School children carry the heaviest burden of intestinal parasitic infection and anemia [10].

While there is a wide variation in the prevalence of anemia among HIV/AIDS patients in different studies all over the world, there is paucity of information on the prevalence and associated risk factors of anemia among pediatric HIV patients in Ethiopia. Pediatric ART started in the country relatively late. This study, therefore, aims to evaluate the magnitude of anemia among pediatric HIV positive patients based on age, gender, HAART status, intestinal parasitic infection, and CD4+ T cell levels.

2. Methods

2.1. Study Setting and Context. A comparative cross-sectional study was conducted in Zewditu Memorial Hospital (ZMH), Addis Ababa, Ethiopia, between August 05 and November 25, 2013. This hospital was selected due to the presence of large numbers of pediatric HIV patients under follow-up care and it is a model ART center as well. The hospital provides many health care services including pediatric HIV testing, counseling, and ART.

2.2. Study Population and Data Collection. One hundred eighty (180) pediatric HIV/AIDS patients (age less than 18 years) were enrolled consecutively. Guardians of patients and those children above 12 years of age were informed about the objective of the study. Then stool specimens were collected from each patient after getting written consent. Structured questionnaire was used to assess independent variables. Complete blood count and CD4+ T cell count, from EDTA whole blood using Cell-Dyn 1800 and FACScalibur, respectively, are routinely performed for patients on follow-up visits in ZMH. Accordingly, CD4+ T cell count and hemoglobin level were taken simultaneously with stool specimen collection. Therefore, no blood specimen was collected for the purpose of this study.

2.3. Specimen Collection and Processing. EDTA anticoagulated whole blood was run on CellDyn 1800 and FACScalibur to determine hemoglobin level and CD4+ T cell count, respectively. Immunosuppression and anemia were defined based on WHO criteria [11] as follows—*mild anemia*: hemoglobin level between 10 and 10.9 g/dL for under 5 and between 11 and 11.9 g/dL for under 18 years of age children; *moderate anemia*: hemoglobin level between 7.0 and 9.9 g/dL for under 5 and between 8.0 and 10.9 g/dL for under 18 years of age children; *severe anemia*: hemoglobin level <7.0 g/dL for

under 5 and <8.0 g/dL for under 18 years of age children; *mild immunosuppression*: CD4+ T lymphocyte counts between 350 and 499 cells/μL for under 18 or between 25 and 35% for under 5 years of age children [12]; *advanced immunosuppression*: CD4+ T lymphocyte counts between 200 and 349 cells/μL for under 18 or between 15 and 25% for under 5 years of age children [12]; *severe immunosuppression*: CD4+ T cell count <200 cells/μL for under 18 or less than 15% for under 5 years of age children [12]. Pediatric refers to children less than 18 years of age. *Magnitude of anemia* refers to severity and prevalence of anemia.

For parasitological analysis, a single stool specimen was collected from each patient using clean, dry, leak proof, and wide-mouthed caps. Direct wet mount, Formol-Ether concentration, and modified Zhiehl-Neelson staining techniques were applied to detect intestinal parasites microscopically. A small portion of the stool specimen was also preserved in 10% formalin to repeat tests whenever required and further analysis [13, 14].

2.4. Statistical Analysis. The data were cleaned, coded, and double-entered using EpiData version 3.1.1. and SPSS software version 16 (SPSS INC, Chicago, IL, USA) was used for data entry and analysis. Binary logistic regression was used to determine the association between anemia and demographic and clinical variables. Multiple logistic regressions were used to control the confounding factors. P values less than 0.05 were taken as statistically significant.

2.5. Ethical Considerations. The study protocol was ethically reviewed and approved by the Departmental Research and Ethical Committee of Addis Ababa University, Department of Medical Laboratory Sciences, and Addis Ababa Health Bureau. Then the Health Bureau sent a letter informing the hospital administrators about the study and hence permission was obtained from Zewditu Memorial Hospital. Data were collected after obtaining written consent from parents/guardians and confidentiality was maintained throughout the study by using codes. The positive results were timely reported to the clinicians for appropriate interventions.

3. Results

3.1. Sociodemographic Characteristics of the Participants. A total of 180 study participants were enrolled. Ninety-eight (54.4%) of them were males and 158 (87.8%) of them were urban residents. The mean age of the participants was 11 ± 3.2 and the median was 11 years ranging from 0.3 to 17 years. Majority (83.9%, 151/180) of the participants were at primary school level (Table 1).

3.2. Magnitude of Anemia and Associated Factors. The total prevalence of anemia was 22.2% (40/180) (Table 1). As summarized in the table, the prevalence of anemia was higher in females (24.4%) and rural residents (41%). Moreover, anemia showed higher incidence in patients aged 6–11 years (25%) and in primary school children (21.2%). When anemia was characterized by severity, mild, moderate, and severe anemia

TABLE 1: Sociodemographic characteristics of pediatric HIV/AIDS patients attending Zewditu Memorial Hospital from August 5, 2013, to November 25, 2013, Addis Ababa, Ethiopia ($N = 180$).

Variables	Anemia		Total N (%)
	Present N (%)	Absent N (%)	
Age group (years)			
<2	1 (50)	1 (50)	2 (1.1)
2–5	2 (33.3)	4 (66.7)	6 (3.3)
6–11	21 (25.3)	62 (74.7)	83 (46.1)
12–18	16 (18)	73 (82)	89 (49.5)
Sex			
Male	20 (20.4)	78 (79.6)	98 (54.4)
Female	20 (24.4)	62 (75.6)	82 (45.6)
Residence			
Urban	31 (19.6)	127 (80.4)	158 (87.8)
Rural	9 (41)	13 (59)	22 (12.2)
Education			
Did not begin	1 (25)	3 (75)	4 (2.2)
Kindergarten	1 (8.3)	11 (91.7)	12 (6.7)
Primary	32 (21.2)	119 (78.8)	151 (83.9)
Secondary	6 (46)	7 (54)	13 (7.2)
Total	**40 (22.2)**	**140 (77.8)**	**180 (100)**

TABLE 2: Frequency distribution of anemia status among anemic pediatric HIV/AIDS patients attending Zewditu Memorial Hospital from August 5, 2013, to November 25, 2013, Addis Ababa, Ethiopia ($N = 40$).

Variables	Mild N (%)	Moderate N (%)	Severe N (%)	Total
Age group (years)				
<2	0 (0)	1 (2.5)	0 (0)	1 (2.5)
2–5	2 (5)	0 (0)	0 (0)	2 (5)
6–11	12 (30)	7 (17.5)	2 (5)	21 (52.5)
12–18	7 (17.5)	9 (22.5)	0 (0)	16 (40)
Gender				
Male	12 (30)	8 (20)	0 (0)	20 (50)
Female	9 (22.5)	9 (22.5)	2 (5)	20 (50)
Education				
Did not begin	0 (0)	1 (2.5)	0 (0)	1 (2.5)
Kindergarten	1 (2.5)	0 (0)	0 (0)	1 (2.5)
Primary	18 (45)	12 (30)	2 (5)	32 (80)
Secondary	2 (5)	4 (10)	0 (0)	6 (15)
Residence				
Urban	18 (45)	13 (32.5)	0	31 (77.5)
Rural	3 (7.5)	4 (10)	2 (5)	9 (22.5)
HAART I				
Yes	3 (7.5)	5 (12.5)	0 (0)	8 (20)
No	18 (45)	12 (30)	2 (5)	32 (80)
WHO stage				
I	3 (7.5)	1 (2.5)	0 (0)	4 (10)
II	16 (40)	10 (25)	0 (0)	26 (65)
III	2 (5)	6 (15)	1 (2.5)	9 (22.5)
IV	0 (0)	0 (0)	1 (2.5)	1 (2.5)
Total	**21 (52.5)**	**17 (42.5)**	**2 (5)**	**40 (100)**

account for 21 (52.5%), 17 (42.5%), and 2 (5.0%) patients, respectively (Table 2).

Among anemic patients, 30% of males had mild anemia while 32.5% of urban residents were moderately anemic. Severe anemia was absent in patients classified under WHO HIV/AIDS stages I and II. HAART experienced patients had higher incidence of moderate anemia (12.5%) unlike HAART naïve patients who had the highest incidence of mild anemia (45%) (Table 2).

More than half (54.8%) of those with advanced immunosuppression were anemic and severe anemia was also more prevalent in these groups (Figure 1). Figure 1 also shows that anemia was more prevalent in patients with mild immunosuppression. Both moderate and severe anemia showed higher prevalence in advanced immunosuppression while mild anemia was high in patients with mild immunosuppression.

Twenty-four (60%) of all anemic patients had CD4+ T cell count below 350 cells/μL. Seventy-nine (43.9%) of the participants were HAART experienced patients. Among 40 anemic patients, 32 (80%) of them were HAART naïve. Mild (17.8%) and moderate (11.8%) anemia were more prevalent in HAART naïve patients (Table 2) and anemia was comparatively more prevalent and severe in HAART naïve patients (31.7%) ($P < 0.05$). Majority of the study participants, 123 (68.3%), were at WHO HIV/AIDS clinical stage II followed by clinical stage I (19.4%). Anemia was more prevalent in WHO clinical stages II and III patients, even though these stages

were not independent risk factors to cause anemia ($P > 0.05$). Among 40 anemic patients, 28 (70%) were infected with intestinal parasites. Anemia significantly increased in those patients infected with intestinal parasites ($P < 0.05$) (Table 3).

In binary logistic regression, gender and age group do not show any significant association with anemia ($P > 0.05$), but WHO HIV/AIDS stage II (COR, 95% CI: 0.5 (0.1, 0.92), $P < 0.05$), absence of HAART (COR, 95% CI: 2.1 (1.1, 2.7), $P < 0.01$), rural residence (COR, 95% CI: 0.4 (0.1, 0.9), $P < 0.05$), primary school (COR, 95% CI: 3.2 (1.1, 10), $P < 0.05$), CD4 T cell count < 350 cells/μL (COR, 95% CI: 2.5 (1.01, 4.1), $P < 0.01$), and infection with intestinal parasites (COR, 95% CI: 4.5 (1.2, 5.3), $P < 0.01$) showed significant association with the presence of anemia (Table 3).

After being adjusted with multinomial logistic regression, only absence of HAART (AOR, 95% CI: 2.3 (1.3, 4.7), $P < 0.05$), low CD4 T cell count <350 cells/μL (AOR, 95% CI: 3.8 (1.6, 9.4), $P < 0.05$), and infection with intestinal parasites (AOR, 95% CI: 2.7 (1.1, 7.2), $P < 0.05$) were significantly associated with anemia (Table 3). Therefore, pediatric

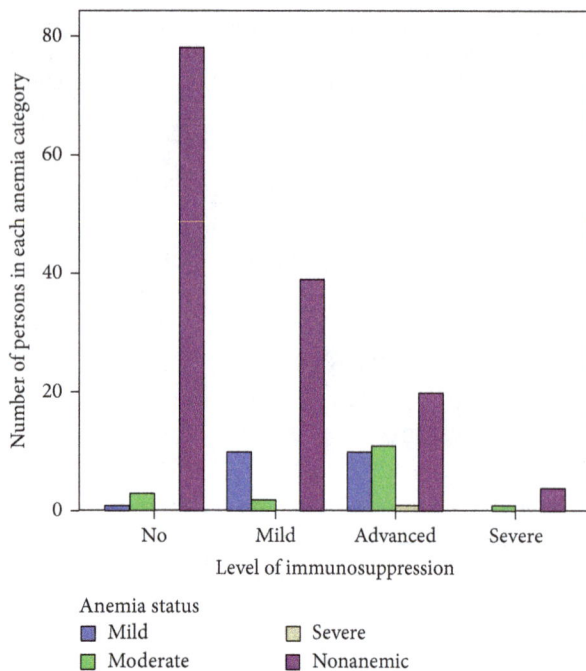

Figure 1: Distribution of anemia status by level of immunosuppression in Zewditu Memorial Hospital, from August 5, 2013, to November 25, 2013, Addis Ababa, Ethiopia.

HIV/AIDS patients without HAART, infected with intestinal parasites, and having low CD4+ T cell counts had 2.3, 2.7, and 3.8 times more likelihood of being anemic compared to their counterparts, respectively (Table 3).

One-way ANOVA analysis showed that there was significant difference in mean hemoglobin concentration between and within the groups of presence of intestinal parasites, CD4+ T cell category, and HAART status (Table 4).

4. Discussion

Anemia in children can be caused by iron deficiency and by health factors such as parasite infections. Genetic disorders such as the hemoglobinopathies and thalassemias are also implicated in some parts of the world. School children carry the heaviest burden of intestinal parasitic infection and anemia [10].

The observed prevalence of anemia in this study (22.2%) is very low compared to a study done in Tanzania (77.4%) [15], Northeastern Nigeria (57.5%) [16], Gondar (70.1%) [17], in Northwest Ethiopia (35%) [18], and Ghana (46%) [19] but is comparable to a study done in Jimma (21.9%) [20] and Southwest Ethiopia (23.1%) [21]. The possible explanation to this low prevalence might be due to low prevalence of helminthes in this study, better follow-up, and better awareness of participants about anemia and being urban residents.

The respective 21 (52.5%) and 17 (42.5%) mild and moderate anemia observed in this study are higher than a study

in Tanzania [15] where mild and moderate anemia account for 28.4% and 32.1%, respectively. Furthermore severe anemia (5.0%) is higher than a study in North West Ethiopia (1.3%) [18]. This difference might be due to geographic difference as most of them used more than one study area, age difference as our participants are pediatric and anemia can be caused by different factors including nutrition in children, and sample size difference as our sample size is smaller than the previous studies which may increase the prevalence. Unlike studies from North West Ethiopia [18] and Tanzania [15], anemia was not significantly associated with gender in the present study which might be due to comparable number of both genders participated in this study. Moreover, mild and moderate anemia were more prevalent in advanced immunosuppression which is in agreement with a study done in Jimma [20].

Similar to the previous studies done in North West Ethiopia [18], Ghana [19], Jimma [20], Addis Ababa [22], and Northeastern Nigeria [16], the prevalence of anemia was significantly associated with lower CD4+ T cell levels but different from a study in West Africa [23] where CD4+ T cell count was not significant predictor of anemia.

The prevalence of anemia was found to be higher among rural residents, even though residence was not an independent predictor of anemia unlike a study done in Jimma [20] where rural residence was associated with significantly increased anemia. This higher prevalence of anemia in rural residents might be due to the fact that those participants residing in rural areas might not have adequate information about nutrition and other factors that could cause anemia.

Intestinal parasitic infections, lower CD4+ T cell count, and being HAART naïve were identified as significant predictors of anemia. Patients with intestinal parasitic infections had 2.7 times more risk of developing anemia compared to those without infections ($P = 0.048$, 95% CI: 1.1–7.2). The risk of developing anemia in patients with low CD4 count was 3.8 times more than those with higher CD4 count of >350 cells/μL ($P = 0.03$, 95% CI: 1.6–9.4). On the other hand HAART naïve patients had 2.3 times more likelihood of being anemic than their counterparts. This may indicate that the likelihood of anemia increases with immunologic deterioration and with the advancement of HIV-related disease in the absence of HAART. This result is comparable with a study done in Southwest Ethiopia [21].

5. Conclusion

The prevalence of anemia in pediatric patients was significantly high in this study. The prevalence and severity of anemia was significantly increased in HAART naïve patients, those infected by intestinal parasites, and in immunosuppressed HIV patients. In conclusion, this study has shown that HAART initiation, anthelminthic medication, and regular checkup of CD4 count might have benefit in reducing anemia in HIV positive pediatric patients. Therefore, further longitudinal studies with long-term follow-up are needed to explore more on the causes of anemia and the pattern of hemoglobin changes with associated factors in HIV positive persons in resource limited settings.

TABLE 3: Association of risk factors with anemia in pediatric HIV/AIDS patients attending Zewditu Memorial Hospital from August 5, 2013, to November 25, 2013, Addis Ababa, Ethiopia (N = 180).

Variables	Anemia		COR (95% CI)	P	AOR (95% CI)	P
	Present N (%)	Absent N (%)				
WHO S						
I	4 (10)	31 (22.2)	1		1	
II	27 (67.5)	96 (68.6)	0.5 (0.1, 0.92)	0.008*	0.3 (0.01, 1.1)	0.4
III	9 (22.5)	11 (7.8)	0.2 (0.04, 0.6)	0.2	1.2 (0.1, 3.2)	0.1
IV	0 (0)	2 (1.4)	0 (0, 0)	1.00	0.1 (0, 1.3)	0.9
HAART I						
Yes	8 (20)	71 (50.7)	1		1	
No	32 (80)	69 (49.3)	2.1 (1.1, 2.7)	0.001*	2.3 (1.3, 4.7)	0.048*
Residence						
Urban	31 (19.6)	127 (80.4)	1		1	
Rural	9 (41)	13 (59)	0.4 (0.1, 0.9)	0.03*	0.6 (0.2, 2.3)	0.5
Edu. s.						
NB	1 (25)	3 (75)	2.6 (0.2, 32)	0.5		
KG	1 (8.3)	11 (91.7)	9.4 (0.9, 96)	0.3		
Prim.	32 (21.2)	119 (78.8)	3.2 (1.1, 10)	0.05*	0.3 (0.06, 1.3)	0.09
Secon.	6 (46)	7 (54)	1		1	
CD4						
<350	24 (60)	24 (17)	2.5 (1.01, 4.1)	0.00*	3.8 (1.6, 9.4)	0.03*
>350	16 (40)	116 (83)	1		1	
IPs						
Present	28 (70)	40 (28.6)	4.5 (1.2, 5.3)	0.00*	2.7 (1.1, 7.2)	0.048*
Absent	12 (30)	100 (71.4)	1		1	
Age group						
<2	1 (50)	1 (50)	0.2 (0.01, 3.7)	0.3		
2–5	2 (33.3)	4 (66.7)	0.4 (0.07, 2.6)	0.36		
6–11	21 (25.3)	62 (74.7)	0.6 (0.3, 1.30)	0.25		
12–18	16 (18)	73 (82)	1			
Sex						
Male	20 (20.4)	78 (79.6)	1			
Female	20 (24.4)	62 (75.6)	0.8 (0.4, 1.6)	0.5		

*Significant at P value <0.05, AOR: adjusted odds ratio, COR: crude odds ratio, WHO S: WHO HIV/AIDS stage, HAART I: HAART initiation, P: P value, IPs: intestinal parasites, Edu. s: educational status, KG: kindergarten, Prim.: primary, Secon.: secondary, NB: did not begin, CD4: CD4 T cell count (cells/μL).

TABLE 4: One-way ANOVA analysis of hemoglobin concentration among pediatric HIV/AIDS patients attending Zewditu Memorial Hospital from August 5, 2013, to November 25, 2013, Addis Ababa, Ethiopia.

Variables	Mean square		F	P value
	Within groups	Between groups		
Gender	2.9	0.95	0.32	0.6
HAART status	2.7	59	25.6	0.04
CD4 category	2.6	71	29.2	0.02
Infection with intestinal parasites	2.5	88	35.8	0.00

Conflict of Interests

All authors declare that they have no conflict of interests associated with the publication of this paper.

Authors' Contributions

Hylemariam Mihiretie conceived and designed the experiments, performed the experiments, analyzed the data, contributed reagents, materials, and analysis tools, and wrote the paper. Bineyam Taye and Aster Tsegaye assisted with design, analysis, and interpretation of data and provided critical review of the paper. Hylemariam Mihiretie, Bineyam Taye, and Aster Tsegaye read and approved the final paper and provided critical appraisal.

Acknowledgments

This study was funded by Addis Ababa University, Ethiopia. The authors would like to thank the Addis Ababa University for financial and administrative support, all study participants for their cooperation, and administrative and laboratory staff of Zewditu Memorial Hospital especially Dr. Aster Shewa-amare, for all the support to carry out this study.

References

[1] W. K. B. A. Owiredu, L. Quaye, N. Amidu, and O. Addai-Mensah, "Prevalence of anaemia and immunological markers among Ghanaian HAART-naïve HIV-patients and those on HAART," *African Health Sciences*, vol. 11, no. 1, pp. 2–15, 2011.

[2] World Health Organization, *Worldwide Prevalence of Anemia 1993–2005*, WHO, 2008.

[3] R. J. Harris, J. A. C. Sterne, S. Abgrall et al., "Prognostic importance of anaemia in HIV type-1-infected patients starting antiretroviral therapy: collaborative analysis of prospective cohort studies," *Antiviral Therapy*, vol. 13, no. 8, pp. 959–967, 2008.

[4] O. Ifudu, "Maximizing response to erythropoietin in treating HIV-associated anemia," *Cleveland Clinic Journal of Medicine*, vol. 68, no. 7, pp. 643–648, 2001.

[5] M. F. Miller, J. H. Humphrey, P. J. Iliff et al., "Neonatal erythropoiesis and subsequent anemia in HIV-positive and HIV-negative Zimbabwean babies during the first year of life: a longitudinal study," *BMC Infectious Diseases*, vol. 6, article 1, 2006.

[6] K.-A. Kreuzer and J. K. Rockstroh, "Pathogenesis and pathophysiology of anemia in HIV infection," *Annals of Hematology*, vol. 75, no. 5-6, pp. 179–187, 1997.

[7] J. C. J. Calis, M. B. van Hensbroek, R. J. de Haan, P. Moons, B. J. Brabin, and I. Bates, "HIV-associated anemia in children: a systematic review from a global perspective," *AIDS*, vol. 22, no. 10, pp. 1099–1112, 2008.

[8] G. Ebissa, N. Deyessa, and S. Biadgilign, "Predictors of early mortality in a cohort of HIV-infected children receiving high active antiretroviral treatment in public hospitals in Ethiopia," *AIDS Care*, pp. 1–8, 2015.

[9] M. A. Doukas, "Human immunodeficiency virus associated anemia," *Medical Clinics of North America*, vol. 76, no. 3, pp. 699–709, 1992.

[10] S. D. Fernando, H. Goonethilleke, K. H. Weerasena et al., "Geohelminth infections in a rural area of Sri Lanka," *Southeast Asian Journal of Tropical Medicine and Public Health*, vol. 32, no. 1, pp. 23–26, 2001.

[11] WHO, *Hemoglobin Concentrations for the Diagnosis of Anemia and Assessment of Severity, Vitamin and Mineral Nutrition Information System*, World Health Organization, Geneva, Switzerland, 2011.

[12] WHO, *Interim WHO Clinical Staging of HIV/AIDS and HIV/AIDS Case Definitions for Surveillance in African Region*, WHO/HIV, 2005.

[13] M. Cheesbrough, *District Laboratory Practices in Tropical Countries. Part 1*, Cambridge University Press, Cambridge, UK, 1999.

[14] H. Mohammed, *Modified Ziehl-Neelson Method*, vol. 11, The Ethiopian Health & Nutrition Research Institute (EHNRI), 2010.

[15] A. Johannessen, E. Naman, S. G. Gundersen, and J. N. Bruun, "Antiretroviral treatment reverses HIV-associated anemia in rural Tanzania," *BMC Infectious Diseases*, vol. 11, article 190, 2011.

[16] B. Denue, I. Kida, H. Hamagabdo, A. Dayar, and M. Sahabi, "Prevalence of anemia and immunological markers in HIV-infected patients on highly active antiretroviral therapy in Northeastern Nigeria," *Infectious Diseases Research and Treatment*, vol. 6, pp. 25–33, 2013.

[17] M. Alem, T. Kena, N. Baye, R. Ahmed, and S. Tilahun, "Prevalence of anemia and associated risk factors among adult HIV patients at the anti-retroviral therapy clinic at the University of Gondar Hospital, Gondar, Northwest Ethiopia," *Scientific Reports*, vol. 2, article 3, 2013.

[18] Y. Wondimeneh, D. Muluye, and G. Ferede, "Prevalence and associated factors of thrombocytopenia among HAART-naive HIV positive patients at Gondar university hospital, northwest Ethiopia," *BMC Research Notes*, vol. 7, article 5, 2014.

[19] O. Wkba, L. Quaye, N. Amidu, and O. Addai-Mensah, "Prevalence of anaemia and immunological markers among Ghanaian HAART-naïve HIV-patients and those on HAART," *African Health Sciences*, vol. 11, no. 1, pp. 2–15, 2011.

[20] M. Abebe and F. Alemseged, "Hematologic abormalities among children on Haart, in Jimma University Specialized Hospital, Southwestern Ethiopia," *Ethiopian Journal of Health Sciences*, vol. 19, no. 2, 2009.

[21] L. Gedefaw, T. Yemane, Z. Sahlemariam, and D. Yilma, "Anemia and risk factors in HAART naïve and HAART experienced HIV positive persons in South West Ethiopia: a comparative study," *PLoS ONE*, vol. 8, no. 8, Article ID e72202, 2013.

[22] A. Adane, K. Desta, A. Bezabih, A. Gashaye, and D. Kassa, "HIV-associated anaemia before and after initiation of antiretroviral therapy at Art Centre of Minilik II Hospital, Addis Ababa, Ethiopia," *Ethiopian Medical Journal*, vol. 50, no. 1, pp. 13–21, 2012.

[23] L. A. Renner, F. Dicko, F. Kouéta et al., "Anaemia and zidovudine-containing antiretroviral therapy in paediatric antiretroviral programmes in the IeDEA Paediatric West African Database to evaluate AIDS," *Journal of the International AIDS Society*, vol. 16, Article ID 18024, 2013.

11

The Cost-Effectiveness of Continuous Erythropoiesis Receptor Activator Once Monthly versus Epoetin Thrice Weekly for Anaemia Management in Chronic Haemodialysis Patients

Omar Maoujoud,[1,2] Samir Ahid,[1] Hocein Dkhissi,[3] Zouhair Oualim,[4] and Yahia Cherrah[1]

[1]Research Team of Pharmacoepidemiology & Pharmacoeconomics, Medical and Pharmacy School,
 Mohammed V University, Madinat Al Irfane, 10000 Rabat, Morocco
[2]Department of Nephrology & Dialysis, Military Hospital Agadir, 20450 Agadir, Morocco
[3]Meknes Dialysis Center (on Behalf of Moroccan Society of Nephrology), 33150 Meknes, Morocco
[4]IdrissAlakbar Dialysis Center (on Behalf of the Scientific Committee, Moroccan Society of Nephrology), 12470 Rabat, Morocco

Correspondence should be addressed to Omar Maoujoud; maoujoud@gmail.com

Academic Editor: Eitan Fibach

Introduction. The aim of this study was to compare the cost-effectiveness of continuous erythropoietin receptor activator (CERA) once monthly to epoetin beta (EpoB) thrice weekly to maintain haemoglobin (Hb) within the range 10.5–12 g/dL. *Methods.* Prospective cohort study and cost-effectiveness analysis. Chronic haemodialysis patients (CHP), being treated with EpoB, were selected for two periods of follow-up: period 1, maintaining prior treatment with EpoB, and period 2, conversion to CERA once monthly. Hb concentrations and costs were measured monthly. Health care payer perspective for one year was adopted. *Results.* 75 CHP completed the study, with a mean age of 52.9 ± 14.3 years. Baseline Hb was 11.14 ± 1.18 g/dL in EpoB phase and 11.46 ± 0.79 g/dL in CERA phase; we observed a significant increase in the proportion of patients successfully treated (Hb within the recommended range), 65.3% versus 70.7%, *p*: 0.008, and in the average effectiveness by 4% (0.55 versus 0.59). Average cost-effectiveness ratios were 6013.86 and 5173.64$, with an ICER CERA to EpoB at −6457.5$. *Conclusion.* Our health economic evaluation of ESA use in haemodialysis patients suggests that the use of CERA is cost-effective compared with EpoB.

1. Introduction

The incidence and prevalence of patients with chronic kidney disease (CKD) are growing worldwide [1, 2]. In patients with CKD, the kidneys are unable to produce enough erythropoietin to stimulate adequate production of red blood cells, causing renal anaemia [3, 4]; in addition, this anaemia is associated with reduced quality of life, high morbidity, and mortality in chronic haemodialysis patients (CHP) [5, 6]; it is commonly managed using erythropoiesis stimulating agents (ESA) [7–9]. The class of ESA includes epoetin alpha, epoetin beta (EpoB), darbepoetin, and the pegylated erythropoietin continuous erythropoiesis receptor activator (CERA) [10–12]. ESA such as epoetin alfa and EpoB require frequent administration (from three times weekly to once weekly) [13], while

darbepoetin alfa can be administered once weekly or once every 2 weeks, to maintain stable Hb levels within the desired target range [14]. CERA has been recently introduced in the Moroccan market to provide correction of renal anaemia, which has unique pharmacologic properties, acting differently than short-acting EpoB at the erythropoietin receptor level [15], with a long serum half-life, allowing for once-a-month dosing. Several studies have suggested that CHP can be readily switched from short-acting ESA to CERA, but the health outcomes for patients and the effects on cost have not been extensively investigated.

The purpose of this study was to carry out a cost-effectiveness analysis (CEA) to evaluate the impact of switching patients from their current short-acting ESA therapy to CERA once monthly in a real-world setting, in this order;

we conducted a multicenter prospective observational study, to compare the cost-effectiveness of CERA once monthly to treatment with EpoB thrice weekly in Moroccan haemodialysis patients.

2. Patients and Methods

Patients were screened at 3 haemodialysis centers in Morocco from January to December 2013; all participating centers used EpoB (Recormon; Hoffmann-La Roche Ltd., Basel, Switzerland) thrice weekly to treat their ESRD patients who had renal anaemia. To be included in the study, CHP were required to meet the following criteria: adult patients (≥18 years of age) with chronic renal anaemia, on chronic haemodialysis therapy with the same mode of dialysis for at least 12 weeks before, $Kt/V \geq 1.2$, baseline Hb concentration between 10.5 and 12 g/dL; stable baseline Hb concentration, continuous subcutaneous maintenance EpoB therapy with the same dosing interval for at least 8 weeks (no change of the weekly dosage), adequate iron status defined as serum ferritin ≥200 ng/mL, or transferrin saturation ≥20%. Patients were excluded from the study when they had received an organ transplant, chemotherapy, or surgery, because they may have become anaemic for reasons other than CKD.

2.1. Study Design.
The conversion from EpoB to CERA (methoxy polyethylene glycol-epoetin beta; Mircera; Hoffmann-La Roche Ltd., Basel, Switzerland) once monthly was already decided by the health care payer policy, who is the provider of erythropoietin stimulating agents for all patients, and was planned after a period of 6 months. Both EpoB and CERA have already been approved for renal anaemia in CHP and got the market authorization. Selected patients were not required to undergo any additional medical interventions, tests, or procedures, as they were receiving usual dialysis care and treated for renal anaemia following national and international guidelines. CHP that complied with the inclusion criteria were selected for a follow-up over two periods: the first period during six months (months −6 to 0), maintaining prior treatment with EpoB thrice weekly, and the second for six months (months 0 to 6), after changing treatment to CERA once monthly.

2.2. Anaemia Treatment Protocol.
All enrolled patients received EpoB or CERA subcutaneously at the end of the dialysis session. The frequency of administration was 3 times a week for EpoB, and every four weeks for CERA, EpoB dosages were adjusted to maintain Hb within the recommended range 10.5–12 g/dL, at intervals of 1 to 2 weeks. Dosages were decreased by 25% for Hb increases >1 g/dL/month, versus previous level, and increased by 25% for Hb decreases >1 g/dL/month. The starting dose of CERA was based on the previous weekly dose of EpoB in the week before conversion. For patients who previously received <8000 UI of EpoB per week; the starting dose of CERA was 120 μg, 200 μg when previous weekly EpoB was in the range 8000–16 000 IU, and 360 μg when previous weekly EpoB was >16 000 IU. Doses for all patients were to be adjusted so that haemoglobin

concentrations would remain within a target range of 10.5–12 g/dL. During the follow-up, CERA dosages were decreased by 25% for Hb increases >1 g/dL/month, versus previous level, and increased by 25% for Hb decreases >1 g/dL/month, according to protocol and not more often than once monthly. Iron supplementation (iron sucrose) was to be initiated or intensified according to centre practice in cases of iron deficiency (serum ferritin <100 μg/L or transferrin saturation <20%) and discontinued in patients who had serum ferritin levels >800 μg/L or transferring saturation >50%.

2.3. Dialysis Protocol.
All patients were on haemodialysis therapy using the AK 200 ULTRA-S dialysis machine (Gambro AB, Lund, Sweden). Ultrapure water was used for preparation of dialysis fluid and bicarbonate was provided from powder cartridges. Treatment time ranged from 4 h to 5 h per session, three times a week, with high-flux synthetic dialyser (UF-coefficient >20 mL/mmHg/h, surface area 1.4 to 2.1 m^2). Anticoagulation was performed with low molecular weight heparin and consisted of a single dose of of 3000 to 4000 units of enoxaparin. The ultrafiltration rate was programmed to reach the patient's optimal dry weight and ranged from 500 mL/h to 900 mL/h. Water treatment system consisted of double reverse osmosis, classic pretreatment (softener, activated carbon, and microfiltration), distribution loop with permanent water circulation, and direct delivery to dialysis machines.

2.4. Assessments.
Based on Nephrology Moroccan clinical practice guidelines [16], it is assumed that CHP treated with EpoB or CERA are monitored every 4 weeks, and the following laboratory parameters were gathered at baseline and then monthly until the end of the study: Hb, white blood cell (WBC) count, red blood cell (RBC) count, hematocrit (Hct), and platelet count, iron storage status: serum iron, and transferrin saturation (TSAT), ferritin, and biochemical profile: serum intact parathyroid hormone (iPTH), C-reactive protein (CRP), protein, albumin, total cholesterol, triglyceride, uric acid, high-density lipoprotein (HDL), low-density lipoprotein (LDL), glucose, blood urea nitrogen (BUN), creatinine (Cr), sodium (Na), potassium (K), calcium (Ca), and phosphate (P).

2.5. Cost-Effectiveness Analysis.
The cost-effectiveness analysis (CEA) was conducted from the healthcare payer perspective, and we applied decision analytic techniques to evaluate the average and incremental cost-effectiveness of EpoB and CERA in the treatment of anaemia. Key model inputs included clinically relevant effectiveness measures, which was measured by the clinical success rate of treatment (CSR), defined as the proportion of patients successfully achieving the Hb target as well as drug acquisition costs for both treatments considered. Model outputs were expected cost-effectiveness ratio and the incremental cost-effectiveness ratio (ICER) that represents the additional cost and effectiveness obtained, when CERA regime is compared to the EpoB regime. In this order, we considered the effectiveness and cost in terms of Hb level achieved during the two periods of six months of follow-up. Two Hb ranges were considered: 10,5

to 12 g/dL (the recommended range), higher than 12 g/dL or lower than 10,5 g/dL. Measurements of Hb were performed every 4 weeks during the study period; the mean of six consecutive measures at each phase of the study was used to categorize patients on the two groups considering Hb ranges. In our analysis, the CSR was calculated at two time periods: (1) from month −6 to month 0 for EpoB and (2) from month 0 to month 6 for CERA. Costs were calculated for each patient in the 2 periods of the study, based on 24-week drug acquisition costs, and these patient-specific costs were averaged across patients within the same range of Hb.

The cost-effectiveness ratio was expressed as the mean 1-year drug costs per one per cent of EPoB or CERA patients successfully treated during the defined time period:

Average cost-effectiveness ratio of treatment

$$= \frac{\text{Average Cost of treatment}}{\text{Average Effectiveness treatment}}. \quad (1)$$

The average cost-effectiveness ratio was then compared between EpoB and CERA.

The ICER was defined as the difference in mean 1-year cost between EpoB and CERA divided by the difference in average effectiveness between the two treatments:

ICER (Cera versus EpoB)

$$= \frac{\text{COST Cera} - \text{COST EpoB}}{\text{EFFECTIVENESS Cera} - \text{EFFECTIVENESS EpoB}}. \quad (2)$$

2.6. Perspective, Timeframe, and Source of Cost Data. A health care payer perspective was adopted, for a time horizon of one year. We considered real market costs approved by the Moroccan Agency on Medical Insurance (ANAM). All costs were collected every 3 months, reported in Moroccan dirhams (MAD), then converted to US Dollar ($) (1 US Dollar = 9,297 MAD), and were inflated to 2013 costs using the consumer price index for health care goods in Morocco. A discount rate of 3% was applied to both costs and utilities. All analyses were performed using TreeAge Pro 2015 (TreeAge Software, Williamstown, MA).

2.7. Assumptions. It was assumed that there is no change in hospitalization attributable to both treatments, that patients make no extra doctor visits due to CERA or EpoB, as they visit the hospital for dialysis irrespective of the treatment regimen for anaemia, and that surveillance costs are assumed to be the same for both treatments.

2.8. Sensitivity Analysis and Monte Carlo Simulation. One-way and two-way sensitivity analyses were performed by varying baseline estimates for costs, effectiveness within a range of potentially reasonable values, and evaluating whether these changes modify the conclusions reached. Probabilistic sensitivity analysis was performed using Monte Carlo simulation (MCS) to explore overall uncertainty in the model, by creating 50,000 samples, for which expected values were calculated. Normal distributions were used for relative and baseline risks. Log-normal distributions were applied to the costing estimates.

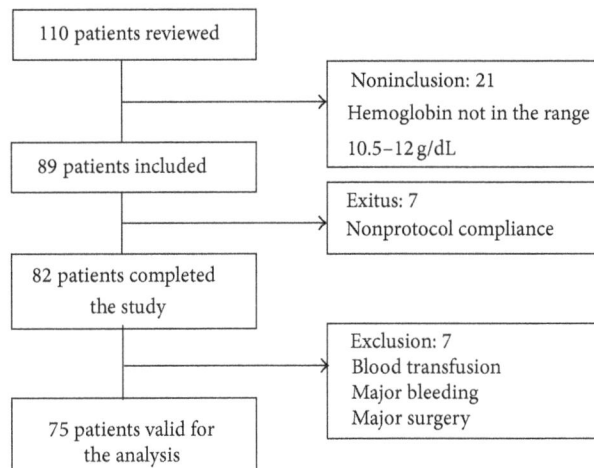

FIGURE 1: Patients included in the study.

2.9. Statistical Analysis. Results are expressed as percentages for discrete variables, medians, and interquartile ranges for nonnormally distributed continuous variables, and mean ± standard deviation for normally distributed continuous variables. All statistical analyses were performed using the statistical package for social sciences (SPSS) software 17.0 (SPSS, Chicago, IL, USA), and comparisons of groups were performed by Mann-Whitney or Wilcoxon test depending on the variable distributions. The study was powered to detect an incremental cost-effectiveness ratio between CERA and EpoB of less than a nominated critical threshold of three times 2013 Moroccan *per capita* gross domestic product. As almost all developing countries, there is no incremental cost-effectiveness threshold in Morocco, being considered as ideal for the acceptance of a given health intervention. So, we used the value established by the World Health Organization's Commission on Macroeconomics and Health, corresponding to three times the per capita gross domestic product (GDP), as a threshold for cost-effectiveness. According to the World Bank, the 2013 per capita GDP value was 3092$. For this reason, if a health procedure presents an ICER lower than 9186$ in Morocco, it may be considered as being cost-effective. Therefore, it was calculated that a total sample size of 70 would be sufficient to detect a 15% decrease in average cost-effectiveness ratio associated with CERA in comparison to EpoB with 80% power at *p*: 0.05.

3. Results

3.1. Patient Cohort Characteristics. We screened a total of 110 patients; 89 of them complied with the inclusion criteria (Figure 1); screen failures were due to an Hb not in the recommended range. In total, 82 patients have completed the study and 75 were valid for the analysis (48 (64.9%) men and 27 (35.1%) women), with a mean age of a mean age of 52.9 ± 14.3 years; the most common reasons for exclusion were active bleeding (major trauma, gastric ulcer bleeding, or surgery). Table 1 summarizes demographic and baseline characteristics of valid patients, diabetic nephropathy was

TABLE 1: Baseline demographic and clinical characteristics of the haemodialysis population.

Parameters	
Patients (n)	75
Age (years)	56.6 ± 11.77
Male (%)	48 (64.9%)
Primary renal disease n (%)	
Diabetes	22 (28.2)
Glomerulonephritis	10 (12.8)
Unknown	24 (30.7)
Vascular	12 (15.3)
Others	10 (12.8)
Vascular access n (%)	
Fisulta	70 (93)
Catheter	5 (7)
Viral hepatitis B or C n (%)	0
Patients on antihypertensive therapy n (%)	35 (46.66)
Statins n (%)	31 (41.33)
Time on dialysis (months)	75.2 ± 25.6
Predialysis systolic BP (mmHg)	138 ± 21.6
Predialysis diastolic BP (mmHg)	81 ± 2,6
Dry weight (kg)	68.2 ± 7.6
Haemoglobin (g/dL)	10.91 ± 1.56
Albumin (g/L)	3.9 ± 0.82
C-reactive protein (mg/L)	5.25 [1.9–11.6]
Ferritin (ng/mL)	392.64 ± 250
Transferrin saturation (%)	29.5 ± 5.4
Kt/V	1.25 [1.06–1.57]
Dialysis session length	243.7 ± 15.6
Intact parathyroid hormone (pg/mL)	362.7 [170.9–521.2]
Calcium (mg/dL)	9.39 ± 0.71
Phosphate (mg/dL)	4.33 ± 1.83
Cholesterol (mg/dL)	166.2 ± 49.2
LDL	94.34 ± 33.2
HDL	40.79 ± 20.6
Triglyceride (mg/dL)	130.5 ± 23.6

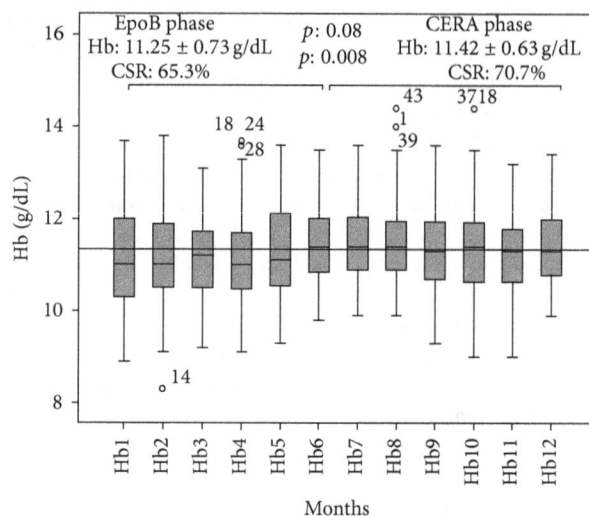

FIGURE 2: Evolution of mean Hb concentration during the two phases of the study. Hb: hemoglobin, EpoB recombinant human erythropoietin beta, CERA: continuous erythropoietin receptor activator, and CSR: clinical success rate (HB within the target 10,5–12 g/dL).

the most common cause of renal disease (28.2%), and 65.4% of the patients had a history of cardiovascular disease. Vascular access was an arteriovenous fistula in the majority of patients 70 (93%), and 5 patients were treated via a permanent catheter.

3.2. Efficacy Evaluation. Baseline Hb level was 11.14 ± 1.18 g/dL in EpoB phase and 11.46±0.79 g/dL in CERA phase; there was a nonsignificant increase in mean Hb level after conversion to CERA (11.25 ± 0.73 versus 11.42 ± 0.63 g/dL p: 0.08), but we observed a significant increase in the proportion of patients successfully treated (CSR 65.3% versus 70.7% p: 0.008). Furthermore, the proportion of patients with Hb < 10.5 g/dL was 14% in EpoB phase and 7% in CERA phase, and the proportion of patients with Hb > 12 g/dL was 12% and 15%, respectively, without need of blood transfusions during the two periods of follow-up. The average effectiveness

rose by 4% (0.55 versus 0.59). Monthly evolution of Hb during the two phases of the study is reported in Figure 2.

3.3. EPO and Iron Requirements. The mean weekly dose during the EpoB period was 6104 ± 3178 ui and was 106.4 ± 50.1 μg/month in the CERA phase; there was no significant difference in the proportions of patients receiving IV iron during the two periods of follow-up (87.5% and 89.1%, resp., p: 0.23), and conversion from EpoB to CERA did not result in statistically significant change in mean serum ferritin, TSAT, or iron dose as reported in Table 2. There were no significant differences between EpoB and CERA periods in terms of dialysis doses (Kt/v 1.26 ± 0.4 versus 1.27 ± 0.1, p: 0.1) and duration of HD sessions (244.5 ± 12.4 versus 243.5 ± 11.4 mn, p: 0.34), also there were no significant changes in inflammatory parameters: serum C-reactive protein (3.3 ± 1.1 versus 3.7 ± 0.9 mg/L, p: 0.11) and albumin levels (3.8 ± 1.8 versus 4.1 ± 0.7 g/L, p: 0.21). Patients with permanent central venous catheter had a nonsignificant higher dose of ESA in comparison to patient with arteriovenous fistula (6107.5 ui versus 6101.2 ui, p: 0.1) for EpoB and (110.4 versus 102.5, p: 0.2) for CERA.

3.4. Cost Effectiveness Analysis. Decision tree framework is presented in Figure 3(a), with CERA and EpoB branches, and the rolled back model with calculations is presented in Figure 3(b). Costs, effectiveness, and incremental associated with CERA administration to CHP, compared to EpoB, are summarized in Table 3. Based on 6-month drug acquisition cost, the mean per patient cost was 1644.2 ± 859.4$ for EpoB and 1515.5 ± 713$ for CERA, projected annual per patient costs were 3288.49±1718.9$ and 3030.19±1426$, respectively, with a cost saving associated with CERA at −258.3$. Average annual effectiveness estimated by the model was 0.55 for

(a)

(b)

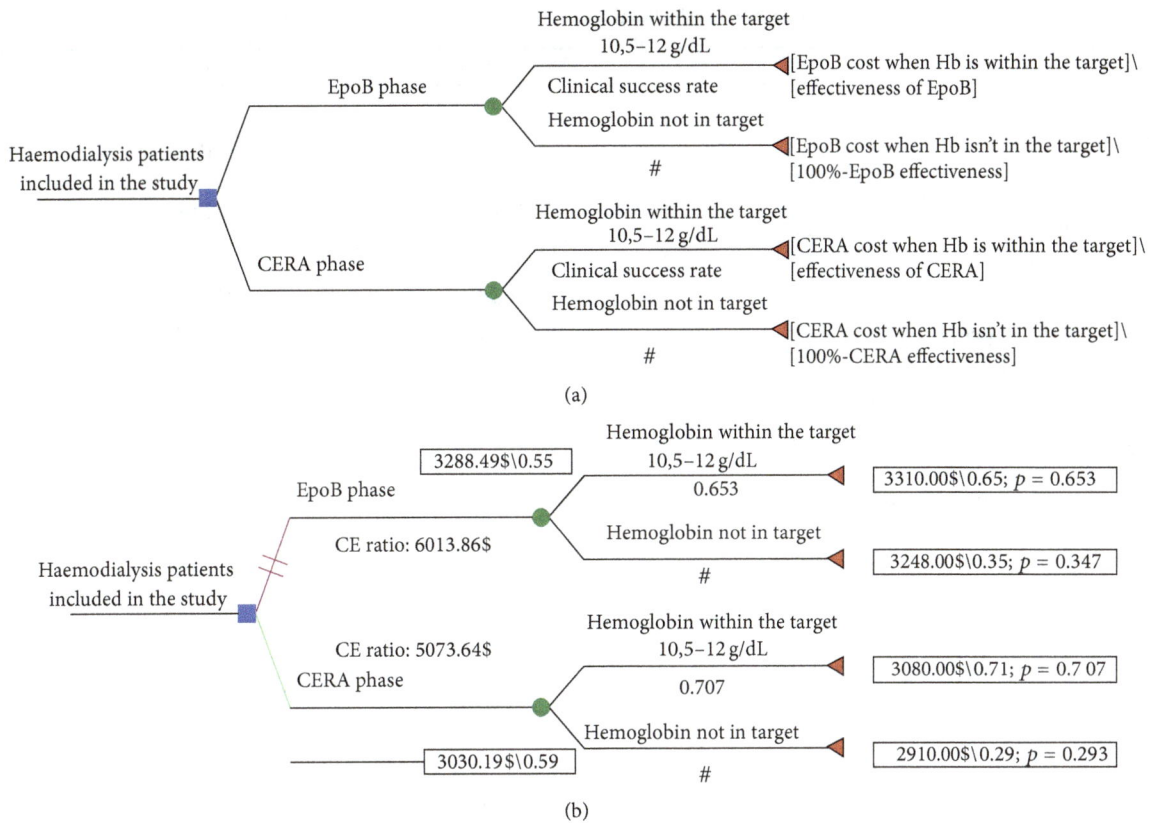

FIGURE 3: (a) Decision tree framework. (b) Results of cost-effectiveness analysis after roll-back calculation. EpoB: recombinant human erythropoietin beta, CERA: continuous erythropoietin receptor activator, CE ration: cost-effectiveness ratio.

TABLE 2: Anaemia management during the study.

Parameters	EpoB phase	CERA phase	p
n	75	75	
Hemoglobin g/dL	11.25 ± 0.73	11.42 ± 0.63	0.08
Transferrin saturation %	28.4	29.2	0.35
Ferritin ng/mL	288.5	299.3	0.2
IV iron %	87.5	89.1	0.23
IV iron dosage mg/month	110,5 ± 11.2	116,3 ± 13.3	0.11
ESA dose	6104 ± 3178 ui	106.4 ± 50.1 μg	
CSR n %	49 (65.3)	53 (70.7)	0.008
Hb > 12 g/dL n (%)	12 (16)	15 (20)	0.001
Hb < 10.5 g/dL n (%)	14 (18.7)	7 (9.3)	0.001

CSR: clinical success rate Hb within the range 10.5–12 g/dL.
ESA: erythropoietin stimulating agent.
Hb: haemoglobin.
EpoB: epoetin beta.
CERA: continuous erythropoietin receptor activator.

EpoB and 0.59 for CERA, and average cost-effectiveness ratios were 6013.86$ and 5173.64$, respectively, with an ICER at −6457.5$ per one per cent of patients successfully treated, so the treatment with EpoB was dominated by CERA as shown in the cost-effectiveness diagram Figure 4.

3.5. Sensitivity Analyses and Monte Carlo Simulation. We performed one-way and multiway sensitivity analysis, the ICERs did not change significantly, despite application of variation rates of ±10% in each of the parameters of cost and effectiveness individually, and clinically implausible changes in variables were required to significantly improve the cost effectiveness EpoB in comparison to CERA. The results of probabilistic sensitivity analysis by Monte Carlo simulation based on 50000 random iterations are shown in Figure 5. The scatterplot illustrates the robustness of the model. Analysis of the results shows that 100% of the points are in the lower right hand portion of the graph (best effectiveness and lower cost), demonstrating that CERA remained more effective, less costly, and hence the dominant treatment compared to EpoB. Also, the robustness of the calculated ICER was confirmed by MCS as shown in Figure 6.

4. Discussion

The present study found that CERA is more cost-effective than EpoB, making it the dominant treatment for the management of anaemia in chronic haemodialysis patients. To our knowledge, this work is the first to evaluate the cost-effectiveness of CERA prospectively in a real-life practice.

TABLE 3: Cost-effectiveness analysis of the study.

Parameters	EpoB	CERA	p
N	75	75	
Patients successfully treated n (%) Hb 10.5–12 g/dL	49 (65.3)	53 (70.7)	0.008
Patients not successfully treated n (%) Hb > 12 or Hb < 10.5 g/dL	26 (34.7)	22 (29.3)	0.001
Drug costs $			
Mean 6-month drug cost per patient	1644.2 ± 859.4	1515.5 ± 713	0.03
Mean 1-year drug cost per patient	3288.49	3030.19	0.03
Incremental 1-year cost Cera versus EpoB $	—	−258.3	
Average effectiveness	0.55	0.59	
Incremental effectiveness Cera versus EpoB $	—	+0.04	
Average cost-effectiveness ratio $/per one per cent of patients successfully treated	6013.86	5173.64	
ICER Cera versus EpoB $/per one per cent of patients successfully treated		−6457.5	

ESA: erythropoietin stimulating agent.
Hb: haemoglobin.
EpoB: epoetin beta.
CERA: continuous erythropoietin receptor activator.
ICER: incremental cost-effectiveness ratio.

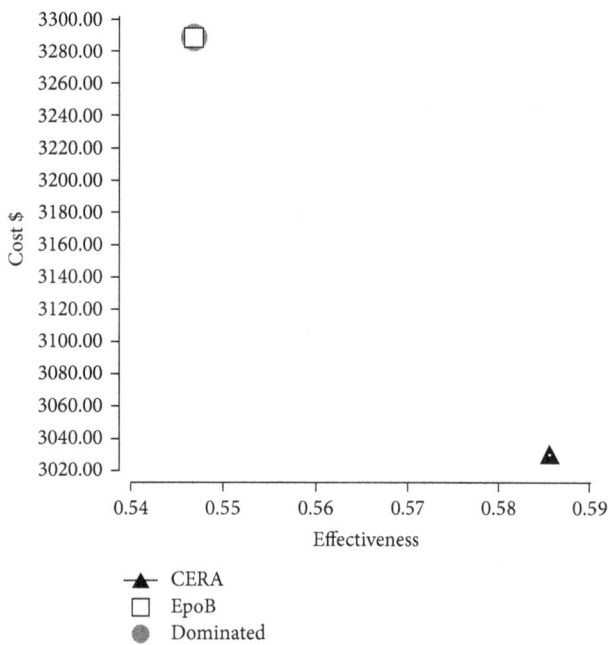

FIGURE 4: Cost-effectiveness diagram. EpoB is dominated by CERA since it is more costly and less effective.

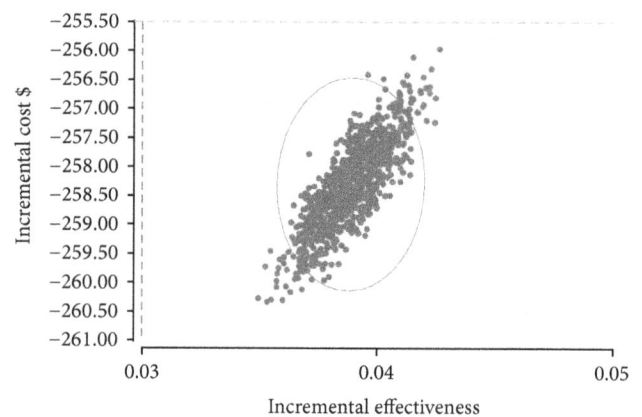

FIGURE 5: Results of Monte Carlo simulation of incremental cost and effectiveness scatter plot of CERA versus EpoB, based on 50000 random iterations of cost-effectiveness model.

As demonstrated in the recent review published by Schmid [14], the literature query of studies dealing with the cost or the cost-effectiveness of CERA was poor; only 18 publications were included in his analysis, most of the available data was from meeting abstracts (eleven), and only seven published studies were in peer-reviewed journals. Majority of included studies were retrospectives, and reported data were only about cost of therapy after a switch to CERA from single-center experiences. Gonzalez et al. [17] reported in a meeting abstract a CEA of CERA compared to erythropoietin alpha, on the base of a decision tree model that simulated the treatment costs and outcomes in Mexican haemodialysis patients. In this study, the clinical success rate (patients within 11–12.5 Hb/dL levels) when using CERA versus EPO-alpha showed significant difference (86.79% versus 50.48% resp., $p < 0.0001$), treatment care cost per year for CERA was $2,776.13 versus $2,907.88 for erythropoietin alpha ($p < 0.0001$), and the cost-effectiveness plane indicates that CERA is a highly cost-effective therapy, with a probability of 0.60 to be cost saving and 0.99 of probability of being cost effective. In another study published as an abstract, aimed to determine the cost-effectiveness of anaemia treatment in dialysis patients for Brazilian Public Health System [18], using

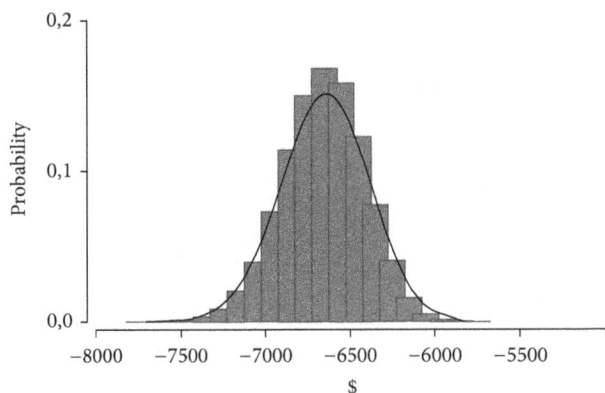

FIGURE 6: Probabilistic sensitivity analysis of ICER distribution of CERA versus EpoB. The analysis confirmed the robustness of the model, based on 50 000 random iteration; the ICER remain within the range of calculated ICER $\pm$ 10%.

a Markov model of a hypothetical cohort of dialysis patients treated with CERA or epoetin for four years, the model showed that epoetin treatment was more cost-effective than CERA treatment. Unfortunately, it was not possible to evaluate the methodology of both previous publications and there concordance with international guidelines for CEA studies [19]. Considering only the cost of treatment; 3 cost-minimisation studies reported as meeting abstracts confirm our finding of cost saving after switch to CERA from another short acting EPO; Bezditko et al. [20] estimated the cost reduction about 5–35%, based on decision tree analysis. In his pharmacoeconomic evaluation of maintenance treatment of anaemia, in Ukrainians haemodialysis patients, the average costs of CERA treatment per patient on haemodialysis were $173/week (intravenous route of administration) and $130/week (subcutaneous route of administration) and average costs for using the shorter-acting EpoB drugs were $267–194/week and $133–182/week, respectively. Franz et al. [21], in a Swiss multicenter prospective observational study, analysed data of dialysis patients treated with ESA over a period of 12 months. After the switch to CERA from treatment with either darbepoetin alfa or epoetin alfa/beta, the cost of ESA treatment decreased by 14% and patients maintained stable Hb values in the first 6 months after conversion. In contrast, Albero Molina et al. [22] reported a +66.4% increasing cost after switch to CERA, in a 6-month prospective follow-up of 17 haemodialysis patients, with stable dose of subcutaneous EpoB average costs/patient/month: EpoB (£174.30 ± £85.40) versus CERA (£290.10 ± £69.00). In another Spanish study, Escudero-Vilaplana et al. [23] reported similar cost increase after switch to CERA from EpoB £103.2 versus £147.5. In our analysis, the cost reduction related to CERA can partially be explained by the lower doses required after conversion from EpoB. Initial dose was calculated according to manufacturer guidelines, and during the follow-up doses adjustments were permitted according to Hb evolution. We believe that this work is the first to report data related to CERA use in such North African ethnic population, similarly to our finding in another Mediterranean population, authors reported low dose requirement of CERA (mean monthly dose was

112.4 ± 76.78 μg) to maintain Hb in the range 10–12 g/dL [24]. Also, low dose requirement in CERA phase can be explained by an increase in iron use in terms of proportion of patients receiving iron, serum ferritin, TSAT, and mean iron doses, but this improvement did not reach statistical significance in comparison to EpoB period. Of note, majority of available data suggests cost saving after conversion to CERA, rather than cost increase; it was difficult to have a conclusion from these previous studies. Since they were surrounded by considerable uncertainty and unavailable full-text articles, few abstracts reported information about baseline and evolution of Hb, ESA doses, median cost/patient, and iron status, and majority of analyses were based on hypothetical cohorts rather than real-life follow-up. For this reasons, we have tried in our analysis to follow the guidelines of the International Society for Pharmacoeconomics and Outcomes Research (ISPOR), health economic evaluation publication guidelines, and Consolidated Health Economic Evaluation Reporting Standards (CHEERS) [19]. Results from a number of previous studies suggested that adoption of a once-monthly ESA could provide considerable time savings for dialysis centers [25–27], in our study; we did not consider healthcare personnel time associated with routine anaemia management tasks, since we adopted the health care payer perspective. However, our study has some limitations. First, the perspective was that of a health-care payer and not a societal one, and as such we did not include indirect costs such as loss of productivity and travel costs. The absence of evidence that ESA use increases employment rats in haemodialysis patients makes it unlikely that adopting societal perspective would have changed our results [5, 28, 29]. Secondly, we considered only drugs acquisition costs, without including other direct medical costs such as hospitalization, medications, and consultations; however, previous research indicated that these additional cost components would be similar between CERA and EpoB [30]. In our CEA, we considered the effectiveness in terms of Hb target reached, rather than a hard end point like mortality or change in quality of life (QOL), the initial design of the study was not appropriate to evaluate the cost per quality adjusted life year (QALY), and the short duration of follow-up was not adequate to expect a significant change in QOL or in mortality related to conversion to CERA. For this reason, we adopted a valid surrogate marker such as the CSR, since a strong correlation between QOL and Hb levels in CHP is admitted now.

In summary, this medicoeconomic evaluation of ESA use in haemodialysis patients suggests that administering CERA once monthly is cost-effective when the health care perspective is employed. We performed our study in accordance with current anaemia management guidelines in haemodialysis patients, and following Health Economic Evaluation Reporting Standards. These data would assist health care decision makers and services reimbursement authorities as they aim to provide the most cost-effective treatments to patients.

Ethical Approval

All procedures performed in studies involving human participants were in accordance with the ethical standards of the institutional and/or national research committee and with the 1964 Helsinki Declaration and its later amendments or comparable ethical standards. The study was performed with informed consent, and following all guidelines for experimental investigations, required by the Institutional Review Board of which all authors are affiliated to.

Consent

Informed consent was obtained from all individual participants included in the study.

Disclosure

Partial data on this paper has been presented as a poster at the World Congress of Nephrology, Organized by the International Society of Nephrology: Cape Town, South Africa, March 2015, Poster no. SAT-451.

Conflict of Interests

The authors declare that they have no conflict of interests.

Acknowledgment

This work has been supported by Medical and Pharmacy School, Mohammed V University, Rabat, Morocco.

References

[1] W. McClellan, S. L. Aronoff, W. K. Bolton et al., "The prevalence of anemia in patients with chronic kidney disease," *Current Medical Research and Opinion*, vol. 20, no. 9, pp. 1501–1510, 2004.

[2] C.-Y. Hsu, "Epidemiology of anemia associated with chronic renal insufficiency," *Current Opinion in Nephrology and Hypertension*, vol. 11, no. 3, pp. 337–341, 2002.

[3] P. A. Marsden, "Treatment of anemia in chronic kidney disease—strategies based on evidence," *The New England Journal of Medicine*, vol. 361, no. 21, pp. 2089–2090, 2009.

[4] J. Jordan, J. Breckles, V. Leung, M. Hopkins, and M. Battistella, "Conversion from epoetin alfa to darbepoetin alfa: effects on patients' hemoglobin and costs to Canadian dialysis centres," *Canadian Journal of Hospital Pharmacy*, vol. 65, no. 6, pp. 443–449, 2012.

[5] R. W. Evans, B. Rader, and D. L. Manninen, "The quality of life of hemodialysis recipients treated with recombinant human erythropoietin. Cooperative Multicenter EPO Clinical Trial Group," *The Journal of the American Medical Association*, vol. 263, no. 6, pp. 825–830, 1990.

[6] S. Li, R. N. Foley, and A. J. Collins, "Anemia, hospitalization, and mortality in patients receiving peritoneal dialysis in the United States," *Kidney International*, vol. 65, no. 5, pp. 1864–1869, 2004.

[7] F. Locatelli, R. L. Pisoni, C. Combe et al., "Anaemia in haemodialysis patients of five European countries: association with morbidity and mortality in the Dialysis Outcomes and Practice Patterns Study (DOPPS)," *Nephrology Dialysis Transplantation*, vol. 19, no. 1, pp. 121–132, 2004.

[8] H. C. Rayner, R. L. Pisoni, J. Bommer et al., "Mortality and hospitalization in haemodialysis patients in five European countries: results from the Dialysis Outcomes and Practice Patterns

Study (DOPPS)," *Nephrology Dialysis Transplantation*, vol. 19, no. 1, pp. 108–120, 2004.

[9] "References," *Kidney International Supplements*, vol. 2, no. 4, pp. 331–335, 2012.

[10] N. W. Levin, S. Fishbane, F. V. Cañedo et al., "Intravenous methoxy polyethylene glycol-epoetin beta for haemoglobin control in patients with chronic kidney disease who are on dialysis: a randomised non-inferiority trial (MAXIMA)," *The Lancet*, vol. 370, no. 9596, pp. 1415–1421, 2007.

[11] I. C. Macdougall, R. Walker, R. Provenzano et al., "C.E.R.A. Corrects anemia in patients with chronic kidney disease not on dialysis: results of a randomized clinical trial," *Clinical Journal of the American Society of Nephrology*, vol. 3, no. 2, pp. 337–347, 2008.

[12] F. Dellanna, R. E. Winkler, F. Bozkurt et al., "Dosing strategies for conversion of haemodialysis patients from short-acting erythropoiesis stimulating agents to once-monthly C.E.R.A.: experience from the MIRACEL study," *International Journal of Clinical Practice*, vol. 65, no. 1, pp. 64–72, 2011.

[13] C. E. Halstenson, M. Macres, S. A. Katz et al., "Comparative pharmacokinetics and pharmacodynamics of epoetin alfa and epoetin beta," *Clinical Pharmacology and Therapeutics*, vol. 50, no. 6, pp. 702–712, 1991.

[14] H. Schmid, "Cost-effectiveness of continuous erythropoietin receptor activator in anemia," *ClinicoEconomics and Outcomes Research*, vol. 6, pp. 319–330, 2014.

[15] I. C. Macdougall, R. Robson, S. Opatrna et al., "Pharmacokinetics and pharmacodynamics of intravenous and subcutaneous continuous erythropoietin receptor activator (C.E.R.A.) in patients with chronic kidney disease," *Clinical Journal of the American Society of Nephrology*, vol. 1, no. 6, pp. 1211–1215, 2006.

[16] SMN, *Moroccan Society of Nephrology Guidelines RBMP. ALD 17(Insuffisance Renal Chronique Terminale)*, SMN, 2011.

[17] P. Gonzalez, E. Gomez, and J. Vargas, "PSY25 Renal Anemia (RA) treatment in Mexican public health care institutions: an evaluation of the costs and consequences," *Value in Health*, vol. 12, no. 7, pp. A379–A380, 2009.

[18] F. H. C. V. Silva, C. M. D. M. Vianna, and F. V. C. Silva, "PUK3 Cost-effectiveness of anemia treatment in dialysis patients in Brazil," *Value in Health*, vol. 14, no. 7, p. A570, 2011.

[19] D. Husereau, M. Drummond, S. Petrou et al., "Consolidated health economic evaluation reporting standards (CHEERS)—explanation and elaboration: a report of the ISPOR health economic evaluation publication guidelines good reporting practices task force," *Value in Health*, vol. 16, no. 2, pp. 231–250, 2013.

[20] N. Bezditko, L. Iakovlieva, O. Mishchenko, O. Gerasymova, and O. Kyrychenko, "PUK24 Pharmacoeconomic aspects of use of erythropoietin drugs in patients on hemodialysis in Ukraine," *Value in Health*, vol. 15, no. 7, p. A459, 2012.

[21] S. Franz, C. Jäger, and T. Gauthier, "Hemoglobin levels and development of ESA dose in hemodialysis patients after conversion to CERA: a multicenter observational study," *Swiss Medical Weekly*, vol. 139, no. 45-46, supplement 178, p. 8S, 2009.

[22] M. D. Albero Molina, R. López-Menchero Martínez, C. del Pozo Fernández, L. Álvarez Fernández, and L. Sánchez Rodríguez, "Eficiencia de la administración mensual subcutánea de metoxi-polietilenglicol epoetina β (Mircera) en pacientes estables en hemodiálisis previamente tratados con eritropoyetina-Eficiencia de la administración sc mensual de MIRCERA en pacientes en HD," *Diálisis y Trasplante*, vol. 34, no. 3, pp. 93–100, 2013.

[23] V. Escudero-Vilaplana, C. Martínez-Nieto, J. M. López-Gómez, A. Vega-Martínez, J. M. Bellón-Cano, and M. Sanjurjo-Sáez, "Erythropoiesis-stimulating agents in anaemia due to chronic kidney disease: a cost-minimization analysis," *International Journal of Clinical Pharmacy*, vol. 35, no. 3, pp. 463–468, 2013.

[24] N. Duman, A. Uyanik, A. Unsal et al., "Once-monthly continuous erythropoietin receptor activator (CERA) for haemoglobin maintenance in haemodialysis patients with chronic renal anaemia," *Clinical Kidney Journal*, vol. 7, no. 5, pp. 464–469, 2014.

[25] U. Saueressig, J. T. C. Kwan, E. De Cock, and C. Sapède, "Healthcare resource utilization for anemia management: current practice with erythropoiesis-stimulating agents and the impact of converting to once-monthly C.E.R.A.," *Blood Purification*, vol. 26, no. 6, pp. 537–546, 2008.

[26] E. De Cock, F. Dellanna, K. Khellaf et al., "Time savings associated with C.E.R.A. once monthly: a time-and-motion study in hemodialysis centers in five European countries," *Journal of Medical Economics*, vol. 16, no. 5, pp. 648–656, 2013.

[27] W. F. J. Klatko, "Time and motion study of anaemia management with erythropoiesis stimulating agents in haemodialysis units in Poland," *Journal of Health Policy and Outcomes Research*, vol. 2, no. 1, pp. 126–132, 2013.

[28] N. W. Levin, "Quality of life and hematocrit level," *American Journal of Kidney Diseases*, vol. 20, no. 1, supplement 1, pp. 16–20, 1992.

[29] M. Tonelli, W. C. Winkelmayer, K. K. Jindal, W. F. Owen Jr., and B. J. Manns, "The cost-effectiveness of maintaining higher hemoglobin targets with erythropoietin in hemodialysis patients," *Kidney International*, vol. 64, no. 1, pp. 295–304, 2003.

[30] F. M. Clement, S. Klarenbach, M. Tonelli, N. Wiebe, B. Hemmelgarn, and B. J. Manns, "An economic evaluation of erythropoiesis-stimulating agents in CKD," *American Journal of Kidney Diseases*, vol. 56, no. 6, pp. 1050–1061, 2010.

12

Prevalence of Anemia and Associated Factors among Pregnant Women in an Urban Area of Eastern Ethiopia

Kefyalew Addis Alene[1] and Abdulahi Mohamed Dohe[2]

[1] *Institute of Public Health, College of Medicine and Health Sciences, University of Gondar, P.O. Box 196, Gondar, Ethiopia*
[2] *Somali Regional Health Bureau, P.O. Box 238, Jijiga, Ethiopia*

Correspondence should be addressed to Kefyalew Addis Alene; kefadis@gmail.com

Academic Editor: Bruno Annibale

This research work presents the magnitude of anemia and its determinant factors among pregnant women. As far as this research is done in the eastern part of Ethiopia, where there is a different cultural issue related to pregnancy and dietary habit, it will help the researchers to know the problem in different parts of the country.

1. Background

Anemia, defined as a decreased concentration of blood hemoglobin, is one of the most common nutritional deficiency diseases observed globally and affects more than a quarter of the world's population [1–8]. It is a major public health problem affecting all ages of the population with its highest prevalence among children under five years of age and pregnant women [2, 3]. Globally, anemia affects 1.62 billion people (25%), among which 56 million are pregnant women [1, 2].

Anemia during pregnancy is considered severe when hemoglobin concentration is less than 7.0 g/dL, moderate when hemoglobin falls between 7.0–9.9 g/dL, and mild from 10.0-11 g/dL [2–4]. Anemia during pregnancy is a major cause of morbidity and mortality of pregnant women in developing countries and has both maternal and fetal consequences [9–13]. It is estimated that anemia causes more than 115,000 maternal and 591,000 perinatal deaths globally per year [3].

In developing countries, the cause of anemia during pregnancy is multifactorial and includes nutritional deficiencies of iron, folate, and vitamin B12 and also parasitic diseases, such as malaria and hookworm. The relative contribution of each of these factors to anemia during pregnancy varies greatly by geographical location, season, and dietary practice. In Sub-Saharan Africa, iron and folate deficiencies are the most common causes of anemia in pregnant women [14]. Anemia has a variety of converging contributing factors including nutritional, genetic, and infectious disease factors; however, iron deficiency is the cause of 75% of anemia cases [2, 5, 8–15]. Iron deficiency anemia affects the development of the nation by decreasing the cognitive development of children and productivity of adults [2, 10].

Seventeen percent of Ethiopian women in the reproductive age group are anemic and 22% of these women are currently pregnant [16]. Despite its known effect on the population, there is very little data available in the study area. Therefore, this study is aimed at determining the prevalence of anemia in pregnant women and identifying its associated factors in the Somali Region of Eastern Ethiopia.

2. Methods

2.1. Study Setting and Design. A community based cross-sectional study was conducted from April to May 2013 in Gode town, Eastern Ethiopia.

2.2. Study Population. The study population consisted of a sample of pregnant women who were residing in the town during the study period. Those pregnant women who were not long-term residents of the city (less than 6 months) were excluded.

2.3. Sampling Procedures.

Sample size was determined based on single population proportion formula using Epi info version 7 with a 95% CI, 5% margin of error, and assumption that 22% of pregnant women are anemic [16]. Assuming a 10% nonresponse rate and a design effect of 2, a total sample size of 581 pregnant women was required. Multistage sampling technique was used to select the study participants. Four kebeles (villages) were selected from 6 kebeles using the randomized method. A proportional allocation was employed to obtain the sample size from each kebele. The starting point was randomly selected and a systematic random sampling method was used to select the study participants.

2.4. Data Collection.

Data were collected using pretested interviewer administered questionnaire, which contains sociodemographic characteristics (age, education, occupation, marital status, and others), obstetric and gynecological history (trimester, gravidity, parity, ANC follow up, iron supplementation, and others), and dietary factors (type of stable diet, meal frequency, and intake of meat, tea, egg, and milk and milk products).

Blood hemoglobin concentration was measured using a HemoCue Hb 301, a precalibrated instrument designed for the measurement of hemoglobin concentration. Venous blood was drawn, through microcuvettes, and inserted into the HemoCue and the result was recorded. Mid upper arm circumference (MUAC) of the mothers was measured and recorded as an independent variable.

2.5. Data Processing and Analyses.

Data were analyzed using SPSS version 20. Description of means, frequencies, proportions, and rates of the given data for each variable was calculated. Bivariate analysis was done to see the association of each independent variable with the outcome variable. Those variables having P value less than 0.2 were entered into the multivariate logistic regression model to identify the effect of each independent variable with the outcome variables. A P value of less than 0.05 was considered statistically significant, and adjusted odds ratio with 95% CI was calculated to determine association.

2.6. Ethical Consideration.

Ethical clearance was obtained from the Institutional Review Board of the University of Gondar. An official letter was obtained for Somali Regional Health Bureau and Gode City Administration Health Office and letters were prepared for the local authority of the selected kebeles. Written informed consent was obtained from each study participant after they were introduced to the purpose of the study and informed about their rights to interrupt the interview at any time. Confidentiality was maintained at all levels of the study. Mothers found to be anemic were referred to the nearest health center or hospital and the referral process was facilitated.

3. Results

3.1. Socioeconomic and Demographic Characteristics.

Out of a total sample size (581) 577 pregnant women were included and there was a nonresponse rate of 0.7%. The mean ages of the mothers at present, at marriage, and at first pregnancy were 27.01 (±5.97), 17.52 (±2.10), and 18.38 (±2.32) years, respectively. Majority of the mothers were married (97.2%), Somali (98.9%), and Muslim (99.1%).

The average family size, number of pregnancies, deliveries, and children of the households were 6.9 (±2.86), 4.98 (±2.62), 3.83 (±2.55), and 3.61 (±2.38), respectively. About 261 (45.2%) of the mothers were in their second trimester, 247 (24.8%) were in the third trimester, and the remaining 69 (12.0%) were in the first trimester.

Most of the mothers were illiterate 507 (87.9%) and housewives 499 (86.5%). The family's main sources of income were salaried jobs 301 (52.2%), private business 101 (17.5%), and remittance 52 (9%). More than half of the respondents 355 (61.5%) were at or below the middle wealth quintile (Table 1).

3.2. History of Malaria and Intestinal Parasite.

Of the 577 respondents, 88 (15.3%) had a known history of intestinal parasite, 548 (95.0%) said they were using insecticide treated bed net (ITNs), and 366 (63.4%) had a known history of malaria. Of those with a known history of intestinal parasite 7 (8%) were infected during the current pregnancy, 39 (44.3%) were infected 1–3 months before the current pregnancy, and the remaining 42 (47.8%) were infected more than four months prior to the current pregnancy. Similarly, from those with known history of malaria 37 (10.1%) were infected during the current pregnancy, 131 (35.8%) were infected 1–3 months before current pregnancy, and the remaining 198 (54.1%) were infected more than four months before current pregnancy.

3.3. Environmental and Housing Characteristics of the Study Subjects.

Of the 577 respondents 211 (36.6%) were living in a rented house, and the remaining 366 (63.4%) owned the house. Four hundred fifty one (78.2%) had private latrine, but only 26 (4.5%) had piped water. Only 18 (3.1%) had tap water, and only 2 (0.3%) had public tap water as their main source of drinking water. Half (56.5%) of the study participants obtained drinking water from a protected well/tanker and the remaining 231 (40%) drank water from arriver. Also, only 34 (5.9%) of the respondents had a farm or garden to cultivate and assist them in meeting their nutritional needs.

3.4. Behavioral Characteristics and Nutritional Status of Respondents.

The most reported staple diet of the household was rice and spaghetti 504 (87.3%). More than half, 382 (66.2%), of the respondents eat three times per day.

The majority of the respondents 570 (98.8%) said they drink tea and 444 (77.9%) of them drink tea before meals, and 339 (59.5%) of them have tea more than two times per day. Five hundred fifty four (96%) and 384 (66.6%) had eaten meat and used fruits more than twice per week, respectively.

TABLE 1: Sociodemographic characteristics of pregnant women at Gode town, Somali Region, Eastern Ethiopia, May 2013.

Variables	Frequency ($N = 577$) Number (%)
Age of the mother	
≤20	62 (10.7)
21–25	137 (23.7)
26–30	187 (32.4)
31–35	122 (21.1)
>35	69 (12.0)
Marital status	
Married	561 (97.2)
Divorced	13 (2.3)
Widowed	3 (0.5)
Religion	
Muslim	572 (99.1)
Christian	5 (0.9)
Ethnicity	
Somali	570 (98.8)
Amhara	5 (0.9)
Oromo	1 (0.2)
Others	1 (0.2)
Educational status	
Unable to read and write	476 (82.5)
Read and write only	31 (5.4)
Primary school (1–8)	37 (6.4)
Secondary school	8 (1.4)
College and above	25 (4.3)
Occupation	
Housewife	499 (86.5)
Government employee	34 (5.9)
Business	44 (7.6)
Family Size	
<5	134 (23.2)
5–7	211 (36.6)
≥8	232 (40.2)
Age at marriage	
<16	198 (34.3)
16–18	283 (49.0)
≥19	96 (16.6)
Source of income	
Salary	301 (52.2)
Business	101 (17.5)
Remittance	52 (9.0)
Others	123 (21.3)
Wealth index (Quintiles)	
Lowest	114 (19.8)
Second	127 (22.0)
Middle	114 (19.8)
Fourth	104 (18.0)
Highest	118 (20.5)

More than half of the respondents, 348 (60.3%), said they use egg less than once per month, but 312 (54.1%) use milk and milk products daily, and 416 (72.1%) had eaten between 5 and 8 food groups in the last 24 hours prior to the interview.

Of the 577 respondents 177 (30.7%) reported involvement in physical work with 27 (15.3%) and 30 (16.9%) of them reporting very heavy and heavy physical work, respectively. One hundred seven (18.5%) reported consuming forbidden foods and 196 (34%) have reported eating charcoal or clay during pregnancy. More than half of 347 (60.1%) said they had visited a health facility for antenatal care (ANC) with 56 (16.1%), 116 (33.4%), and 175 (50.4%) of them reporting an initial ANC visit, a second ANC visit, and more than two ANC visits during a pregnancy. More than half of 388 (67.2%) reported receiving iron supplementation during the current pregnancy.

Nutritional status was evaluated by MUAC and 575 of the respondents were measured (excluding 2 with incomplete MUAC), and 29 (5%) had MUAC of less than 21 cm, 228 (39.7%) had MUAC between 21 and 23 cm, and the remaining 318 (55.3%) had an MUAC within normal limits (>23 cm) (Table 2).

3.5. Prevalence of Anemia. From the total 577 respondents 328 (56.8%) were anemic (95% CI: 52.9–60.8), 7 (1.2%) of them were severely anemic, 154 (26.7%) were moderately anemic, and 167 (28.9%) were mildly anemic. The mean hemoglobin level was 10.79 (±1.47) g/dL. More than half (76.8%) of the anemic study participants were from large families (>5 family members). Most of them (80.7%) were multiparous (≥2) and multigravidous (≥3). Majorities were married at age 18 years or younger (82.9%). Most of them (58.5%) were at or below the middle wealth quintile and were illiterate (89.9%).

3.6. Factors Associated with Anemia. Multivariate logistic regression analysis revealed that trimester of current pregnancy, iron supplementation during pregnancy, wealth quintile, number of pregnancies, and MUAC were significantly associated with anemia in the study population (Table 4).

Pregnant women in the third and second trimesters were 3.32 (95% CI 1.84–6.0) and 2.87 (95% CI 1.61–5.17) times more likely to be affected by anemia as compared to pregnant women in the first trimester, respectively. Similarly, those pregnant women who had 3–5 pregnancies were 1.95 times more likely to be anemic, compared with those who had less than 3 pregnancies (AOR =1.95 (95% CI=1.19–3.19)).

Pregnant women who were not taking iron supplementation during pregnancy were 1.54 more likely to develop anemia (AOR = 1.54 (95% CI = 1.04–2.27)).

Pregnant women in the second wealth quintile were 57% (AOR = 0.43, 95% CI: 0.24–0.76) less likely to develop anemia, compared with those in the lowest wealth quintile. Similarly, pregnant women with MUAC ≥ 23 were 59% less likely to be anemic compared with those with MUAC < 23 (AOR = 0.41 (95% CI: 0.27–0.63)) (Table 3).

4. Discussion

More than half (56.8%) of the pregnant women studied were anemic. This figure is lower than the prevalence of anemia in

TABLE 2: Maternal characteristics of pregnant women at Gode Town, Somali Region, Eastern Ethiopia, May 2013.

Variables	Frequency ($N = 577$) Number (%)
Trimester	
First trimester	69 (12.0)
Second trimester	261 (45.2)
Third trimester	247 (42.8)
Age at first pregnancy (years)	
<17	126 (21.8)
17–19	270 (46.8)
≥20	181 (31.4)
Number of pregnancies	
<3	166 (20.1)
3–5	228 (39.5)
≥6	233 (40.4)
Number of deliveries (parity)	
<2	121 (21.0)
2–4	237 (41.1)
≥5	219 (38)
Number of Children	
<2	126 (21.8)
2–4	247 (42.8)
≥5	204 (35.4)
Child spacing	
Yes	42 (7.3)
No	535 (92.7)
Antenatal care	
Yes	347 (60.1)
No	230 (39.9)
ANC during current pregnancy ($n = 347$)	
Yes	322 (92.8)
No	25 (7.2)
Frequency of ANC (347)	
First ANC	56 (16.1)
Second ANC	116 (33.4)
Third ANC	175 (50.4)

TABLE 3: Dietary habits and nutritional status of pregnant women at Gode Town, Somali Region, Eastern Ethiopia, May 2013.

Variables	Frequency ($N = 577$) Number (%)
Stable diet	
Rice and spaghetti	504 (87.3)
Maize and sorghum	68 (11.8)
Others	5 (0.9)
Meal frequency	
More than three times	120 (20.8)
Three times	382 (66.2)
Two times	63 (10.9)
One time	12 (2.1)
Meat frequency	
One a week	137 (23.7)
Twice a week	267 (46.3)
More than twice per week	150 (26)
Once per month	7 (1.2)
Less than one time per month	16 (2.8)
Drinking tea	
Yes	570 (98.8)
No	7 (1.2)
Time for drinking tea ($N = 570$)	
Before meal	444 (77.9)
After Meal	126 (22.1)
Fruit frequency	
Every day	28 (4.9)
Once a week	67 (11.6)
Twice a week	178 (30.8)
More than twice per week	111 (19.2)
Once per month	70 (12.1)
Less than once per month	348 (60.3)
Egg frequency	
Every day	25 (4.3)
Once a week	65 (11.3)
Twice a week	48 (8.3)
More than twice per week	21 (3.6)
Once per month	70 (12.1)
Less than once per month	348 (60.3)
Milk and milk product frequency	
More than two times per day	312 (54.1)
Once per day	160 (27.7)
Once per week	43 (7.5)
Less than once per week	62 (10.7)
Food groups eaten in 24 hours	
1–4	141 (24.4)
5–8	416 (72.1)
>8 food groups	20 (3.5)
Physical work	
Yes	177 (30.7)
No	400 (69.3)
Forbidden foods for pregnancy	
Yes	107 (18.5)
No	470 (81.5)

pregnant women of some other developing countries such as India and Pakistan [4, 15]. This may be due to the inclusion of more rural villages in the studies from Pakistan and India, which were not included in this study. This finding is much higher than the national prevalence of anemia in pregnant women, which is 22% [16], and also higher than the prevalence noted from the 2011 Ethiopian Demographic Health Survey (EDHS) report, which found that 30.4% of

TABLE 3: Continued.

Variables	Frequency ($N = 577$) Number (%)
Eating charcoal and clay	
Yes	196 (34)
No	381 (66)
Iron supplementation	
Yes	388 (67.2)
No	189 (32.8)
Nutritional status (MUAC) ($n = 575$)	
<21 cm	29 (5)
21–23 cm	228 (39.7)
>23 cm	318 (55.3)

Ethiopians were anemic [8]. This discrepancy could be due to the exclusion of agropastoralist zones and the time gap between the current study and the 2011 EDHS.

Gravidity and age of current pregnancy (trimester) were important variables, which have shown a significant association with anemia in the current study. The risk of developing anemia increases with the age of pregnancy (trimester). The risk of developing anemia was higher in third and second trimester when compared with those in the first trimester. This finding is consistent with a study done in Saudi Arabia, which found that the prevalence of anemia is higher in the third trimester in comparison with first trimester [11], and another study conducted in India, which also indicated that the prevalence of anemia was higher in pregnant women in the third and second trimesters [10]. Additionally, studies conducted in Malaysia, Vietnam, and Nepal found that increased gestational age is significantly associated with the risk of developing anemia [6, 17, 18]. This could be due to the fact that when the gestational age increases the mother becomes weak and the iron in the blood is shared with the fetus in the womb therefore decreasing the iron binding capacity of the mother's blood.

The other important variable significantly associated with anemia is number of pregnancies (gravidity). The risk of developing anemia in pregnant women with 3–5 pregnancies is increased when compared with those who had less than 3 pregnancies. This finding is consistent with studies conducted in Saudi Arabia and India, which found that increased number of pregnancies and deliveries is positively associated with the risk of developing anemia [10, 11]. This could be due to the loss of iron and other nutrients during increased and repeated pregnancies and also the possibility of sharing of resources with the fetus. However, other studies conducted in Ethiopia and Nepal did not find association between gravidity and anemia [8, 18]. This could be due to the difference in sociocultural characteristics of the study populations.

Similarly the wealth status of the household was significantly associated with the development of anemia. Increased wealth quintiles from lowest to second lowest reduce the risk of developing anemia by 57%. This finding is consistent with the findings from other studies in low and middle-income countries, which found that the risk of anemia among women living in the lowest wealth quintile was increased when compared with those living in the fourth and fifth wealth quintiles. A study done in India showed that pregnant women from lower socioeconomic classes were at increased risk of developing anemia compared with those in higher socioeconomic classes [2, 10]. This could be due to the fact that those from lower socioeconomic status (SES) lack the ability to purchase the quality or quantity of foods compared with those from higher SES.

Many other studies on anemia in pregnancy conducted in Ethiopia, Pakistan, Nepal, Vietnam, and Malaysia [5, 6, 8, 17, 18] did not consider the effect of wealth index. This could be because the wealth index is calculated from different household assets.

Two other variables with significant association with anemia were iron supplementation during pregnancy and MUAC level. The risk of developing anemia increased in pregnant women who did not receive iron supplementation during pregnancy when compared with those who received iron supplementation. This finding is consistent with the findings from studies in Vietnam and India, which indicated that lack of iron supplementation is among the most significant risk factors for developing anemia during pregnancy [6, 10]. This is likely due to the fact that the requirement of iron increases for pregnant women compared with nonpregnant women, and if they do not receive iron supplementation, the iron they ingest from food sources is not adequate to meet their needs. The finding contrasts with a study done at Pakistan, which found that women who reported consuming iron supplementation had a significantly lower hemoglobin concentration. This may be due to a difference in methodology between the studies.

MUAC less than 23 is found to increase the risk of developing anemia. The current study has shown that pregnant women with MUAC ≥ 23 had 59% less risk of developing anemia. This finding is consistent with a study done in Nepal, which found that MUAC > 23.6 significantly decreased risk of developing anemia [18]. This can be explained by the fact that undernourished pregnant women have a higher probability of being micronutrient deficient and therefore iron deficient and anemic.

Other independent variables which are not significant factors in this study but found to be significant by other studies reviewed include age of the mother, age at pregnancy, age at marriage, number of deliveries, number of children, family size, educational status of the mother, and occupation of the mother [5, 9, 14]. This could be due to the difference between sociocultural and behavioral characteristics of the community in this study and previous studies.

This study was conducted at the community level and considered altitude as an independent variable to assess anemia. Limitations include the cross-sectional nature of the study and using patient report rather than laboratory data for the identification of previous malarial and parasitic infections. Also, the study did not include rural residents.

TABLE 4: Factors associated with anemia among pregnant women in Gode town, Somali Region, Eastern Ethiopia; May 2013.

Variables	Anemia status		COR (95% CI)	AOR (95% CI)
	Anemic	Normal		
Trimester				
First trimester	24	45	1.00	1.00
Second trimester	155	106	*2.74 (1.58–4.77)*	*2.87 (1.61–5.17)*
Third trimester	149	98	*2.85 (1.63–4.98)*	**3.32 (1.84–6.00)**
Parity				
<2	63	58	*1.00*	
2–4	150	87	*1.59 (1.02–2.47)*	
≥5	115	104	*1.02 (0.65–1.59)*	
Family size				
<5	76	58	*1.00*	
5–7	135	76	*1.29 (0.84–1.98)*	
≥8	117	115	*1.75 (1.19–2.56)*	
Forbidden foods				
Yes	70	37	*1.00*	
No	258	212	*0.64 (0.41–0.99)*	
ANC				
Yes	184	163	*1.00*	
No	144	86	*0.74 (0.52–1.05)*	
Iron supplementation during pregnancy				
Yes	207	181	1.00	1.00
No	121	68	0.72 (0.45–1.15)	**1.54 (1.04–2.27)**
24 hr recall food groups				
1–4	94	47	1.00	
5–8	224	192	0.58 (0.39–0.87)	
>8	10	10	0.50 (0.2–1.29)	
Wealth index				
Lowest	49	65	1.00	1.00
Second	78	49	0.40 (0.24–0.68)	**0.43 (0.24–0.76)**
Middle	65	49	0.85 (0.50–1.43)	0.989 (0.57–1.72)
Fourth	59	45	0.71 (0.42–1.20)	0.69 (0.39–1.21)
Highest	77	41	0.70 (0.41–1.20)	0.67 (0.37–1.19)
Gravidity				
<3	59	57	1.00	1.00
3–5	148	80	1.79 (1.14–2.82)	**1.95 (1.19–3.19)**
≥6	121	112	1.04 (0.67–1.63)	1.14 (0.7–1.85)
MUAC				
<23	107	44	1.00	1.00
≥23	219	205	0.44 (0.30–0.66)	**0.41 (0.27–0.63)**

5. Conclusion

The prevalence of anemia among pregnant women in this study was high compared with women in other areas of Ethiopia. Trimester of current pregnancy, wealth quintile, gravidity, iron supplementation, and MUAC were found to be significantly associated with anemia. Iron supplementation and special care during late pregnancy are recommended to reduce anemia. Further research on risk factors of anemia, which include rural residents, should be conducted to strengthen and broaden these findings.

Conflict of Interests

The authors declare that there is no conflict of interests regarding the publication of this paper.

Authors' Contribution

Kefyalew Addis Alene and Abdulahi Mohamed Dohe participated in all steps of the study from its commencement to writing it up. They have reviewed and approved the submission of the paper. These authors contributed equally to this work.

References

[1] WHO/CDC, *Worldwide Prevalence of Anemia 1993–2005: WHO Global Database on Anemia*, WHO Press, Geneva, Switzerland, 2008.

[2] Y. Balarajan, U. Ramakrishnan, E. Özaltin, A. H. Shankar, and S. V. Subramanian, "Anaemia in low-income and middle-income countries," *The Lancet*, vol. 378, no. 9809, pp. 2123–2135, 2011.

[3] S. Salhan, V. Tripathi, R. Singh, and H. S. Gaikwad, "Evaluation of hematological parameters in partial exchange and packed cell transfusion in treatment of severe anemia in pregnancy," *Anemia*, vol. 2012, Article ID 608658, 7 pages, 2012.

[4] B. Esmat, R. Mohammad, S. Behnam et al., "Prevalence of iron deficiency anemia among iranian pregnant women; a systematic review and meta-analysis," *Journal of Reproduction and Infertility*, vol. 11, no. 1, pp. 17–24, 2010.

[5] N. Baig-Ansari, S. H. Badruddin, R. Karmaliani et al., "Anemia prevalence and risk factors in pregnant women in an urban area of Pakistan," *Food and Nutrition Bulletin*, vol. 29, no. 2, pp. 132–139, 2008.

[6] R. Aikawa, N. C. Khan, S. Sasaki, and C. W. Binns, "Risk factors for iron-deficiency anaemia among pregnant women living in rural Vietnam," *Public Health Nutrition*, vol. 9, no. 4, pp. 443–448, 2006.

[7] A. A. Khalafallah and A. E. Dennis, "Iron deficiency anaemia in pregnancy and postpartum: pathophysiology and effect of oral versus intravenous iron therapy," *Journal of Pregnancy*, vol. 2012, Article ID 630519, 10 pages, 2012.

[8] J. Haidar, "Prevalence of anaemia, deficiencies of iron and folic acid and their determinants in ethiopian women," *Journal of Health, Population and Nutrition*, vol. 28, no. 4, pp. 359–368, 2010.

[9] M. Akhtar and I. Hassan, "Severe Anemia during late pregnancy," *Case Reports in Obstetrics and Gynecology*, vol. 2012, Article ID 485452, 3 pages, 2012.

[10] R. G. Vivek, A. B. Halappanavar, P. R. Vivek, S. B. Halki, V. S. Maled, and P. S. Deshpande, "Prevalence of Anemia and its epidemiological," *Determinants in Pregnant Women*, vol. 5, no. 3, pp. 216–223, 2012.

[11] S. S. Elzahrani, "Prevalence of iron deficiency anemia among pregnant women attending antenatal clinics at Al-Hada Hospital," *Canadian Journal on Medicine*, vol. 3, no. 1, pp. 10–14, 2012.

[12] N. Raza, I. Sarwar, B. Munazza, M. Ayub, and M. Suleman, "Assessment of iron deficiency in pregnant women by determining iron status," *Journal of Ayub Medical College Abbottabad*, vol. 23, no. 2, pp. 36–40, 2011.

[13] S. Brooker, P. J. Hotez, and D. A. P. Bundy, "Hookworm-related anaemia among pregnant women: a systematic review," *PLoS Neglected Tropical Diseases*, vol. 2, no. 9, article e291, 2008.

[14] S. J. Baker and E. M. DeMaeyer, "Nutritional anemia: Its understanding and control with special reference to the work of the world health organization," *American Journal of Clinical Nutrition*, vol. 32, no. 2, pp. 368–417, 1979.

[15] G. S. Toteja, P. Singh, B. S. Dhillon et al., "Prevalence of anemia among pregnant women and adolescent girls in 16 districts of India," *Food and Nutrition Bulletin*, vol. 27, no. 4, pp. 311–315, 2006.

[16] Ethiopia, *Demographic and Health Survey*, Central Statistics Agency, Addis Ababa, Ethiopia, 2011.

[17] Federal Democratic Republic of Ethiopia Population Census Commission, *The 2007 Population and Housing census of Ethiopia Results for Somali Region Statistical Report*, Central Statistical Agency, Addis Ababa, Ethiopia, 2010.

[18] Z. Makhoul, D. Taren, B. Duncan et al., "Risk factors associated with anemia, iron deficiency and iron deficiency anemia in rural Nepali pregnant women," *Southeast Asian Journal of Tropical Medicine and Public Health*, vol. 43, no. 3, pp. 735–745, 2012.

13

Validity of Palmar Pallor for Diagnosis of Anemia among Children Aged 6–59 Months in North India

Arun Kumar Aggarwal, Jaya Prasad Tripathy, Deepak Sharma, and Ajith Prabhu

School of Public Health, Postgraduate Institute of Medical Education and Research, Chandigarh 160012, India

Correspondence should be addressed to Arun Kumar Aggarwal; aggak63@gmail.com

Academic Editor: Eitan Fibach

Introduction. The Integrated Management of Childhood and Neonatal Illness (IMNCI) recommends the use palmar pallor to diagnose anaemia. Earlier studies to validate palmar pallor as clinical sign for anaemia were largely done in African context. There was a need to test validity of palmar pallor to detect anemia in different settings. *Objective.* To study the validity and interobserver agreement of palmar pallor examination to diagnose anemia in children under 5 years of age in India. *Methods.* In a village in Northern India, hemoglobin estimation was done for 80 children using cyanomethemoglobin method. Two examiners, a physician and a health worker, trained in IMNCI evaluated children for palmar pallor. Sensitivity and specificity and Kappa statistics were calculated. *Results.* Health worker diagnosed palmar pallor with sensitivity of 30.8–42.8% and specificity of 70–89%. Similar figures for doctor were 40–47% and 60–66%, respectively. Kappa agreement between a health worker and a physician was 0.48 (95% CI = 0.298–0.666) and then increased to 0.51 when categories of severe pallor and mild pallor were merged. *Conclusion.* While using palmar pallor as clinical sign for anaemia, children with no pallor should also be followed up closely for possible detection of missed cases during follow-up.

1. Introduction

Anemia is a major public health problem in India with almost 7 in 10 children aged 6–59 months being anemic [1]. The Integrated Management of Childhood Illness (IMCI) recommends the use of simple clinical sign like palmar pallor to diagnose anemia [2]. This recommendation was based mainly on the studies where purpose was to identify severe anemia with hemoglobin (Hb) <5 grams and moderate anemia with Hb 5–<8 grams [3]. Validity of anemia detection may differ in different settings due to differences in the prevalence of anemia rates, different causes of anemia, and many other factors like different skin pigmentation and so forth that can influence interpretation of palmar pallor. The data about the validity of palmar pallor assessment for detection of anemia from different settings may help improve global understanding about the method of detection. The aim of the present study was thus to study the validity and interobserver agreement of palmar pallor examination to diagnose anemia in children under 5 years of age in India.

2. Methodology

In India, every village has Anganwadi centre (AWC), where children of age 6 months–5 years come every morning for 3-4 hours. They are given supplementary food items, immunization, nonformal preschool education, and periodic health check-ups. The study was carried out in a village in northern Haryana, India, with a population of 2500 and two AWCs. A team comprised of a doctor, laboratory technicians, and an attendant visited both of the AWCs on a scheduled day and time. All children aged 6 months–5 years were recruited into the study. Some children who did not report to the AWC were contacted at their homes.

Informed consent was obtained from the parents/guardian to collect capillary blood samples for Hb estimation from their children. A total of 80 children were available in these centres. Trained laboratory technicians obtained blood drop from finger prick by following standard aseptic technique and prepared dried blood sample on filter paper.

TABLE 1: Validity of doctor and health worker's classification of palmar pallor against different haemoglobin cutoff levels.

	Sensitivity %	Specificity %	Accuracy %	ROC (95% CI)
HB cutoff for anaemia in grams for validation of doctor's classification				
<5	42.8	60.3	58.7	0.51 (0.31–0.72)
<6	43.7	60.9	57.5	0.52 (0.38–0.66)
<7	47.1	65.2	57.5	0.56 (0.45–0.67)
<8	41.1	62.5	47.5	0.52 (0.39–0.63)
<9	40.8	66.7	43.7	0.54 (0.36–0.71)
<10	41	100	42.5	0.70 (0.65–0.76)
HB cutoff for anaemia in grams for validation of health workers classification				
<5	42.8	71.2	68.7	0.57 (0.36–0.77)
<6	31.2	70.3	62.5	0.51 (0.38–0.64)
<7	41.2	78.3	62.5	0.59 (0.49–0.70)
<8	35.7	83.3	50.0	0.59 (0.49–0.69)
<9	32.4	88.9	38.7	0.60 (0.48–0.73)
<10	30.8	100	32.5	0.65 (0.60–0.70)

In the laboratory, analysis of hemoglobin levels was done by cyanomethemoglobin method using dried blood sample (DBS), within 10 days of receipt of the sample. These dried blood samples on the filter paper were transferred to the test tubes, and the blood sample was extracted using Drabkin's solution. Subsequently, these samples were subjected to laboratory analysis using cyanomethemoglobin method, as used in DLHS4 survey. The laboratory was set up and standardized under DLHS-4 survey and had successfully followed all internal and external quality assurance protocols.

Anemia was defined using different cutoff points to make it compatible with the existing studies and as per the national clinical protocols. Anemia is defined as hemoglobin level <11.0 g/dL and severe anemia as <7.0 g/dL. However, original validation studies had used cutoff of <5 grams for severe anemia and <8 grams for moderate anemia.

Two examiners, a physician and a health worker, previously trained in IMNCI, evaluated clinical signs for these children. The physician was postgraduate in specialty of community medicine and the health worker was graduate working as health worker in village-based health post for more than 10 years. Each examiner was blinded to the other. Pallor was defined as *"some palmar pallor"* if the skin of the child's palm was pale and *"severe palmar pallor"* if the skin of the palm was very pale or so pale that it looked white. Kappa statistics was used to measure the level of agreement between the two examiners. Kappa agreement was also calculated by clubbing the categories of "severe palmar pallor" and "some palmar pallor" as a single category *"pallor."*

Standard measures of a diagnostic test like sensitivity and specificity were also calculated. Single clinical category "pallor" was used to undertake the validation analysis. Validation indices were calculated with this clubbed category using different laboratory cutoffs of Hb levels. Area under ROC curve was also ascertained.

3. Results

Out of the 80 children examined, 47 (59%) were males. The age of the children ranged from 6 months to 5 years with mean age of 2.7 years (SD = 1.5). The mean hemoglobin level was 7.0 mg/dL (SD = 1.47) ranging from 4 to 11 mg/dL. Among the children examined, 34 (42.4%) had severe anemia with hemoglobin levels <7 mg/dL, 45 (56.3%) had mild-moderate anemia (7–10.9 mg/dL), whereas only one child (1.3%) had no anemia (≥11 mg/dL).

A health worker could diagnose palmar pallor with sensitivity ranging from 30.8 to 42.8% and specificity from 70 to 89% (excluding extreme value), at different cutoffs of Hb levels. Similar figures for doctor were 40–47% and 60–66%, respectively. Receiver operating curve (ROC) for different cutoffs and both health worker and doctor ranged from 0.51 to 0.75. It was the highest (0.65–0.70) at Hb cutoff of <10 grams (Table 1).

The level of agreement between pallor assessment by a health worker and a physician was found to be 0.482 (95% CI = 0.298–0.666) with weighted Kappa being 0.48. Kappa agreement improved to 0.51 when single category of "pallor" was used to assess the agreement (Table 2).

4. Discussion

Our study revealed glaringly very high anemia rate among children 6 months–5 years of age, who were apparently not sick and were attending to the "AWCs." This may be because of the fact that these centres cater to the poorest section of the society, where anemia rate is expected to be high. High rates of asymptomatic anaemia have been reported in other studies as well, in this part of the world [1, 4, 5].

We found that the sensitivity of palmar pallor was low and specificity was moderate at different cutoffs of Hb levels, used for defining anemia. Variable results have been reported in

TABLE 2: Interrater agreement among doctor and health worker to diagnose palmar pallor.

Doctor's classification	Health workers classification			Total
	No pallor	Some pallor	Severe pallor	
No pallor	43 (89.6)	5 (10.4)	0	48
Some pallor	11 (39.3)	16 (57.1)	1 (3.6)	28
Severe pallor	2 (50.0)	1 (25.0)	1 (25.0)	4

Kappa 0.48 (0.09), $P < 0.001$. Agreement 75%, expected 51.7%.
Clubbing some pallor and severe pallor as single category pallor.
Kappa agreement: 0.51 (std. error 0.1), $P < 0.001$. Agreement 77.5%, expected 54%.

other studies for classification of anaemia. Montresor et al. [6] and Desai et al. [7] reported a low sensitivity (20–37%) and high specificity (84–91%) of clinical diagnosis. Zucker et al. found that sensitivity for defining severe anemia using cutoff of Hb <5 grams was 60% [8]. In our study sensitivity was 42.8% using the same cutoffs. Luby et al. reported 93% sensitivity for the detection of severe anemia and 66% for moderate anemia [9]. In a meta-analysis, sensitivity of clinical pallor signs ranged from 29.2% to 80.9%. Palmar pallor assessment had the highest pooled sensitivity (80.9%) at hemoglobin < 8 g/dL whereas pooled sensitivity was much lower (39.2%) at hemoglobin threshold level <11 g/dL [3]. We also found similar results; however, differential in sensitivities at different Hb cutoffs was less.

Use of palmar pallor for detection of anaemia in the IMCI guidelines was based on the experience of these African studies, with the understanding that, in resource restraint countries, detection of palmar pallor even at modest level of sensitivity and specificity would be lifesaving for many children. Many authors have argued to improve validity of palmar pallor by combining with other clinical signs [10–15], but these have their own limitations. Therefore, in Indian rural setting, where asymptomatic anemia rate is very high, IMNCI guidelines to detect palmar pallor may still be useful for initiating early treatment for childhood anemia. As per the results of this study, health workers will classify 30% children as "some anemia" or "severe anemia." All these children will get the therapeutic iron dose correctly, with or without referral. However, 70% children will be labelled as having "no pallor," who otherwise had some degree of anemia in all but one case. As per IMNCI guidelines these children will also receive dietary counseling and prophylactic iron administration. Second examination by a doctor in such cases is likely to alter the decision from "no pallor" to "pallor" in 13 (16%) cases. But considering comparable sensitivities of health worker and doctor for detection of severe pallor, when laboratory Hb estimation is taken as gold standard, actual contribution of doctor for case detection is likely to be less. It can be argued that in such a setting with very high anemia rate all children may be given therapeutic iron dosage. However, in the absence of any clinical sign of anemia, administration of therapeutic dose of iron may be unethical. Thus we propose that, in settings where it is not possible to do Hb estimations, palmar pallor assessments may be done as per the existing IMNCI protocols. Children with "no pallor" should also be

followed up closely and frequently for possible detection of pallor or some other clinical symptom at some later date.

Some limitations of the study are worth noticing. Many factors could have led to variability in validity of the anaemia classification with palmar pallor. Skin colour and palmar pigmentation could vary in different countries. Cleanliness of palms can be a hindering factor for observation. It is likely that sick children who were brought to OPDs or who were examined indoors in other validation studies had clean palms, whereas, in our study, children were examined in their play centres and their hands were likely to be dusty. The effect of extremes of surrounding temperature on palmar blood circulation also cannot be ruled out. A different method of Hb estimation can also account for the variability. It is well documented that HemoCue method as used in some studies gives higher Hb values compared to cyanomethemoglobin method used in our study [16, 17].

Thus, while more research is needed to explore other simple, accurate methods of hemoglobin estimation in high prevalence settings like India, palmar pallor assessment will continue to be useful in early treatment of anemia with the caution that children with "no pallor" should also be followed up closely.

Conflict of Interests

The authors declare that there is no conflict of interests regarding the publication of this paper.

References

[1] International Institute for Population Sciences and Macro International, *National Family Health Survey (NFHS-3), 2005-06: India*, vol. 1, IIPS, Mumbai, India, 2007.

[2] "Integrated management of childhood illness: conclusions. WHO Division of Child Health and Development," *Bulletin of the World Health Organization*, vol. 75, supplement 1, pp. 119–128, 1997.

[3] J. P. Chalco, L. Huicho, C. Alamo, N. Y. Carreazo, and C. A. Bada, "Accuracy of clinical pallor in the diagnosis of anemia in children: a meta-analysis," *BMC Pediatrics*, vol. 5, article 46, 2005.

[4] A. Zhao, Y. Zhang, Y. Peng et al., "Prevalence of anemia and its risk factors among children 6–36 months Old in Burma," *The American Journal of Tropical Medicine and Hygiene*, vol. 87, no. 2, pp. 306–311, 2012.

[5] S. Hercberg, *Children in the Tropics: Iron and Folate-Deficiency Anemia*, International Children's Center, Paris, France, 1990.

[6] A. Montresor, M. Albonico, N. Khalfan et al., "Field trial of a haemoglobin colour scale: an effective tool to detect anaemia in preschool children," *Tropical Medicine & International Health*, vol. 5, no. 2, pp. 129–133, 2000.

[7] M. R. Desai, P. A. Phillips-Howard, D. J. Terlouw et al., "Recognition of pallor associated with severe anaemia by primary caregivers in western Kenya," *Tropical Medicine and International Health*, vol. 7, no. 10, pp. 831–839, 2002.

[8] J. R. Zucker, B. A. Perkins, H. Jafari, J. Otieno, C. Obonyo, and C. C. Campbell, "Clinical signs for the recognition of children with moderate or severe anaemia in western Kenya," *Bulletin of the World Health Organization*, vol. 75, no. 1, pp. 97–102, 1998.

[9] S. P. Luby, P. N. Kazembe, S. C. Redd et al., "Using clinical signs to diagnose anaemia in African children," *Bulletin of the World Health Organization*, vol. 73, no. 4, pp. 477–482, 1995.

[10] H. D. Kalter, G. Burnham, P. R. Kolstad et al., "Evaluation of clinical signs to diagnose anaemia in Uganda and Bangladesh, in areas with and without malaria," *Bulletin of the World Health Organization*, vol. 75, no. 1, pp. 103–111, 1998.

[11] M. G. N. Spinelli, J. M. P. Souza, S. B. de Souza, and E. H. Sesoko, "Reliability and validity of palmar and conjunctival pallor for anemia detection purposes," *Revista de Saude Publica*, vol. 37, no. 4, pp. 404–408, 2003.

[12] T. Getaneh, T. Girma, T. Belachew, and S. Teklemariam, "The utility of pallor detecting anemia in under five years old children," *Ethiopian Medical Journal*, vol. 38, no. 2, pp. 77–84, 2000.

[13] L. Muhe, B. Oljira, H. Degefu, S. Jaffar, and M. W. Weber, "Evaluation of clinical pallor in the identification and treatment of children with moderate and severe anaemia," *Tropical Medicine & International Health*, vol. 5, no. 11, pp. 805–810, 2000.

[14] I. H. Thaver and L. Baig, "Anaemia in children: part I. Can simple observations by primary care provider help in diagnosis?" *Journal of the Pakistan Medical Association*, vol. 44, no. 12, pp. 282–284, 1994.

[15] C. F. Ingram and S. M. Lewis, "Clinical use of WHO haemoglobin colour scale: validation and critique," *Journal of Clinical Pathology*, vol. 53, no. 12, pp. 933–937, 2000.

[16] X. Zhao and S.-A. Yin, "Comparison of HemoCue with cyanmethemoglobin method for estimating hemoglobin," *Wei Sheng Yan Jiu*, vol. 32, no. 5, pp. 495–497, 2003.

[17] R. Saxena and R. Malik, "Comparison of HemoCue method with the cyanmethemoglobin method for estimation of hemoglobin," *Indian Pediatrics*, vol. 40, no. 9, p. 917, 2003.

14

Validation of the WHO Hemoglobin Color Scale Method

Leeniyagala Gamaralalage Thamal Darshana and Deepthi Inoka Uluwaduge

Medical Laboratory Sciences Unit, Department of Allied Health Sciences, Faculty of Medical Sciences,
University of Sri Jayewardenepura, Gangodawila, Nugegoda 10250, Sri Lanka

Correspondence should be addressed to Leeniyagala Gamaralalage Thamal Darshana; darshana0031@gmail.com

Academic Editor: Eitan Fibach

This study was carried out to evaluate the diagnostic accuracy of WHO color scale in screening anemia during blood donor selection in Sri Lanka. A comparative cross-sectional study was conducted by the Medical Laboratory Sciences Unit of University of Sri Jayewardenepura in collaboration with National Blood Transfusion Centre, Sri Lanka. A total of 100 subjects participated in this study. Hemoglobin value of each participant was analyzed by both WHO color scale method and cyanmethemoglobin method. Bland-Altman plot was used to determine the agreement between the two methods. Sensitivity, specificity, predictive values, false positive, and negative rates were calculated. The sensitivity of the WHO color scale was very low. The highest sensitivity observed was 55.55% in hemoglobin concentrations >13.1 g/dL and the lowest was 28.57% in hemoglobin concentrations between 7.1 and 9.0 g/dL. The mean difference between the WHO color scale and the cyanmethemoglobin method was 0.2 g/dL (95% confidence interval; 3.2 g/dL above and 2.8 g/dL below). Even though the WHO color scale is an inexpensive and portable method for field studies, from the overall results in this study it is concluded that WHO color scale is an inaccurate method to screen anemia during blood donations.

1. Introduction

Anemia is a public health problem that affects both developed and developing countries. Pregnant women and young children are the most affected groups by its overwhelming effects. Hemoglobin concentration is considered as the most reliable indicator of anemia than the clinical findings [1]. The World Health Organization (WHO) color scale method is an inexpensive method for estimating hemoglobin concentration from a drop of blood by means of a color scale [2]. The color scale comprises a small card with six shades of red that represent hemoglobin levels at 4, 6, 8, 10, 12, and 14 g/dL, respectively [3]. Although many absorbent papers were tested, it was concluded that the Whatman 31 ET paper gave the best results with regular round stain of a limited spread. The color standards are printed in a continuous row without any separation and are mounted on a rigid white polyvinyl chloride or polypropylene sheet or thick card with a neutral pale-grey matt background. Estimation of the hemoglobin is done by matching the blood sample with the color standards through circular apertures which are placed in the center of each color standard [4]. The WHO color scale was primarily designed for anemia screening in obstetrical management, pediatric clinics, malaria and hookworm control programs, blood transfusion donor selection, and epidemiological surveys [2, 5, 6].

WHO color scale is a semiqualitative method and over the years it has been a useful tool in identifying anemia in field studies. Efficiency in terms of cost, accuracy, and time makes it an important resource in primary health care settings in developing countries. At present WHO color scale is the most widely used method for detecting anemia in settings where there is no laboratory. It performs better than clinical diagnosis alone in detecting mild to moderate anemia. However color scale's detecting ability is reduced as anemia becomes more severe [7].

Sensitivity and specificity of WHO color scale were very high in laboratory based studies but reduced considerably in field studies [7]. A comparative cross-sectional study done in Ethiopia showed a very low sensitivity in detecting anemia among pregnant mothers [5]. Sensitivity for the hemoglobin values <9 g/dL was 42.9% and for values <10 g/dL was 33.3%

whereas sensitivity for the hemoglobin values <11 g/dL was 43.5%. However specificity remained relatively high in all three categories [5]. Underestimation of the high hemoglobin levels is also reported by Montresor et al. in a field study conducted to detect the anemia among preschool children in Zanzibar [6]. High number of false positives is another problem associated with the WHO color scale. Barduagni et al. have reported very low positive predictive value (PPV) for the color scale (26.7%) in a study which assessed the prevalence of anemia among school children in Northern Egypt suggesting that high number of healthy individuals can be labeled as anemic [8]. Similar results were reported by van den Broek et al. in a study assessing the potential of WHO color scale in anemia screening of pregnant mothers. Positive predictive values were very low for hemoglobin concentrations of ≤8 g/dL and ≤6 g/dL (11.1% and 15.8%, resp.) giving large amounts of false positives as anemic [9].

The predonation assessment of the blood donor hemoglobin is the best approach to determine the iron-status of the donor. Hemoglobin screening prior to blood donation is essential to safeguard anemic individuals from blood donating and protects returning donors from donation-induced iron deficiency [10]. WHO color scale is a common tool that is used to screen anemia during blood donation because of its simplicity [1]. However, some issues have been raised regarding its screening accuracy. Shahshahani and Amiri have reported relatively low sensitivity for the WHO color scale (54.5%) in a study which screened individuals prior to blood donation in Iran. Hemoglobin levels measured by color scale were significantly lower (0.32 ± 0.65 g/dL; $P < 0.001$) than the levels measured by the standard method [11]. In Sri Lanka too WHO color scale is the mostly used tool to screen anemia prior to blood donation. The present study was undertaken to evaluate the diagnostic accuracy of WHO color scale in screening anemia during blood donor selection in Sri Lanka.

2. Materials and Methods

A comparative cross-sectional study was conducted by the Medical Laboratory Sciences Unit of University of Sri Jayewardenepura in collaboration with National Blood Transfusion Centre, Sri Lanka. Study subjects were chosen from the donors who were attending above center and the data was collected between January and April 2010. Informed written consents were obtained from each and every participant prior to the inclusion. Ethical clearances were obtained in written statements form Ethical Review Committee of University of Sri Jayewardenepura and National Blood Transfusion Centre, Sri Lanka. A total of 100 subjects were selected as the participants for the study.

Finger pricked blood was used to measure the color scale hemoglobin value. A blood drop was placed on the test strip provided with the color scale and after waiting for 30 seconds the color of the blood spot was immediately matched against the given color standards (4, 6, 8, 10, 12, and 14 g/dL) and the corresponding value was recorded. Venous blood (2 mL) was collected from each subject into

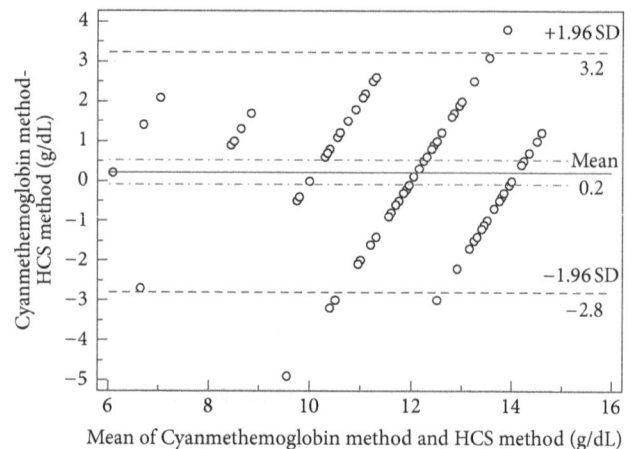

FIGURE 1: Bland-Altman plot for the haemoglobin colour scale compared with the reference method (cyanmethemoglobin method).

EDTA (ethylenediamine tetraacetic acid) containers for the laboratory assessments. Internationally recommended (gold standard) cyanmethemoglobin method was used to determine the reference hemoglobin concentrations of the blood samples [12]. Anticoagulated venous blood (20 μL) was mixed with Drabkin's diluting fluid (5 mL) and after 5 minutes absorbance was taken at 540 nm by using a Labomed UV-VIS AUTO-UV-2602 spectrophotometer. Hemoglobin concentration was measured from a previously prepared standard curve with a hemoglobin standard (concentration of 660 mg/L to 250 times diluted blood of 16.5 g/dL). All the laboratory procedures including preparation of dilutions, absorbance reading, and measuring of hemoglobin concentration from the standard curve were done by single qualified laboratory technician to avoid the operator bias. Laboratory reference hemoglobin value was recorded in g/dL to one single decimal point and WHO color scale results were compared with the laboratory reference readings. Sensitivity, specificity, positive predictive value, and negative predictive values were measured. Bland-Altman plot and proximities of the color scale value to the reference value were obtained (Figure 1). All the statistical analyses were done by using Microsoft Office Excel 2007 and SPSS software version 12.0.

3. Results

Subjects were divided into five categories depending on their reference hemoglobin concentrations (Table 1). Sensitivity and the specificity of the WHO color scale remained low in all five categories; however, the sensitivity showed tendency to increase slightly when the hemoglobin concentration is increasing. Positive predictive value was very low in severe-moderate anemic regions (2.08%, in 5–7 g/dL; 4.44%, in 7.1–9 g/dL) indicating high rate of false positives at very low hemoglobin concentrations. Contrastingly, negative predictive value of the color scale remained relatively high in severe to mild anemic regions.

WHO color scale readings of 53 subjects out of 100 were within the range of the reference hemoglobin value ±1.0.

TABLE 1: Reliability of WHO color scale with the reference method (cyanmethemoglobin method).

Hemoglobin concentration (g/dL)	5–7	7.1–9	9.1–11	11.1–13	>13.1
Specificity %	52.04	53.76	52.94	49.01	50.68
Sensitivity %	50	28.57	46.66	55.10	55.55
Positive prediction %	2.08	4.44	14.89	50.94	29.41
Negative prediction %	98.08	90.9	84.90	53.19	75.51

TABLE 2: Proximity of the test results to the reference method (cyanmethemoglobin method).

	Proximity to reference hemoglobin (g/dL)			
	±1.0	±1.1–2.0	±2.1–3.0	± >3.0
Number of subjects	53	30	12	05

Color scale results of the other 47 subjects were deviated from the reference value ±1.0. Seventeen subjects (17) had their hemoglobin values deviated from reference value ±2.0 (Table 2).

The mean difference value for the two methods (WHO color scale and cyanmethemoglobin method) was 0.2 g/dL. The limits of agreements for the two methods given by Bland-Altman plot were shown as the mean difference ±1.96 standard deviation. The limits of agreements for the WHO color scale were 2.8 g/dL below and 3.2 g/dL above.

4. Discussion

Sensitivity and specificity are two of the very important parameters required by a screening test to be validated. Diagnostic ability of a test method highly depends on these parameters. In the present study we observed low sensitivity and specificity values for all five hemoglobin concentrations (Table 1). Although slight increase in the sensitivity was observed when the hemoglobin concentration is increasing, that too was relatively low (55.55%) being the maximum sensitivity observed. The lowest sensitivity (28.57%) was observed in moderate anemic region (7.1–9 g/dL) and this result is somewhat similar to Gies et al. who have reported the lowest sensitivity (33.3%) of color scale for hemoglobin concentration <10 g/dL region indicating the poor accuracy of color scale in low hemoglobin concentrations [5].

In the present study, we observed low positive predictive values for the color scale. Lowest positive predictive value (2.08%) was observed in severe anemic (hemoglobin 5–7 g/dL) category. This implies high number of healthy nonanemic individuals can be diagnosed as anemic individuals. Our positive predictive value (4.44% for hemoglobin 7.1–9 g/dL) is even lower than van den Broek et al. who have reported positive predictive value (11.1%) for a similar hemoglobin range (≤8 g/dL) [9].

WHO color scale, at best, can measure hemoglobin value ±1 g/dL of reference hemoglobin value. Any value given by color scale outside this range would be inaccurate. In the present study only 53% of the data procured the appropriate range. Almost half of the values (47%) given by color scale

being different from more than ±1 g/dL of reference value imply the poor performance of the color scale in field studies.

When examining the diagnostic accuracy of a test method (in this case WHO color scale) examining the agreement between test method and the gold standard method is vital. Bland-Altman plot was designed to measure the agreement and establish a limit of agreement of two test methods [13]. Therefore we used Bland-Altman plot to compare the agreement between the color scale and the reference instead of correlation coefficient or regression analysis. According to the results obtained from Bland-Altman plot the limits of agreement (the scattering area in which 95% of data are distributed) were 2.8 g/dL below and 3.2 g/dL above demonstrating a wide range of agreement (6 g/dL) for the color scale which is poor and unacceptable. The agreement would have been acceptable if it were 2 g/dL as ±1 g/dL change in color scale result to the reference value can be acceptable. Similar results were reported in a study done in England in which the limits of agreement for the WHO color scale were 3.50 g/dL below and 3.11 g/dL above and the range of agreement was slightly higher (6.61 g/dL) than the present study [14].

In the present study overall performance of the WHO color scale is not satisfactory. Interobserver variation could be a factor for the poor accuracy of the color scale. In this study color scale readings were taken by 3 public health inspectors who were working at the National Blood Transfusion Centre. Reading of the color scale under faded light or under weak light and the discoloration could be the factors interfering with the reading of color scale. Although it was made with Whatman 31 ET special chromatographic paper, there is a tendency to discoloration of the paper as it becomes older. This could substantially affect the reading of the color scale.

5. Conclusion

The WHO color scale is an inexpensive, portable, and easy method to screen anemia. Although its accuracy remains high in laboratory based studies, when it comes to field studies the accuracy becomes questionable. It was developed to be an alternative of the clinical evaluation of anemia and not of a spectrophotometer, but whenever a spectrophotometer is available that method should be preferred to the WHO color scale method in measuring the hemoglobin level. For the areas where spectrophotometers are not available clinical evaluation could be better than the WHO color scale. In future studies large sample numbers are recommended to obtain better results.

Conflict of Interests

The authors declare that there is no conflict of interests regarding the publication of this paper.

Acknowledgments

The authors gratefully acknowledge the support given by the director and the staff of National Blood Transfusion

Centre, Sri Lanka, and the staff of Medical Laboratory Sciences Unit, Faculty of Medical Sciences of University of Sri Jayewardenepura.

References

[1] World Health Organization, *Worldwide Prevalence of Anaemia 1993–2005, WHO Global Database on Anaemia*, WHO, Geneva, Switzerland, 2008.

[2] S. M. Lewis, G. J. Stott, and K. J. Wynn, "An inexpensive and reliable new haemoglobin colour scale for assessing anaemia," *Journal of Clinical Pathology*, vol. 51, no. 1, pp. 21–24, 1998.

[3] World Health Organization, *Haemoglobin Colour Scale: Practical Answer to a vital Need*, Department of Blood Safety and Clinical Technology, WHO, Geneva, Switzerland, 2001.

[4] G. J. Stott and S. M. Lewis, "A simple and reliable method for estimating haemoglobin," *Bulletin of the World Health Organization*, vol. 73, no. 3, pp. 369–373, 1995.

[5] S. Gies, B. J. Brabin, M. A. Yassin, and L. E. Cuevas, "Comparison of screening methods for anaemia in pregnant women in Awassa, Ethiopia," *Tropical Medicine and International Health*, vol. 8, no. 4, pp. 301–309, 2003.

[6] A. Montresor, M. Albonico, N. Khalfan et al., "Field trial of a haemoglobin colour scale: an effective tool to detect anaemia in preschool children," *Tropical Medicine and International Health*, vol. 5, no. 2, pp. 129–133, 2000.

[7] J. Critchley and I. Bates, "Haemoglobin colour scale for anaemia diagnosis where there is no laboratory: a systematic review," *International Journal of Epidemiology*, vol. 34, no. 6, pp. 1425–1434, 2005.

[8] P. Barduagni, A. S. Ahmed, F. Curtale, M. Raafat, and L. Soliman, "Performance of Sahli and colour scale methods in diagnosing anaemia among school children in low prevalence areas," *Tropical Medicine and International Health*, vol. 8, no. 7, pp. 615–618, 2003.

[9] N. R. van den Broek, C. Ntonya, E. Mhango, and S. A. White, "Diagnosing anaemia in pregnancy in rural clinics: assessing the potential of the haemoglobin colour scale," *Bulletin of the World Health Organization*, vol. 77, no. 1, pp. 15–21, 1999.

[10] World Health Organization, *Blood Donor Selection: Guidelines on Assessing Donor Suitability for Blood Donation*, WHO, Geneva, Switzerland, 2012.

[11] H. J. Shahshahani and F. Amiri, "Validity of hemoglobin color scale in blood donor screening based on Standard Operating Procedures of Iranian Blood Transfusion Organization," *Sci J Blood Transfus Organ*, vol. 5, no. 4, pp. 281–286, 2009.

[12] B. J. Bain, I. Bates, and S. M. Lewis, *Dacie and Lewis Practical Haematology*, Churchill Livingstone, Philadelphia, Pa, USA, 11th edition, 2011.

[13] J. M. Bland and D. G. Altman, "Statistical methods for assessing agreement between two methods of clinical measurement," *The Lancet*, vol. 1, no. 8476, pp. 307–310, 1986.

[14] J. J. Paddle, "Evaluation of the Haemoglobin colour scale and comparison with the HemoCue haemoglobin assay," *Bulletin of the World Health Organization*, vol. 80, no. 10, pp. 813–816, 2002.

15

Hematological Indices for Differential Diagnosis of Beta Thalassemia Trait and Iron Deficiency Anemia

Aysel Vehapoglu,[1] Gamze Ozgurhan,[2] Ayşegul Dogan Demir,[1] Selcuk Uzuner,[1] Mustafa Atilla Nursoy,[1] Serdar Turkmen,[3] and Arzu Kacan[4]

[1] Department of Pediatrics, School of Medicine, Bezmialem Vakif University, 34093 Istanbul, Turkey
[2] Department of Pediatrics, Suleymaniye Obstetrics and Gynecology Hospital, 34010 Istanbul, Turkey
[3] Department of Biochemistry, Istanbul Training and Research Hospital, 34098 Istanbul, Turkey
[4] Department of Pediatrics, Istanbul Training and Research Hospital, Istanbul, Turkey

Correspondence should be addressed to Aysel Vehapoglu; ayvahap@hotmail.com

Academic Editor: Bruno Annibale

Background. The two most frequent types of microcytic anemia are beta thalassemia trait (β-TT) and iron deficiency anemia (IDA). We retrospectively evaluated the reliability of various indices for differential diagnosis of microcytosis and β-TT in the same patient groups. *Methods.* A total of 290 carefully selected children aged 1.1–16 years were evaluated. We calculated 12 discrimination indices in all patients with hemoglobin (Hb) values of 8.7–11.4 g/dL. None of the subjects had a combined case of IDA and β-TT. All children with IDA received oral iron for 16 weeks, and HbA2 screening was performed after iron therapy. The patient groups were evaluated according to red blood cell (RBC) count; red blood distribution width index; the Mentzer, Shine and Lal, England and Fraser, Srivastava and Bevington, Green and King, Ricerca, Sirdah, and Ehsani indices; mean density of hemoglobin/liter of blood; and mean cell density of hemoglobin. *Results.* The Mentzer index was the most reliable index, as it had the highest sensitivity (98.7%), specificity (82.3%), and Youden's index (81%) for detecting β-TT; this was followed by the Ehsani index (94.8%, 73.5%, and 68.3%, resp.) and RBC count (94.8%, 70.5%, and 65.3%). *Conclusion.* The Mentzer index provided the highest reliabilities for differentiating β-TT from IDA.

1. Introduction

Anemia resulting from lack of sufficient iron to synthesize hemoglobin is the most common hematological disease in infants and children. It has been estimated that 30% of the global population suffers from iron deficiency anemia (IDA), and most of those affected live in the developing countries. Microcytic anemia in a case of thalassemia results from impaired globin chain synthesis and decreased hemoglobin (Hb) synthesis, resulting in microcytosis and hypochromia; 1.5% of the world's population carries genes for β-thalassemia [1]. Individuals with the beta thalassemia trait (β-TT) are usually asymptomatic and may be unaware of their carrier status unless diagnosed by testing. β-TT is the most common type of hemoglobinopathy transmitted by heredity. It is estimated that about 50% of the world's population with β-TT

are in Southeast Asia; it is also common in the Mediterranean region, the Middle East, Southeast Asia, Southwest Europe, and Central Africa [2]. Due to the migration and intermarriage of different ethnic populations, β-TT is found in people with no obvious ethnic connection to the disorder.

A definitive differential diagnosis between β-TT and IDA is based on the result of HbA$_2$ electrophoresis, serum iron levels, and a ferritin calculation [3]. Electronic cell counters have been used to determine red cell indices as a first indicator of β-TT. The purpose of using indices to discriminate anemia is to detect subjects who have a high probability of requiring appropriate follow-up and to reduce unnecessary investigative costs. Since 1970, a number of complete blood count indices have been proposed as simple and inexpensive tools to determine whether a blood sample is more suggestive of β-TT or IDA [4–12]. Most of these articles include

TABLE 1: Hematological and biochemical date of study groups.

	β-TT (n: 154)		IDA (n: 136)	
	Range	Mean ± SD	Range	Mean ± SD
Hb (g/dL) total	9–11.46	10.39 ± 0.69	8.7–11.42	10.23 ± 0.95
RBC ($\times 10^6$/L)	4.34–6.54	5.56 ± 0.4	3.45–6.33	4.84 ± 0.59
MCV (fL)	52.1–71	60.11 ± 3.49	45.3–79.53	67.49 ± 7.14
MCH (pg)	16.3–23.8	18.9 ± 1.37	13.65–27.7	21.33 ± 3.09
RDW (%)	13.9–24.63	16.76 ± 1.83	12.5–28.66	17.4 ± 3.48
SI (μg/dL)	20–194	76.6 ± 29.2	4.6–31.2	23.74 ± 9.48
SIBC (μg/dL)	257–472	339 ± 40.47	279–495	392 ± 41.74
TS (%)	5.5–55.2	22.88 ± 8.7	0.9–8.7	6.1 ± 2.6
Ferritin (ng/mL)	11.2–96	33.75 ± 22.9	1.1–11.2	7.54 ± 3.2

β-TT: beta thalassemia trait; IDA: iron deficiency anemia; Hb: hemoglobin; RBC: red blood cell; MCV: mean corpuscular volume; MCH: mean corpuscular hemoglobin; RDW: red blood cell distribution width; SI: serum iron; SIBC: serum iron binding capacity; TS: transferrin saturation.

adults but very few data are available on children. An ideal discrimination index has high sensitivity and specificity; that is, it can detect the maximum number of patients with β-TT (high sensitivity) while eliminating patients with IDA (high specificity). In this study, we compared the ability of different 12 indices to distinguish β-TT from IDA by calculating their sensitivity, specificity, and Youden's index values.

2. Material and Methods

We retrospectively analyzed 290 children with microcytic anemia (mean age: 6.2 ± 4.2 years; range: 1.1–16 years). Samples were obtained from 121 boys and 169 girls with no clinical symptoms of acute or chronic inflammation or infectious diseases. None of them had received a transfusion or had an acute bleeding episode in the previous month. The samples were obtained during the course of routine analysis and collected in EDTA anticoagulant tubes. Red blood cell (RBC) count and red blood cell distribution width (RDW) were assessed on a Siemens Advia 2120 Hematology Analyzer. Serum iron (SI), serum iron binding capacity, serum ferritin, and HbA$_2$ values were determined in all children. HbA$_2$ was detected by high-performance liquid chromatography (Shimadzu LC-MS). SI and total iron binding capacity (TIBC) were determined calorimetrically (Siemens Advia 2400 Chemistry Analyzer), and ferritin was measured by immunoassay using a Siemens Advia XP Analyzer. Transferrin saturation was calculated as the ratio of SI to TIBC. The hematological and biochemical data of the groups are evaluated before iron replacement regimen. Those are shown in Table 1. Iron deficiency modulates HbA$_2$ synthesis, resulting in reduced HbA$_2$ levels in patients with IDA [13, 14]. The increase in HbA$_2$ levels (>3.5%) is the most significant parameter for identifying beta thalassemia carriers. Patients with β-TT and concomitant iron deficiency may show normal HbA$_2$ levels. Therefore, none of the subjects in the present study had both IDA and β-TT. All children with IDA received oral iron (3–5 mg/kg/day) for 16 weeks. HbA$_2$ screening was performed after completion of the 16-week iron replacement regimen.

A total of 154 children were confirmed to have β-TT. The β-TT group consisted of children with Hb levels of 9–11.46 g/dL, mean corpuscular volume (MCV) < 80 fL at age > 6 years or MCV < 70 fL at age < 6 years, serum iron level > 30 μg/dL, transferrin saturation > 16%, serum ferritin level > 12 ng/dL, and HbA$_2$ > 3.5%. A total of 136 children were confirmed to have IDA with serum ferritin levels ≤ 12 ng/dL. The IDA group consisted of children with Hb levels of 8.7–11.4 g/dL, mean corpuscular volume (MCV) < 80 fL at age > 6 years or MCV < 70 fL at age < 6 years, serum iron level < 30 μg/dL, transferrin saturation < 16%, and serum ferritin level ≤ 12 ng/dL. Children with Hb levels < 8.7 g/dL were excluded because these cases of severe anemia are not confused with β-TT in daily practice. None of the subjects of the present study had a combined case of β-TT and IDA. The combined cases were excluded from the early stages of the evaluation study.

The 12 discrimination indices used in the evaluation were calculated and are summarized in Table 2. Sensitivity, specificity, positive predictive value (PPV), negative predictive value (NPV), and Youden's index were calculated for each measure as follows:

$$\text{Sensitivity} = \left[\frac{\text{true positive}}{(\text{true positive} + \text{false negative})} \right] \times 100,$$

$$\text{Specificity} = \left[\frac{\text{true negative}}{(\text{true negative} + \text{false positive})} \right] \times 100,$$

$$\text{PPV} = \frac{\text{true positive}}{(\text{true positive} + \text{false positive})} \times 100,$$

$$\text{NPV} = \frac{\text{true negative}}{(\text{true negative} + \text{false negative})} \times 100,$$

$$\text{Youden's index} = (\text{sensitivity} + \text{specificity}) - 100.$$

$$(1)$$

2.1. Statistical Analysis. Data were analyzed with computerized statistical package for social sciences (SPSS) version 15.0. An independent sample t-test was performed to detect differences between the two groups of anemic children.

TABLE 2: Different RBC indices and mathematical formulas used to differentiate between β-TT and IDA.

Hematological index	Formula
Mentzer index (MI) (1973)	MCV/RBC
RDWI (1987)	MCV × RDW/RBC
Shine and Lal (S and L) (1977)	MCV × MCV × MCH/100
Srivastava (1973)	MCH/RBC
Green and King (G and K) (1989)	MCV × MCV × RDW/Hb × 100
Sirdah (2007)	MCV − RBC − (3 × Hb)
Ehsani (2005)	MCV − (10 × RBC)
England and Fraser (E and F) (1973)	MCV − (5 × Hb) − RBC − 3.4
Ricerca (1987)	RDW/RBC
MDHL (1999)	(MCH/MCV) × RBC
MCHD (1999)	MCH/MCV

MDHL index: mean density of Hb/liter of blood; MCHD index: mean cell Hb density.

P values < 0.05 were considered significant. The differential values for each discrimination index were applied as defined in the original published reports: red blood distribution width index (RDWI), Mentzer index [4], the Shine and Lal index [5], the England and Fraser index [6], the Srivastava index [7], the Green and King index [8], the Ricerca et al. index [9], and the Sirdah et al. index [10]. The Ehsani et al. index [11], mean density of hemoglobin per liter of blood (MDHL), mean cell hemoglobin density (MCHD) [12], and RBC count were evaluated and compared. The values of each index required to distinguish between β-TT and IDA and the number and proportion of correctly identified patients (true positives) calculated using these indices are shown in Table 3. Sensitivity, specificity, PPV, NPV, and Youden's index values for each index needed to distinguish between β-TT and IDA are shown in Table 4.

3. Results

Hb values in the β-TT group were 10.39 ± 0.69, and those in the IDA group were 10.23 ± 0.95 (P > 0.05). MCV was 60.11 ± 3.49 and MCHD was 18.9 ± 1.37 in the β-TT group, and these values were lower than those in the IDA group (67.49 ± 7.14 and 21.3 ± 3.09, respectively; P < 0.05). The RDWI values were increased in both groups: 17.4 ± 3.48 in the IDA group and 16.76 ± 1.83 in patients with β-TT (P > 0.05). Red cell values at various ages of study groups are shown in Table 5.

RBC count was higher in the β-TT (5.56 ± 0.4) group than that in the IDA (4.84 ± 0.59; P < 0.05). A high erythrocyte count (RBC > $5.0 \times 10^6/\mu$L) is a common feature of IDA and β-TT. The RBC count is one of the most accurate indices available. The RBC count provided the best sensitivity (94.8%) but had low specificity (70.5%), and Youden's index was 65.3%.

As indicated in Table 4, none of the indices studied demonstrated 100% precision in recognizing β-TT. The Ricerca et al. and the Shine and Lal indices demonstrated the highest sensitivity (100%) but had low specificities for correctly identifying IDA (14.7%) and β-TT (10.2%). Therefore, according to our results, these indices cannot be used as screening tools for β-TT, as using them could result in a significant number of false-negative results. The England and Fraser index had the lowest sensitivity of 66.2%, and identification was wrong in about 28% of β-TT cases. The England and Fraser and the Mentzer indices demonstrated the highest specificities at 85.3% and 82.3%, respectively. Furthermore, Table 4 shows the highest and lowest PPV, which were found for the Mentzer index (86.3%) and the Shine and Lal (55%) and MCHL indices (55%), respectively. The Shine and Lal and the Ricerca et al. indices demonstrated the highest NPV at 100%, and MCHD had the lowest NPV at 52.7%. Additionally, Table 4 shows that the highest and lowest Youden's index values belonged to the Mentzer index (81%) and MCHD (5.8%). None of the indices was completely sensitive or specific in distinguishing β-TT and IDA.

The Mentzer index showed good sensitivity, specificity, and Youden's index values of 98.7%, 82.3%, and 81%, respectively. When the Mentzer index was calculated, 264 children with microcytic anemia (91%) were correctly diagnosed. Youden's index showed the following ranking with respect to the indices' ability to distinguish between β-TT and IDA: Mentzer index > Ehsani et al. index > RBC count > Sirdah et al. index > RDWI > Srivastava index > Green and King index > England and Fraser index > MDHL > Ricerca et al. index > Shine and Lal index > MCHD. The difference between the results of all of these indices and the gold standard (HbA$_2$) was significant (P < 0.001).

4. Discussion

β-TT and IDA are among the most common types of microcytic anemia encountered by pediatricians. Distinguishing β-TT from IDA has important clinical implications because each disease has an entirely different cause, prognosis, and treatment. Thalassemia is endemic in Turkey. Misdiagnosis of β-TT has consequences for potential homozygous offspring. Up to now, many investigators have used different mathematical indices to distinguish β-TT from IDA using only a complete blood count. This process helps to select appropriate individuals for a more detailed examination; however, no study has found 100% specificity or sensitivity for any of these RBC indices. Our data (Table 1) showed significant differences between the hematological and biochemical parameters of β-TT and IDA children except for Hb and RDW, but these differences were not reflected in the indices' reliability in differential diagnosis of β-TT and IDA. RBC count has been considered a valuable index [15], but we showed that RBC count had only 70.5% specificity and 65.3% Youden's index. In the 290 children with microcytic anemia, 186 children (64.1%) had a high RBC count (RBC count > $5.0 \times 10^6/\mu$L) at the time of diagnosis. However, the frequency of high RBC count was 29.4% in children with IDA. It seems that RBC alone was not a reliable tool for distinguishing β-TT from IDA. Elevated RBC count might be associated with

TABLE 3: Results obtained from each discrimination index and correctly identified number of the children.

Indices (cutoffs)	β-TT (n: 154)	IDA (n: 136)	Total number of correctly diagnosed children	Correctly diagnosed (%)
Mentzer				
β-TT < 13	152	24	264 (152 + 112)	91
IDA > 13	2	112		
RBC count ($\times 10^6$/L)				
β-TT > 5	146	40	242 (146 + 96)	83.4
IDA < 5	8	96		
RDWI				
β-TT < 220	128	32	232 (128 + 104)	80
IDA > 220	26	104		
Shine and Lal				
β-TT < 1530	154	122	168 (154 + 14)	57.9
IDA > 1530	0	14		
Srivastava				
β-TT < 3.8	132	38	230 (132 + 98)	79.3
IDA > 3.8	22	98		
Green and King				
β-TT < 65	128	36	228 (128 + 100)	78.6
IDA > 65	26	100		
Sirdah				
β-TT < 27	132	28	240 (132 + 108)	82.7
IDA > 27	22	108		
Ehsani				
β-TT < 15	146	36	246 (146 + 100)	84.8
IDA > 15	8	100		
England and Fraser				
β-TT < 0	102	20	218 (102 + 116)	75
IDA > 0	52	116		
Ricerca				
β-TT < 4.4	154	116	174 (154 + 20)	60
IDA > 4.4	0	20		
MDHL				
β-TT > 1.63	118	36	198 (118 + 80)	68.2
IDA < 1.63	36	80		
MCHD				
β-TT > 0.3045	120	98	158 (120 + 38)	54.4
IDA < 0.3045	34	38		

erythrocytosis. We observed that the RBC count increased at the initiation of iron therapy in patients with IDA and decreased by the end of therapy. A similar observation was made by Aslan and Altay, who reported an elevated RBC count in 61% of cases with mild anemia [16].

In a 2010 study, Ferrara et al. demonstrated that RDWI had the highest sensitivity (78.9%), that the England and Fraser index had the highest specificity and highest Youden's index (99.1 and 64.2%, resp.), and that the Green and King index had the highest efficiency (80.2%) in 458 children with mild microcytic anemia aged 1.8–7.5 years [17].

AlFadhli et al. compared nine discriminant functions in patients with microcytic anemia and measured validity using Youden's index. Youden's index considers both sensitivity and specificity and provides an appropriate measure of validity for

a particular question or technique. They showed that the England and Fraser index had the highest Youden's index value (98.2%) for correctly differentiating β-TT and IDA, whereas the Shine and Lal index was ineffective for differentiating microcytic anemia [18]. According to our data, the Mentzer index had the highest Youden's index for correctly distinguishing β-TT and IDA at 81%. When the Mentzer index was calculated, 91% of children with microcytic anemia were correctly diagnosed. The England and Fraser and the Shine and Lal indices had the lowest Youden's index values of 51.4% and 10.2%, respectively.

In 2009, Ehsani et al. showed that the best discrimination index according to Youden's criteria was the Mentzer index (90.1%), followed by the Ehsani et al. index (85.5%). In their study, the Mentzer and Ehsani et al. indices were able to

TABLE 4: Sensitivity, specificity, positive predictive value (PPV), negative predictive value (NPV), and Youden's index of twelve indices to discriminate between β-TT and IDA in 290 children.

Indices	Sensitivity (%)	Specificity (%)	PPV (%)	NPV (%)	Youden's index
Mentzer					
β-TT	98.7	82.3	86.3	98.2	81
IDA	82.3	98.7	98.2	86.3	
RBC count					
β-TT	94.8	70.5	78.4	92.3	65.3
IDA	70.5	94.8	92.3	78.4	
RDWI					
β-TT	83.1	76.4	80	80	59.5
IDA	76.4	83.1	80	80	
Shine and Lal					
β-TT	100	10.2	55	100	10.2
IDA	10.2	100	100	55	
Srivastava					
β-TT	85.7	72	77.6	81.6	57.7
IDA	72	85.7	81.6	77.6	
Green and King					
β-TT	83.1	73.5	77.6	79.3	56.6
IDA	73.5	83.1	79.3	77.6	
Sirdah					
β-TT	85.7	79.4	82.5	83	65
IDA	79.4	85.7	83	82.5	
Ehsani					
β-TT	94.8	73.5	80.2	92.5	68.3
IDA	73.5	94.8	92.5	80.2	
England and Fraser					
β-TT	66.2	85.3	83.6	69	51.4
IDA	85.3	66.2	69	83.6	
Ricerca					
β-TT	100	14.7	57	100	14.7
IDA	14.7	100	100	57	
MDHL					
β-TT	76	58.8	76.6	69	34.8
IDA	58.8	76	69	76.6	
MCHD					
β-TT	77.9	27.9	55	52.7	5.8
IDA	27.9	77.9	52.7	55	

correctly diagnose 94.7% and 92.9% of cases, respectively, and both are easy to calculate [11]. Similar results (Mentzer index: sensitivity, 90.9%; specificity, 80.3%) were found by Ghafouri et al. [19]. Their results overlapped those of our study.

Rahim and Keikhaei examined the diagnostic accuracy of 10 indices in 153 patients with β-TT and 170 patients with IDA. According to Youden's index, the Shine and Lal index and RBC count showed the greatest diagnostic value in patients < 10 years (89% and 82%, resp.). They found that the Mentzer index had 85% sensitivity, 93% specificity, and 79% Youden's index [20].

In 2007, Ntaios et al. reported that the Green and King index was the most reliable index, as it had the highest sensitivity (75.06%), efficiency (80.12%), and Youden's index

(70.86%) for detecting β-TT [21]. A similar result for the Green and King index (Youden's index, 80.9%) was found by Urrechaga et al. [2]. However, studies in pediatric age groups are scarce, and their results are conflicting. It may be that interpopulation differences in the effectiveness of various RBC indices for discriminating β-TT from IDA could be attributed to differences in the mutation spectrum of the thalassemia disease in different populations [22].

The diagnosis of β-TT involves measuring the HbA_2 concentration of lysed RBCs via HPLC. The HbA_2 analysis is considered the gold standard for diagnosing thalassemia. Several studies have shown that iron deficiency directly affects the rates of HbA_2 synthesis in bone marrow; therefore, 16–20 weeks of iron therapy should be instituted, after which

TABLE 5: Red cell values at various ages of study groups and mean and lower limit of normal (−2 SD).

Age	Hemoglobin (g/dL) Mean ± SD (range)	Hemoglobin (g/dL) Mean and lower limit of normal (−2 SD)	MCV (fL) Mean ± SD (range)	MCV (fL) Mean and lower limit of normal (−2 SD)
Female				
0.5–2 years	10.06 ± 0.73 (9.0–11.4)	12.0 (10.5)	63.79 ± 4.24 (56.62–69.74)	78 (70)
2–6 years	10.17 ± 0.74 (8.9–11.6)	12.5 (11.5)	62.09 ± 5.42 (49.0–69.90)	81 (75)
6–12 years	10.42 ± 0.78 (8.9–11.4)	13.5 (11.5)	62.80 ± 5.80 (53.4–77.3)	86 (77)
12–18 years	10.15 ± 0.99 (8.9–11.6)	14.0 (12.0)	65.71 ± 5.23 (56.8–71.9)	90 (78)
Male				
0.5–2 years	10.16 ± 0.74 (8.9–11.3)	12.0 (10.5)	69.90 ± 3.85 (57.0–69.4)	78 (70)
2–6 years	10.38 ± 0.75 (8.9–11.5)	12.5 (11.5)	60.92 ± 5.0 (52.0–69.7)	81 (75)
6–12 years	10.72 ± 0.71 (9.0–11.4)	13.5 (11.5)	63.25 ± 6.03 (56.7–74.3)	86 (77)
12–18 years	10.78 ± 0.78 (8.9–11.4)	14.5 (13.0)	62.46 ± 3.59 (59.6–68.7)	88 (78)

Hb: hemoglobin; MCV: mean corpuscular volume; SD: standard deviation.
From [24].

a repeat serum iron with electrophoresis is done to confirm improvement in the HbA_2 levels [23].

5. Conclusion

In conclusion, the cell-count-based indices, particularly the Mentzer index, are easily available and reliable methods for detecting β-TT. According to our results, the percentage of correctly diagnosed patients was the highest with the Mentzer index (91%) followed by the Ehsani et al. index (84.8%). The third highest one was RBC count (83.4%). Cell-count-based parameters and formulas, particularly the MCV and RBC counts and their related indices (Mentzer index and Ehsani et al. index), have good discrimination ability in diagnosing β-TT.

Ethical Approval

Signed informed consent was obtained from the parents of study subjects. The study was done according to the rules of the Local Ethics Committee of Faculty of Medicine, Bezmialem Vakif University, Turkey.

Conflict of Interests

The authors declare that there is no conflict of interests regarding the publication of this paper.

References

[1] D. A. Rathod, A. Kaur, V. Patel et al., "Usefulness of cell counter-based parameters and formulas in detection of β-thalassemia trait in areas of high prevalence," *American Journal of Clinical Pathology*, vol. 128, no. 4, pp. 585–589, 2007.

[2] E. Urrechaga, L. Borque, and J. F. Escanero, "The role of automated measurement of RBC subpopulations in differential diagnosis of microcytic anemia and β-thalassemia screening," *American Journal of Clinical Pathology*, vol. 135, no. 3, pp. 374–379, 2011.

[3] C. Thomas and L. Thomas, "Biochemical markers and hematologic indices in the diagnosis of functional iron deficiency," *Clinical Chemistry*, vol. 48, no. 7, pp. 1066–1076, 2002.

[4] W. C. Mentzer Jr., "Differentiation of iron deficiency from thalassaemia trait," *The Lancet*, vol. 1, no. 7808, p. 882, 1973.

[5] I. Shine and S. Lal, "A strategy to detect β thalassaemia minor," *The Lancet*, vol. 1, no. 8013, pp. 692–694, 1977.

[6] J. M. England and P. M. Fraser, "Differentiation of iron deficiency from thalassaemia trait by routine blood-count," *The Lancet*, vol. 1, no. 7801, pp. 449–452, 1973.

[7] P. C. Srivastava, "Differentiation of thalassemia minor from iron deficiency," *The Lancet*, vol. 2, pp. 154–155, 1973.

[8] R. Green and R. King, "A new red cell discriminant incorporating volume dispersion for differentiating iron deficiency anemia from thalassemia minor," *Blood Cells*, vol. 15, no. 3, pp. 481–495, 1989.

[9] B. M. Ricerca, S. Storti, G. d'Onofrio et al., "Differentiation of iron deficiency from thalassaemia trait: a new approach," *Haematologica*, vol. 72, no. 5, pp. 409–413, 1987.

[10] M. Sirdah, I. Tarazi, E. Al Najjar, and R. Al Haddad, "Evaluation of the diagnostic reliability of different RBC indices and formulas in the differentiation of the β-thalassaemia minor from iron deficiency in Palestinian population," *International Journal of Laboratory Hematology*, vol. 30, no. 4, pp. 324–330, 2008.

[11] M. A. Ehsani, E. Shahgholi, M. S. Rahiminejad, F. Seighali, and A. Rashidi, "A new index for discrimination between iron deficiency anemia and beta-thalassemia minor: results in 284 patients," *Pakistan Journal of Biological Sciences*, vol. 12, no. 5, pp. 473–475, 2009.

[12] O. A. Telmissani, S. Khalil, and T. R. George, "Mean density of hemoglobin per liter of blood: a new hematologic parameter with an inherent discriminant function," *Laboratory Haematology*, vol. 5, pp. 149–152, 1999.

[13] A. Mosca, R. Paleari, G. Ivaldi, R. Galanello, and P. C. Giordano, "The role of haemoglobin A(2) testing in the diagnosis of thalassaemias and related haemoglobinopathies," *Journal of Clinical Pathology*, vol. 62, no. 1, pp. 13–17, 2009.

[14] E. J. Harthoorn-Lasthuizen, J. Lindemans, and M. M. A. C. Langenhuijsen, "Influence of iron deficiency anaemia on

haemoglobin A(2) levels: possible consequences for β-thalassaemia screening," *Scandinavian Journal of Clinical and Laboratory Investigation*, vol. 59, no. 1, pp. 65–70, 1999.

[15] A. Demir, N. Yaralı, T. Fısgın, F. Duru, and A. Kara, "Most reliable indices in differentiation between thalassemia trait and iron deficiency anemia," *Pediatrics International*, vol. 44, no. 6, pp. 612–616, 2002.

[16] D. Aslan and Ç. Altay, "Incidence of high erythrocyte count in infants and young children with iron deficiency anemia: reevaluation of an old parameter," *Journal of Pediatric Hematology/Oncology*, vol. 25, no. 4, pp. 303–306, 2003.

[17] M. Ferrara, L. Capozzi, R. Russo, F. Bertocco, and D. Ferrara, "Reliability of red blood cell indices and formulas to discriminate between β thalassemia trait and iron deficiency in children," *Hematology*, vol. 15, no. 2, pp. 112–115, 2010.

[18] S. M. AlFadhli, A. M. Al-Awadhi, and D. AlKhaldi, "Validity assessment of nine discriminant functions used for the differentiation between Iron deficiency anemia and thalassemia minor," *Journal of Tropical Pediatrics*, vol. 53, no. 2, pp. 93–97, 2007.

[19] M. Ghafouri, L. Mostaan Sefat, and L. Sharifi, "Comparison of cell counter indices in differention of beta thalassemia trait and iron deficiency anemia," *The Scientific Journal of Iranian Blood Transfusion Organization*, vol. 2, no. 7, pp. 385–389, 2006.

[20] F. Rahim and B. Keikhaei, "Better differential diagnosis of iron deficiency anemia from beta-thalassemia trait," *Turkish Journal of Hematology*, vol. 26, no. 3, pp. 138–145, 2009.

[21] G. Ntaios, A. Chatzinikolaou, Z. Saouli et al., "Discrimination indices as screening tests for β-thalassemic trait," *Annals of Hematology*, vol. 86, no. 7, pp. 487–491, 2007.

[22] C. Rosatelli, G. B. Leoni, T. Tuveri et al., "Heterozygous β-thalassemia: relationship between the hematological phenotype and the type of β-thalassemia mutation," *American Journal of Hematology*, vol. 39, no. 1, pp. 1–4, 1992.

[23] I. El-Agouza, A. Abu Shahla, and M. Sirdah, "The effect of iron deficiency anaemia on the levels of haemoglobin subtypes: possible consequences for clinical diagnosis," *Clinical and Laboratory Haematology*, vol. 24, no. 5, pp. 285–289, 2002.

[24] P. R. Dallman, "Blood and blood-forming tissue," in *Pediatrics*, A. Rudolph, Ed., Appleton-Century-Crofts, Norwalk, Conn, USA, 16th edition, 1977.

16

Prevalence and Predictors of Maternal Anemia during Pregnancy in Gondar, Northwest Ethiopia: An Institutional Based Cross-Sectional Study

Mulugeta Melku,[1] Zelalem Addis,[2] Meseret Alem,[3] and Bamlaku Enawgaw[4]

[1] *Department of Hematology, School of Biomedical and Laboratory Sciences, College of Medicine and Health Sciences, University of Gondar, P.O. Box 196, 6200 Gondar, Ethiopia*

[2] *Department of Medical Microbiology, School of Biomedical and Laboratory Sciences, College of Medicine and Health Sciences, University of Gondar, 6200 Gondar, Ethiopia*

[3] *Department of Immunology and Molecular Biology, School of Biomedical and Laboratory Sciences, College of Medicine and Health Sciences, University of Gondar, 6200 Gondar, Ethiopia*

[4] *Department of Hematology, School of Biomedical and Laboratory Sciences, College of Medicine and Health Sciences, University of Gondar, 6200 Gondar, Ethiopia*

Correspondence should be addressed to Mulugeta Melku; mulugeta.melku@gmail.com

Academic Editor: Aurelio Maggio

Background. Anaemia is a global public health problem which has an eminence impact on pregnant mother. The aim of this study was to assess the prevalence and predictors of maternal anemia. *Method.* A cross-sectional study was conducted from March 1 to April 30, 2012, on 302 pregnant women who attended antenatal care at Gondar University Hospital. Interview-based questionnaire, clinical history, and laboratory tests were used to obtain data. Bivariate and multivariate logistic regression was used to identify predictors. *Result.* The prevalence of anemia was 16.6%. Majority were mild type (64%) and morphologically normocytic normochromic (76%) anemia. Anemia was high at third trimester (18.9%). Low family income (AOR [95% CI] = 3.1 [1.19, 8.33]), large family size (AOR [95% CI] = 4.14 [4.13, 10.52]), *hookworm* infection (AOR [95% CI] = 2.72 [1.04, 7.25]), and *HIV* infection (AOR [95% CI] = 5.75 [2.40, 13.69]) were independent predictors of anemia. *Conclusion.* The prevalence of anemia was high; mild type and normocytic normochromic anemia was dominant. Low income, large family size, *hookworm* infection, and HIV infection were associated with anemia. Hence, efforts should be made for early diagnosis and management of *HIV* and *hookworm* infection with special emphasis on those having low income and large family size.

1. Background

Anaemia is a global public health problem affecting both developing and developed countries with major consequences for human health as well as social and economic development which results in a loss of billions of dollars annually [1–3]. According to the 2008 World Health Organization (WHO) report, anaemia affected 1.62 billion (24.8%) people globally [2]. It had an estimated global prevalence of 42% in pregnant women and is a major cause of maternal mortality [4, 5]. In Africa, 57.1% of the pregnant women were anemic. Moreover, anemia in pregnant women is a severe

public health problem in Ethiopia; 62.7% of pregnant women were anemic [2]. Although the prevalence varies widely in different settings and accurate data are often lacking, in resource-limited areas terribly significant proportions of women of childbearing age particularly pregnant are anaemic [3]. Geographically, those living in Asia and Africa are at the greatest risk [1].

The effect of anemia during pregnancy on maternal and neonatal life ranges from varying degrees of morbidity to mortality. As many studies elucidated, severe anemia (Hg < 7 g/L) during pregnancy has been associated with major maternal and fetal complications. It increases the risk of preterm delivery [6, 7], low birth weight [6–9], intrauterine fetal death [7], neonatal death [10], maternal mortality [11], and infant mortality [12].

Anemia is multifactorial in etiology; the disease is thought to be mainly caused by iron deficiency in developing countries. In sub-Saharan Africa where iron deficiency is common, the prevalence of anemia has often been used as a proxy for iron deficiency anemia (IDA) [3]. Other micronutrient deficiency (vitamins A and B12, riboflavin, and folic acid) has also been a cause of anemia during pregnancy [13]. Likewise, Infectious diseases such as malaria, helminthes infestations, and HIV are also implicated with high prevalence of anemia in sub-Saharan Africa [14, 15]. There was also a considerable variation in the prevalence of pregnancy anemia because of the differences in socioeconomic conditions, lifestyles, and health seeking behaviors of different population across different countries and cultures and obstetrics and gynecological related condition of pregnant mothers [16–41].

Since anaemia during pregnancy has a deleterious consequences, WHO adopted reducing maternal mortality as one of the three health-related millennium development goals so that international community is committing within this framework to reduce maternal mortality by three quarter at the end of 2015 [42]. Anemia prevalence data remains an important indicator of public health since anemia is related to morbidity and mortality in the population groups usually considered to be the most vulnerable like pregnant women. At a global level, anemia prevalence is a useful indicator to assess the impact of widespread or highly effective interventions and to track the progress made towards the goal of reducing anemia during pregnancy [43]. Anemia prevalence study is also useful to monitor the progress of reproductive health [2]. Despite the efforts made to reduce the burden, its prevalence has not been studied yet comprehensively in developing countries. Thus, the objective of this study was to determine the prevalence and predictors of anemia among pregnant women who attended ANC in Gondar University Hospital.

2. Methods

2.1. Study Population, Sample Size, and Sampling Procedure.
The study population was pregnant mothers attending antenatal care (ANC) at Gondar University Teaching Hospital. The hospital is found in Gondar town under Amhara regional state of Ethiopia which is located at 750 Km far from Addis Ababa, the capital city of Ethiopia, to the Northwest part of the country. The town is situated at an altitude of 2100 to 2870 meters above the sea level. According to the 2007 Ethiopian census report, Gondar has a total population of 206 and 987 and more than half (108, 902) of them are females [44].

A single population proportion formula, $[n = (Z\alpha/2)^2 p(1 - p)/d^2]$, was used to estimate the sample size. However, due to the lack of previous studies about the prevalence of anemia during pregnancy in this particular area, 50% prevalence was used for calculation. By reviewing the records of daily flow of pregnant women for ANC utilization, about 1410 pregnant women were estimated

to visit ANC clinic during the study period. Since the population during the study period was below 10,000, the sample correction formula was applied. Then, a total of 302 pregnant women who attended ANC service were selected using systematic random sampling technique from their sequence of ANC visit in the period between March and April, 2012, for two months.

2.2. Data Collection.
A face-to-face interview using structured pretested questionnaire was employed to obtain data about sociodemographic, obstetric, and gynecological, dietary intake, and medical conditions of pregnant mothers. As for the current pregnancy, intake of haematinics, gestational age, ante partum hemorrhage, and dietary intake were documented. Blood pressure, weight, and height were measured and body mass index (BMI) was calculated as (weight (kg)/height (m^2)). Women were then categorized into four groups according to their BMI as follows: underweight (BMI $\leq 20 \text{ kg/m}^2$), normal ($20 \text{ kg/m}^2 \leq \text{BMI} \leq 24.9 \text{ kg/m}^2$), overweight (BMI of $25 \text{ kg/m}^2 \leq \text{BMI} \leq 29.9 \text{ kg/m}^2$), and obese (BMI $\geq 30 \text{ kg/m}^2$) [23]. A total of 6 mL venous blood sample was obtained from each participant. Of this, 3 mL of it was drawn into ethylene diamine tetraacetic acid tube for complete blood count whereas the remaining 3 mL was drawn to plane tube for serological tests. Participants were also requested to give fresh stool sample for parasitological examination of intestinal parasitosis.

2.3. Laboratory Analysis.
Complete blood count including red blood cell count, hemoglobin concentration (Hgb), mean cell volume (MCV), mean cell hemoglobin (MCH), and mean cell hemoglobin concentration (MCHC), platelet count, and white blood cell count were carried out using SYXMEX KX-21 haematology analyzer (Sysmex Corporation Kobe, Japan). A thin and thick blood film had been prepared and stained with Giemsa stain for the detection and speciation of *Plasmodium* parasite species. Stool wet mount was prepared using saline and/or iodine and examined microscopically for identification of intestinal helminthes and protozoa parasitosis. All stool samples were processed within 30 minutes of collection. Serum and/or plasma samples were tested for HIV following the current HIV1/2 testing algorism using KHB (Shanghai Kehua bio-engineering Co., LTD., China), Statpack (Chembio Diagnostic Systems, Inc., New york, USA), and Uni-gold (Trinity Biotech Plc, Bray, Ireland). Syphilis reactivity was also tested using RPR test (Human GmbH-Wiesbaden, Germany) as per the manufacturer's instruction and recommendation.

2.4. Assessment of Anemia.
Hgb cutoff value adjusted to sea level altitude was used to define anemia on the basis of gestational age and to classify the degree of severity using WHO criteria. The Hgb value less than 11.0 g/dL at first and third trimesters and less than 10.5 g/dL at second trimester was used to define anemia. Based on the severity, women with Hgb value of ($10 \text{ g/dL} \leq \text{Hgb} < 11 \text{ g/dL}$) at first and third trimesters and ($10 \text{ g/dL} \leq \text{Hgb} < 10.5 \text{ g/dL}$) at second trimester were classified as mild anemic. Pregnant

women who had a Hgb value of ($7\,\text{g/dL} \leq \text{Hgb} < 10\,\text{g/dL}$) and ($\text{Hgb} < 7\,\text{g/dL}$) were categorized as moderate and severe anemic, respectively, regardless of their gestational age [45]. Manufacturer references were used to define the normal ranges for MCV (80.0–100.0 fl), MCH (27.0–33.5 pg), and MCHC (32.0–36.0 g/dL).

2.5. Data Processing and Analysis. Data were entered to EPI info version 3.5.3 and then transferred to SPSS version 20 statistical package for analysis. Descriptive and summary statistics were carried out using percentages and mean ± SD and were presented in tables and graphs. Binary logistic regression analysis was conducted to evaluate the difference in anemia prevalence across the relevant variables. Odds ratio, Chi-square, and 95% CI for odds ratio were computed to assess the strength of association and statistical significance in bivariate analysis. Independent variables having *P* less than or equal to 0.2 in univariate analysis were included in multivariate analysis to control confounders in regression models. Variables having *P* value less than 0.05 in multivariate binary logistic regression model were considered to be statistically significant.

2.6. Ethical Clearance. The study was approved by institutional review board of University of Gondar. The purpose and importance of the study were explained to each study participants. Written consent was obtained from each woman. To ensure confidentiality of participants, information, anonymous typing was used whereby the name of the participants and any participants' identifier were not written on the questionnaire, and, also during the interview to keep the privacy, they were interviewed alone. Results were communicated with clinicians working in ANC unit for appropriate management.

3. Result

3.1. Characteristics of the Study Participants. A total of 302 pregnant women with a mean (±SD) age of 26.47 ± 5.24 years were included in the study. The majority 242 (80.1%), 284 (94%), 250 (82.8%), and 194 (64.2%) were urban dwellers, married, had attended primary school and above, and house wives by occupation, respectively. The average monthly income of the participants was 1860 Ethiopian Birr (EB) and 147 (48.7%) were living with three to four family members (Table 1).

Concerning obstetrical history, 57.3% were multigravida, of whom 52.7% had an interpregnancy interval of more than or equal to 24 months and 23.7% experienced abortion. Nearly 70% of the study participants were at third trimester. Assessment of medical condition of the participant revealed that 72.5% had a normal BMI, 95.4% had no history of chronic diseases, and 4.6% had history of previous surgery. Laboratory investigation showed that 10.3% and 26.5% of the participants were reactive for HIV and infected with one or more than one intestinal parasites, respectively. *A. lumbricoides* (34.1%), *hookworm* (25.3%), and *E. histolytica/dispar* (17.2%) were the predominant parasites found (Table 2).

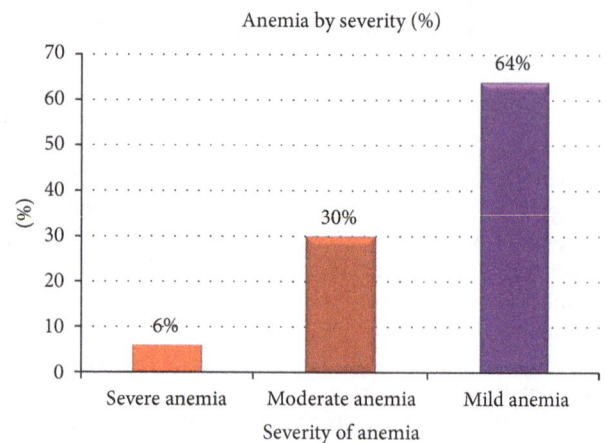

FIGURE 1: Percentage of anemia by severity among anemic pregnant women (*n* = 50).

The dietary habit and nutritional assessment revealed 19.8% did not take animal products in their current pregnancy, and 42.4% had a habit of eating green vegetables on monthly and above basis. About 80.1% had a habit of drinking coffee and tea after meal (data not shown). In their current pregnancy, 44.7%, 41.4%, and 7.3% took iron sulfate, folic acid, and multivitamin tables as nutritional supplement, respectively (Table 3).

3.2. Prevalence and Predictors of Anemia. The mean Hgb level of pregnant women was 11.96 ± 1.37 g/dL (range: 5.85–17.05 g/dL) and the overall prevalence of maternal anemia was 16.6% (*n* = 50). Of the anemic women, 6%, 30%, and 64% were severely, moderately, and mildly anemic, respectively (Figure 1).

Based on red blood cell morphologic classification of anemia, of the total anemic pregnant mothers, 76% had normocytic normochromic anemia and 14% had microcytic hypochromic type of anemia (Table 4).

High prevalence of anemia was observed in those pregnant women who were living with more than four family members (36.4%), illiterate (25.7%), and whose monthly family income < 1000EB (22%) (Table 1). In addition, high prevalence rate of anemia was found among mothers who were HIV seropositive (38.7%), infected with *hookworm* (34.8%), underweighted (30%), with more than four gravidae (32.3%), having chronic disease (27.3%), and at 3rd trimester (18.9%) (Table 2).

The prevalence of anemia among those who had a habit of eating animal products in their food stuff, not having a habit of eating vegetable, and who take tea/coffee after meal was 17.8%, 22.4%, and 15.3%, respectively. About 18.6% and 17.5% pregnant women who did not take iron sulphate and folate as nutritional therapy, respectively, were anemic (Table 3).

In bivariate analysis illiteracy, low monthly family income, large family size, underweight, gravidity, *hookworm* infection, and HIV seropositivity were significantly associated with maternal anemia. But in multivariate logistic regression analysis controlling the possible cofounders, only

TABLE 1: Sociodemographic characteristics of pregnant women and prevalence of anemia by sociodemographic characteristics (n = 302).

Variable	Anemia		Total (%)	COR (95% CI)
	Yes	No		
Age				
year	23 (15.8)	123 (84.2)	146 (48.3)	1
25–29 years	13 (15.9)	69 (84.1)	82 (27.2)	1.01 (0.48, 2.11)
≥30 years	14 (18.9)	60 (81.1)	74 (24.5)	1.25 (0.6, 2.60)
Residence				
Rural	11 (18.3)	49 (81.7)	60 (19.9)	1.17 (0.56, 2.45)
Urban	39 (16.1)	203 (83.9)	242 (80.1)	1
Marital status				
Married	47 (16.5)	237 (83.5)	284 (94)	1
Others*	3 (16.7)	15 (83.3)	18 (6)	1.01 (0.28, 3.62)
Maternal educational status				
Illiterate	18 (25.7)	52 (71.3)	70 (23.2)	3.31 (1.29, 8.54)*
Primary school	5 (9.4)	48 (90.6)	53 (17.5)	0.997 (0.30, 3.33)
Secondary school	20 (19)	85 (81)	105 (34.8)	2.25 (0.89–5.65)
Tertiary	7 (9.5)	67 (90.5)	74 (24.5)	1
Occupation				
House wife	38 (19.6)	156 (80.4)	194 (64.2)	2.27 (0.91, 5.67)
Government employed	6 (9.7)	56 (90.3)	62 (20.5)	1
Other**	6 (13)	40 (87)	46 (15.2)	1.4 (0.42, 4.65)
Family monthly income				
EB	30 (21.9)	107 (78.1)	137 (45.4)	3.22 (1.28, 8.13)*
1000–2575 EB	14 (15.6)	76 (84.4)	90 (29.8)	2.12 (0.77, 5.81)
EB	6 (8)	69 (92)	75 (24.8)	1
Family size				
≤2	16 (13.10)	106 (86.9)	122 (40.4)	
3-4	22 (15)	125 (85)	147 (48.7)	1.17 (0.58, 2.34)
≥5	12 (36.4)	21 (63.6)	33 (10.9)	3.79 (1.56, 9.17)*

Significant (P < 0.05) in bivariate analysis; other include single, divorced, and widowed; other** include private employed, farmers, merchants, and students.

low monthly family income (AOR = 3.15, 95% CI: 1.19, 8.33), large family size (AOR = 4.13, 95% CI: 1.62, 10.52), *hookworm* infection (AOR = 5.75, 95% CI: 2.40, 13.69), and HIV seropositivity (AOR = 2.72, 95% CI: 1.014, 7.25) remained being independent predictors of pregnancy anemia (Table 5).

4. Discussion

The overall prevalence of anemia was 16.6% (95%CI (12.6, 20.6)). This prevalence was comparable to studies conducted in Trinidad and Tobago (15.3%) [16], Thailand (20.1%) [17], Zurich (18.5%) [45], Hawassa (15.3%) [39], and Gondar town (22%) [46].

The prevalence is considerably lower than previous study reports from Malaysia (35%), Jordan (34.7%), Vietnam (43.2%), Southeastern Nigeria (76.9%), Eastern Sudan (62.6%), and Jimma, Ethiopia (38.2%) [22, 23, 25, 35, 38, 41]. The possible reason for the difference may be resulted from geographical variation of factors across different areas. In addition, lower prevalence can be attributed to gradual improvement of life style and living standards and health seeking behavior by the effort of government to achieve the

Millennium development goal aimed to reduce the maternal mortality by three-quarter by year 2015. In support of this argument, the prevalence of anemia in women of age 15–49 years had decreased from 27% in 2005 to 17% by the year 2011 in Ethiopia [47].

In this study, mild anemia was common followed by moderate anemia. This is consistent with reports from Africa and elsewhere in the world [23, 25, 29, 31, 39]. This study tried to demonstrate the common morphological characteristic of anemia among pregnant mothers. Of the total anemic pregnant women, 76% had normocytic normochromic anemia followed by microcytic hypochromic type which is in agreement with a report from Turkey [18] and Azezo, Gondar town [46].

This study demonstrated that mothers who have low monthly family income were three times more likely to be anemic as compared to those with high monthly family income. This is in agreement with some studies [24, 29] and contradicted to other reports [22, 23, 40, 41]. According to the 2007 Ethiopian central statistical agency household income consumption and expenditure survey, more than 57% of the total expenditure is spent on food [48]. Moreover, in

TABLE 2: The prevalence of anemia according to the obstetrics and medical factors (n = 302).

Variable	Anemic		Total (%)	COR (95% CI)
	Yes (%)	No (%)		
Gravidity				
Primigravidae	15 (11.6)	114 (88.4)	129 (42.7)	1
Secundigravidae	11 (14.3)	66 (85.7)	77 (25.5)	1.27 (0.55, 2.92)
3-4 gravidae	14 (21.5)	51 (78.5)	65 (21.5)	2.09 (0.94, 4.65)
≥5 gravidae	10 (32.3)	21 (67.7)	31 (10.3)	3.62 (1.43, 9.17)*
History of abortion				
Yes	8 (19.5)	33 (80.5)	41 (23.7)	0.94 (0.391, 2.27)
No	27 (20.4)	105 (79.6)	132 (76.3)	1
Interpregnancy interval				
1st pregnancy	15 (11.6)	114 (88.4)	129 (42.7)	1
	2 (14.3)	12 (85.7)	14 (4.6)	1.27 (0.26, 6.21)
≥24 months	33 (20.8)	126 (79.2)	159 (52.7)	2 (1.03, 3.86)
Gestational age				
1st trimester	1 (12.5)	7 (87.5)	8 (2.6)	1
2nd	12 (12.2)	86 (87.8)	98 (32.5)	0.98 (0.11, 8.62)
3rd	37 (18.9)	159 (81.1)	196 (64.9)	1.63 (0.19, 13.65)
Body mass index				
Underweight	9 (30)	21 (70)	30 (10)	2.42 (1.03, 5.64)*
Normal and above	41 (15.1)	231 (84.9)	272 (90)	1
Presence of chronic disease				
Yes	4 (27.3)	11 (72.7)	14 (4.6)	1.4 (0.38, 5.21)
No	47 (16.3)	241 (83.7)	288 (95.4)	1
Presence of peptic ulcer disease				
Yes	20 (18.3)	89 (81.7)	109 (36.1)	1.22 (0.66, 2.27)
No	30 (15.5)	163 (84.5)	193 (63.9)	1
History of previous surgery				
Yes	2 (14.3)	12 (85.7)	14 (4.6)	0.83 (0.181, 3.84)
No	48 (16.7)	240 (83.3)	288 (95.4)	1
Malaria attack in current pregnancy				
Yes	3 (20)	12 (80)	15 (5)	1.28 (0.347, 4.7)
No	47 (16.4)	240 (83.6)	287 (95)	1
Hookworm infection				
Yes	8 (34.8)	15 (65.2)	23 (7.6)	3.01 (1.20, 7.52)*
No	42 (15.1)	237 (84.9)	279 (92.4)	1
HIV infection				
Reactive	12 (38.7)	19 (61.3)	31 (10.3)	3.87 (1.74, 8.62)*
Nonreactive	38 (14)	233 (86)	271 (89.7)	1
Syphilis				
Reactive	3 (27.3)	8 (72.7)	11 (3.6)	1.95 (0.5, 7.61)
Nonreactive	47 (16.2)	244 (83.8)	291 (96.4)	1

*Significant (P < 0.05) in bivariate analysis. Chronic disease comprises hypertension, kidney disease, cardiac problems, and diabetes mellitus.

this study, 80% of study participants were from urban area suggesting that they are food net buyers. As income is low, the expenditure for food becomes low. Besides, due to food price inflation, the purchasing power of income is low. So, low income groups did not get adequate nutrition and thereby low family income groups were at risk of anemia.

According to the results of our study, pregnant mothers who had been living within a family of more than four members were more likely to be anemic compared to those living with ≤ 2 family members. Nevertheless, in Jordan [23], there was no significant difference of anemia prevalence between groups of pregnant mothers living with varying family sizes. This difference may be attributed as in Jordan case; the study was undertaken in rural district where there was not great variation in family size and income. But, in this study, 80% of pregnant women were in urban areas having

TABLE 3: Prevalence of anemia in relation to dietary habit, ANC followup, and nutrient supplementation at their current pregnancy period (n = 302).

Variable	Anemia		Total (N = 302)	COR (95% CI)
	Yes	No		
Eating meat and animal products				
Yes	43 (17.8)	199 (82.2)	242 (80.1)	1
No	7 (11.7)	53 (88.3)	60 (19.9)	0.61 (0.26, 1.44)
Eating green leafy vegetables				
Yes	39 (15.4)	214 (84.6)	253 (83.8)	1.00
No	11 (22.4)	38 (77.6)	49 (16.2)	1.6 (0.75, 3.372)
Taking fruit after meal				
Yes	34 (16.6)	172 (83.5)	206 (68.2)	1
No	16 (16.7)	80 (83.3)	96 (31.8)	1.012 (0.53, 1.94)
Taking coffee or tea immediately after meal				
Yes	37 (15.3)	205 (84.7)	242 (80.1)	0.65 (0.32, 1.32)
No	13 (21.7)	47 (78.3)	60 (19.9)	1
ANC followup during current pregnancy				
Yes	28 (16.1)	146 (83.9)	174 (57.6)	1
No	22 (17.2)	106 (82.8)	128 (42.4)	1.08 (0.59, 1.99)
Iron sulphate table intake in current pregnancy				
Yes	19 (14.1)	116 (85.9)	135 (44.7)	1
No	31 (18.6)	136 (81.4)	167 (55.3)	1.39 (0.75, 2.59)
Folic acid intake in current pregnancy				
Yes	19 (15.2)	106 (84.8)	125 (41.4)	1
No	31 (17.5)	146 (82.5)	177 (58.6)	1.19 (0.64, 2.2)
Multivitamin intake in current pregnancy				
Yes	3 (13.6)	19 (86.4)	22 (7.3)	1
No	47 (16.8)	233 (83.2)	280 (92.7)	1.28 (0.36, 4.49)

TABLE 4: Distribution of morphologic type anemia among study participants.

Morphologic type of cells	Anemic status		
	Anemic	Not anemic	Total
	n (%)	n (%)	n (%)
Microcytic hypochromic (MCV < 80 fl, MCH < 27 pg)	8 (16%)	1 (0.4%)	9 (3.0%)
Normocytic Normochromic (MCV and MCH within the normal value)	38 (76%)	235 (93.2%)	273 (90.4%)
Macrocytic normochromic (MCV > 100 fl, MCH (27 pg < MCH < 33.5 pg))	2 (4%)	5 (1.98%)	7 (2.3%)
Other combinations	2 (4%)	11 (4.37%)	13 (4.3%)
Total	50 (16.6%)	252 (83.4%)	302 (100%)

varying income levels and 20% in rural areas with varying family size.

This study also showed that the proportion of anemia among pregnant women who had been infected with HIV was significantly higher compared to those noninfected that is six times at higher risk. This is in line with previous studies [29, 31–33, 35]. This increased prevalence of anemia among HIV seropositive pregnant women may be explained by the fact that HIV infection is associated with lower serum folate, vitamin B12, and ferritin in pregnancy [31]. In addition, Anemia in HIV/AIDS patients may arise from a number of causes, including deregulation of the host immune system leading to destruction or inhibition of hematopoietic cells [49].

In our study, *hookworm* has increased the risk of being anemic and this finding was consistent with other studies [26, 41, 46]. This is because adult *hookworm* parasites attach and injure upper intestinal mucosa and also ingest blood. This brings about gastrointestinal blood loss and induces depletion of iron, folic acid, and vitamin B12 that ultimately anemia [13, 50].

Even though it was not statistically significant in multivariate logistic regression (but significant in bivariate analysis), multigravida and grand gravida had high odds for anemia as compared to primigravidae. Likewise, studies in Malaysia [22], Burkina Faso [29], Sudan [38], and Jimma [41] reported that gravidity did not have statistically significant contribution for difference in anemia prevalence.

TABLE 5: Multivariate binary logistic regression analysis of pregnancy anemia with predictor variables ($n = 302$).

Variables	Anemia		Total	OR (95% CI)	
	Yes	No		COR (95% CI)	AOR (95% CI)
Maternal educational status					
Illiterate	18 (25.7)	52 (74.3)	70	**3.31 (1.29, 8.54)**	0.61 (0.14, 2.68)
Primary	5 (9.4)	48 (90.6)	53	0.997 (0.30, 3.33)	0.37 (0.08, 1.73)
Secondary	20 (19)	85 (81)	105	2.25 (0.89–5.65)	0.99 (0.30, 3.22)
Tertiary	7 (9.5)	67 (90.5)	74	1	1
Family income/month					
Low (<1000 birr)	30 (21.9)	107 (78.1)	137	3.22 (1.28, 8.13)	3.15 (1.19, 8.33)*
Medium (1000–2575 birr)	14 (15.6)	76 (84.4)	90	2.12 (0.77, 5.81)	1.80 (0.62, 5.18)
High (>2575 birr)	6 (8)	69 (92)	75	1	1
Family size					
≤2	16 (13.1)	106 (86.9)	122	1	1
3-4 members	22 (15)	125 (85)	147	1.17 (0.58, 2.34)	1.03 (0.49, 2.13)
≥5 members	12 (36.4)	21 (63.6)	33	3.78 (1.56, 9.17)	4.13 (1.62, 10.52)**
Body mass index					
Underweight (<20 kg/m^2)	9 (30)	21 (70)	30	**2.42 (1.03, 5.64)**	2.27 (0.83, 6.21)
Normal and above (≥20 kg/m^2)	41 (15.1)	231 (84.9)	272	1	1
Gravidity					
Primigravidae	15 (11.6)	114 (88.4)	129	1	1
Secungravidae	11 (14.3)	66 (85.7)	77	1.27 (0.55, 2.91)	1.1 (0.37, 3.08)
3-4 gravidae	14 (21.5)	51 (78.5)	65	2.09 (0.94, 4.65)	2.19 (0.68, 6.99)
≥5 gravidae	10 (32.3)	21 (67.7)	31	**3.62 (1.43, 9.17)**	1.87 (0.31, 11.36)
Hookwarm					
Yes	8 (34.8)	15 (65.2)	23	3.01 (1.2, 7.52)	2.72 (1.01, 7.25)*
No	42 (15.1)	237 (84.9)	279	1	1
HIV					
Yes	12 (38.7)	19 (61.3)	31	3.9 (1.74, 8.62)	5.75 (2.4, 13.69)***
No	38 (14)	233 (86)	271	1	1

Bold numerical values indicate significant in bivariate but not in multivariate analysis. *Significant ($P < 0.05$), **significant ($P < 0.01$), and ***highly significant ($P < 0.001$) in multivariate analysis.

Despite this, a study from Trinidad and Tiago, multigravida had significantly increased likelihood of being anemic than primigravidae [16]. The disparity may be as a result of sociodemographic characteristic difference between study participants. In this study, participants who were multigravida had the following characteristics. 90% had normal and above BMI, 78% were urban residents, and 50% of them had middle and high monthly family income. These situations may reduce the risk of anemia in multigravida pregnant mothers participated in this study.

In this study, supplementation of iron sulphate, folic acid, and multivitamin during the current pregnancy period did not significantly reduce the prevalence of anemia as compared to those who did not take these supplementations. The finding was in contradiction with other studies [19–21, 25, 26, 28]. The possible reason may be that, in anemic pregnant women, these nutritional supplements were more likely to be prescribed as an intervention for management of anemia in their previous ANC visit. This needs a further study to explicitly explain how much effective the current WHO nutritional supplementation recommendation program is being implemented for prevention and control of anaemia in pregnant women [51].

4.1. Limitations of the Study. One of the limitation of this study is the nature of the study design its self, being as a cross-sectional study design, it does not show which preceded anemia or risk factors. Due to constraint of time and resource, stool concentration technique and parasite density were not done so we could not assess the impact of parasite load on the severity of anemia. In addition to this, the low sensitivity of wet mount to detect parasite in patient with low parasite load may underestimate the prevalence of intestinal parasite and alter odds ratio. The other limitation is that this study was conducted at tertiary care hospital located at Gondar town and majority of the study participants were urban residents. But many of the pregnant women in that district were living in rural areas where access to antenatal facilities is limited, so the prevalence of anemia would have been even more if the study was done in the general population.

5. Conclusion

In conclusion, the prevalence of anemia among pregnant women was high especially at third trimester. Mild type of anemia was the commonest one. Morphologically, the predominant type of anemia was normocytic normochromic, followed by microcytic hypochromic anemia. Low family income, high family size, *hookworm* infection, and living with HIV/AIDS were the main predictors of maternal anemia. To reduce the prevalence, there is a need to strengthen health care seeking behavior of women to ensure early diagnosis and management of HIV, hookworm, anemia, and other medical conditions. There is also a need to encourage family planning, and design policies and strategies pertinent to reduction of anemia in low income groups. A large community based study needs to be done to determine the prevalence and predictors of anemia in the general population of pregnant women. Besides, further studies using micronutrient assay techniques which are sensitive for the detection of latent anemia before the change of RBC morphology and indices takes place have to be conducted.

Conflict of Interests

The authors declare that there is no conflict of interests regarding the publication of this paper.

Authors' Contribution

Mulugeta Melku participated in designing the study, performed the data collection and statistical analysis, and was a lead author of the paper. Zelalem Addis, Meseret Alem, and Bamlaku Enawgaw participated in designing the study and helped in drafting the paper. All authors read and approved the final paper.

Acknowledgments

The authors thank all midwives and laboratory staffs who heartfully participated during data collection and laboratory analysis activities. The authors are also grateful to thank pregnant women for their voluntary participation in our study. Lastly, they would like to thank the University of Gondar and Gondar University Hospital for financial and logistics supports.

References

[1] E. McLean, M. Cogswell, I. Egli, D. Wojdyla, and B. De Benoist, "Worldwide prevalence of anaemia, WHO Vitamin and Mineral Nutrition Information System, 1993–2005," *Public Health Nutrition*, vol. 12, no. 4, pp. 444–454, 2009.

[2] WHO, *Worldwide Prevalence of Anaemia 1993–2005: WHO Global Database on Anaemia*, WHO, Geneva, Switzerland, 2008.

[3] WHO and UNICEF, *Focusing on Anaemia: Towards an Integrated Approach for Effective Anaemia Control*, WHO, Geneva, Switzerland, 2004.

[4] Y. Balarajan, U. Ramakrishnan, E. Özaltin, A. H. Shankar, and S. V. Subramanian, "Anaemia in low-income and middle-income countries," *The Lancet*, vol. 378, no. 9809, pp. 2123–2135, 2011.

[5] WHO, UNICEF, UNFPA, and World Bank, *Maternal Mortality in 2005: Estimates Developed by WHO, UNICEF, UNFPA and World Bank*, WHO, Geneva, Switzerland, 2007.

[6] F. W. Lone, R. N. Qureshi, and F. Emanuel, "Maternal anaemia and its impact on perinatal outcome," *Tropical Medicine and International Health*, vol. 9, no. 4, pp. 486–490, 2004.

[7] F. W. Lone, R. N. Qureshi, and F. Emmanuel, "Maternal anaemia and its impact on perinatal outcome in a tertiary care hospital in Pakistan," *Eastern Mediterranean Health Journal*, vol. 10, no. 6, pp. 801–807, 2004.

[8] H. S. Lee, M. S. Kim, M. H. Kim, Y. J. Kim, and W. Y. Kim, "Iron status and its association with pregnancy outcome in Korean pregnant women," *European Journal of Clinical Nutrition*, vol. 60, no. 9, pp. 1130–1135, 2006.

[9] F. Bodeau-Livinec, V. Briand, J. Berger et al., "Maternal anemia in Benin: prevalence, risk factors, and association with low birth weight," *The American Journal of Tropical Medicine and Hygiene*, vol. 85, no. 3, pp. 414–420, 2011.

[10] T. Kousar, Y. Memon, S. Sheikh, S. Memon, and R. Sehto, "Risk factors and causes of death in Neonates," *Rawal Medical Journal*, vol. 35, no. 2, pp. 205–208, 2010.

[11] B. J. Brabin, M. Hakimi, and D. Pelletier, "An analysis of anemia and pregnancy-related maternal mortality," *Journal of Nutrition*, vol. 131, no. 2, pp. 604S–615S, 2001.

[12] T. Marchant, J. A. Schellenberg, R. Nathan et al., "Anaemia in pregnancy and infant mortality in Tanzania," *Tropical Medicine and International Health*, vol. 9, no. 2, pp. 262–266, 2004.

[13] Sight and Life, "Nutritional Anemia," SIGHT AND LIFE Press, 2007, http://www.sightandlife.org/fileadmin/data/Books/Nutritional_anemia_book.pdf.

[14] S. Ouédraogo, G. K. Koura, K. Accrombessi, F. Bodeau-Livinec, A. Massougbodji, and M. Cot, "Maternal anemia at first antenatal visit: prevalence and risk factors in a malaria-endemic area in Benin," *The American Journal of Tropical Medicine and Hygiene*, vol. 87, no. 3, pp. 418–424, 2012.

[15] K. Tolentino and J. F. Friedman, "An update on anemia in less developed countries," *The American Journal of Tropical Medicine and Hygiene*, vol. 77, no. 1, pp. 44–51, 2007.

[16] E. O. Uche-Nwachi, A. Odekunle, S. Jacinto et al., "Anaemia in pregnancy: associations with parity, abortions and child spacing in primary healthcare clinic attendees in Trinidad and Tobago," *African Health Sciences*, vol. 10, no. 1, pp. 66–70, 2010.

[17] B. Sukrat and S. Sirichotiyakul, "The prevalence and causes of anemia during pregnancy in Maharaj Nakorn Chiang Mai Hospital," *Journal of the Medical Association of Thailand*, vol. 89, supplement 4, pp. S142–S146, 2006.

[18] L. Karaoglu, E. Pehlivan, M. Egri et al., "The prevalence of nutritional anemia in pregnancy in an east Anatolian province, Turkey," *BMC Public Health*, vol. 10, article 329, 2010.

[19] M.-J. A. Brian, S. D. Leary, G. D. Smith, H. J. McArdle, and A. R. Ness, "Maternal anemia, iron intake in pregnancy, and offspring blood pressure in the avon longitudinal study of parents and children," *The American Journal of Clinical Nutrition*, vol. 88, no. 4, pp. 1126–1133, 2008.

[20] E. Fujimori, A. P. S. Sato, S. C. Szarfarc et al., "Anemia in Brazilian pregnant women before and after flour fortification with iron," *Revista de Saude Publica*, vol. 45, no. 6, pp. 1027–1035, 2011.

[21] S. Thirukkanesh and A. M. Zahara, "Compliance to vitamin and mineral supplementation among pregnant women in urban and rural areas in Malaysia," *Pakistan Journal of Nutrition*, vol. 9, no. 8, pp. 744–750, 2010.

[22] J. Haniff, A. Das, L. T. Onn et al., "Anemia in pregnancy in Malaysia: a cross-sectional survey," *Asia Pacific Journal of Clinical Nutrition*, vol. 16, no. 3, pp. 527–536, 2007.

[23] L. Al-Mehaisen, Y. Khader, O. Al-Kuran, F. Abu Issa, and Z. Amarin, "Maternal anemia in rural Jordan: room for improvement," *Anemia*, vol. 2011, Article ID 381812, 7 pages, 2011.

[24] R. Ayub, N. Tariq, M. M. Adil, M. Iqbal, T. Jaferry, and S. R. Rais, "Low haemoglobin levels, its determinants and associated features among pregnant women in Islamabad and surrounding region," *Journal of the Pakistan Medical Association*, vol. 59, no. 2, pp. 86–89, 2009.

[25] Q. Zhang, Z. Li, and C. V. Ananth, "Prevalence and risk factors for anaemia in pregnant women: a population-based prospective cohort study in China," *Paediatric and Perinatal Epidemiology*, vol. 23, no. 4, pp. 282–291, 2009.

[26] R. Aikawa, N. C. Khan, S. Sasaki, and C. W. Binns, "Risk factors for iron-deficiency anaemia among pregnant women living in rural Vietnam," *Public Health Nutrition*, vol. 9, no. 4, pp. 443–448, 2006.

[27] A. J. Rodríguez-Morales, R. A. Barbella, C. Case et al., "Intestinal parasitic infections among pregnant women in Venezuela," *Infectious Diseases in Obstetrics and Gynecology*, vol. 2006, Article ID 23125, 2006.

[28] D. A. Khan, S. Fatima, R. Imran, and F. A. Khan, "Iron, folate and cobalamin deficiency in anaemic pregnant females in tertiary care centre at Rawalpindi," *Journal of Ayub Medical College, Abbottabad*, vol. 22, no. 1, pp. 17–21, 2010.

[29] N. Meda, L. Mandelbrot, M. Cartoux, B. Dao, A. Ouangré, and F. Dabis, "Anaemia during pregnancy in Burkina Faso, West Africa, 1995-96: prevalence and associated factors," *Bulletin of the World Health Organization*, vol. 77, no. 11, pp. 916–922, 1999.

[30] D. Geelhoed, F. Agadzi, L. Visser et al., "Severe anemia in pregnancy in rural Ghana: a case-control study of causes and management," *Acta Obstetricia et Gynecologica Scandinavica*, vol. 85, no. 10, pp. 1165–1171, 2006.

[31] C. C. Dim and H. E. Onah, "The prevalence of anemia among pregnant women at booking in Enugu, South Eastern Nigeria," *Journal of Obstetrics and Gynaecology*, vol. 26, no. 8, pp. 773–776, 2006.

[32] O. Adesina, A. Oladokun, O. Akinyemi, T. Akingbola, O. Awolude, and I. Adewole, "Risk of anaemia in HIV positive pregnant women in Ibadan, South West Nigeria," *African Journal of Medicine and Medical Sciences*, vol. 40, no. 1, pp. 67–73, 2011.

[33] M. D. Dairo and T. O. Lawoyin, "Socio-demographic determinants of anaemia in pregnancy at primary care level: a study in urban and rural Oyo State, Nigeria," *African Journal of Medicine and Medical Sciences*, vol. 33, no. 3, pp. 213–217, 2004.

[34] D. J. VanderJagt, H. S. Brock, G. S. Melah, A. U. El-Nafaty, M. J. Crossey, and R. H. Glew, "Nutritional factors associated with anaemia in pregnant women in northern Nigeria," *Journal of Health, Population and Nutrition*, vol. 25, no. 1, pp. 75–81, 2007.

[35] C. J. Uneke, D. D. Duhlinska, and E. B. Igbinedion, "Prevalence and public-health significance of HIV infection and anaemia among pregnant women attending antenatal clinics in southeastern Nigeria," *Journal of Health, Population and Nutrition*, vol. 25, no. 3, pp. 328–335, 2007.

[36] E. A. Achidi, A. J. Kuoh, J. T. Minang et al., "Malaria infection in pregnancy and its effects on haemoglobin levels in women from a malaria endemic area of Fako Division, South West Province, Cameroon," *Journal of Obstetrics and Gynaecology*, vol. 25, no. 3, pp. 235–240, 2005.

[37] T. Marchant, J. R. M. Armstrong Schellenberg, T. Edgar et al., "Anaemia during pregnancy in southern Tanzania," *Annals of Tropical Medicine and Parasitology*, vol. 96, no. 5, pp. 477–487, 2002.

[38] I. Adam, A. H. Khamis, and M. I. Elbashir, "Prevalence and risk factors for anaemia in pregnant women of eastern Sudan," *Transactions of the Royal Society of Tropical Medicine and Hygiene*, vol. 99, no. 10, pp. 739–743, 2005.

[39] S. Gies, B. J. Brabin, M. A. Yassin, and L. E. Cuevas, "Comparison of screening methods for anaemia in pregnant women in Awassa, Ethiopia," *Tropical Medicine and International Health*, vol. 8, no. 4, pp. 301–309, 2003.

[40] S. Desalegn, "Prevalence of anaemia in pregnancy in Jima town, Southwestern Ethiopia," *Ethiopian Medical Journal*, vol. 31, no. 4, pp. 251–258, 1993.

[41] T. Belachew and Y. Legesse, "Risk factors for anemia among pregnant women attending antenatal clinic at Jimma University Hospital, southwest Ethiopia," *Ethiopian Medical Journal*, vol. 44, no. 3, pp. 211–220, 2006.

[42] United Nation, *United Nations Millennium Declaration: Resolution Adopted By the Geneal Assembly*, United Nation, Newyork, NY, USA, 2000.

[43] World Health Organization, "The World Health Report 2002: Reducing risks, promoting healthy life," 2002, http://www.who.int/whr/2002/en/whr02_en.pdf.

[44] CSA, *Summary and Statistical Report of the 2007 Population and Housing Census: Population Size By Age and Sex*, CSA, Addis Ababa, Ethiopia, 2008.

[45] WHO, *Haemoglobin Concentrations For the Diagnosis of Anaemia and Assessment of Severity, Vitamin and Mineral Nutrition Information System*, WHO, Geneva, Switzerland, 2011.

[46] M. Alem, B. Enawgaw, A. Gelaw, T. Kena, M. Seid, and Y. Olkeba, "Prevalence of anemia and associated risk factors among pregnant women attending antenatal care in Azezo Health Center Gondar town, Northwest Ethiopia," *Journal of Interdisciplinary Histopathology*, vol. 1, no. 3, pp. 137–144, 2013.

[47] CSA, *Ethiopia Demographic and Health Survey: Preliminary Report*, CSA, Addis Ababa, Ethiopia, 2011.

[48] CSA, *Household Income, Consumption and Expenditure (HICE) Survey 2004/5. Volume I: Analytical Report*, CSA, Addis Ababa, Ethiopia, 2007.

[49] D. H. Henry and J. A. Hoxie, "Hematologic manifestation of AIDS," in *Hematology: Basic Principles and Practices*, R. Hofman, E. Benz, S. Shattil et al., Eds., pp. 2585–2628, Churchill Livingstone, New York, NY, USA, 5th edition, 2008.

[50] S. Brooker, P. J. Hotez, and D. A. P. Bundy, "Hookworm-related anaemia among pregnant women: a systematic review," *PLoS Neglected Tropical Diseases*, vol. 2, no. 9, article e291, 2008.

[51] UNICEF, UNU, and WHO, *Iron Deficiency Anemia: Assessment, Prevention, and Control*, WHO, Geneva, Switzerland, 2001.

17

A Retrospective Study Investigating the Incidence and Predisposing Factors of Hospital-Acquired Anemia

Peter C. Kurniali,[1,2,3] **Stephanie Curry,**[1,2] **Keith W. Brennan,**[1,2] **Kim Velletri,**[1] **Mohammed Shaik,**[3] **Kenneth A. Schwartz,**[3] **and Elise McCormack**[1,2]

[1]*Department of Medicine, Roger Williams Medical Center, Providence, RI, USA*
[2]*Department of Medicine, Boston University School of Medicine, Boston, MA, USA*
[3]*Division of Hematology Oncology, Michigan State University and Breslin Cancer Center, 401 W. Greenlawn Avenue, Lansing, MI 48910, USA*

Correspondence should be addressed to Peter C. Kurniali; peter.kurniali@hc.msu.edu

Academic Editor: Duran Canatan

Hospitalized patients frequently have considerable volumes of blood removed for diagnostic testing which could lead to the development of hospital-acquired anemia. Low hemoglobin levels during hospitalization may result in significant morbidity for patients with underlying cardiorespiratory and other illnesses. We performed a retrospective study and data was collected using a chart review facilitated through an electronic medical record. A total of 479 patients who were not anemic during admission were included in analysis. In our study, we investigated the incidence of HAA and found that, between admission and discharge, 65% of patients dropped their hemoglobin by 1.0 g/dL or more, and 49% of patients developed anemia. We also found that the decrease in hemoglobin between admission and discharge did not differ significantly with smaller phlebotomy tubes. In multivariate analysis, we found that patients with longer hospitalization and those with lower BMI are at higher risk of developing HAA. In conclusion, our study confirms that hospital-acquired anemia is common. More aggressive strategies such as reducing the frequency of blood draws and expanding the use of smaller volume tubes for other laboratory panels may be helpful in reducing the incidence of HAA during hospitalization.

1. Introduction

Hospitalized patients frequently have considerable volumes of blood removed for diagnostic testing which may drop their hemoglobin and could lead to the development of hospital-acquired anemia (HAA) [1]. Although the cause of anemia associated with hospitalization is likely multifactorial, iatrogenic anemia due to phlebotomy has been described [1–3]. Low hemoglobin levels during hospitalization may result in significant morbidity for patients with underlying cardiorespiratory and other illnesses [2]. Packed red blood cell transfusion is usually required when the patients become symptomatic or when hemoglobin level is less than 7 g/dL, depending upon comorbid diseases. Blood products transfusion has the risks, including infectious and noninfectious complications [4–6]. Several strategies have been proposed in an attempt to reduce the risk of anemia due to phlebotomy, such as utilizing smaller volume blood tubes for diagnostic testing. However, there is limited research investigating whether a reduction in the size of the phlebotomy tube will reduce the incidence of anemia.

The primary objective of the study was to investigate the incidence of HAA. The impact of reducing the volume of blood taken from hospital patients by using smaller volume phlebotomy tubes on the decrease in hospitalized patients hemoglobin was investigated as a secondary objective. We hypothesized that, following the change in size to a smaller tube, the decrease in hemoglobin during hospitalization will be diminished when compared to a time period before use of the smaller volume tube was initiated.

2. Methods

2.1. Data Sources. A retrospective study on patients admitted to Roger Williams Medical Center (RWMC) in Providence, RI, was performed on hospital admissions between January 2011 and October 2011.

2.2. Reduction of Phlebotomy Tubes. On May 16, 2011, a new smaller phlebotomy tube was implemented at RWMC. The hospital changed the size of the tube used for collecting a basic metabolic panel (BMP) from an 8.5 mL tube (BD 367988) to a 4.5 mL tube (BD 367962), a reduction in volume of 4 mL. This permitted delineation of two separate study groups: those hospitalized before (group A) and those hospitalized after (group B) implementation of reduced volume blood collection tubes. Comparing these two groups allowed us to assess whether the volume of the phlebotomy tube affects the drop in hemoglobin for hospitalized patients.

2.3. Eligibility Criteria. We reviewed charts from patients admitted to the general internal medical floor at RWMC between January 2011 and October 2011. Patients over age of 18 admitted to internal medicine service during this period were included in the study. In order to determine whether the decrease in hemoglobin was related to the hospitalization or to their underlying illness, certain patients who met the following criteria were excluded from the study. Those patients who had acute medical conditions that may cause or contribute to the decrease in hemoglobin (including gastrointestinal bleeding, transfusion dependent anemia, a previous history of anemia, hemolysis, hemorrhagic stroke, retroperitoneal bleed, chronic kidney disease/dialysis, or any hematologic malignancy) or were treated with medications that may affect hemoglobin levels (including iron or erythropoietin or chemotherapy) were excluded. Those who had central or peripherally inserted central line placement, who received blood transfusion during hospitalization, and who were hospitalized for less than 2 days or were triaged to surgical, intensive care unit (ICU), cardiac care unit (CCU), and step-down unit (a transition unit for patients who were treated in the ICU or CCU) were also excluded. We also exclude patients who had hemoglobin in the anemic range (less than 13 g/dL for males and less than 12 g/dL for females according to the WHO criteria) on hospital admission.

2.4. Statistical Analysis. Data was collected using a chart review facilitated through an electronic medical record. Statistical analysis was done using chi-square test for categorical variable and *t*-test for numerical variable. Patients characteristics were compared based on age group (<65 years and ≥65 years) (Table 1).

In the first part of analysis, the incidence of anemia in hospitalized patients was analyzed using chi-square test. In the second part of analysis, the factors which can predict drop in hemoglobin were assessed using multiple regression analysis using drop of hemoglobin (continuous variable) as a dependent variable and age, race, body mass index (BMI), length of stay, BUN/creatinine, tube size (groups A

TABLE 1: Baseline characteristics of the patients.

	<65	≥65	P value
Patients who meet the inclusion criteria	224	255	
Sex			0.002
M	103 (46%)	83 (33%)	
F	121 (54%)	172 (67%)	
Race			0.001
Caucasian	167	231	
AA	21	7	
Hispanic	25	13	
Other	11	4	
Length of stay	2.92 ± 1.3	3.25 ± 1.6	0.01
Comorbidities			0.001
0	69	16	
1	57	45	
2	44	81	
3	33	55	
≥4	21	58	
Admission BUN	14.9 ± 6.5	22.07 ± 10	0.001
Admission creatinine	0.85 ± 0.2	0.94 ± 0.3	0.0009
BUN/creatinine ratio	18.05 ± 8.6	23.7 ± 8.17	0.0001

and B), and comorbidities (hypertension, diabetes mellitus, coronary artery disease, cerebrovascular disease, chronic kidney disease, dyslipidemia, peripheral arterial disease) as independent variables. We used backward selection technique, and the best-fit model was selected after adjusting all the confounding variables. The level of significance was set at $P < 0.05$ for variable in final model. Data were analyzed using the SAS 9.3 (the SAS Corporation, Inc., Cary, NC). Graphics were developed using Prism 6.04 (GraphPad Software, Inc., La Jolla, CA).

3. Results

3.1. Characteristics of the Patients. From January 2011 to October 2011, a total of 4206 hospitalizations to general medical floor were reviewed and 621 hospitalizations met the inclusion criteria. A total of 142 patients out of 621 patients were found to have hemoglobin in the anemic range on hospital admission and were excluded from the analysis. A total of 479 patients who were not anemic during admission were included in the analysis. The effect of a smaller volume phlebotomy tube on the incidence of HAA was evaluated in two groups (276/479 in group A and 203/479 in group B) (Figure 1).

Patients were characterized based on their sex, demographic, comorbidities, length of hospitalization, and kidney function. Patients that were elderly (defined as age ≥ 65) had more comorbidities, longer hospitalizations, and a higher incidence of dehydration on admission (Table 1).

3.2. The Drop in Hemoglobin after Hospitalization. After exclusion of patients who were anemic on admission, there

TABLE 2: Multilinear regression analysis: factors influencing the drop of hemoglobin in hospitalized patients.

Independent variable	β-estimate ($\pm$SE)	Number of patients used in analysis	P value
Age $\geq$65 y versus <65 y	0.166 ($\pm$0.097)	479	0.08
Male versus female	−0.058 ($\pm$0.098)	479	0.55
BMI	−0.014 ($\pm$0.005)	479	**0.005***
Length of stay	0.067 ($\pm$0.030)	479	**0.02***
BUN/CR	−0.005 ($\pm$0.005)	479	0.35
Group A versus B	−0.162 ($\pm$0.094)	479	0.08
Comorbidities (<3 versus $\geq$3)	−0.020 ($\pm$0.100)	479	0.77
White versus others	0.484 ($\pm$0.276)	479	0.08
African American versus others	0.541 ($\pm$0.330)	479	0.10
Hispanic versus others	0.490 ($\pm$0.316)	479	0.12

*Statistically significant.

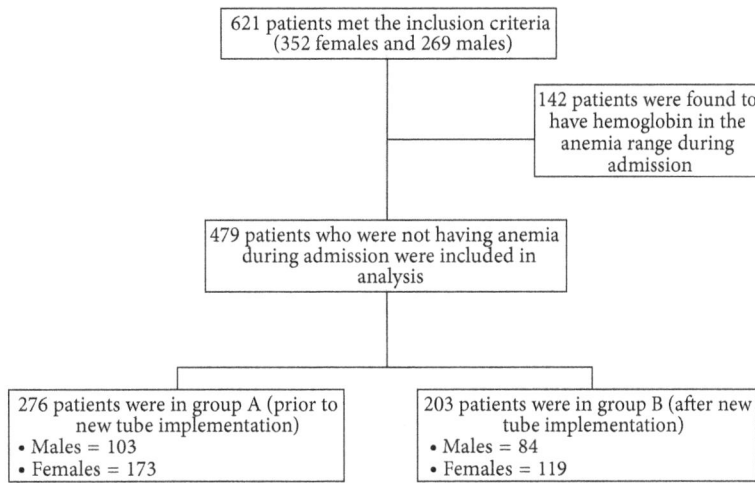

FIGURE 1: Patients enrollments and selections—detailed.

were 479 patients, 39 percent men (186/479) and 61 percent women (293/479). Between admission and discharge, 65% of patients (310/479 patients) dropped their hemoglobin by 1.0 g/dL or more, 63% of the men (118/186 patients) and 66% of the women (192/293 patients).

Upon discharge, 49% of patients (234/479) developed anemia. On average, patients dropped their hemoglobin from 13.8 (on admission) to 12.4 gm/dL (on discharge) (Figure 2(a)). Among this group, 37% (86/234) were men and 63% (148/234 patients) were women. The hemoglobin in men dropped from 14.45 to 13 gm/dL ($P < 0.0001$), while, in women, it dropped from 13.39 to 12.05 gm/dL ($P < 0.0001$) (Figure 2(b)). However, the difference in the rate of anemia by gender was not significant ($P = 0.36$). On average, men and women dropped their hemoglobin by 1.4 and 1.3 g/dL, respectively.

An age-group analysis showed that 54% (138 out of 255) of patients aged $\geq$ 65 years became anemic during hospitalization compared to 42% (96 out of 224) of patients aged < 65 years ($P = 0.01$).

3.3. Difference in Change of Hemoglobin before and after Decreased Volume Tube Implementation. Eleven percent of

blood draws in this hospital included BMP, in which the volume of phlebotomy tube was reduced from 8 cc to 4 cc. The decrease in hemoglobin between admission and discharge did not differ significantly between group A and group B (1.44 ± 1.09 versus 1.29 ± 0.92, $P = 0.214$) (Figure 2(c)).

3.4. Multivariate Analysis of the Drop in Hemoglobin. We performed multiple linear regression analysis on patients to evaluate factors contributing to the drop in hemoglobin. Even though elderly patients had a higher incidence of HAA compared to the younger counterparts, after adjusting with other factors, such as comorbidities and body mass index, the difference was not statistically significant. After adjusting the age, sex, length of hospitalization, BUN/creatinine ratio on admission (to evaluate the effect of dehydration), comorbidities, and BMI, we found that the two main factors which can predict the drop in hemoglobin in hospitalized patients were the length of stay and BMI. One-day increase in length of hospital stay decreases the hemoglobin by 0.06 ($\pm$0.03) mg/dL under the assumption that the other variables are held constant. Using the same statistical constraints, an increase in BMI by 10 would decrease the drop of hemoglobin by 0.1 mg/dL (Table 2).

(a)

(b)

(c)

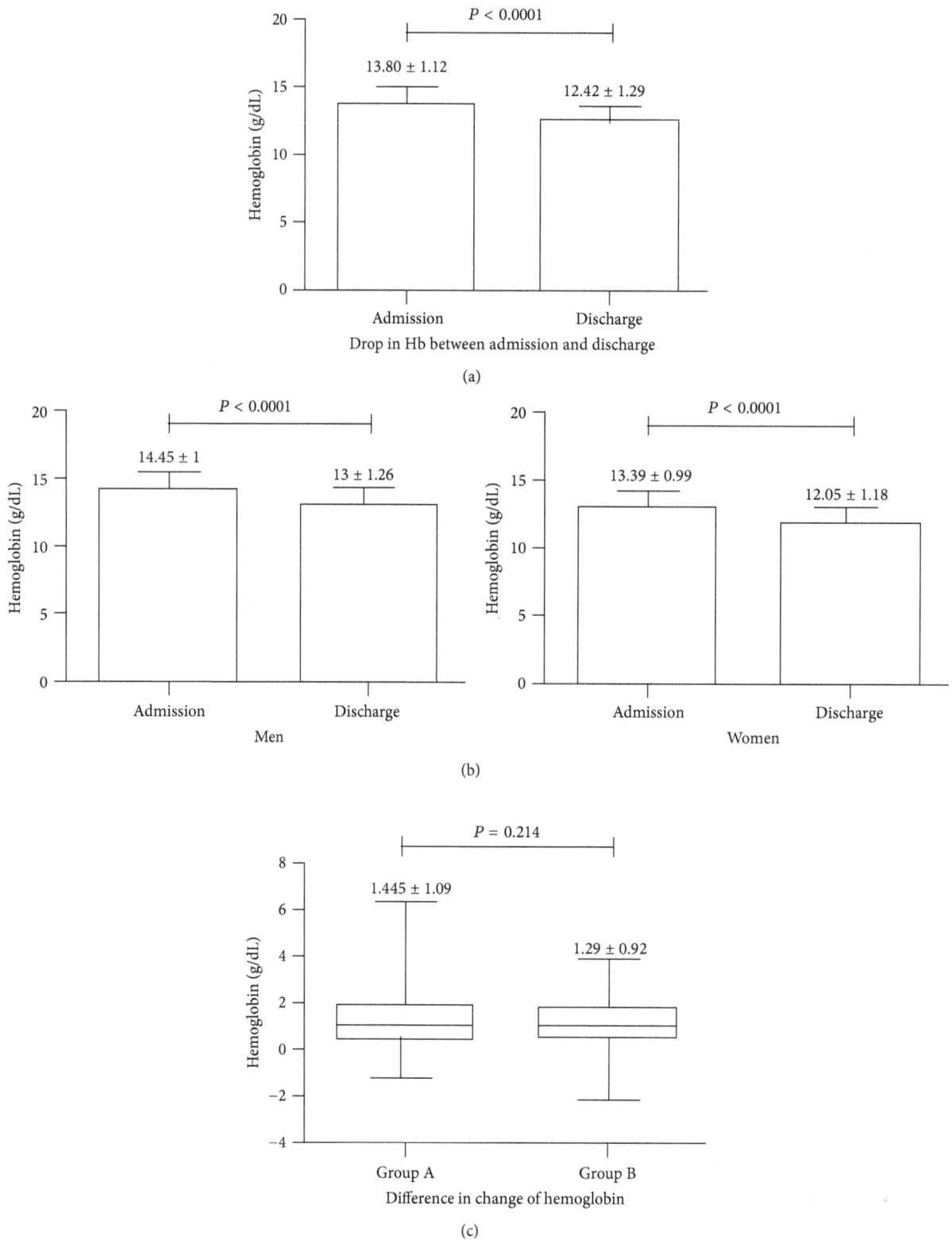

FIGURE 2: Difference in change and reduction of hemoglobin before and after smaller tube implementation. Hemoglobin dropped significantly between admission and discharge (Figure 2(a)). The drop in hemoglobin between admission and discharge by sex categorization. Both men and women dropped their hemoglobin significantly (Figure 2(b)). Implementation of smaller tube did not significantly reduce the change in hemoglobin (Figure 2(c)).

4. Discussion

There have been few studies evaluating incidence of anemia during admission to a general medical floor. Our study is the first to demonstrate that decreasing the volume of blood used for phlebotomy failed to decrease the incidence and severity of HAA. Hospitalization is associated with a significant decrease in hemoglobin. In our study, about 65 percent of patients dropped their hemoglobin by at least 1 gm/dL or more, and 45 percent of patients became anemic during hospitalization. Patients who had longer hospitalization and those who had lower BMI had a greater decrease in hemoglobin.

Patients admitted to the hospital may also have dehydration due to their medical conditions. These patients often received intravenous hydration, which may cause hemodilution leading to a reduction in hemoglobin [7, 8]. In our study, BUN/creatinine ratio, which is considered a surrogate indicator for hydration status, did not have significant effect on drop of hemoglobin.

The mechanism of hospital-acquired anemia may depend upon the amount of blood draws for diagnostic studies as well as decreased red cell production secondary to the patients associated comorbidities. The patients primary illness could include inflammation or infection with a decreased RBC production commonly referred to as the anemia of chronic disease. The high frequency of anemia developing during hospitalization suggests that both decreased production and high volume of blood withdrawn for diagnostic purposes contribute to the anemia.

The results of our study were similar to previous studies showing that length of stay is an important predictor for the development of HAA [9]. The reported incidence of HAA from previous studies varies from 25% to 74%, depending on the study population (i.e., acute coronary syndrome and kidney disease) [3, 9–11].

Our findings supported the theory that the amount of blood drawn correlates with the development of HAA. The longer the patients were hospitalized, the more likely they would have increased amounts of blood draws. Using smaller volume tubes for BMP, which constituted only 11% of blood draws in this institution, did not significantly affect the drop of hemoglobin. However, the effect might have been significant if the smaller tube was applied to a larger proportion of blood drawn (i.e., complete blood count or cardiac enzymes).

Potential limitations of this study are that it was retrospective and did not include serial measurements of reticulocytes as an index of red cell production. We also did not measure the exact amount of blood lost during phlebotomy as well as the frequency of phlebotomy and timing in each patient. This study was performed in single institution and may not be applicable to other clinical centers. We are aware of variability for the development of HAA among medical institutions. A recent study showed that teaching institutions had a lower risk of HAA [12].

In conclusion, our study confirms that hospital-acquired anemia is common. Almost half of our studied hospitalized patients developed HAA. Patients with longer hospitalization and those with lower BMI are at higher risk of developing HAA. More aggressive strategies, such as reducing the frequency of blood draws and expanding the use of smaller volume tubes for other laboratory panels, may be helpful in reducing the incidence of HAA during hospitalization. It is important for physicians to be aware of HAA and to reduce unnecessary blood draws that may contribute to the high incidence of HAA.

Disclosure

Dr. Kurniali was a medical resident at Roger Williams Medical Center/Boston University School of Medicine when the study was conducted. The authors had access to the data and a role in writing the paper.

Conflict of Interests

The authors declare that there is no conflict of interests regarding the publication of this paper.

Acknowledgments

This project was presented at the American College of Physician Rhode Island Associate Day as an oral presentation on May 3, 2012, and updated data was presented at the American Society of Hematology annual meeting on December 7, 2013, as a poster presentation.

References

[1] P. Thavendiranathan, A. Bagai, A. Ebidia, A. S. Detsky, and N. K. Choudhry, "Do blood tests cause anemia in hospitalized patients? The effect of diagnostic phlebotomy on hemoglobin and hematocrit levels," *Journal of General Internal Medicine*, vol. 20, no. 6, pp. 520–524, 2005.

[2] L. Pabla, E. Watkins, and H. A. Doughty, "A study of blood loss from phlebotomy in renal medical inpatients," *Transfusion Medicine*, vol. 19, no. 6, pp. 309–314, 2009.

[3] A. C. Salisbury, K. J. Reid, K. P. Alexander et al., "Diagnostic blood loss from phlebotomy and hospital-acquired anemia during acute myocardial infarction," *Archives of Internal Medicine*, vol. 171, no. 18, pp. 1646–1653, 2011.

[4] P. C. Hébert, "Anemia and red cell transfusion in critical care. Transfusion Requirements in Critical Care Investigators and the Canadian Critical Care Trials Group," *Minerva Anestesiologica*, vol. 65, no. 5, pp. 293–304, 1999.

[5] P. C. Hébert, G. Wells, M. A. Blajchman et al., "A multicenter, randomized, controlled clinical trial of transfusion requirements in critical care. Transfusion Requirements in Critical Care Investigators, Canadian Critical Care Trials Group," *The New England Journal of Medicine*, vol. 340, no. 6, pp. 409–417, 1999.

[6] S. V. Rao, J. G. Jollis, R. A. Harrington et al., "Relationship of blood transfusion and clinical outcomes in patients with acute coronary syndromes," *Journal of the American Medical Association*, vol. 292, no. 13, pp. 1555–1562, 2004.

[7] M. Rasouli, A. M. Kiasari, and S. Arab, "Indicators of dehydration and haemoconcentration are associated with the prevalence and severity of coronary artery disease," *Clinical and*

Experimental Pharmacology and Physiology, vol. 35, no. 8, pp. 889–894, 2008.

[8] S. M. Shirreffs, "Markers of hydration status," *The Journal of Sports Medicine and Physical Fitness*, vol. 40, no. 1, pp. 80–84, 2000.

[9] C. G. Koch, L. Li, Z. Sun et al., "Hospital-acquired anemia: prevalence, outcomes, and healthcare implications," *Journal of Hospital Medicine*, vol. 8, no. 9, pp. 506–512, 2013.

[10] O. Meroño, M. Cladellas, L. Recasens et al., "In-hospital acquired anemia in acute coronary syndrome. Predictors, in-hospital prognosis and one-year mortality," *Revista Espanola de Cardiologia*, vol. 65, no. 8, pp. 742–748, 2012.

[11] J. S. Choi, Y. A. Kim, Y. U. Kang et al., "Clinical impact of hospital-acquired anemia in association with acute kidney injury and chronic kidney disease in patients with acute myocardial infarction," *PLoS ONE*, vol. 8, no. 9, Article ID e75583, 2013.

[12] A. C. Salisbury, K. J. Reid, A. P. Amin, J. A. Spertus, and M. Kosiborod, "Variation in the incidence of hospital-acquired anemia during hospitalization with acute myocardial infarction (Data from 57 US Hospitals)," *American Journal of Cardiology*, vol. 113, no. 7, pp. 1130–1136, 2014.

18

An Etiologic Profile of Anemia in 405 Geriatric Patients

Tabea Geisel,[1,2] Julia Martin,[1,2] Bettina Schulze,[3] Roland Schaefer,[4]
Matthias Bach,[3] Garth Virgin,[5] and Jürgen Stein[1,2,6]

[1] Crohn Colitis Center Rhein-Main, 60594 Frankfurt/Main, Germany

[2] Institute of Nutritional Science, University of Giessen, 35392 Giessen, Germany

[3] St. Elisabethen Krankenhaus, 60487 Frankfurt/Main, Germany

[4] Krankenhaus Sachsenhausen, Teaching Hospital of the J. W. von Goethe University Frankfurt/Main,
 60594 Frankfurt/Main, Germany

[5] Vifor Pharma Deutschland GmbH, 81379 Munich, Germany

[6] Department of Gastroenterology and Nutritional Medicine, Krankenhaus Sachsenhausen,
 Teaching Hospital of the J. W. von Goethe University Frankfurt/Main, 60594 Frankfurt/Main, Germany

Correspondence should be addressed to Jürgen Stein; j.stein@em.uni-frankfurt.de

Academic Editor: Donald S. Silverberg

Background. Anemia is a common condition in the elderly and a significant risk factor for increased morbidity and mortality, reducing not only functional capacity and mobility but also quality of life. Currently, few data are available regarding anemia in hospitalized geriatric patients. Our retrospective study investigated epidemiology and causes of anemia in 405 hospitalized geriatric patients. *Methods.* Data analysis was performed using laboratory parameters determined during routine hospital admission procedures (hemoglobin, ferritin, transferrin saturation, C-reactive protein, vitamin B12, folic acid, and creatinine) in addition to medical history and demographics. *Results.* Anemia affected approximately two-thirds of subjects. Of 386 patients with recorded hemoglobin values, 66.3% were anemic according to WHO criteria, mostly (85.1%) in a mild form. Anemia was primarily due to iron deficiency (65%), frequently due to underlying chronic infection (62.1%), or of mixed etiology involving a combination of chronic disease and iron deficiency, with absolute iron deficiency playing a comparatively minor role. *Conclusion.* Greater awareness of anemia in the elderly is warranted due to its high prevalence and negative effect on outcomes, hospitalization duration, and mortality. Geriatric patients should be routinely screened for anemia and etiological causes of anemia individually assessed to allow timely initiation of appropriate therapy.

1. Introduction

Iron deficiency is the most prevalent nutritional deficiency worldwide. This metal ion is an essential element in a variety of physiological processes in human beings, including the production of energy in the brain. Iron is also an enzymatic cofactor in the synthesis of neurotransmitters and myelin and is well known for being especially important as a means of oxygen transportation [1]. The main consequence of iron deficiency is anemia, a common condition and significant problem in the older population. However, many physicians continue to neglect the significance of anemia as a serious clinical condition in the elderly [2]. While decreased

hemoglobin levels were previously largely considered a normal consequence of aging, there is now evidence that anemia is associated with an increased risk for morbidity and mortality [3, 4]. According to hemoglobin (Hb) cut-off levels defined by the World Health Organization (WHO) (<12 g/dL for females, <13 g/dL for males) [5], anemia is present in 10% of women and 11% of men over the age of 65, increasing to 20% of women and 26% of men over 85 [6]. An even higher prevalence is seen in hospitalized patients, of whom approximately 40–50% have been found to be anemic [7]. The primary consequences of anemia, even mild anemia in which hemoglobin values are only marginally reduced (>9.5 g/dL), are the impairment of functional capacities and a reduced quality of life [8–10]. Furthermore, in elderly persons, anemia can impair physical performance and mobility, thus increasing the risk of falls. An association between anemia in older adults and mortality has been observed in several studies, even in the absence of concomitant illness. In elderly patients, anemia is often overlooked, despite the fact that it has been shown to have potentially serious consequences [2–5, 10].

Data describing the prevalence and causes of anemia in hospitalized geriatric populations are rare and incongruent. Our aim was therefore to determine the epidemiology and etiology of anemia in a hospitalized geriatric population in Germany.

2. Methods

2.1. Study Design. In this German study, all patients who were admitted between March 2010 and March 2011 to the Geriatric Clinic of the St. Elisabethen Krankenhaus in Frankfurt, Germany, and whose medical records were available were included. The data was analyzed retrospectively.

Patients included in the study were aged 65 years or over. The presence of anemia was defined according to criteria issued by the WHO: hemoglobin (Hb) <12 g/dL for females and <13 g/dL for males. Hb values on admission were available for 386 of the 405 patients (95.3%) and three grades of anemia severity were differentiated: severe (Hb < 8 g/dL), moderate (Hb 8 to <9.5 g/dL), and mild (Hb ≥ 9.5 g/dL). In addition, patient data were assessed for routinely determined levels of serum iron (in 92.6% of patients), serum ferritin (95.6%), transferrin saturation (TSAT) (99.0%), vitamin B_{12} (91.9%), folic acid (88.1%), CRP (96.8%), and serum creatinine (99.51%).

2.1.1. Definition of Anemia Classification

Anemia Associated with Iron Deficiency. Patients with Hb levels under 12 g/dL (women) and 13 g/dL (men) and a TSAT value <20% were considered to have anemia associated with iron deficiency. Three subcategories were defined.

(i) Anemia related to absolute iron deficiency (iron deficiency anemia, IDA) was characterized by a decreased serum ferritin level (<30 μg/mL) in combination with low serum CRP levels (≤0.5 mg/dL).

(ii) Anemia caused by inflammation (AI) was defined by high ferritin levels (>100 μg/mL) and increased CRP (≥0.5 mg/dL).

(iii) Patients with ferritin levels between 30 μg/mL and 100 μg/mL and high CRP levels (≥0.5 mg/dL) were classified as having mixed anemia (IDA/AI).

Anemia due to Factors Other Than Iron Deficiency. Patients with Hb levels under 12 g/dL (women) and 13 g/dL (men) and a TSAT value ≥ 20% were considered to have anemia caused by factors other than iron deficiency. Four subcategories were defined.

(i) Anemia secondary to cobalamin deficiency was diagnosed if the serum level was <150 pg/mL.

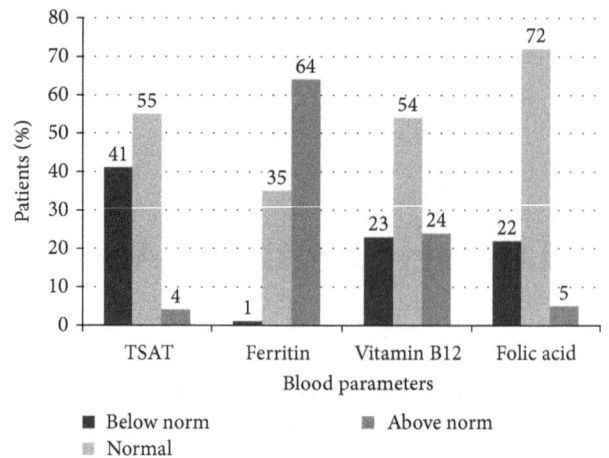

FIGURE 1: Anemia-related laboratory parameters at time of admission (TSAT = transferrin saturation).

(ii) Anemia secondary to folic acid deficiency was diagnosed if the serum level was <2 μg/L.

(iii) Anemia of chronic renal insufficiency (CRI) was classified by creatinine values >1.2 mg/dL in females and >1.5 mg/dL in males [11–13].

(iv) Anemia secondary to other etiologies was defined as unexplained anemia (UA) [6]. See Figure 1.

2.2. Statistical Analysis. The primary objective of this study was to determine the prevalence of anemia and of different etiological subtypes of anemia in a hospitalized geriatric patient population.

Descriptive statistics were attained through the calculation of arithmetical means, standard deviations, and minimum and maximum values of all data. To test the significance of all categorical variables, the Chi-squared test (Pearson) was performed. Arithmetical means were calculated with t-tests for dependent and independent samples, and correlations were determined using the Spearman Rho method. All outcomes with a minimum of $P < 0.05$ were considered significant. Missing values were disregarded in all statistical tests. All statistical analyses were performed using IBM SPSS Statistics 20SPSS statistical software.

3. Results

During the period studied, 405 patients (116 men and 289 women) who were admitted to the geriatric clinic had medical records available and were therefore included in the study. The average age was 83.6 ± 6.9 years (range 65–101 years). The patients were divided into three observational groups according to age: 65 to 75 years, 76 to 85 years, and over 85 years of age, representing 12.10%, 36.79%, and 51.11% of the study population, respectively.

The most frequent main causes of hospitalization in this geriatric patient group were fractures (39.4%, $n = 150$), cardiovascular disease (18.4%, $n = 70$), and disturbances of gait and mobility (16.8%, $n = 64$). Other reasons for

TABLE 1: Anemia subtypes according to main reason for hospitalization.

	All patients $n = 368$ $n\,(\%^*)$	All anemic patients $n = 241$ $n\,(\%^{*1})$	IDA $n\,(\%^{*1})$	IDA/AI $n\,(\%^{*1})$	AI $n\,(\%^{*1})$	B$_{12}$/folic acid deficiency $n\,(\%^{*1})$	Renal anemia $n\,(\%^{*1})$	UA $n\,(\%^{*1})$
Fractures	150 (40.76)	110 (43.90)	0 (0)	9 (8.18)	31 (28.18)	8 (7.27)	10 (9.09)	52 (47.27)
Cardiovascular disease	70 (19.02)	40 (57.14)	3 (7.50)	6 (15.00)	15 (37.50)	3 (7.50)	7 (17.50)	6 (15.00)
Disturbance of gait and mobility	64 (17.39)	26 (40.63)	1 (3.85)	5 (19.23)	3 (11.54)	2 (7.69)	5 (19.23)	10 (38.46)
Digestive tract diseases	15 (4.08)	13 (86.67)	1 (7.69)	2 (15.38)	4 (30.77)	2 (15.38)	4 (30.77)	0 (0)
Disorders of the musculoskeletal apparatus	14 (3.80)	13 (92.86)	0 (0)	1 (7.69)	3 (23.08)	3 (23.08)	6 (46.15)	0 (0)
Neoplasma	14 (3.80)	10 (71.43)	0 (0)	1 (10)	6 (60.00)	2 (20)	1 (10)	0 (0)
Infectious diseases	9 (2.45)	7 (77.78)	1 (14.29)	2 (28.57)	2 (28.57)	1 (14.29)	1 (14.92)	0 (0)
Injuries	9 (2.45)	4 (44.44)	0 (0)	2 (50.00)	0 (0)	1 (25.00)	1 (25)	0 (0)
Other reasons	23 (6.25)	18 (78.26)	1 (5.56)	3 (16.67)	4 (22.22)	2 (11.11)	4 (22.22)	4 (22.22)
		241 (100)	7 (2.90^{*2})	31 (12.86^{*2})	68 (28.22^{*2})	24 (9.96^{*2})	39 (16.18^{*2})	72 (29.88^{*2})

*Relating to all hospitalized patients.
^{*1}Relating to all anemic patients with this diagnosis.
^{*2}Relating to all anemic patients.

TABLE 2: Iron parameters in all patients subdivided into age groups.

	Number of patients		Mean ± SD		Median		Min.		Max.	
	Female	Male	Female	Male	Female	Male	Female	Male	Female	Male
Hb (g/dL)										
65–75 years	33	21	11.67 ± 3.01	11.84 ± 2.05	11.5	11.6	9	8.5	19.5	16.5
76–85 years	97	59	11.58 ± 2.24	11.91 ± 1.81	11.6	11.4	8.1	9.1	19.7	16.2
>85 years	149	29	11.30 ± 2.0	11.94 ± 1.97	11.4	12.4	8.1	8.9	16.9	16.2
Serum iron (mg/dL)										
65–75 years	32	19	3.53 ± 1.93	5.05 ± 3.08	3	5	1	1	8	9
76–85 years	97	57	4.15 ± 2.36	4.26 ± 2.117	4	5	1	1	9	8
>85 years	142	27	4.7 ± 2.38	3.85 ± 2.37	5	4	1	1	9	8
Serum ferritin (μg/L)										
65–75 years	35	22	184.14 ± 206.62	371.36 ± 232.83	116	314	29	41	1131	905
76–85 years	94	58	262.38 ± 263.06	336.71 ± 284.13	201.5	253	18	56	2026	1435
>85 years	149	27	262.38 ± 263.06	336.56 ± 291.14	212	216	7	38	1352	1250
TSAT (%)										
65–75 years	36	22	18.64 ± 12.35	18.18 ± 9.39	15	18.5	4	4	60	35
76–85 years	100	61	20.44 ± 12.39	21.44 ± 11.61	18	20	3	6	87	67
>85 years	153	30	19.62 ± 10.03	20.97 ± 14.41	17	18	5	6	52	79
CRP (mg/dL)										
65–75 years	35	22	4.77 ± 6.29	1.47 ± 1.85	2.3	0.65	0.2	0.2	28.7	7.4
76–85 years	127	82	4.77 ± 6.29	2.19 ± 4.02	1.7	0.95	0	0.2	28.7	30
>85 years	151	28	3.88 ± 6.08	1.7 ± 0.7	1.9	0.7	0	0	49	9.8

admission were digestive tract diseases (3.9%, $n = 15$), disorders of the musculoskeletal apparatus (3.7%, $n = 14$), neoplasms (3.7%, $n = 14$), infectious diseases (2.4%, $n = 9$), and injuries (2.4%, $n = 9$), with a further 6.0% ($n = 23$) admitted for other reasons.

Table 1 shows the distribution of these conditions according to specific anemia subtypes. On average, the patients had eight additional diagnoses concurrent to the primary diagnosis, and mean duration of stay in the clinic of all study subjects was 22 days. The main demographic characteristics of the patients are summarized in Table 2.

Of those hospitalized patients whose Hb values at admission were available ($n = 386$), 66.3% (74.8% of men and 62.9% of women) were anemic. There was no correlation between age and Hb level. While only four patients (1.5%) were found to be severely anemic, 37 (13.5%) had moderate anemia and the remaining 85.1% were categorized as having mild anemia.

The total number of patients diagnosed with anemia was 237, of whom 154 (65.0%) were defined as having iron deficiency anemia, with TSAT values <20%. Absolute IDA was found in only 7 (4.6%) of these patients, while 33 (21.4%) had a combination of IDA and AI. The majority of patients with IDA ($n = 95$, 61.7%) were diagnosed with AI, indicated by high CRP and ferritin levels.

Decreased levels of vitamin B_{12} or folic acid were determined as the cause of anemia in 30 patients (5.9% and 6.8%, resp.). In a further 46 (19.4%) study subjects, anemia was found to be the result of chronic renal insufficiency. The remaining patients fell into none of these categories and were therefore classified as having "unexplained anemia."

The mean serum ferritin level of 315.7 μg/L fell within the normal reference range. Serum ferritin values were, however, increased in the majority of study subjects (64%), while 35% were found to have normal serum ferritin levels.

4. Discussion

Anemia is a common condition in the elderly, especially in hospitalized geriatric patients, and is known to be associated with increased morbidity and mortality. The present study was specifically aimed at investigating the epidemiology and etiology of anemia in a hospitalized geriatric population. Blood samples were retrospectively analyzed for the purpose of the study.

The most striking conclusion drawn is the high prevalence of anemia across the board in elderly patients admitted to hospital owing to a wide range of different disorders. Two-thirds of the patients studied were found to be anemic on admission. Although one other study, also focusing on geriatric inpatients, has shown a similar prevalence of anemia [7], most research involving elderly subjects has found the prevalence to be lower [6, 10, 14]. This discrepancy may be accountable to the fact that, in contrast to the current study with its population of hospitalized elderly patients, most other studies have examined ambulant patients or older people in the community [15, 16]. Geriatric persons with health problems severe enough to result in hospital admission are more likely than the geriatric population as a whole to suffer from acute infection and also to have an increased risk of blood loss due to surgery. Thus, hospitalized patients are at a higher risk of developing anemia [17]. Anemia was found in most cases to be mild, with an Hb level > 10 g/dL, in accordance with previously published results [6, 18]. However, even mild anemia is frequently associated with negative outcomes with regard to mortality and morbidity in the elderly [2, 19] and should therefore not be accepted as a normal physiological response to the aging process. Furthermore, the etiological origins of anemia must be determined in all cases in order to facilitate the choice and implementation of effective therapy. It might be seen as a limitation of the present study that reasons for hospital admission were not taken into account. However, we

deliberately chose to include all geriatric patients admitted to our clinic, independent of grounds for hospitalization, in order to gain a broader perspective on the prevalence and causes of anemia in elderly patients.

No statistically significant correlation was detected between patients' age and Hb values. This is not in keeping with results of previous research, which have suggested an age-related decrease in Hb levels [6]. Again, this may relate to the specific elderly population included, since all study subjects had serious health issues (and thus, presumably, an increased risk of anemia), whereas in the geriatric population as a whole, the prevalence of serious illness increases with age. Thus, in terms of general state of health, the older the hospitalized patients are, the more representative they can be considered to be of the general population in that age group. As a consequence, what might be considered an innate "bias" of our population towards seriously ill patients (in comparison to studies involving nonhospitalized geriatric persons) is not independent of age, but probably more pronounced in the context of the younger geriatric population.

Determination of the underlying cause of anemia in geriatric persons is complicated by comorbidity and polypharmacy, which are particularly common among the elderly [5]. This must also be taken into account when classifying and comparing the results.

Nonetheless, anemia in the elderly can generally be categorized into four major types: anemia related to nutrient deficiencies (iron, cobalamin, and folic acid), anemia related to chronic inflammation, anemia due to renal insufficiency, and unexplained anemia [6].

Of 237 patients considered to be anemic, 154 (65.0%) had TSAT values <20% and were therefore diagnosed with iron deficiency anemia. In terms of the classification of anemia, the most common etiological subtypes were anemia of inflammation or a mixed form resulting from AI and IDA. Only a few studies have investigated the etiologic profile of anemia in hospitalized patients in the age range from 65 to 101 years [7, 14]. Comparing our results to previous studies is complicated by differences in anemia classification. However, inflammation seems to be the predominant cause of anemia in the observed population, with nutritive factors playing only a limited role [14]. In elderly persons, the causes of anemia vary depending on their clinical setting. AI and IDA are, however, the most common forms of anemia both in community-dwelling and in hospitalized geriatric patients [14]. In our study, IDA was less prevalent than expected in light of results obtained in prior studies.

Only 4.6% of our study subjects with iron deficiency-associated anemia were found to have absolute iron deficiency anemia (IDA), in comparison to 17% in previous reports [6, 20]. A possible explanation for this discrepancy might be the higher mean age (83.6 years) of our patients compared to populations of similar studies, whose mean ages were between 77 and 80 years [13, 21]. Furthermore, we had a high number of comorbidities in our study population. A recent study with a comparable prevalence of comorbidities disclosed an IDA rate of 31% [7].

Sixty-two percent of patients with iron deficiency-related anemia were diagnosed with AI. Petrosyan et al. reported a similar prevalence rate (60%) of AI in a comparable study population [7]. Prevalence rates in community-dwelling elderly persons, however, may be considerably lower. For example, the NHANES (National Health and Nutrition Examination Survey) III demonstrated a prevalence of 24% for this type of anemia in a community-dwelling elderly population [6]. Considerable differences in prevalence may be accountable to the setting (community-dwelling elderly, nursing home residents, or hospital patients), variations in mean age of the study population, and the resultant respective variations in the number of comorbidities and chronic conditions. While AI predominantly occurs as a consequence of chronic or long-term illness or infection, it is also associated with malignancy and inflammatory disorders. These are conditions whose prevalence increases with advancing age and which are more likely to be encountered in a hospitalized setting. Since fractures were the most frequent main cause of hospitalization in our study population, these patients came into the rehabilitation ward. Since an increase in inflammation parameters (CRP and ferritin) is to be expected under these circumstances, this represents an additional explanation for the high prevalence of AI in our study [22]. Studies of noninstitutionalized older persons have demonstrated higher and lower prevalences of IDA and AI, respectively [21, 23].

In our study, anemia of mixed etiology resulting from iron deficiency and chronic inflammation was also analyzed. Thirty-three patients (21.43%) were found to have combined IDA and AI.

Anemia due to deficiencies of vitamin B_{12} or folic acid was found in 5.91% and 6.75% of patients, respectively. Other studies showed higher prevalence rates of 10–20% for cobalamin and 21% for folic acid deficiency [7, 24, 25]. Guralnik et al. determined anemia secondary to folic acid or cobalamin deficiency in 14% of their elderly population [6]. However, comparison of these results is of limited value, as different diagnostic criteria were used.

Anemia of chronic renal insufficiency (CRI) was defined by creatinine values >1.2 mg/dL in females and >1.5 mg/dL in males. Forty-seven (19.41%) of the elderly patients assessed were found to have CRI-related anemia. While previous studies have reported a prevalence of 8–17.5% for anemia resulting from renal insufficiency, most of these studies used a glomerular filtration rate (GFR) of <30 mL/min as the defining criterion for chronic kidney disease [7, 26, 27]. While GFR is indeed considered a better parameter for the diagnosis of chronic renal insufficiency, the present study, due to its retrospective design, was only able to assess chronic renal illness on the basis of the available creatinine values. The results of the studies are therefore not directly comparable.

The patients that fell into none of the given etiological subgroup categories were therefore classified as having unexplained anemia. Possible underlying mechanisms for unexplained anemia include physiological changes such as higher circulating levels of proinflammatory cytokines, myelodysplasia, decreased androgen levels, and a decrease in the proliferative capacity of bone marrow stem cells [6, 28].

Our study has strengths and limitations. The most limiting factor is the retrospective design of the study. Consequently, only those laboratory parameters which were collected as clinical routine on admission were available to be assessed.

Important strengths of the study are the large study population (n = 405), the wide spectrum of reasons for admission and of underlying disease or condition, and the use of a variety of different iron and inflammation parameters as assessment criteria for the classification of different causes of anemia.

Conclusive evidence from a large number of studies has confirmed that adequate treatment of iron deficiency significantly improves rates of mortality and morbidity in patients suffering from a wide range of conditions, including chronic heart failure [29, 30], coronary heart disease [31], chronic kidney disease [32, 33], cancer [34, 35], and rheumatoid arthritis [36, 37]. Nevertheless, screening and treatment of ID continue to be widely neglected in the routine management of geriatric patients. There is clearly a need for greater awareness of the high prevalence of anemia in the elderly and of its significance in terms of poorer outcomes, prolonged hospital stays, and increased mortality. Our study underlines the importance of routine screening and individual assessment of the etiological causes of anemia in geriatric patients, allowing the timely initiation of optimal and appropriate therapy. In addition, the perioperative administration of intravenous iron is advisable in order to reduce anemia-related complications and minimize transfusion requirements.

Rather than relying on a single biomarker, screening should include a range of parameters including TSAT, serum ferritin, and CRP. A new generation of intravenous iron preparations allows rapid single-session doses of up to 1,000 mg, thus offering an excellent option for effective treatment and prevention of iron deficiency in all patients, including the elderly [38]. Dosage can be calculated using standard calculation methods such as the Ganzoni formula.

Abbreviations

AI: Anemia of inflammation
CRI: Chronic renal insufficiency
CRP: C-reactive protein
GFR: Glomerular filtration rate
IDA: Iron deficiency anemia
NHANES: National Health and Nutrition Examination Survey
TSAT: Transferrin saturation
UA: Unexplained anemia
WHO: World Health Organization.

Conflict of Interests

Tabea Geisel, Julia Martin, and Bettina Schulze have no conflict of interests.

Authors' Contribution

All authors contributed to the concept and design of the work and to the acquisition and interpretation of data. Tabea

Geisel drafted the paper. All authors revised the paper for important intellectual content and approved the final version for publication.

Acknowledgments

The sponsor's role was limited to financial support only. The sponsor took no active part in data collection, data analysis, data interpretation, or paper preparation. The authors would like to thank Janet Collins for proof reading and language support. Garth Virgin is an employee of Vifor Pharma Deutschland GmbH. Roland Schaefer has acted as a consultant for Vifor Pharma Deutschland GmbH. Matthias Bach has received speaker honoraria for Vifor Pharma Deutschland GmbH. Jürgen Stein has received speaker honoraria and is a member of the board of Vifor Pharma Deutschland GmbH.

References

[1] R. R. Crichton, S. Wilmet, R. Legssyer, and R. J. Ward, "Molecular and cellular mechanisms of iron homeostasis and toxicity in mammalian cells," *Journal of Inorganic Biochemistry*, vol. 91, no. 1, pp. 9–18, 2002.

[2] A. R. Nissenson, L. T. Goodnough, and R. W. Dubois, "Anemia: not just an innocent bystander?" *Archives of Internal Medicine*, vol. 163, no. 12, pp. 1400–1404, 2003.

[3] S. D. Denny, M. N. Kuchibhatla, and H. J. Cohen, "Impact of anemia on mortality, cognition, and function in community-dwelling elderly," *American Journal of Medicine*, vol. 119, no. 4, pp. 327–334, 2006.

[4] B. W. J. H. Penninx, M. Pahor, R. C. Woodman, and J. M. Guralnik, "Anemia in old age is associated with increased mortality and hospitalization," *Journals of Gerontology A*, vol. 61, no. 5, pp. 474–479, 2006.

[5] World Health Organization, "Nutritional Anemia: Report of a WHO Scientific Group," *Technical Report Series*, vol. 405, pp. 1–40, 1968.

[6] J. M. Guralnik, R. S. Eisenstaedt, L. Ferrucci, H. G. Klein, and R. C. Woodman, "Prevalence of anemia in persons 65 years and older in the United States: evidence for a high rate of unexplained anemia," *Blood*, vol. 104, no. 8, pp. 2263–2268, 2004.

[7] I. Petrosyan, G. Blaison, and E. Andrés, "Anaemia in the elderly: an aetiologic profile of a prospective cohort of 95 hospitalised patients," *European Journal of Internal Medicine*, vol. 23, pp. 524–528, 2012.

[8] A. A. Lash and S. M. Coyer, "Anemia in older adults," *Medsurg Nursing*, vol. 17, no. 5, pp. 298–305, 2008.

[9] D. R. Thomas, "Anemia and quality of life: unrecognized and undertreated," *Journals of Gerontology A*, vol. 59, no. 3, pp. 238–241, 2004.

[10] W. P. J. den Elzen, J. M. Willems, R. G. J. Westendorp, A. J. M. De Craen, W. J. J. Assendelft, and J. Gussekloo, "Effect of anemia and comorbidity on functional status and mortality in old age: results from the Leiden 85-plus Study," *Canadian Medical Association Journal*, vol. 181, no. 3-4, pp. 151–157, 2009.

[11] G. Weiss and L. T. Goodnough, "Anemia of chronic disease," *New England Journal of Medicine*, vol. 352, no. 10, pp. 1011–1059, 2005.

[12] C. Gasche, A. Berstad, R. Befrits et al., "Guidelines on the diagnosis and management of iron deficiency and anemia in inflammatory bowel diseases," *Inflammatory Bowel Diseases*, vol. 13, no. 12, pp. 1545–1553, 2007.

[13] E. Joosten, W. Pelemans, M. Hiele, J. Noyen, R. Verhaeghe, and M. A. Boogaerts, "Prevalence and causes of anaemia in a geriatric hospitalized population," *Gerontology*, vol. 38, no. 1-2, pp. 111–117, 1992.

[14] M. Tettamanti, U. Lucca, F. Gandini et al., "Prevalence, incidence and types of mild anemia in the elderly: the "Health and Anemia" population-based study," *Haematologica*, vol. 95, no. 11, pp. 1849–1856, 2010.

[15] E. M. Inelmen, M. D'Alessio, M. R. A. Gatto et al., "Descriptive analysis of the prevalence of anemia in a randomly selected sample of elderly people living at home: some results of an Italian multicentric study," *Aging*, vol. 6, no. 2, pp. 81–89, 1994.

[16] M. E. Salive, J. Cornoni-Huntley, J. M. Guralnik et al., "Anemia and hemoglobin levels in older persons: relationship with age, gender, and health status," *Journal of the American Geriatrics Society*, vol. 40, no. 5, pp. 489–496, 1992.

[17] E. A. Price, R. Mehra, T. H. Holmes, and S. L. Schrier, "Anemia in older persons: etiology and evaluation," *Blood Cells, Molecules, and Diseases*, vol. 46, no. 2, pp. 159–165, 2011.

[18] R. Eisenstaedt, B. W. J. H. Penninx, and R. C. Woodman, "Anemia in the elderly: current understanding and emerging concepts," *Blood Reviews*, vol. 20, no. 4, pp. 213–226, 2006.

[19] L. Ferrucci, J. M. Guralnik, S. Bandinelli et al., "Unexplained anaemia in older persons is characterised by low erythropoietin and low levels of pro-inflammatory markers," *British Journal of Haematology*, vol. 136, no. 6, pp. 849–855, 2007.

[20] B. J. Anía, V. J. Suman, V. F. Fairbanks, and L. J. Melton III, "Prevalence of anemia in medical practice: community versus referral patients," *Mayo Clinic Proceedings*, vol. 69, no. 8, pp. 730–735, 1994.

[21] A. A. Merchant and C. N. Roy, "Not so benign haematology: anaemia of the elderly," *British Journal of Haematology*, vol. 156, no. 2, pp. 173–185, 2012.

[22] P. P. Vinha, A. A. Jordão Jr., J. A. Farina Jr., H. Vannucchi, J. S. Marchini, and S. F. D. C. da Cunha, "Inflammatory and oxidative stress after surgery for the small area corrections of burn sequelae," *Acta Cirurgica Brasileira*, vol. 26, no. 4, pp. 320–324, 2011.

[23] O. J. Kirkeby, S. Fossum, and C. Risoe, "Anaemia in elderly patients. Incidence and causes of low haemoglobin concentration in a city general practice," *Scandinavian Journal of Primary Health Care*, vol. 9, no. 3, pp. 167–171, 1991.

[24] L. C. Pennypacker, R. H. Allen, J. P. Kelly et al., "High prevalence of cobalamin deficiency in elderly outpatients," *Journal of the American Geriatrics Society*, vol. 40, no. 12, pp. 1197–1204, 1992.

[25] R. Carmel, R. Green, D. S. Rosenblatt, and D. Watkins, "Update on cobalamin, folate, and homocysteine," *Hematology*, vol. 2003, pp. 62–81, 2003.

[26] A. S. Artz and M. J. Thirman, "Unexplained anemia predominates despite an intensive evaluation in a racially diverse cohort of older adults from a referral anemia clinic," *Journals of Gerontology A*, vol. 66, no. 8, pp. 925–932, 2011.

[27] B. Terrier, M. Resche-Rigon, E. Andres et al., "Prevalence, characteristics and prognostic significance of anemia in daily practice," *QJM*, vol. 105, no. 4, Article ID hcr230, pp. 345–354, 2012.

[28] L. Ferrucci, R. D. Semba, J. M. Guralnik et al., "Proinflammatory state, hepcidin, and anemia in older persons," *Blood*, vol. 115, no. 18, pp. 3810–3816, 2010.

[29] M. Kapoor, M. D. Schleinitz, A. Gemignani, and W. C. Wu, "Outcomes of patients with chronic heart failure and iron deficiency treated with intravenous iron: a meta-analysis," *Cardiovascular & Hematological Disorders-Drug Targets*, vol. 13, pp. 35–44, 2013.

[30] E. A. Jankowska, S. von Haehling, S. D. Anker, I. C. Macdougall, and P. Ponikowski, "Iron deficiency and heart failure: diagnostic dilemmas and therapeutic perspectives," *European Heart Journal*, vol. 34, pp. 816–829, 2013.

[31] N. S. Belousova, S. A. Il'ina, G. É. Chernogoriuk, and L. I. Tiukalova, "The influence of correction of iron metabolism and erythron characteristics in mild iron deficiency states on clinical manifestations of coronary heart disease," *Klinicheskaia Meditsina*, vol. 90, pp. 41–46, 2012.

[32] G. Wong, K. Howard, E. Hodson, M. Irving, and J. C. Craig, "An economic evaluation of intravenous versus oral iron supplementation in people on haemodialysis," *Nephrology Dialysis Transplantation*, vol. 28, pp. 413–420, 2013.

[33] D. W. Coyne, T. Kapoian, W. Suki et al., "Ferric gluconate is highly efficacious in anemic hemodialysis patients with high serum ferritin and low transferrin saturation. Results of the Dialysis Patients' Response to IV Iron with Elevated Ferritin (DRIVE) study," *Journal of the American Society of Nephrology*, vol. 18, no. 3, pp. 975–984, 2007.

[34] A. Gafter-Gvili, B. Rozen-Zvi, and L. Vidal, "Intravenous iron supplementation for the treatment of chemotherapy-induced anaemia—systematic review and meta-analysis of randomised controlled trials," *Acta Oncologica*, vol. 52, pp. 18–29, 2013.

[35] H. T. Steinmetz, "The role of intravenous iron in the treatment of anemia in cancer patients," *Therapeutic Advances in Hematology*, vol. 3, pp. 177–191, 2012.

[36] E. Bloxham, V. Vagadia, K. Scott et al., "Anaemia in rheumatoid arthritis: can we afford to ignore it?" *Postgraduate Medical Journal*, vol. 87, no. 1031, pp. 596–600, 2011.

[37] W.-S. Chen, C.-Y. Liu, H.-T. Lee et al., "Effects of intravenous iron saccharate on improving severe anemia in rheumatoid arthritis patients," *Clinical Rheumatology*, vol. 31, no. 3, pp. 469–477, 2012.

[38] W. Y. Qunibi, "The efficacy and safety of current intravenous iron preparations for the management of iron-deficiency anaemia: a review," *Arzneimittel-Forschung*, vol. 60, no. 6 a, pp. 399–412, 2010.

19

Intravenous Iron Therapy in Patients with Iron Deficiency Anemia: Dosing Considerations

Todd A. Koch,[1] Jennifer Myers,[2] and Lawrence Tim Goodnough[3]

[1]*Luitpold Pharmaceuticals, Inc., Norristown, PA 19403, USA*
[2]*St. John's University, Jamaica, NY 11439, USA*
[3]*Department of Pathology and Medicine (Hematology), Stanford, CA 94305, USA*

Correspondence should be addressed to Lawrence Tim Goodnough; ltgoodno@stanford.edu

Academic Editor: Bruno Annibale

Objective. To provide clinicians with evidence-based guidance for iron therapy dosing in patients with iron deficiency anemia (IDA), we conducted a study examining the benefits of a higher cumulative dose of intravenous (IV) iron than what is typically administered. *Methods.* We first individually analyzed 5 clinical studies, averaging the total iron deficit across all patients utilizing a modified Ganzoni formula; we then similarly analyzed 2 larger clinical studies. For the second of the larger studies (Study 7), we also compared the efficacy and retreatment requirements of a cumulative dose of 1500 mg ferric carboxymaltose (FCM) to 1000 mg iron sucrose (IS). *Results.* The average iron deficit was calculated to be 1531 mg for patients in Studies 1–5 and 1392 mg for patients in Studies 6-7. The percentage of patients who were *retreated* with IV iron between Days 56 and 90 was significantly ($p < 0.001$) lower (5.6%) in the 1500 mg group, compared to the 1000 mg group (11.1%). *Conclusions.* Our data suggests that a total cumulative dose of 1000 mg of IV iron may be insufficient for iron repletion in a majority of patients with IDA and a dose of 1500 mg is closer to the actual iron deficit in these patients.

1. Introduction

Iron is an essential element and its balance must be maintained for proper physiologic functioning. Blood loss, a major cause of iron deficiency, is highly prevalent (e.g., females with menses and patients with chronic occult gastrointestinal (GI) blood loss) and requires proper diagnosis and management [1–4]. Therapeutic management of IDA is focused primarily on repletion of iron stores [1–4]. While iron deficient individuals without inflammation may respond to oral iron therapy, administration of IV iron is beneficial in many patient populations, including those with inflammation (resulting, e.g., from kidney disease, heart failure, or rheumatological diseases), patients who cannot tolerate oral iron, and patients who are noncompliant with oral iron therapy [5–8]. Even under the best of circumstances, oral iron is not well tolerated, and patients are often nonadherent for a variety of reasons, including intolerable side effects and the need for multiple daily doses [9]. The frequently poor absorption of oral iron, moreover, can contribute to suboptimal patient response.

The hepcidin response in anemic patients having inflammatory conditions, such as inflammatory bowel disease (IBD), inhibits GI absorption of oral iron [10]. Moreover, hepcidin impacts iron homeostasis in patients with concurrent inflammation (e.g., repressed recycling of iron from the reticuloendothelial system and sequestration in bone marrow); this may limit both oral and IV iron supplementation and may serve to explain why such patients remain iron deficient despite multiple courses of therapy [6, 10, 11].

Cancer-related anemia (CRA) has multiple etiologies, including chemotherapy-induced myelosuppression, blood loss, functional iron deficiency, erythropoietin deficiency due to renal disease, and marrow involvement with tumor, among others. The most common treatment options for CRA include iron therapy, erythropoietic-stimulating agents (ESAs), and red cell transfusion. Safety concerns as well as restrictions and reimbursement issues surrounding ESA therapy for CRA have resulted in suboptimal treatment. Many believe that more routine use of IV iron for CRA and chemotherapy-induced anemia (CIA) is appropriate in view of existing

TABLE 1: Potential role of iron therapy in management of anemia [12].

Condition	Expected hepcidin levels	Iron parameters	Iron therapy strategies	Potential hepcidin therapy
Absolute iron deficiency anemia (IDA)	Low	Low TSAT and ferritin	PO or IV if poorly tolerated or malabsorbed	No
Functional iron deficiency (ESA therapy, CKD)	Variable, depending on ±CKD	Low TSAT, variable ferritin	IV	Antagonist (if hepcidin levels are not low)
Iron sequestration (anemia of inflammation (AI))	High	Low TSAT, normal-to-elevated ferritin	IV	Antagonist
Mixed anemia (AI/IDA or AI/functional iron deficiency)	Variable	Low TSAT, low-to-normal ferritin	IV*	Antagonist (if hepcidin levels are not low)

TSAT = transferrin saturation; PO = oral; IV = intravenous; CKD = chronic kidney disease; ESA = erythropoiesis-stimulating agent.
*Mixed anemia is a diagnosis of exclusion without a therapeutic trial of iron.
From [12].

evidence. Oncology patients whose CIA is treated with ESAs, furthermore, respond better to IV iron therapy than to oral supplementation [7, 13–19].

Table 1 illustrates various conditions where IV iron therapy may be warranted.

Despite beneficial effects in a wide range of patients, administration of IV iron may generate oxidative stress and other inflammatory changes, and the risk-benefit profile of IV iron continues to undergo evaluation in renal dialysis patients [20, 21], as well as patients with anemia due to other chronic diseases [22]. The long-term effects of IV iron preparations will require further study in relevant clinical settings, [23] as will the long-term deleterious effects of allogeneic blood transfusions [24–26].

IV iron preparations currently approved in the US are listed in Table 2 [8, 10, 27–36]. Beginning with the first iron dextran product introduced, the recommended cumulative replacement dose for many of these products has been approximately 1000 mg of iron [29–35].

A patient's total body iron deficit can be calculated using the Ganzoni formula (total iron dose = [actual body weight × (15-actual Hb)] × 2.4 + iron stores) [32]. Because many view this formula as inconvenient, it is not consistently used in clinical practice [37]. Although use of the Ganzoni formula is ideally the best way to select dose, it is impractical, partly because product labels state specific dosing regimens. In typical clinical practice, doses are more efficiently chosen based on approved product labels and local protocols, and only in the Dexferrum (iron dextran injection, USP) and INFeD (iron dextran injection, USP) prescribing information is a weight and Hb-based table available to calculate a patient's total iron requirement utilizing similar formula. There are also only a limited number of clinical practice guidelines regarding the use of a total cumulative repletion dose of IV iron in IDA patients, and, as mentioned above, the FDA-approved labeling for many IV iron products recommends a total cumulative dose of approximately 1000 mg. Currently, there is no consensus regarding the most appropriate iron deficit repletion dosing in patients with IDA, partly because

the iron dosing selected for virtually all trials has been based largely on clinical judgment, clinical guidelines in nephrology, or best estimates from past results. In this retrospective study, we systematically explored the iron deficit in patients who received IV iron in clinical studies and examined the potential benefits (i.e., normalization of Hb and time to retreatment with IV iron) of a higher cumulative dose of IV iron than what is typically administered, with the goal of providing clinicians with practical, evidence-based guidance for determining iron dosing requirements in a wide range of patients with IDA.

2. Materials and Methods

In this study, we used the same population recruited from previous clinical trials [38–44]. These studies adhered to US federal regulations and were performed in accordance with the Declaration of Helsinki and lastly protocols and informed consent forms were approved by local or national institutional review boards. All participants in these studies provided written informed consent. Patient records/information were anonymized and deidentified prior to analysis.

In Studies 1–5 (summarized below), each patient's iron deficit (mg) had been originally calculated and dose of iron administered, according to a modified Ganzoni formula: subject weight in kg × [15-current Hb g/dL] × 2.4 + 500, as specified in each study protocol. The Ganzoni formula had been modified for use in these studies to help alleviate any potential for iron overload in subjects who had a transferrin saturation (TSAT) >20% and ferritin >50 ng/mL at study entry. For these subjects, a conservative estimate was made, and the additional 500 mg from the formula to replete iron stores was not added to the total iron requirement. Each study administered IV iron (ferric carboxymaltose, FCM) as a total cumulative dose to randomized patients based upon the iron deficit so calculated. In analyzing each study, we utilized the baseline iron deficits for each patient using the same method and then averaged the total iron deficit across patients. These clinical studies examined IDA in postpartum

TABLE 2: Current FDA-approved intravenous iron preparations [8, 10, 27–36].

Trade name	Dexferrum (iron dextran injection, USP)	INFeD (iron dextran injection, USP)	Ferrlecit (sodium ferric gluconate complex in sucrose injection)	Venofer (iron sucrose injection, USP)	Feraheme (ferumoxytol)	Injectafer (ferric carboxymaltose injection)
Manufacturer	American Regent, Inc.	Actavis Pharma, Inc.	Sanofi-Aventis	American Regent, Inc.	AMAG Pharmaceuticals	American Regent, Inc.
Test dose	Yes	Yes	No	No	No	No
Black box warning	Yes	Yes	No	No	Yes	No
FDA-approved indications	Iron deficiency where oral iron administration is unsatisfactory or impossible	Iron deficiency where oral iron administration is unsatisfactory or impossible	Iron deficiency anemia in adult and pediatric CKD patients receiving hemodialysis and receiving ESAs	IDA in adult and pediatric patients with non-dialysis-dependent, hemodialysis dependent, and peritoneal dialysis-dependent CKD	IDA in adult patients with CKD	IDA in adult patients who have intolerance to oral iron or have had unsatisfactory response to oral iron or adult patients with non-dialysis-dependent CKD
Total cumulative dose	Dependent on patient's total iron requirement	Dependent on patient's total iron requirement	1000 mg	1000 mg	1020 mg	1500 mg

CKD = chronic kidney disease; ESA = erythropoiesis-stimulating agent; IDA = iron deficiency anemia.
American Regent, Inc., is the human drug division of Luitpold Pharmaceuticals, Inc., Shirley, NY.

TABLE 3: Average calculated iron deficit dose in clinical Studies 1–5.

Study	Patient population	Calculated mean iron deficit based on the modified Ganzoni formula[*] (mg)	Standard deviation	Number of patients
(1) van Wyck et al., 2007 [38]	Postpartum	1458	330	182
(2) van Wyck et al., 2009 [39]	Heavy uterine bleeding	1608	383	251
(3) Seid et al., 2008 [40]	Postpartum	1539	351	143
(4) Barish et al., 2012 [41]	IDA various etiologies	1520	342	348
(5) Hussain et al., 2013 [42]	IDA various etiologies	1508[**]	359	161
Overall mean		1531	NC	1085

IDA = iron deficiency anemia; NC = not calculated.
[*] Patients randomized to receive IV iron based on a calculated iron deficit.
[**] Including all randomized patients.
Data on file, Luitpold Pharmaceuticals, Inc.

patients, patients with heavy uterine bleeding (HUB), non-dialysis-dependent chronic kidney disease (NDD-CKD), GI disorders, and other underlying conditions.

Following are short descriptions of each study:

(1) Comparison of the safety and efficacy of IV iron (FCM) and oral iron (ferrous sulfate) in patients with postpartum anemia ($N = 361$) [38], NCT00396292.

(2) Comparison of the safety and efficacy of IV iron (FCM) and oral iron (ferrous sulfate) in the treatment of IDA secondary to HUB ($N = 477$) [39], NCT00395993.

(3) Comparison of the safety and efficacy of IV iron (FCM) and oral iron (ferrous sulfate) in the treatment of postpartum patients ($N = 291$) [40], NCT00354484.

(4) Comparison of the safety and tolerability of IV iron (FCM) and standard medical care (oral and IV iron) in treating IDA of various etiologies ($N = 708$) [41], NCT00703937.

(5) Comparison of the safety and tolerability of IV iron (FCM) and iron dextran in treating IDA of various etiologies ($N = 160$) [42], NCT00704028.

Following review of Studies 1–5, two larger studies (6 and 7) that utilized 1500 mg IV iron (as specified in the protocols) were examined. Although the modified Ganzoni formula was *not* specified in the protocols to determine dose requirements in these 2 studies, we did apply the formula to determine each patient's baseline iron deficit in a separate retrospective *post hoc* analysis of each study. We then averaged the total iron deficit across patients. Additionally, Study 7 compared the safety and efficacy of 1500 mg of IV iron (as FCM) to 1000 mg of IV iron (as iron sucrose [IS]) examining any potential efficacy or safety difference between the two dosing regimens.

A short summary of Studies 6 and 7 follows:

(6) Comparison of 1500 mg IV iron (FCM) with oral iron and IV iron standard of care (SoC) therapy (as determined by the investigator) in patients with IDA of various etiologies who had an unsatisfactory response to oral iron or were deemed inappropriate for oral iron [43], NCT00982007.

(7) Comparison of the safety and efficacy of 1500 mg (FCM) to 1000 mg of IV iron (IS) in patients with IDA and NDD-CKD [44], NCT00981045.

Statistical Analysis. Baseline iron deficits in each clinical study were calculated for all subjects who were randomized to receive IV iron. In Study 5 [42], iron deficits were calculated for all subjects, as the comparator (iron dextran) was also dosed based on the modified Ganzoni formula and was summarized with descriptive statistics. For the iron deficit calculations performed for Studies 6 and 7, all subjects in the Safety Population were included. The iron deficits were averaged and the standard deviation was generated.

For Study 7, the Safety Population consisted of all subjects who received a dose of randomized treatment. The intent-to-treat (ITT) population for evaluating all efficacy endpoints consisted of all subjects from the Safety Population who received at least 1 dose of randomized study medication and had at least 1 postbaseline Hb assessment. Treatment assignments were analyzed according to the actual treatment received. The differences between 1500 mg and 1000 mg for time-to-event variables in Study 7 were assessed with the point estimate and 95% CI for the hazard ratio calculated from a Cox proportional hazards model. Treatment group differences were assessed using the Cox proportional hazards model with treatment as a fixed factor. In addition, p values for treatment differences were provided from the log-rank test. Time-to-event variables are displayed descriptively as Kaplan-Meier curves.

All statistical tests were *post hoc* with no adjustment to type I error for multiple comparisons.

3. Results

The average total iron deficits for patients in the 7 cited trials are summarized in Tables 3 and 4. The overall average total iron deficit in the initial 5 clinical trials was 1531 mg (Table 3). Total iron requirements among patients in each cohort in Studies 6 and 7 are summarized in Table 4. In Study 6, the average calculated iron deficit (Cohorts 1 and 2) was 1496 mg.

TABLE 4: Average calculated iron deficit dose in clinical Studies 6 and 7.

Study	Patient population	Treatment group	Calculated mean iron deficit based on the modified Ganzoni formula (mg)	Standard deviation	Number of patients	Total mean
Study 6	IDA of various etiologies	Cohort 1 (A): 1500 mg IV iron	1340	356	246	1496 mg
		Cohort 1 (B): oral iron	1344	360	253	
		Cohort 2 (C): 1500 mg IV iron	1600	446	252	
		Cohort 2 (D): IV SoC	1703	482	245	
Study 7 (REPAIR-IDA)	NDD-CKD	1500 mg IV iron	1355	401	1275	1352 mg
		1000 mg IV iron	1349	403	1285	
Overall mean			1392	NC	3556	

IDA = iron deficiency anemia; NDD-CKD = non-dialysis-dependent chronic kidney disease; SoC = standard of care; NC = not calculated.
Data on file, Luitpold Pharmaceuticals, Inc.

TABLE 5: Retreatment between Days 56–90 in clinical Study 7 (Safety Population).

	1500 mg IV iron ($n = 1276$)	1000 mg IV iron ($n = 1285$)	p value
N (%) patients retreated	71 (5.6%)	142 (11.1%)	$p < 0.001$

Data on file, Luitpold Pharmaceuticals, Inc.

TABLE 6: Hb >12 g/dL and end of treatment (Day 56) from clinical Study 7 (ITT population).

	1500 mg IV iron ($n = 1249$)	1000 mg IV iron ($n = 1244$)	p value
N (%) patients with Hb >12.0 g/dL	265 (24.4%)	169 (15.6%)	$p = 0.001$

Hb = hemoglobin; ITT = intent-to-treat.
Data on file, Luitpold Pharmaceuticals, Inc.

TABLE 7: Subjects with Hb >11 g/dL, 12 g/dL, or Hb change ≥1 g/dL in Study 7 anytime from randomization to end of study (Safety Population).

	1500 mg IV iron ($n = 1276$)	1000 mg IV iron ($n = 1244$)	Hazard ratio (95% CI)
N (%) of patients with Hb >11 g/dL	557 (56.1%)	504 (51.1%)	1.15 (1.02–1.30)
N (%) of patients with Hb >12 g/dL	358 (28.6%)	251 (20.0%)	1.44 (1.23–1.70)
N (%) of patients with Hb change ≥1 g/dL	610 (48.7%)	513 (41.0%)	1.27 (1.13–1.43)

Hb = hemoglobin.
Data on file, Luitpold Pharmaceuticals, Inc.

In Study 7, the average calculated iron deficit for patients receiving either 1500 mg or 1000 mg was 1352 mg. Overall, the average total iron deficit for clinical Studies 6 and 7 was 1392 mg.

In Study 7, study participants were randomized to receive either two 750 mg doses of IV iron (FCM) 7 days apart or IS 200 mg administered in up to 5 infusions over 14 days. The primary efficacy endpoint was the mean change in Hb from baseline to highest reported Hb (from baseline to Day 56). Patients were followed up for safety to Day 120. The mean total dose of iron received was 1464 mg in the 1500 mg group and 963 mg in the 1000 mg group. Mean baseline Hb values were 10.31 g/dL for the 1500 mg group and 10.32 g/dL for the 1000 mg group.

In this study, the mean increase in Hb overall was 1.13 g/dL in the 1500 mg group and 0.92 g/dL in the 1000 mg group (95% CI, 0.13–0.28), meeting the prespecified endpoint of noninferiority of 1500 mg to 1000 mg. Additionally, as evidenced by the 95% CI not including 0, 1500 mg was superior to 1000 mg in increasing Hb.

The proportion of patients in the 1500 mg group who were *retreated* with IV iron between Days 56 and 90 (Safety Population) was significantly ($p < 0.001$) lower, 71/1276 (5.6%), than the 142/1285 (11.1%) patients who required retreatment in the 1000 mg group (Table 5). Figure 1 displays the time from Day 56 to additional IV iron when comparing 1500 mg to 1000 mg.

Post hoc analyses of patients with Hb >12 g/dL at end of treatment (Day 56) and time to first Hb >11 g/dL and >12 g/dL and Hb increase ≥1 g/dL were conducted. The proportion of patients with Hb >12 g/dL at the end of treatment (baseline to Day 56) was 265/1249 in the 1500 mg group (24.4%) and 169/1244 in the 1000 mg group (15.6%), $p = 0.001$ (Table 6).

Patients who received 1500 mg IV iron were also more likely to achieve Hb >11 g/dL, Hb >12 g/dL, or an increase in Hb ≥1 g/dL compared with those receiving 1000 mg (Table 7).

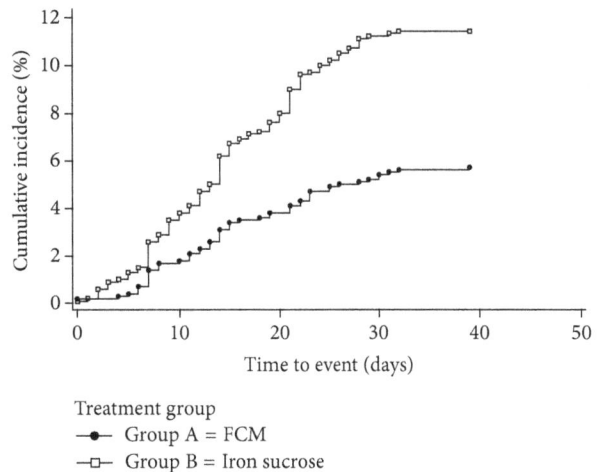

FIGURE 1: The time to additional intravenous (IV) iron after Day 56 comparing 1500 mg to 1000 mg IV iron in the Safety Population of Study 7. Data on file, Luitpold Pharmaceuticals, Inc.

Furthermore, the times to first Hb >11 g/dL and >12 g/dL and to Hb increases ≥1 g/dL were all statistically significantly shorter for the 1500 mg group than for the 1000 mg group ($p = 0.013$, $p < 0.001$, and $p < 0.001$, resp.). Figure 2 presents the Kaplan-Meier analysis for time to first Hb >12 g/dL.

The 1500 mg total cumulative dose had a similar safety profile to that of 1000 mg of IS, demonstrating that 50% more iron in the form of FCM can be administered while maintaining a safety profile comparable to that of IS [44].

4. Discussion

In the US, it has become common practice to administer a cumulative dose of approximately 1000 mg of IV iron (in

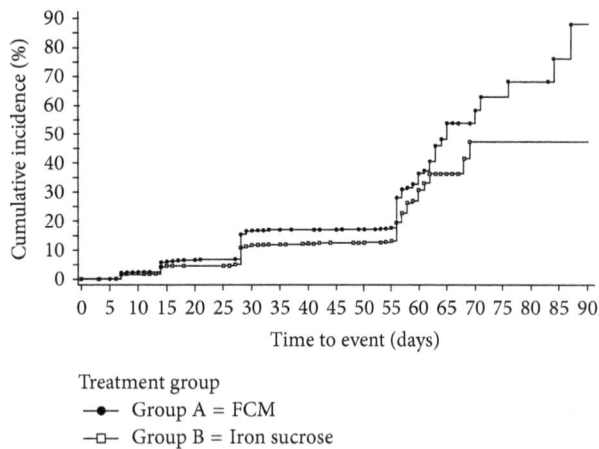

FIGURE 2: The time from randomization to first hemoglobin >12 g/dL in patients who received 1500 mg IV iron and patients who received 1000 mg from Study 7, $p < 0.001$. Day 56 is the last study visit, and at the discretion of the investigator, patients were allowed to be retreated with additional IV iron between Days 56 and 90. Data on file, Luitpold Pharmaceuticals, Inc.

divided doses) for the treatment of IDA. This is due, in large part, to the use of IV iron in nephrology. Both the Kidney Disease Outcomes Quality Initiative (KDOQI), initially developed in 1996, and the more recent Kidney Disease: Improving Global Outcomes (KDIGO) practice guidelines provide recommendations for the treatment of IDA utilizing IV iron. In the randomized controlled trials reviewed to develop the guidelines, a cumulative dose of 1000 mg of IV iron was utilized [45, 46]. Although that has now become the standard therapeutic dose for iron deficiency of various etiologies in light of a wealth of safety and efficacy data, it may not provide repletion of iron that is sufficient to alleviate the iron deficient state, thereby necessitating retreatment or creating the potential for a subtherapeutic response.

Despite these recommendations, in many clinical situations the treatment of IDA with IV iron has not been limited to a cumulative dose of 1000 mg. In oncology patients, for example, the National Comprehensive Cancer Network (NCCN) states that if the calculated dose exceeds 1000 mg, the remaining dose may be given after 4 weeks if the Hb response is inadequate [47].

Additionally, in two randomized controlled trials involving IV iron supplementation in oncology patients, a total of up to 3000 mg iron was administered in weekly doses of 100 mg [48]. In another prospective, randomized, controlled trial, patients with chemotherapy-related anemia received cumulative doses of IV iron ranging from 1000 to 3000 mg [7].

Guidelines for the management of IDA in inflammatory bowel disease (IBD), moreover, recommend IV iron as the preferred route of administration and state that anemic IBD patients rarely present with total iron deficits below 1000 mg. These guidelines recommend use of the Ganzoni formula to estimate iron replacement needs, and in controlled trials, up to 3600 mg of iron sucrose has been administered safely (up

to TSAT >50%) [49]. A 2011 review by Gozzard [50] further highlights numerous clinical situations requiring doses of IV iron above a cumulative dose of 1000 mg. Congruent with evidence reported in the international IBD guidelines, the article states that cumulative doses up to 3600 mg of IV iron may be administered safely in these patients. The review also suggests that higher doses of IV iron may overcome impaired iron absorption associated with hepcidin blockade in this patient population. In another multiple-dose, phase II/III study of IDA patients with GI disorders, mean total cumulative doses of 1800 mg IV iron were administered [51]. Clinical evidence also indicates that iron requirements of 1000 to 1500 mg or higher may be required in patients with NDD-CKD to attain target ferritin and Hb levels, up to 1600 mg may be required in obstetric patients, and as much as 2000 mg may be needed in patients with heavy or abnormal menstrual bleeding [50].

To help determine the optimal means of administering these higher doses, it is important to note that the degradation kinetics, and therefore the safety, of parenteral iron products are directly related to the molecular weight and stability of the iron complex [52–56].

Complexes can be generally classified as labile or robust (kinetic variability, i.e., how fast the ligands coordinated to the iron can be exchanged) and weak or strong (thermodynamic variability, i.e., how strongly the ligands are bound to the iron and thus how much energy is required to dissociate a ligand from the iron) or any intermediate state [52]. The reactivity of each complex correlates inversely with its molecular weight; larger complexes are less prone to release significant amounts of labile iron or react directly with transferrin [53, 54]. Type I complexes such as iron dextran preparations (INFeD Dexferrum) or FCM (Injectafer) have a high molecular weight and a high structural homogeneity and thereby deliver iron from the complex to transferrin in a regulated way via macrophage endocytosis and subsequent controlled export [52, 55]. They also bind iron tightly as nonionic polynuclear iron(III) hydroxide and do not release large amounts of iron ions into the blood. Such complexes can be administered intravenously and are clinically well tolerated even when administered at high doses. For less stable iron complexes, the maximum single doses are significantly lower and the administration times are drastically longer [54, 56].

FCM is a stable type I polynuclear iron(III) hydroxide carbohydrate complex that prevents the partial release of iron to serum ferritin observed with IS, allowing administration of high doses, since this iron is available only via reticuloendothelial processing [37, 57, 58]. FCM can be administered as a single 750 mg dose via a slow IV push injection over 7.5 minutes or as an IV infusion over at least 15 minutes. The second dose is administered at least 7 days later for a recommended cumulative dose of 1500 mg iron [36]. Use of high doses reduces the number of infusions, enabling the possibility of cost reductions compared to multiple administrations [59–62].

In our study, a modified Ganzoni formula was used to calculate total iron deficits in patients from 5 clinical studies involving FCM. After analyzing each study individually, we found the overall average iron deficit in those trials to be 1531 mg, suggesting that patients having IDA of various etiologies may benefit from a higher cumulative dose of IV iron than what is typically administered in clinical practice utilizing most of the currently available IV iron formulations.

Using the same modified Ganzoni formula, total iron deficits were also calculated in our *post hoc* analyses of the 2 larger studies (6 and 7) involving patients with IDA secondary to numerous underlying disorders, including HUB, GI diseases, and CKD. In Study 6, the average calculated iron deficit was 1496 mg. In Study 7, the average calculated iron deficit for patients receiving either 1500 mg IV iron, as FCM, or 1000 mg of IS was 1352 mg. The lower figure may be due to higher baseline ferritin and TSAT values in the CKD population, as 29% of the patients did not have the 500 mg of iron stores included in their iron deficit when it was calculated using the modified Ganzoni formula. Overall, the average calculated iron deficit in patients from Studies 6 and 7 was 1392 mg.

Data from Study 7 reinforced the benefits of higher IV iron dosing such that significantly fewer patients who received a total cumulative dose of 1500 mg of iron required IV iron retreatment during the follow-up period (Days 56–90) than those who received a total cumulative dose of 1000 mg. In addition, patients who received 1500 mg of iron achieved their first Hb >11 g/dL and >12 g/dL and a ≥1 g increase in Hb faster than those who received 1000 mg. This finding suggests that patients given 1000 mg may not be receiving a full repletion dose of iron compared to those given 1500 mg. Study 6 was not similarly analyzed because of confounders (i.e., small sample size and lack of consistent dosing for comparators). Despite patients in Cohort D (IV SoC) of that study having the highest mean calculated iron deficit (1703 mg), the mean amount of iron they received was paradoxically only 812 mg. This discrepancy between deficit and treatment in patients who received IV SoC may be due, in part, to convenience factors associated with the IV SoC dosing available to the investigators during the study, as well as the lack of practical guidance for determining iron dosing requirements.

In a study that compared the Ganzoni calculated dose to a simplified dose regimen, it was found that adherence was higher with the simplified dosing and resulted in better efficacy outcomes [59]. As a result, standard of care in Europe has moved from the Ganzoni calculation to a simple dosing scheme. In the US, most of the IV iron has a simple dosing scheme and the Ganzoni formula is not utilized as frequently, our study suggests that the simplified dosing scheme most often utilized may not fully replete the iron stores of the majority of patients.

Although the results of our study suggest that a total cumulative dose of IV iron greater than 1000 mg may be appropriate for many patients with IDA (we are aware of no similar published analyses), there are some limitations to consider. Parts of our analyses were retrospective in nature, and further prospective research will be needed to establish the long-term efficacy and safety of these higher total cumulative doses of IV iron. The population analyzed from Study 7 was limited to patients with CKD. Other etiologies of IDA may respond differently in relation to IV iron. In addition, most of the studies that evaluated the Ganzoni formula included patients with IDA resulting

from a variety of disease states. Also while, to the author's knowledge significant efficacy differences between similar cumulative doses of the various IV iron products have not been demonstrated, a future prospective study comparing various doses of the same product in a homogenous patient population would remove any product or population related bias that may have occurred in our study. It may be beneficial to observe whether higher or lower total cumulative doses of the same IV iron are more efficacious for patients with specific IDA etiologies.

5. Conclusions

Our study suggests that a total cumulative dose of 1000 mg of IV iron may be insufficient for iron repletion in the majority of patients with IDA and that a dose of 1500 mg is closer to the actual iron deficit in these patients. Additionally, 1500 mg of iron resulted in a more rapid, robust Hb response, allowed more patients to reach target Hb levels, and required a longer mean time to retreatment with additional IV iron compared to 1000 mg of iron. Our analysis and review of the literature suggest that 1500 mg of IV iron is more suitable for iron repletion in many patients with IDA compared to the commonly utilized dose of 1000 mg of IV iron. Further studies to confirm appropriate dose requirements in various patient populations are warranted.

Conflict of Interests

Lawrence Tim Goodnough is a consultant for Luitpold Pharmaceuticals, Inc. Jennifer Myers was an employee of Luitpold Pharmaceuticals, Inc. Todd A. Koch is an employee of Luitpold Pharmaceuticals, Inc.

Acknowledgments

The authors would like to thank David Morris, Ph.D. degree, for statistical input during the preparation of this paper, Andy He, PharmD, for publication management, and Aesculapius Consulting, Inc., for the editorial services.

References

[1] L. T. Goodnough, "The new age of iron: evaluation and management of iron-restricted erythropoiesis," *Seminars in Hematology*, vol. 46, no. 4, pp. 325–327, 2009.

[2] B. Annibale, G. Capurso, A. Chistolini et al., "Gastrointestinal causes of refractory iron deficiency anemia in patients without gastrointestinal symptoms," *The American Journal of Medicine*, vol. 111, no. 6, pp. 439–445, 2001.

[3] P. L. Acher, T. Al-Mishlab, M. Rahman, and T. Bates, "Iron-deficiency anaemia and delay in the diagnosis of colorectal cancer," *Colorectal Disease*, vol. 5, no. 2, pp. 145–148, 2003.

[4] D. Raje, H. Mukhtar, A. Oshowo, and C. Ingham Clark, "What proportion of patients referred to secondary care with iron deficiency anemia have colon cancer?" *Diseases of the Colon and Rectum*, vol. 50, no. 8, pp. 1211–1214, 2007.

[5] M. Auerbach, J. A. Pappadakis, H. Bahrain, S. A. Auerbach, H. Ballard, and N. V. Dahl, "Safety and efficacy of rapidly

administered (one hour) one gram of low molecular weight iron dextran (INFeD) for the treatment of iron deficient anemia," *American Journal of Hematology*, vol. 86, no. 10, pp. 860–862, 2011.

[6] L. T. Goodnough, E. Nemeth, and T. Ganz, "Detection, evaluation, and management of iron-restricted erythropoiesis," *Blood*, vol. 116, no. 23, pp. 4754–4761, 2010.

[7] M. Auerbach, H. Ballard, J. R. Trout et al., "Intravenous iron optimizes the response to recombinant human erythropoietin in cancer patients with chemotherapy-related anemia: a multicenter, open-label, randomized trial," *Journal of Clinical Oncology*, vol. 22, no. 7, pp. 1301–1307, 2004.

[8] M. Auerbach, "Ferumoxytol as a new, safer, easier-to-administer intravenous iron: yes or no?" *The American Journal of Kidney Diseases*, vol. 52, no. 5, pp. 826–829, 2008.

[9] J. Bonnar, A. Goldberg, and J. A. Smith, "Do pregnant women take their iron?" *The Lancet*, vol. 1, no. 7592, pp. 457–458, 1969.

[10] G. Weiss and L. T. Goodnough, "Anemia of chronic disease," *The New England Journal of Medicine*, vol. 352, no. 10, pp. 1011–1059, 2005.

[11] N. C. Andrews, "Anemia of inflammation: the cytokine-hepcidin link," *Journal of Clinical Investigation*, vol. 113, no. 9, pp. 1251–1253, 2004.

[12] L. T. Goodnough and A. Shander, "Current status of pharmacologic therapies in patient blood management," *Anesthesia & Analgesia*, vol. 116, no. 1, pp. 15–34, 2013.

[13] D. H. Henry, N. V. Dahl, M. Auerbach, S. Tchekmedyian, and L. R. Laufmane, "Intravenous ferric gluconate significantly improves response to epoetin alfa versus oral iron or no iron in anemic patients with cancer receiving chemotherapy," *Oncologist*, vol. 12, no. 2, pp. 231–242, 2007.

[14] M. Hedenus, G. Birgegard, P. Nasman et al., "Addition of intravenous iron to epoetin beta increases hemoglobin response and decreases epoetin dose requirement in anemic patients with lymphoproliferative malignancies: a randomized multicenter study," *Leukemia*, vol. 21, no. 4, pp. 627–632, 2007.

[15] L. Bastit, A. Vandebroek, S. Altintas et al., "Randomized, multicenter, controlled trial comparing the efficacy and safety of darbepoetin alfa administered every 3 weeks with or without intravenous iron in patients with chemotherapy-induced anemia," *Journal of Clinical Oncology*, vol. 26, no. 10, pp. 1611–1618, 2008.

[16] A. Gafter-Gvili, D. P. Steensma, and M. Auerbach, "Should the ASCO/ASH guidelines for the use of intravenous iron in cancer- and chemotherapy-induced anemia be updated?" *Journal of the National Comprehensive Cancer Network*, vol. 12, no. 5, pp. 657–664, 2014.

[17] J. A. Gilreath, D. D. Stenehjem, and G. M. Rodgers, "Diagnosis and treatment of cancer-related anemia," *American Journal of Hematology*, vol. 89, no. 2, pp. 203–212, 2014.

[18] M. Auerbach, A. S. Liang, and J. Glaspy, "Intravenous iron in chemotherapy and cancer-related anemia," *Community Oncology*, vol. 9, no. 9, pp. 289–295, 2012.

[19] J. D. Rizzo, M. Brouwers, P. Hurley, J. Seidenfeld, M. R. Somerfield, and S. Temin, "American Society of Clinical Oncology/American Society of Hematology clinical practice guideline update on the use of epoetin and darbepoetin in adult patients with cancer," *Journal of Oncology Practice*, vol. 6, no. 6, pp. 317–320, 2010.

[20] D. S. Silverberg, A. Iaina, G. Peer et al., "Intravenous iron supplementation for the treatment of the anemia of moderate to severe chronic renal failure patients not receiving dialysis," *American Journal of Kidney Diseases*, vol. 27, no. 2, pp. 234–238, 1996.

[21] R. S. Hillman and P. A. Henderson, "Control of marrow production by the level of iron supply," *Journal of Clinical Investigation*, vol. 48, no. 3, pp. 454–460, 1969.

[22] R. L. Jurado, "Iron, infections, and anemia of inflammation," *Clinical Infectious Diseases*, vol. 25, no. 4, pp. 888–895, 1997.

[23] K. Bishu and R. Agarwal, "Acute injury with intravenous iron and concerns regarding long-term safety," *Clinical Journal of the American Society of Nephrology*, supplement 1, pp. S19–S23, 2006.

[24] L. T. Goodnough, J. H. Levy, and M. F. Murphy, "Concepts of blood transfusion in adults," *The Lancet*, vol. 381, no. 9880, pp. 1845–1854, 2013.

[25] D. R. Spahn and L. T. Goodnough, "Alternatives to blood transfusion," *The Lancet*, vol. 381, no. 9880, pp. 1855–1865, 2013.

[26] L. T. Goodnough, "Blood management: transfusion medicine comes of age," *The Lancet*, vol. 381, no. 9880, pp. 1791–1792, 2013.

[27] A. Shander, R. K. Spence, and M. Auerbach, "Can intravenous iron therapy meet the unmet needs created by the new restrictions on erythropoietic stimulating agents?: report from the Society for the Advancement of Blood Management 2008 Annual Meeting," *Transfusion*, vol. 50, no. 3, pp. 719–732, 2010.

[28] M. Auerbach, L. T. Goodnough, D. Picard, and A. Maniatis, "The role of intravenous iron in anemia management and transfusion avoidance," *Transfusion*, vol. 48, no. 5, pp. 988–1000, 2008.

[29] G. M. Chertow, P. D. Mason, O. Vaage-Nilsen, and J. Ahlmén, "Update on adverse drug events associated with parenteral iron," *Nephrology Dialysis Transplantation*, vol. 21, no. 2, pp. 378–382, 2006.

[30] Dexferrum [package insert], American Regent, Shirley, NY, USA, 2008.

[31] INFeD, *Package Insert*, Watson Pharma, Morristown, NJ, USA, 2009.

[32] A. M. Ganzoni, "Intravenous iron-dextran: therapeutic and experimental possibilities," *Schweizerische Medizinische Wochenschrift*, vol. 100, no. 7, pp. 301–303, 1970.

[33] American Regent, *Venofer [Package Insert]*, American Regent, Shirley, NY, USA, 2012.

[34] Ferrlecit, *Package Insert*, Sanofi-Aventis US, Bridgewater, NJ, USA, 2011.

[35] Feraheme [package insert], AMAG Pharmaceuticals, Lexington, Mass, USA, 2015.

[36] American Regent, *Injectafer [Package Insert]*, American Regent, Shirley, NY, USA, 2013.

[37] S. Kulnigg, S. Stoinov, V. Simanenkov et al., "A novel intravenous iron formulation for treatment of anemia in inflammatory bowel disease: the ferric carboxymaltose (FERINJECT) randomized controlled trial," *The American Journal of Gastroenterology*, vol. 103, no. 5, pp. 1182–1192, 2008.

[38] D. B. van Wyck, M. G. Martens, M. H. Seid, J. B. Baker, and A. Mangione, "Intravenous ferric carboxymaltose compared with oral iron in the treatment of postpartum anemia: a randomized controlled trial," *Obstetrics and Gynecology*, vol. 110, no. 2, pp. 267–278, 2007.

[39] D. B. van Wyck, A. Mangione, J. Morrison, P. E. Hadley, J. A. Jehle, and L. T. Goodnough, "Large-dose intravenous ferric carboxymaltose injection for iron deficiency anemia in heavy

uterine bleeding: a randomized, controlled trial," *Transfusion*, vol. 49, no. 12, pp. 2719–2728, 2009.

[40] M. H. Seid, R. J. Derman, J. B. Baker, W. Banach, C. Goldberg, and R. Rogers, "Ferric carboxymaltose injection in the treatment of postpartum iron deficiency anemia: a randomized controlled clinical trial," *American Journal of Obstetrics & Gynecology*, vol. 199, no. 4, pp. 435.e1–435.e7, 2008.

[41] C. F. Barish, T. Koch, A. Butcher, D. Morris, and D. B. Bregman, "Safety and efficacy of intravenous ferric carboxymaltose (750 mg) in the treatment of iron deficiency anemia: two randomized, controlled trials," *Anemia*, vol. 2012, Article ID 172104, 9 pages, 2012.

[42] I. Hussain, J. Bhoyroo, A. Butcher, T. A. Koch, A. He, and D. B. Bregman, "Direct comparison of the safety and efficacy of ferric carboxymaltose versus iron dextran in patients with iron deficiency anemia," *Anemia*, vol. 2013, Article ID 169107, 10 pages, 2013.

[43] J. E. Onken, D. B. Bregman, R. A. Harrington et al., "A multicenter, randomized, active-controlled study to investigate the efficacy and safety of intravenous ferric carboxymaltose in patients with iron deficiency anemia," *Transfusion*, vol. 54, no. 2, pp. 306–315, 2014.

[44] J. E. Onken, D. B. Bregman, R. A. Harrington et al., "Ferric carboxymaltose in patients with iron-deficiency anemia and impaired renal function: the REPAIR-IDA trial," *Nephrology Dialysis Transplantation*, vol. 29, no. 4, pp. 833–842, 2014.

[45] National Kidney Foundation. KDOQI, "Clinical practice guidelines and clinical practice recommendations for anemia in chronic kidney disease," *American Journal of Kidney Diseases*, vol. 47, supplement 3, pp. S1–S145, 2006.

[46] Kidney Disease: Improving Global Outcomes (KDIGO) Anemia Work Group, "KDIGO clinical practice guideline for anemia in chronic kidney disease," *Kidney International Supplements*, vol. 2, no. 4, pp. S279–S335, 2012.

[47] National Comprehensive Cancer Network (NCCN), *Clinical Practice Guidelines in Oncology. Cancer- and Chemotherapy-Induced Anemia. Version 2*, NCCN, 2015.

[48] M. Aapro, A. Österborg, P. Gascón, H. Ludwig, and Y. Beguin, "Prevalence and management of cancer-related anaemia, iron deficiency and the specific role of I.V. iron," *Annals of Oncology*, vol. 23, no. 8, pp. 1954–1962, 2012.

[49] C. Gasche, A. Berstad, R. Befrits et al., "Guidelines on the diagnosis and management of iron deficiency and anemia in inflammatory bowel diseases," *Inflammatory Bowel Diseases*, vol. 13, no. 12, pp. 1545–1553, 2007.

[50] D. Gozzard, "When is high-dose intravenous iron repletion needed? Assessing new treatment options," *Drug Design, Development and Therapy*, no. 5, pp. 51–60, 2011.

[51] P. Geisser and V. Rumyantsev, "Pharmacodynamics and safety of ferric carboxymaltose: a multiple-dose study in patients with iron-deficiency anaemia secondary to a gastrointestinal disorder," *Arzneimittelforschung*, vol. 60, no. 6, pp. 373–385, 2010.

[52] R. R. Crichton, B. Danielson, and P. Geisser, *Iron Therapy with Special Emphasis on Intravenous Administration*, UNI-MED, Bremen, Germany, 4th edition, 2008.

[53] B. G. Danielson, "Structure, chemistry, and pharmacokinetics of intravenous iron agents," *Journal of the American Society of Nephrology*, vol. 15, no. 2, pp. S93–S98, 2004.

[54] P. Geisser, M. Baer, and E. Schaub, "Structure/histotoxicity relationship of parenteral iron preparations," *Drug Research*, vol. 42, no. 12, pp. 1439–1452, 1992.

[55] S. Beshara, H. Lundqvist, J. Sundin et al., "Pharmacokinetics and red cell utilization of iron(III) hydroxide-sucrose complex in anaemic patients: a study using positron emission tomography," *British Journal of Haematology*, vol. 104, no. 2, pp. 296–302, 1999.

[56] P. Geisser and S. Burckhardt, "The pharmacokinetics and pharmacodynamics of iron preparations," *Pharmaceutics*, vol. 3, no. 1, pp. 12–33, 2011.

[57] M. Malone, C. Barish, A. He, and D. Bregman, "Comparative review of the safety and efficacy of ferric carboxymaltose versus standard medical care for the treatment of iron deficiency anemia in bariatric and gastric surgery patients," *Obesity Surgery*, vol. 23, no. 9, pp. 1413–1420, 2013.

[58] K. A. Lyseng-Williamson and G. M. Keating, "Ferric carboxymaltose: a review of its use in iron-deficiency anaemia," *Drugs*, vol. 69, no. 6, pp. 739–756, 2009.

[59] R. Evstatiev, P. Marteau, T. Iqbal et al., "FERGIcor, a randomized controlled trial on ferric carboxymaltose for iron deficiency anemia in inflammatory bowel disease," *Gastroenterology*, vol. 141, no. 3, pp. 846.e2–853.e2, 2011.

[60] X. Calvet, M. À. Ruíz, A. Dosal et al., "Cost-minimization analysis favours intravenous ferric carboxymaltose over ferric sucrose for the ambulatory treatment of severe iron deficiency," *PLoS ONE*, vol. 7, no. 9, Article ID e45604, 2012.

[61] F. Gomollón and J. P. Gisbert, "Current management of iron deficiency anemia in inflammatory bowel diseases: a practical guide," *Drugs*, vol. 73, no. 16, pp. 1761–1770, 2013.

[62] A. A. Khalafallah and A. E. Dennis, "Iron deficiency anaemia in pregnancy and postpartum: pathophysiology and effect of oral versus intravenous iron therapy," *Journal of Pregnancy*, vol. 2012, Article ID 630519, 10 pages, 2012.

20

Effect of Maternal Iron Deficiency Anemia on the Iron Store of Newborns in Ethiopia

Betelihem Terefe,[1] Asaye Birhanu,[2] Paulos Nigussie,[3] and Aster Tsegaye[2]

[1]Department of Hematology and Immunohematology, University of Gondar, Gondar, Ethiopia
[2]School of Medical Laboratory Science, Addis Ababa University, Addis Ababa, Ethiopia
[3]Ethiopian Health and Nutrition Research Institute (EHNRI), Addis Ababa, Ethiopia

Correspondence should be addressed to Betelihem Terefe; betch.nym@gmail.com

Academic Editor: Aurelio Maggio

Iron deficiency anemia among pregnant women is a widespread problem in developing countries including Ethiopia, though its influence on neonatal iron status was inconsistently reported in literature. This cross-sectional study was conducted to compare hematologic profiles and iron status of newborns from mothers with different anemia status and determine correlation between maternal and neonatal hematologic profiles and iron status in Ethiopian context. We included 89 mothers and their respective newborns and performed complete blood count and assessed serum ferritin and C-reactive protein levels from blood samples collected from study participants. Maternal median hemoglobin and serum ferritin levels were 12.2 g/dL and 47.0 ng/mL, respectively. The median hemoglobin and serum ferritin levels for the newborns were 16.2 g/dL and 187.6 ng/mL, respectively. The mothers were classified into two groups based on hemoglobin and serum ferritin levels as iron deficient anemic (IDA) and nonanemic (NA) and newborns of IDA mothers had significantly lower levels of serum ferritin ($P = 0.017$) and hemoglobin concentration ($P = 0.024$). Besides, newborns' ferritin and hemoglobin levels showed significant correlation with maternal hemoglobin ($P = 0.018$; $P = 0.039$) and ferritin ($P = 0.000$; $P = 0.008$) levels. We concluded that maternal IDA may have an effect on the iron stores of newborns.

1. Background

Iron deficiency (ID) is the most important cause of nutritional anemia and is the most common micronutrient deficiency worldwide, especially in developing countries [1]. Pregnant women are particularly vulnerable to ID because of the increased metabolic demands imposed by pregnancy involving a growing placenta, fetus, and maternal tissues, coupled with associated dietary risks [2].

In developing countries including Ethiopia, pregnant women commonly begin gestation with depleted or low body iron stores which might make them prone to developing iron deficiency anemia (IDA) [3]. Frequently, the anemia is severe in degree and it coexists with maternal malnutrition [3]. Under these situations, the competing demands of mother and fetus may disturb the normal maternal-fetal iron homeostasis [3–5]. This may have a resultant effect both on

the mother and on the fetus, such as premature delivery, intrauterine growth retardation, and neonatal and perinatal death [6]. As the main source of iron for infants until the age of 6 months is the iron endowed from maternal circulation [7], it is logical to question the extension of the effect of maternal IDA on the fetus during and beyond its stay in the womb.

In spite of many researches conducted on this specific issue, consistent findings were not evident. Some have reported the negative impact of maternal IDA on iron stores of newborns [3, 5, 8–11], while others could not find any relationship in between [12–14]. Most of the studies have used serum ferritin as a measurement of iron store, but this serum ferritin has one known drawback as it is an acute phase reactant (APR); it increases during infection, including sub-clinical infections [15]. Therefore in this study, we incorporated another APR that is C-reactive protein

(CRP) test to minimize the bias that can be caused due to infection and tried to determine the effect of IDA on the iron store of term newborns.

2. Methods

This study was conducted from December 2011 to February 2012 in Obstetrics and Gynecology Department of St. Paul's hospital, Addis Ababa, Ethiopia. Mothers who had bleeding during pregnancy, preterm delivery (<37 weeks), multiple pregnancy, eclampsia, diabetes mellitus, heart, kidney, lung disease, and hematologic disease were excluded.

A total of 101 mothers and their respective newborns were included first. However, 12 of them were withdrawn from the study because they had anemia other than IDA. Therefore, the final sample comprised 89 mothers and their respective newborns.

Sociodemographic characteristics of study participants were collected using pretested questionnaires and blood samples were collected at the median cubital vein of the mothers during the process of labor and at the placental end of the umbilical cord. Pairs of samples were collected from each mother and cord using K_3EDTA test tubes (for complete blood counting, CBC) and test tubes with serum gel separator (for ferritin determination and CRP measurement).

CBC and ferritin concentrations were analyzed using Cell-dyn 1800 (Abbott Laboratories, Abbott Park, Illinois) and fully automated Cobas e 411 (Roche Diagnostics GmbH, D-68298 Mannheim, Germany), respectively. CRP was determined by a qualitative slide agglutination test using Cromatest (Linear Chemicals SL, Barcelona, Spain). The instruments were calibrated before the beginning of analyses. Precision test was carried out to assure reproducibility of results provided by the Cell-dyn 1800 analyzer and it was within the acceptable limit stated by the manufacturer. In addition, commercial quality control samples were included in every session of analyses for both CBC enumeration and serum ferritin level determination. Three levels of whole blood controls (high, medium, and low), two levels of plasma control (low, normal), and serum control (positive and negative) were used for CBC ferritin and CRP determinations, respectively. Levy-Jennine (LJ) charts were plotted and the controls were within the 2SD limits with no shifts or drifts detected.

We entered the data from the analyzers and questionnaire into Microsoft Excel and analyzed it using MedCalc Software Version 12.1.4. D'Agostino-Pearson test was used to check the normality of data distribution. Since all of the analytes studied were not normally distributed, nonparametric tests were applied. Frequencies, percentages, medians, and interquartile ranges (IQR) were computed to summarize the data. In order to compare quantitative and qualitative variables between the groups, Mann-Whitney and Chi-square tests were applied, respectively. Association of maternal and newborns parameters were assessed by spearman's correlation. P value of <0.05 was considered as statistically significant in all analyses.

The study protocol was approved by the Research Ethics Review Committees of Addis Ababa University and St. Paul's Hospital. In addition, informed verbal consents were collected from the mothers.

3. Result

3.1. Description of the Sociodemographic and Obstetric Data of Study Participants. We included 89 mothers with their respective newborns. The median age of the mothers was 23 years (IQR = 21–27 years). As clearly presented in Table 1, about one-third of the mothers (34.8%; n = 31) had educational level above secondary school, while 29.2% (n = 26) of the mothers were illiterates. Housewives were dominant and accounted for 75.3% (n = 67) of the participants.

The majority of mothers were primiparous (64.0%; n = 57), and also were attending antenatal care (ANC) during their pregnancy. Those mothers who have been taking iron during their pregnancy accounted for 58.4% (n = 52) (Table 1).

Most of the babies were delivered through vaginal delivery (78.7%; n = 70) and the proportion of male (49.4%; n = 44) and female (50.6%; n = 45) newborns were almost equal. The babies had median weight of 3100 g (IQR = 2800–3400 g) and a few (12.4%; n = 11) had low birth weight (Table 1).

3.2. Hematological and Ferritin Status of Mothers and Their Newborns. The median hemoglobin and serum ferritin levels for the mothers were 12.2 g/dL (IQR = 11.3–12.9 g/dL) and 45.5 ng/mL (IQR = 26.8–80.34 ng/mL), respectively (Table 2). The median hemoglobin and serum ferritin levels for the newborns were 16.2 g/dL (IQR = 15.0–17.2 g/dL) and 191.5 ng/mL (IQR = 140.5–264.8 ng/mL), respectively (Table 2). Table 2 also summarizes the median and the IQRs of other studied CBC parameters among mothers and their newborns.

3.3. Grouping Study Participants. The mothers were grouped into two categories, NA and IDA based on hemoglobin and serum ferritin concentrations. We used 11 g/dL as cutoff value for maternal hemoglobin concentration after altitude corrections as per World Health Organization (WHO) recommendation [16]. Similarly, the cutoff value for maternal ferritin level was set at 15 ng/mL for those mothers who were not reactive to CRP test and 30 ng/mL for those mothers who were reactive to CRP test in order to balance the effect of infection as recommended by the WHO [15].

Then, mothers showing low hemoglobin concentration (<11 g/dL) and low ferritin level (<15 ng/mL or <30 ng/mL as per their CRP reaction status) were grouped under IDA. Mothers with normal hemoglobin concentration (≥11 g/dL) were classified as NA. Accordingly, 21 mothers (23.6%) were grouped under IDA category while the rest 68 mothers (76.4%) were grouped under NA category. Prevalence of anemia, median differences in hemoglobin, and ferritin levels among newborns of mothers in the two categories were computed and presented in Table 3.

3.4. Correlations between Mothers and Newborns Laboratory Parameters. The newborns ferritin level has significant correlation with hemoglobin (r_s = 0.25, P = 0.018) and ferritin (r_s = 0.38, P < 0.001) levels of their mothers (Table 4). In addition, the newborns hemoglobin had significant correlation with hemoglobin (r_s = 0.22, P = 0.039) and ferritin

TABLE 1: Summary of sociodemographic and obstetric characteristics of mothers and their newborns gender and weight attending at St. Paul's Hospital, Addis Ababa.

Characteristics	Total ($n = 89$) frequency (%)	IDA ($n = 21$) frequency (%)	NA ($n = 68$) frequency (%)	P value*
Maternal age				
≤24 yrs	52 (58.4%)	11 (52.4%)	41 (60.3%)	0.700
>24 yrs	37 (41.6%)	10 (47.6%)	27 (39.7%)	
Maternal education level				
No education	26 (29.2%)	6 (28.6%)	20 (29.4%)	
Primary school	19 (21.4%)	6 (28.6%)	13 (19.1%)	0.805
Secondary school	13 (14.6%)	3 (14.2%)	10 (14.7%)	
Above secondary school	31 (34.8%)	6 (28.6%)	25 (36.8%)	
Maternal occupation				
Housewives	67 (75.3%)	16 (76.2%)	51 (75.0%)	0.858
Employed	22 (24.7%)	5 (23.8%)	17 (25.0%)	
Parity				
Primiparous	57 (64.0%)	12 (57.1%)	45 (66.2%)	0.621
Multiparous	32 (36.0%)	9 (42.9%)	23 (33.8%)	
Delivery				
Vaginal	70 (78.7%)	17 (81.0%)	53 (77.9%)	0.992
Cesarean section	19 (21.3%)	4 (19.0%)	15 (22.1%)	
ANC followup				
Yes	79 (88.8%)	17 (81.0%)	62 (91.2%)	0.367
No	10 (11.2%)	4 (19.0%)	6 (8.8%)	
Iron intake during pregnancy				
Yes	52 (58.4%)	10 (47.6%)	42 (61.8%)	0.370
No	37 (41.6%)	11 (52.4%)	26 (38.2%)	
Newborns' gender				
Female	45 (50.6%)	10 (47.6%)	35 (51.5%)	0.953
Male	44 (49.4%)	11 (52.4%)	33 (48.5%)	
Weight of newborns				
Normal birth weight	78 (87.6%)	19 (90.5%)	59 (86.8%)	0.942
Low birth weight	11 (12.4%)	2 (9.5%)	9 (13.2%)	

IDA = iron deficient anemic; NA = nonanemic. *Data are from the Chi-square test.

(r_s = 0.28, P = 0.008) levels of their mothers (Table 4); additionally the newborns hemoglobin showed significant correlation with mothers mean corpuscular hemoglobin (MCH) and mean corpuscular hemoglobin concentration (MCHC) values (Table 4).

4. Discussion

In our study, we determined that maternal IDA may have an effect on the iron stores of newborns as hemoglobin (P = 0.025) and ferritin concentrations (P = 0.027) were significantly lower in newborns delivered from IDA mothers than newborns delivered from NA mothers (Table 3 and Figure 1). These findings were in accordance with previous reports elsewhere [3, 8, 17, 18]. However, there are also findings in contrary to the present study which showed that iron accretion in the fetus was independent of maternal iron status [12–14].

The disagreements might be raised due to differences in cutoff value for serum ferritin (<10 ng/mL, which has low sensitivity), failure to incorporate tests that rule out infection (which may mask the actual ferritin status) [13], and differences in condition of study participants including mothers who were taking iron supplementation during pregnancy, which may have masked the relationship of maternal and newborns iron status [14].

It is well established that serum ferritin is an indicator of the level of body iron sores [19]. Thus, the significantly lower level of ferritin in newborns delivered from IDA mothers compared to NA mothers suggests reduced iron stores in these newborns. Additionally, the newborns delivered from IDA mothers had a significantly lower concentration of hemoglobin than newborns from NA mothers that might contribute for a decreased amount of recycled heme iron resultantly decreasing its contribution for the iron pool. Here, we were not surprised to see no statistically significant

TABLE 2: Hematological profile and ferritin status of mothers and their newborns at St. Paul's Hospital, Addis Ababa ($n = 89$).

Parameters	Median (IQR)[a]		P value*
	Mothers	Newborns	
Hemoglobin (g/dL)	12.2 (11.2–12.9)	16.2 (15.0–17.2)	<0.001
Mean cell volume (fL)	90.0 (88.1–93.5)	105.5 (102.7–109.7)	<0.001
Mean cell hemoglobin (pg)	30.7 (30.2–31.8)	37.3 (36.2–38.2)	<0.001
Mean cell hemoglobin concentration (%)	34.2 (33.9–34.8)	35.0 (34.3–35.8)	<0.001
Red cell distribution width (%)	14.1 (13.5–14.9)	16.3 (15.6–17.1)	<0.001
Serum ferritin (ng/mL)	47.0 (26.5–79.7)	187.6 (140.0–264.7)	<0.001

IDA = iron deficient anemic; NA = nonanemic. [a]IQR, 25th to 75th quartiles, *data are from Mann-Whitney test.

TABLE 3: Hematological profile and ferritin status of newborns by anemia and iron status of their mothers[a] at St. Paul's Hospital, Addis Ababa ($n = 89$).

Parameters	Group median (IQR)[b]		P value
	IDA ($n = 21$)	NA ($n = 68$)	
Hgb (g/dL)	15.6 (14.8–16.4)	16.7 (15.5–17.6)	**0.024***
MCV (fL)	105.1 (101.6–108.4)	105.9 (103.0–109.9)	0.588*
MCH (pg)	37.0 (35.9–38.1)	37.5 (36.4–38.3)	0.344*
MCHC (%)	35.0 (33.9–35.4)	35.1 (34.3–35.9)	0.227*
RDW (%)	16.0 (15.5–16.5)	16.4 (15.7–17.3)	0.080*
Ferritin (ng/mL)	138.9 (105.0–211.7)	200.7 (151.4–265.3)	**0.017***
Frequency (%) of anemia	3 (14.3%)	5 (7.9%)	0.593**

Hgb = hemoglobin; MCV = mean cell volume; MCH = mean cell hemoglobin; MCHC = mean cell hemoglobin concentration; RDW = red cell distribution width. [a]IDA = iron deficient anemic; NA = nonanemic. [b]IQR, 25th to 75th quartiles. *Data are from Mann-Whitney test. **Data are from the Chi-square test.

TABLE 4: Spearman's correlation coefficients (r) comparing hematological profile and ferritin status of mothers and their respective newborns at St. Paul's Hospital, Addis Ababa ($n = 89$).

Newborns parameters	Mother's parameters r_s (P value)					
	Hgb	MCV	MCH	MCHC	RDW	Ferritin
Hgb	0.22[a]	0.09	0.23[a]	0.35[c]	−0.00	0.28[b]
MCV	0.06	−0.03	−0.03	−0.05	−0.08	0.12
MCH	0.15	0.02	0.09	0.14	−0.06	0.10
MCHC	0.16	0.24[a]	0.31[b]	0.39[c]	−0.02	0.04
RDW	−0.01	−0.19	−0.16	0.04	0.03	0.01
Ferritin	0.25[a]	0.10	0.13	0.11	−0.21	0.38[c]

Hgb = hemoglobin; MCV = mean cell volume; MCH = mean cell hemoglobin; MCHC = mean cell hemoglobin concentration; RDW = red cell distribution width. [a]P value < 0.05, [b]P value < 0.01, and [c]P value < 0.001.

difference in prevalence of anemia among newborns of the two groups of mothers ($P = 0.593$). This is because visible difference that can be evidenced in the form of anemia is not expected at such an early stage in life [7]. However, later in life, anemia prevalence could be different among newborns from the two groups of mothers since newborns are highly dependent on the stored iron acquired from the mother during pregnancy till the age of 6 months [20, 21]. Therefore, the significantly lower ferritin level and hemoglobin concentration in newborns delivered from IDA mothers compared to NA mothers may make them prone to iron deficiency and

anemia in early infancy. This may have serious consequences on cognitive development and cellular immunity [22].

The evidence presented in this study also denotes that all the hematological and ferritin parameters studied were markedly higher in newborns than in their mothers. Similar findings were also documented in previous studies [3, 5, 8–11]. The higher ferritin levels in newborns can be explained by the existence of active transfer of iron across placenta from mother to the fetus [23]. Also, it can be due to the upregulation of transferrin receptor synthesis in the case of iron deficiency, which enables placenta to compete more effectively for circulating transferrin iron with erythroid marrow of the pregnant mothers intending adequate iron supply of the growing fetus [7, 11, 24].

In this study, newborns ferritin level has significant correlation with hemoglobin and ferritin levels of mothers. In addition, the newborns hemoglobin had significant correlation with hemoglobin and ferritin levels of mothers. Several investigators have determined the correlation between hemoglobin and ferritin parameters of newborns and their mothers; however, the results vary from study to study. Kumar et al., for example, have showed that maternal ferritin levels had significant correlations with Hgb levels ($r_s = +0.488$; $P < 0.001$) and ferritin ($r_s = +0.440$; $P < 0.001$) in cord blood [3]. Singla et al. have also found that maternal serum ferritin was significantly correlated with cord blood Hgb ($r_s = +0.390$, $P < 0.01$) and cord serum ferritin ($r_s = +0.523$; $P < 0.001$) [8]. The relatively lower correlation observed in this study compared to the two studies may be due to the absence of any severe anemia cases in our study, while there were severe anemia cases in the two studies.

In this study, we determined that the deleterious effect of maternal IDA may extend beyond pregnancy, in an Ethiopian context. This suggests the need for strengthening strategy to improve the maternal iron status. Improving the nutritional status of pregnant women could have a positive impact on improving the iron status of the mothers and also their newborns. The other option might be delayed clamping of the umbilical cord after birth for improving the iron status of young infants [25].

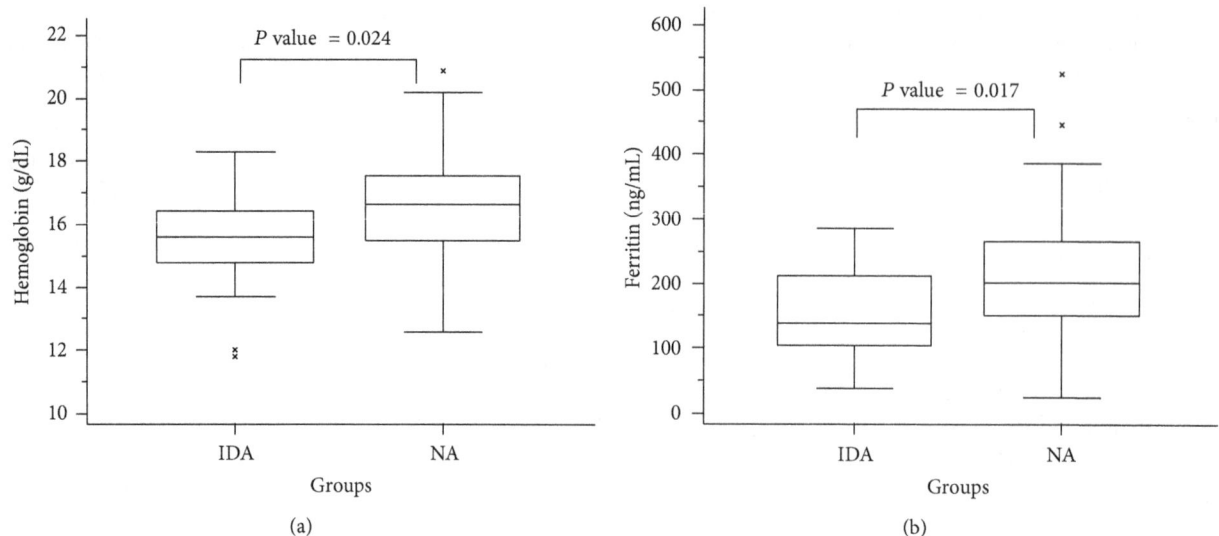

FIGURE 1: Box plots of hematological profile and ferritin parameters in newborns according to anemia and iron status of the mothers. IDA = iron deficient anemic; NA = nonanemic. P values are from the Mann-Whitney test.

5. Conclusion

Median hemoglobin and ferritin concentrations were significantly lower in newborns delivered from IDA mothers compared to NA mothers. Additionally newborns hemoglobin and ferritin concentration had a significant correlation with hemoglobin and ferritin concentration of the mothers. Based on these findings we can conclude that maternal IDA may have an effect on the iron stores of newborns.

Conflict of Interests

The authors declare that they have no competing interests.

Authors' Contribution

Betelihem Terefe, Asaye Birhanu, and Aster Tsegaye have participated in the conception and design of the study. Betelihem Terefe and Paulos Nigussie have participated in the selection of study participants. Betelihem Terefe and Paulos Nigussie have participated in the laboratory analysis and acquisition of data. All authors have participated in preparing and critically reviewing the draft paper. All authors also have read and approved the final paper.

Acknowledgments

The authors would like to thank Addis Ababa University for the financial support and Paul's Hospital Laboratory for their Cell-dyn 1800 reagent supply. The authors thank the study participants for their kind collaboration.

References

[1] A. Krafft, R. Huch, and C. Breymann, "Impact of parturition on iron status in nonanaemic iron deficiency," *European Journal of Clinical Investigation*, vol. 33, no. 10, pp. 919–923, 2003.

[2] M. F. Picciano, "Pregnancy and lactation: physiological adjustments, nutritional requirements and the role of dietary supplements," *Journal of Nutrition*, vol. 133, no. 6, pp. 1997S–2002S, 2003.

[3] A. Kumar, A. K. Rai, S. Basu, D. Dash, and J. S. Singh, "Cord blood and breast milk iron status in maternal anemia," *Pediatrics*, vol. 121, no. 3, pp. e673–e677, 2008.

[4] A. M. Siddappa, R. Rao, J. D. Long, J. A. Widness, and M. K. Georgieff, "The assessment of newborn iron stores at birth: a review of the literature and standards for ferritin concentrations," *Neonatology*, vol. 92, no. 2, pp. 73–82, 2007.

[5] R. A. El-Farrash, E. Abdel Rahman Ismail, and A. Shafik Nada, "Cord blood iron profile and breast milk micronutrients in maternal iron deficiency anemia," *Pediatric Blood & Cancer*, vol. 58, no. 2, pp. 233–238, 2012.

[6] T. O. Scholl, "Iron status during pregnancy: setting the stage for mother and infant," *The American Journal of Clinical Nutrition*, vol. 81, no. 5, pp. 1218S–1222S, 2005.

[7] C. M. Chaparro, "Setting the stage for child health and development: prevention of iron deficiency in early infancy," *Journal of Nutrition*, vol. 138, no. 12, pp. 2529–2533, 2008.

[8] P. N. Singla, M. Tyagi, R. Shankar, D. Dash, and A. Kumar, "Fetal iron status in maternal anemia," *Acta Paediatrica*, vol. 85, no. 11, pp. 1327–1330, 1996.

[9] D. G. Sweet, G. Savage, T. R. J. Tubman, T. R. J. Lappin, and H. L. Halliday, "Study of maternal influences on fetal iron status at term using cord blood transferrin receptors," *Archives of Disease in Childhood: Fetal and Neonatal Edition*, vol. 84, no. 1, pp. F40–F43, 2001.

[10] S. Ziaei, E. Hatefnia, and G. Togeh, "Iron status in newborns born to iron-deficient mothers," *Iranian Journal of Medical Sciences*, vol. 28, no. 2, pp. 62–64, 2003.

[11] F. Emamghorashi and T. Heidari, "Iron status of babies born to iron-deficient anaemic mothers in an Iranian hospital," *Eastern Mediterranean Health Journal*, vol. 10, no. 6, pp. 808–814, 2004.

[12] C.-T. Wong and N. Saha, "Inter-relationships of storage iron in the mother, the placenta and the newborn," *Acta Obstetricia et Gynecologica Scandinavica*, vol. 69, no. 7-8, pp. 613–616, 1990.

[13] R. Hadipour, A. K. Norimah, B. K. Poh, F. Firoozehchian, R. Hadipour, and A. Akaberi, "Haemoglobin and serum ferritin levels in newborn babies born to anaemic Iranian women: a cross-sectional study in an Iranian Hospital," *Pakistan Journal of Nutrition*, vol. 9, no. 6, pp. 562–566, 2010.

[14] A. de Azevedo Paiva, P. H. C. Rondó, R. A. Pagliusi, M. D. R. D. O. Latorre, M. A. A. Cardoso, and S. S. R. Gondim, "Relationship between the iron status of pregnant women and their newborns," *Revista de Saúde Pública*, vol. 41, no. 3, pp. 321–327, 2007.

[15] WHO, *Serum Ferritin Concentrations for theAssessment of Iron Status and Iron Deficiency in Populations. Vitamin and Mineral Nutrition Information System*, WHO/NMH/NHD/MNM/11.2, World Health Organization, Geneva, Switzerland, 2011, http://www.who.int/vmnis/indicators/serum_ferritin.pdf.

[16] WHO, "Haemoglobin concentrations for the diagnosis of anaemia and assessment of severity," Vitamin and Mineral Nutrition Information System, World Health Organization, Geneva, Switzerland, 2011, (WHO/NMH/NHD/MNM/11.1), http://www.who.int/vmnis/indicators/haemoglobin.pdf.

[17] D. G. Sweet, G. Savage, T. R. J. Tubman, T. R. J. Lappin, and H. L. Halliday, "Study of maternal influences on fetal iron status at term using cord blood transferrin receptors," *Archives of Disease in Childhood: Fetal and Neonatal Edition*, vol. 84, no. 1, pp. F40–F43, 2001.

[18] R. A. El-Farrash, E. A. R. Ismail, and A. S. Nada, "Cord blood iron profile and breast milk micronutrients in maternal iron deficiency anemia," *Pediatric Blood & Cancer*, vol. 58, no. 2, pp. 233–238, 2012.

[19] G. O. Walters, F. M. Miller, and M. Worwood, "Serum ferritin concentration and iron stores in normal subjects," *Journal of Clinical Pathology*, vol. 26, no. 10, pp. 770–772, 1973.

[20] R. Zetterström, "Iron deficiency and iron deficiency anaemia during infancy and childhood," *Acta Paediatrica*, vol. 93, no. 4, pp. 436–439, 2004.

[21] E. E. Ziegler, S. E. Nelson, and J. M. Jeter, "Iron supplementation of breastfed infants from an early age," *The American Journal of Clinical Nutrition*, vol. 89, no. 2, pp. 525–532, 2009.

[22] M. B. Zimmermann and R. F. Hurrell, "Nutritional iron deficiency: seminar," *The Lancet*, vol. 370, no. 9586, pp. 511–520, 2007.

[23] R. Gupta and S. Ramji, "Effect of delayed cord clamping on iron stores in infants born to anemic mothers: a randomized controlled trial," *Indian Pediatrics*, vol. 39, no. 2, pp. 130–135, 2002.

[24] E. J. Harthoorn-Lasthuizen, J. Lindemans, and M. M. A. C. Langenhuijsen, "Does iron-deficient erythropoiesis in pregnancy influence fetal iron supply?" *Acta Obstetricia et Gynecologica Scandinavica*, vol. 80, no. 5, pp. 392–396, 2001.

[25] P. F. van Rheenen and B. J. Brabin, "A practical approach to timing cord clamping in resource poor settings," *British Medical Journal*, vol. 333, no. 7575, pp. 954–958, 2006.

21

Attitudes toward Management of Sickle Cell Disease and Its Complications: A National Survey of Academic Family Physicians

Arch G. Mainous III,[1,2] **Rebecca J. Tanner,**[1] **Christopher A. Harle,**[1] **Richard Baker,**[3] **Navkiran K. Shokar,**[4] **and Mary M. Hulihan**[5]

[1]*Department of Health Services Research, Management and Policy, University of Florida, P.O. Box 100195, Gainesville, FL 32610, USA*
[2]*Department of Community Health and Family Medicine, University of Florida, P.O. Box 100237, Gainesville, FL 32610-0237, USA*
[3]*Department of Health Sciences, University of Leicester, 22-28 Princess Road West, Leicester LE1 6TP, UK*
[4]*Department of Family and Community Medicine, Texas Tech University Health Science Center at El Paso, 9849 Kenworthy Street, El Paso, TX 79924, USA*
[5]*Division of Blood Disorders, CDC, National Center on Birth Defects and Developmental Disabilities, Mail-Stop E87, 1600 Clifton Road, Atlanta, GA 30333, USA*

Correspondence should be addressed to Arch G. Mainous III; arch.mainous@ufl.edu

Academic Editor: Duran Canatan

Objective. Sickle cell disease (SCD) is a disease that requires a significant degree of medical intervention, and family physicians are one potential provider of care for patients who do not have access to specialists. The extent to which family physicians are comfortable with the treatment of and concerned about potential complications of SCD among their patients is unclear. Our purpose was to examine family physician's attitudes toward SCD management. *Methods.* Data was collected as part of the Council of Academic Family Medicine Educational Research Alliance (CERA) survey in the United States and Canada that targeted family physicians who were members of CERA-affiliated organizations. We examined attitudes regarding management of SCD. *Results.* Overall, 20.4% of respondents felt comfortable with treatment of SCD. There were significant differences in comfort level for treatment of SCD patients depending on whether or not physicians had patients who had SCD, as well as physicians who had more than 10% African American patients. Physicians also felt that clinical decision support (CDS) tools would be useful for treatment (69.4%) and avoiding complications (72.6%) in managing SCD patients. *Conclusions.* Family physicians are generally uncomfortable with managing SCD patients and recognize the utility of CDS tools in managing patients.

1. Introduction

Sickle cell disease (SCD) affects millions of people throughout the world and is particularly common among those whose ancestors came from sub-Saharan Africa; Spanish-speaking regions in the Western Hemisphere (South America, the Caribbean, and Central America); Saudi Arabia; India; and Mediterranean countries such as Turkey, Greece, and Italy. It is estimated that SCD affects 90,000 to 100,000 Americans, and sickle cell trait occurs among 1 in 12 African Americans [1].

Patients with sickle cell disease require comprehensive care including preventive interventions, pain management, hydroxyurea, and blood transfusions [2]. Further, complications of transfusions like iron overload are common and have significant consequences like cirrhosis, heart failure, and death [3, 4]. Due to the complex and disabling nature of sickle cell disease, appropriate ambulatory management is critical to avoid acute pain and vasoocclusive episodes and hospitalizations. One estimate has suggested that annually, United States' average hospitalization costs for SCD are $6,223 per hospitalization [5]. Interventions designed to prevent SCD complications and avoid hospitalizations are estimated to have substantial economic benefits, as the discounted lifetime cost of care averages $460,151 per patient with SCD [6].

Translation of evidence from clinical trials into health care delivery for patients with sickle cell disease needs to happen. For example, hydroxyurea, the only currently available FDA-approved medication for preventing complications of sickle cell disease, is effective. The Multicenter Study of Hydroxyurea in Patients with Sickle Cell Anemia, a multicenter landmark randomized controlled trial, clearly demonstrated that use of hydroxyurea by adult patients with sickle cell anemia resulted in a significant reduction in the frequency of pain crises, hospitalizations, and red blood cell transfusions [7]. A nine-year follow-up observational study revealed a reduction in mortality for patients taking hydroxyurea compared to study participants not taking the medication [8]. However, hydroxyurea is underused [9]. In one study at three teaching hospitals in the southeastern United States only 42% of adult SCD patients were taking hydroxyurea [10].

The extent to which family physicians are comfortable implementing such advances in treatment for SCD in clinical practice is unclear. Little information exists on current practice and use of therapies for children and adults with SCD in this setting. There are many factors that could influence a physician's attitudes toward SCD. For example, SCD is more prevalent among African Americans, and so physicians whose practices are comprised of larger proportions of African Americans might be more attuned to issues such as SCD that disproportionately affect their patient population. Physicians who have active patients with SCD may be more familiar and more comfortable with SCD patients and the disease. Physician age is another factor that may influence comfort with managing and treating SCD patients. Younger physicians may have a greater recall of details regarding less common diseases that are infrequently seen in practice. In addition, age may influence interest in use of technology in the clinical encounter. Because of the significant impact on morbidity and mortality and health care costs associated with inappropriate management of SCD [11–14], it is important to better understand current practice. A better understanding of sickle cell management and complication knowledge deficits of physicians will help to drive interventions like clinical decision support CDS systems [15, 16] and primary-specialty physician comanagement programs to improve care for the vulnerable population of people with SCD. Less common diseases such as SCD are prime candidates for CDS tools, as they can support physician knowledge and management of diseases that they do not encounter regularly in practice.

2. Methods

This study is an analysis of a survey conducted as part of the Council of Academic Family Medicine Educational Research Alliance (CERA). CERA is a joint initiative of all four major US academic family medicine organizations (Society of Teachers of Family Medicine (STFM), North American Primary Care Research Group (NAPCRG), Association of Departments of Family Medicine (ADFM), and Association of Family Medicine Residency Directors (AFMRD)).

The investigators submitted questions related to SCD practice and treatment for inclusion in the CERA survey. The survey was designed as an omnibus survey incorporating several distinct subprojects focusing on different topic areas. Practicing physician members of the CERA-affiliated organizations in the United States were identified for participation. Although these organizations are all headquartered in the United States, there are some members from outside the United States. This survey was limited to US based members. Since some individuals were members of multiple organizations, unique individuals were selected for the sampling frame. The study was approved by the American Academy of Family Physicians Institutional Review Board.

The survey was conducted between November, 2013, and January, 2014, and sent to 3158 physicians who are members of Council of Academic Family Medicine organizations. The potential respondents were surveyed electronically with an initial email invitation for participation. The survey was conducted through the infrastructure of STFM. The survey was introduced in an email that included a personalized greeting, a letter signed by the presidents of each of the four participating organizations urging participation, and a link to the survey. Nonrespondents were sent two follow-up emails encouraging participation. As the survey was structured as an omnibus survey, with several subprojects contained within the overall survey, it was possible for respondents to skip questions.

The survey questions for this study were developed following a review of the literature to identify key concepts and issues suggesting the need for additional knowledge. The attitudinal outcomes of interest were physicians' responses to questions related to their "comfort managing sickle cell disease patients," "complication concerns," "willingness to manage patients," and "usefulness of CDS tools".

2.1. Comfort Managing Patients. Comfort with overall management and pain management of SCD patients was assessed using a Likert scale (somewhat/very uncomfortable, neutral, and somewhat/very comfortable). Comfort with managing SCD patients with specific treatment options (red blood cell transfusions, hematopoietic stem cell transplant (HSCT), and hydroxyurea) was assessed as well. These options represent the main treatments available for SCD patients and represent a wide range of usage in practice, from relatively common pain management to the less frequently used HSCT.

2.2. Complication Concerns. Concern for SCD complications was assessed using physician's stated level of concern (somewhat/very unconcerned, neutral, and somewhat/very concerned) for known complications of SCD, including iron overload, stroke, atherosclerosis, and pneumonia.

2.3. Willingness to Comanage Patients with a Specialist. Willingness to comanage an SCD patient was assessed for pediatric and adult patients (somewhat/very likely, neutral, and somewhat/very unlikely).

2.4. Use of Clinical Decision Support Tools on SCD Care. The willingness of a physician to self-manage care of SCD patients with the assistance of a CDS tool was assessed for pediatric and adult patients (somewhat/very unlikely, neutral, and somewhat/very likely). The perceived utility of CDS tools was assessed for diagnosis of SCD, treatment of SCD, and the avoidance of complications (somewhat/very useful, neutral, and somewhat/very not useful).

2.5. Demographics. We collected data on age, race/ethnicity, academic rank, primary physician duty, patient time, time in clinic, proportion of patients who are African American, number of patients with SCD, and proportion of patients with SCD who are under 19 years of age from all survey participants (Table 1).

3. Analysis

We computed descriptive statistics to understand the general practice patterns of the survey respondents and their overall attitudes toward SCD and SCD treatment. We collapsed all of the Likert scale questions into two categories, examining the difference between those who answered the questions with a positive answer (somewhat and very comfortable, likely, and concerned) and respondents who felt neutral or responded negatively. Next, we conducted bivariate analyses with chi-square tests to compare attitudes based on respondents' proportion of African American patients (less than 10% versus 10% or greater), as well as by the presence of SCD patients in the physician's practice, and by physician age (younger than 50 versus 50 and older). We judged statistical significance at $P \leq 0.05$.

4. Results

The overall number of surveys returned was 1060 for a 34% response rate. We analyzed data from the 1042 physicians who responded to at least one question on the SCD section of the survey. Table 1 shows demographic information about these physician respondents. The majority of physicians had no SCD patients, and only 15.9% had more than five SCD patients. Slightly less than half of the surveyed physicians spent 3 or more half-days in clinic. Overall, few physicians had a substantial proportion of African American patients, with only 25.7% reporting 25% or more African American patients. Table 2 shows the bivariate analysis for comfort managing patients, complications concerns, willingness to comanage patients, and thoughts on CDS tools for the full population. Table 3 shows differences between physicians with <10% African American patients and physicians with 10% or more African American patients. Table 4 shows differences between physicians with no active SCD patients and those with active SCD patients. There were no significant differences between groups in relation to perceived utility of CDS for helping direct treatment or avoiding complications. A majority of all groups felt that CDS would be useful.

There were several significant differences between physicians under age 50 and those aged 50 and older. A smaller

TABLE 1: Respondent demographics.

Sample size	1042
Male, %	56.6
Age, %	
Under 40	21.9
40–49	28.8
50–59	30.0
60+	19.3
Race/ethnicity, %	
White	84.2
African American	3.6
Hispanic	3.5
Asian/other	8.8
Rank, %	
Assistant professor	31.9
Associate professor	32.5
Full professor	24.6
Not applicable	11.0
Terminal degree, %	
M.D.	93.5
D.O.	5.7
Other	0.8
Primary duty, %	
Administration	26.4
Clinical teaching	51.5
Research	5.9
Faculty development	1.7
Clinical care	9.6
Nonacademic physician	0.6
Other	4.4
Patient time ≥50%, %	22.8
Time in clinic, %	
<3 half days	50.4
3–6 half days	44.6
7+ half days	5.1
% of patients who are African American, %	
<10%	46.8
10–24%	27.5
25–49%	18.4
50+%	7.3
Number of patients with SCD	
0 patients	59.6
1–4 patients	34.5
5–10 patients	14.5
11+ patients	1.4
% of SCD patients who are under 19 years of age, %	
<10%	56.8
10–24%	18.1
25–49%	14.0
50+%	11.1

percentage of younger physicians were comfortable with overall management of SCD patients (15.7%) compared to

TABLE 2: Physician perceptions of SCD, full sample.

	Full sample
Comfort managing patients	Comfortable
Overall management, %	20.4
RBC transfusions, %	30.8
HSCT, %	0.6
Hydroxyurea treatment, %	20.5
Pain management, %	47.8
Complication concerns	Concerned
Iron overload, %	60.9
Stroke, %	77.6
Atherosclerosis, %	45.9
Pneumonia, %	71.4
Willing to comanage patient with specialist	Likely
Pediatric patients, %	79.7
Adult patients, %	67.8
Impact of CDS on willingness to manage SCD patients	Likely
Pediatric patients, %	25.6
Adult patients, %	34.1
Perceived utility of CDS for SCD patient care	Useful
Diagnosis	22.9
Treatment	69.4
Avoiding complications	72.6

older physicians (25.1%, $P = 0.0002$). A larger percentage of physicians who were older expressed concern for iron overload, with 66.1% expressing concern, in contrast to 55.8% of younger physicians ($P = 0.0009$). A greater percentage of younger physicians were more willing to comanage adult SCD patients (70.8%) than older physicians (64.3%, $P = 0.03$). A greater percentage of younger physicians were willing to independently manage adult SCD patients with the assistance of a CDS tool, with 38.1% of younger physicians indicating an increased likelihood, compared to 29.9% of older physicians ($P = 0.007$). A larger percentage of younger physicians saw the utility of CDS tools, with 72.5% indicating that CDS tools would be useful for the treatment of patients, compared with 66.6% of older physicians ($P = 0.04$). In addition, a greater percentage of younger physicians considered CDS tools useful for avoiding complications than older physicians (77.7% versus 67.2%, $P = 0.0002$).

5. Discussion

The results of this study indicate that academic family physicians have few SCD patients in their patient panel. More importantly, the results indicate that there are concerns among these primary care physicians regarding their ability to manage SCD and its complications. That said, there seems to be general agreement that a CDS tool may play a beneficial role in managing these patients especially among younger physicians.

As might be expected, more frequent interaction with SCD patients or African American patients, those at higher risk for SCD, was associated with greater comfort in managing SCD patients. Age of the physician was related to comfort managing these patients in several important ways. Older physicians appeared more comfortable with treatment and management of a complication like iron overload, potentially reflecting lifetime exposure to this patient population, while younger physicians were more likely to embrace tools that would assist them in managing patients independently.

A CDS for managing SCD received significant endorsement from this sample of academic family physicians. CDS tools have been successfully utilized in the management of care for a number of conditions [15, 16]. It appears that a CDS would have utility for both managing treatment and complications. Younger physicians were more likely to see a CDS to be particularly useful. As electronic health records become more commonplace in primary care the ability to implement a CDS for less common diseases is increased. Although there is evidence of alert fatigue with CDS for common conditions [17], the use of a CDS for SCD would not likely be perceived as an annoyance but rather as a benefit.

This study is the first study to report on family physician's comfort and attitudes with managing SCD. In addition to this strength, there are several limitations to this study. The first is that although the survey is based on a national sample of family physicians, a group that would likely encounter SCD child and adult patients, the group under study is all in academic settings. Consequently, in terms of clinical practice most academic family physicians do not practice full time. This amount of clinical practice may potentially affect their comfort with SCD. Second, even though the sample size allows us to examine responses to more than 1,000 respondents, the response rate of 34% is not exceptionally high. Thus, there may be some bias in the participants based on their comfort and interest in the questions. The low response rate may have been a result of the time of year the survey was sent out, as it was administered during the holiday season. As was clear from the practice characteristics, SCD patients are not common in the patient panels of the respondents. It is possible that individuals with no SCD patients were less likely to participate in a study on managing SCD patients. Finally, the level of training that physicians received for SCD was not assessed. Physician attitudes regarding SCD management are likely to be influenced not only by SCD patients in their care, but also by the amount of SCD-specific training they received.

In conclusion, although academic family physicians recognize issues in their comfort and ability to manage SCD patients they endorse the potential utility of CDS. Future studies could evaluate whether a CDS system could improve the quality of care and control of complications like iron overload for this vulnerable population.

Disclaimer

The findings and conclusions in this report are those of the authors and do not necessarily represent the official position of the Centers for Disease Control and Prevention.

TABLE 3: Physician perceptions of SCD by percentage of patients who are African American.

	Physicians with <10% African American patients	Physicians with ≥10% African American patients	P value
Comfort managing patients	Comfortable	Comfortable	
Overall management, %	12.7	27.0	<0.0001
RBC transfusions, %	25.4	35.6	0.0006
HSCT, %	0.2	1.0	0.14
Hydroxyurea treatment, %	16.1	24.3	0.002
Pain management, %	42.4	52.6	0.001
Complication concerns	Concerned	Concerned	
Iron overload, %	58.6	62.8	0.18
Stroke, %	75.3	79.5	0.12
Atherosclerosis, %	43.5	48.0	0.15
Pneumonia, %	68.0	74.3	0.03
Willing to comanage patient with specialist	Likely	Likely	
Pediatric patients, %	78.2	80.9	0.31
Adult patients, %	69.8	66.0	0.20
Impact of CDS on willingness to manage SCD patients	Likely	Likely	
Pediatric patients, %	24.0	27.0	0.27
Adult patients, %	31.3	36.6	0.08
Perceived utility of CDS for SCD patient care	Useful	Useful	
Diagnosis	27.2	19.2	0.003
Treatment	68.1	70.4	0.45
Avoiding complications	70.2	74.5	0.13

TABLE 4: Physician perceptions of SCD by number of patients with SCD.

	Physicians with no SCD patients	Physicians with 1 or more SCD patients	P value
Comfort managing patients	Comfortable	Comfortable	
Overall management, %	9.8	36.1	<0.0001
RBC transfusions, %	21.8	45.1	<0.0001
HSCT, %	0.2	1.3	0.026
Hydroxyurea treatment, %	14.2	30.4	<0.0001
Pain management, %	39.0	61.7	<0.0001
Complication concerns	Concerned	Concerned	
Iron overload, %	58.5	64.3	0.07
Stroke, %	75.3	80.7	0.04
Atherosclerosis, %	45.4	46.7	0.70
Pneumonia, %	67.3	77.6	0.0004
Willing to comanage patient with specialist	Likely	Likely	
Pediatric patients, %	76.5	84.1	0.003
Adult patients, %	70.1	64.5	0.07
Impact of CDS on willingness to manage SCD patients	Likely	Likely	
Pediatric patients, %	23.5	28.8	0.06
Adult patients, %	30.8	38.7	0.01
Perceived utility of CDS for SCD patient care	Useful	Useful	
Diagnosis	26.9	17.0	0.0003
Treatment	68.9	70.1	0.71
Avoiding complications	72.2	73.2	0.72

Conflict of Interests

The authors declare that there is no conflict of interests regarding the publication of this paper.

Acknowledgments

The authors would like to acknowledge Richard Lottenberg, M.D., for his assistance. This study is funded in part by Cooperative Agreement 1U01DD000754-01 from the Centers for Disease Control and Prevention. The findings and conclusions in this report are those of the authors and do not necessarily represent the official position of the Centers for Disease Control and Prevention.

References

[1] National Heart, Lung, and Blood Institute, *Disease and Conditions Index. Sickle Cell Anemia: Who Is at Risk?* US Department of Health and Human Services, National Institutes of Health, National Heart, Lung, and Blood Institute, Bethesda, Md, USA, 2009.

[2] National Institutes of Health, *The Management of Sickle Cell Disease*, Department of Health and Human Services, National Institutes of Health, National Heart, Lung, and Blood Institute, Bethesda, Md, USA, 2002.

[3] M. A. Blinder, F. Vekeman, M. Sasane, A. Trahey, C. Paley, and M. S. Duh, "Age-related treatment patterns in sickle cell disease patients and the associated sickle cell complications and healthcare costs," *Pediatric Blood and Cancer*, vol. 60, no. 5, pp. 828–835, 2013.

[4] J. Porter and M. Garbowski, "Consequences and management of iron overload in sickle cell disease," *Hematology/the Education Program of the American Society of Hematology*, vol. 2013, no. 1, pp. 447–456, 2013.

[5] C. A. Steiner and J. L. Miller, "Sickle cell disease patients in U.S. hospitals, 2004," HCUP Statistical Brief #21, Agency for Healthcare Research and Quality, Rockville, Md, USA, 2006, http://www.hcup-us.ahrq.gov/reports/statbriefs/sb21.pdf.

[6] T. L. Kauf, T. D. Coates, L. Huazhi, N. Mody-Patel, and A. G. Hartzema, "The cost of health care for children and adults with sickle cell disease," *American Journal of Hematology*, vol. 84, no. 6, pp. 323–327, 2009.

[7] S. Charache, M. L. Terrin, R. D. Moore et al., "Effect of hydroxyurea on the frequency of painful crises in sickle cell anemia. Investigators of the Multicenter Study of Hydroxyurea in Sickle Cell Anemia," *The New England Journal of Medicine*, vol. 332, no. 20, pp. 1317–1322, 1995.

[8] M. H. Steinberg, F. Barton, O. Castro et al., "Effect of hydroxyurea on mortality and morbidity in adult sickle cell anemia: risks and benefits up to 9 years of treatment," *The Journal of the American Medical Association*, vol. 289, no. 13, pp. 1645–1651, 2003.

[9] S. Lanzkron, C. Haywood Jr., J. B. Segal, and G. J. Dover, "Hospitalization rates and costs of care of patients with sickle-cell anemia in the state of Maryland in the era of hydroxyurea," *American Journal of Hematology*, vol. 81, no. 12, pp. 927–932, 2006.

[10] H. Elmariah, M. E. Garrett, L. M. de Castro et al., "Factors associated with survival in a contemporary adult sickle cell disease cohort," *The American Journal of Hematology*, vol. 89, no. 5, pp. 530–535, 2014.

[11] E. Jacob and American Pain Society, "Pain management in sickle cell disease," *Pain Management Nursing*, vol. 2, no. 4, pp. 121–131, 2001.

[12] J. Kanter and R. Kruse-Jarres, "Management of sickle cell disease from childhood through adulthood," *Blood Reviews*, vol. 27, no. 6, pp. 279–287, 2013.

[13] B. Aygun, S. Padmanabhan, C. Paley, and V. Chandrasekaran, "Clinical significance of RBC alloantibodies and autoantibodies in sickle cell patients who received transfusions," *Transfusion*, vol. 42, no. 1, pp. 37–43, 2002.

[14] C. H. Pegelow, R. J. Adams, V. McKie et al., "Risk of recurrent stroke in patients with sickle cell disease treated with erythrocyte transfusions," *The Journal of Pediatrics*, vol. 126, no. 6, pp. 896–899, 1995.

[15] M. S. Player, J. M. Gill, A. G. Mainous III et al., "An electronic medical record-based intervention to improve quality of care for gastro-esophageal reflux disease (GERD) and atypical presentations of GERD," *Quality in Primary Care*, vol. 18, no. 4, pp. 223–229, 2010.

[16] A. G. Mainous III, C. A. Lambourne, and P. J. Nietert, "Impact of a clinical decision support system on antibiotic prescribing for acute respiratory infections in primary care: quasi-experimental trial," *Journal of the American Medical Informatics Association*, vol. 20, no. 2, pp. 317–324, 2013.

[17] A. S. Kesselheim, K. Cresswell, S. Phansalkar, D. W. Bates, and A. Sheikh, "Clinical decision support systems could be modified to reduce "alert fatigue" while still minimizing the risk of litigation," *Health Affairs*, vol. 30, no. 12, pp. 2310–2317, 2011.

22

Efficacy and Safety of Intravenous Ferric Carboxymaltose in Geriatric Inpatients at a German Tertiary University Teaching Hospital: A Retrospective Observational Cohort Study of Clinical Practice

Matthias Bach,[1] **Tabea Geisel,**[2,3] **Julia Martin,**[2,3] **Bettina Schulze,**[1]
Roland Schaefer,[4] **Garth Virgin,**[5] **and Juergen Stein**[2,3,6]

[1]*St. Elisabethen Krankenhaus, 60487 Frankfurt/Main, Germany*

[2]*Interdisciplinary Crohn Colitis Centre Rhein-Main, 60594 Frankfurt/Main, Germany*

[3]*Institute of Nutritional Science, University of Giessen, 35392 Giessen, Germany*

[4]*Krankenhaus Sachsenhausen, Teaching Hospital of the J. W. Goethe University, 60594 Frankfurt/Main, Germany*

[5]*Vifor Pharma Deutschland GmbH, 81379 Munich, Germany*

[6]*Gastroenterology and Clinical Nutrition, Krankenhaus Sachsenhausen, Teaching Hospital of the J. W. Goethe University, 60594 Frankfurt/Main, Germany*

Correspondence should be addressed to Juergen Stein; j.stein@em.uni-frankfurt.de

Academic Editor: Eitan Fibach

Current iron supplementation practice in geriatric patients is erratic and lacks evidence-based recommendations. Despite potential benefits in this population, intravenous iron supplementation is often withheld due to concerns regarding pharmacy expense, perceived safety issues, and doubts regarding efficacy in elderly patients. This retrospective, observational cohort study aimed to evaluate the safety and efficacy of intravenous ferric carboxymaltose (FCM, Ferinject) in patients aged >75 years with iron deficiency anaemia (IDA). Within a twelve-month data extraction period, the charts of 405 hospitalised patients aged 65–101 years were retrospectively analysed for IDA, defined according to WHO criteria for anaemia (haemoglobin: <13.0 g/dL (m)/<12.0 g/dL (f)) in conjunction with transferrin saturation <20%. Of 128 IDA patients screened, 51 (39.8%) received intravenous iron. 38 patient charts were analysed. Mean cumulative dose of intravenous FCM was 784.4 ± 271.7 mg iron (1–3 infusions). 18 patients (47%) fulfilled treatment response criteria (≥1.0 g/dL increase in haemoglobin between baseline and hospital discharge). AEs were mild/moderate, most commonly transient increases of liver enzymes ($n = 5/13.2\%$). AE incidence was comparable with that observed in patients <75 years. No serious AEs were observed. Ferric carboxymaltose was well tolerated and effective for correction of Hb levels and iron stores in this cohort of IDA patients aged over 75 years.

1. Introduction

Iron deficiency is one of the most common nutritional deficiencies in the elderly population as a whole, with a prevalence of approximately 10–15% in persons aged 65 and older and 35% in those aged 85 and above [1, 2]. Anaemia is defined according to World Health Organization (WHO) criteria as a haemoglobin level of <12 g/dL in women and <13 g/dL in men. While some 40–50% of hospitalised patients are anaemic, rates of up to 47% have also been found in patients living in nursing homes [1, 3, 4].

The aetiology of anaemia in the elderly is multifaceted. Major causes are reduced iron absorption as a result of drug interactions, diseases of the digestive tract, and/or chronic inflammation. Depletion of iron stores may also occur as a consequence of (mostly chronic) bleeding [5, 6]. However, anaemia is usually a result of iron deficiency, either absolute or functional (i.e., insufficient supply of iron to the erythroid marrow despite adequate iron stores) [7]. Geisel et al. reported 66% prevalence of anaemia in geriatric inpatients. 65% of cases were associated with iron deficiency (ID), mostly due to chronic infection, or ID combined with anaemia of inflammation (IDA/AI, 21.4%) [3]. While comorbidities and polypharmacy may be contributory factors, nutrition played only a limited role [2].

In the past, reduced haemoglobin levels were widely regarded as a normal consequence of the aging process [8]. However, data clearly show anaemia in the elderly population to be associated with a significantly higher risk of morbidity and mortality, even in the absence of concomitant illness [9, 10]. The impact of anaemia (even mild anaemia) on quality of life can be considerable in terms of energy levels, functional and cognitive capacity, and mobility [11, 12]. Typical anaemia symptoms such as physical weakness, tiredness, or dizziness may increase the risk of falls [13, 14], thus leading to increased hospitalisation and/or mortality [15, 16].

Even latent iron deficiency has been shown to significantly impair cognitive function and physical coordination [11, 17]. Motor deficiencies in older women increase drastically even when haemoglobin levels are in the lower normal range [18], increasing the risk of falls and resultant fractures [19].

In a recent review, Goodnough and Schrier recommend routine initial assessment of iron status in all elderly patients [20] and, once IDA is clearly ascertained, the commencement of oral iron supplementation as a therapeutic trial, aiming to correct anaemia and replenish iron stores. Under oral iron therapy, Hb levels can be expected to rise by a maximum of 1-2 g/dL every two weeks [21]. Replenishment of iron stores requires further supplementation for at least six months after anaemia correction. However, in elderly patients, therapy may be required for a longer period, since functional IDA (anaemia of inflammation, AI) leads to diminished intestinal iron absorption and slower bone marrow response [22, 23]. Adherence is often poor, particularly when patients have to consume numerous medications on a daily basis due to concomitant multimorbidity. Moreover, in geriatric patients, oral iron supplementation is often poorly tolerated, particularly as a result of abdominal discomfort, and poorly absorbed when malabsorptive conditions are present (see above).

Intravenous (i.v.) iron replacement therefore has considerable potential advantages for the treatment of elderly patients with IDA [21, 24]. Most i.v. iron formulations are effective, well tolerated, and associated with a lower incidence of serious adverse reactions (e.g., anaphylaxis) than most clinicians perceive [25–27].

While safety data for i.v. iron supplementation in geriatric patients are scarce, a recent retrospective study by Dossabhoy demonstrated iron dextran to be relatively safe and effective in elderly patients (mean, 70 years) with chronic kidney disease [28].

Ferric carboxymaltose (FCM, Ferinject, Vifor (International) Inc., St. Gallen, Switzerland) is a next-generation, parenteral, dextran-free, strong, and robust iron complex suitable for i.v. administration in individual doses up to 1000 mg and has been demonstrated to be safe and highly effective in the treatment of both mild and severe IDA in a large cohort of patients up to 70 years of age [29]. Apart from two recently published heterogenous chart analyses [28, 30], however, no data exist for patients over 70 years of age. Here, we report results of a monocentric retrospective chart data analysis designed to assess the safety and efficacy of i.v. iron as FCM in a cohort of patients aged over 75 years.

2. Study Design

This report presents a retrospective chart data analysis of patients admitted between March 2010 and March 2011 to the Geriatric Clinic of the St. Elisabethen Krankenhaus in Frankfurt, Germany, whose medical records were available. Aim of the analysis was to investigate the efficacy and safety of ferric carboxymaltose (Ferinject, Vifor Pharma). Data for analysis were extracted from the charts of elderly persons who had been admitted to the rehabilitation unit and treated according to the medical needs of their underlying disease in accordance with therapy requirements published in the German Physician's Circular (GPC). Patient charts included in the analysis were those of patients over 75 years of age with iron deficiency anaemia (IDA) whose hospital stay lasted at least 2 weeks. The 2-week minimum stay was chosen in order to allow time for optimal Hb correction even when i.v. iron was not administered until several days after admission.

Patients with Hb levels below 12 g/dL (women)/13 g/dL (men) and a TSAT value <20% were considered to have anemia associated with iron deficiency. Three subcategories were defined [31, 32]:

(i) Anaemia related to absolute iron deficiency (iron deficiency anaemia, IDA) was characterised by a decreased serum ferritin level (<30 μg/mL) in combination with low serum CRP (<0.5 mg/dL).

(ii) Anaemia caused by inflammation (AI) was defined by high ferritin levels (>100 μg/mL) and increased CRP ($\geq$0.5 mg/dL).

(iii) Patients with ferritin levels between 30 μg/mL and 100 μg/mL and high CRP levels ($\geq$0.5 mg/dL) were classified as having mixed anaemia (IDA/AI).

Patients were subdivided into two age groups, 76–85 years or >85 years, and additionally stratified by baseline ferritin values of $\leq$300 or >300 ng/mL. FCM (500 mg or 1000 mg) was diluted in normal saline and administered i.v. over a 15–25 min period.

Data sets were excluded from analysis if any of the following factors were present: Hb < 8 g/dL, TSAT $\geq$ 20%, or serum albumin < 2.5 g/dL; known hypersensitivity to iron polysaccharide complexes or FCM; vitamin B_{12} or folic acid deficiency; anaemia due to causes other than iron deficiency; iron overload disorders (e.g., haemochromatosis); significant cardiovascular disease (including myocardial infarction during the six months prior to study inclusion); uncontrolled endocrinological or metabolic disorders; active infection, malignancy, or active liver disease.

Primary objective was to assess the safety of i.v. iron supplementation as FCM in hospitalised geriatric patients with anaemia. Secondary objective was to evaluate the efficacy of

TABLE 1: Patient characteristics: main reason for hospitalisation and length of stay.

	All, $n = 38$	76–85 yrs, $n = 17$ (%)	>85 yrs, $n = 21$ (%)
Age (years)	85.9 ± 5.05	81.24 ± 2.94	89.71 ± 2.66
Median (range)	86.5 (76–96)	82.0 (76–85)	90.0 (86–96)
Fractures	18	7	11
Cardiovascular disease	6	4	2
Disturbances of gait and mobility	5	3	2
Digestive tract diseases	2	1	1
Neoplasm	1	0	1
Infectious diseases	3	0	3
Cerebrovascular disease	3	2	1
Hospital stay (d)			
mean ± SD	27.2 ± 8.9	26.9 ± 8.9	27.2 ± 8.9
(median; min–max)	(26; 14–53)	(27; 14–53)	(26; 14–50)

TABLE 2: Baseline iron parameters of all patients aged >75 years, subdivided into age groups.

Age group	Number of patients	Hb (g/dL) mean ± SD (median; min–max)	Ferritin (μg/L) mean ± SD (median; min–max)	TSAT (%) mean ± SD (median; min–max)	CRP (mg/dL) mean ± SD (median; min–max)
76–85 years	17	10.42 ± 0.85 (10.3; 8.8–11.8)	194.52 ± 144.49 (160.0; 21–714)	9.59 ± 3.71 (10.00; 4–17)	7.16 ± 10.33 (4.1; 0.2–49.0)
>85 years	21	11.00 ± 1.52 (10.7; 8.8–13.5)	255.42 ± 208.64 (163.0; 29–796)	9.6 ± 2.78 (10.00; 5–10)	5.49 ± 7.03 (3.6; 0.2–28.7)
All	38	10.74 ± 1.30 (10.5; 8.8–13.5)	228.2 ± 185.24 (161.50; 21–796)	9.61 ± 3.23 (9.6; 4–17)	6.41 ± 9.04 (3.9; 0.2–49.0)

FCM in correcting iron deficiency and increasing Hb levels in this patient population.

2.1. Assessments. Safety and tolerability were assessed by analysing the incidence and severity of adverse events (AEs) at first dose of FCM and their relationship with FCM administration as recorded by the treating physician. Routine clinical laboratory safety parameters, vital signs, and physical parameters were also monitored and documented.

No primary efficacy endpoint was defined. Efficacy was assessed by changes in Hb levels as recorded after dose in patient charts during routine follow-up in the course of inpatient hospital care, and treatment responders were defined by an Hb increase of ≥1.0 g/dL from baseline until discharge from hospital. Laboratory parameters were determined at the local laboratory during the course of hospital care.

2.2. Statistical Analyses. Descriptive statistics were attained by calculation of arithmetical means, standard deviations, medians, and minimum and maximum values of all data. To test significance of all categorical variables, the chi^2-test (Pearson) was performed. Arithmetical means were calculated with t-tests for dependent and independent samples, and correlations were determined using the Spearman Rho method. All outcomes with a minimum of $p < 0.05$ were considered significant. Missing values were disregarded in all statistical tests. All statistical analyses were performed using IBM SPSS Statistics 20SPSS statistical software.

3. Results

Of all subjects whose Hb values were recorded at admission ($n = 386$), 256 (66.3%; men 74.8%, women 62.9%) were anaemic. There was no correlation between age and Hb level. Of these, 154 (60.2%) were defined as having iron deficiency anaemia. Absolute IDA was found in only 7 (4.6%), while the majority were diagnosed with AI (128, 83.1%) or a combination of IDA and AI (19, 12.3%) indicated by high CRP and ferritin levels. Of those with IDA, only 51 (33.1%) received i.v. iron supplementation. After screening of patient records according to the criteria listed above, 38 charts were included in the retrospective analysis (subject characteristics shown in Table 1). Main reasons for noninclusion were a hospital stay shorter than 14 days and/or age below 76 years.

Mean cumulative dose of intravenous FCM was 784.4 ± 271.7 mg iron, administered in one to three infusions. In clinical practice, baseline requirements for replenishment of iron stores are commonly calculated using the Ganzoni formula [33]: total iron deficit = body weight [kg] × (target Hb − actual Hb) [g/L] × 0.24 + iron stores [mg]. Required dosage according to Ganzoni was 478.2–1724.0 mg iron (mean 1105.6 ± 299.2). Patients were, in fact, significantly undertreated, mean actual iron substitution being approximately 30% below the Ganzoni calculation. Table 2 shows baseline iron parameters of subjects. Details of iron supplementation and Hb response are described in Table 3.

3.1. Safety. Intravenous iron as FCM was well tolerated, without clinically significant AEs. The most common AEs

TABLE 3: Amount of iron supplementation and Hb response.

Age group	Calculated iron requirement (mg) mean ± SD (median; min–max)	Supplemented iron (mg) mean ± SD (median; min–max)	Number of infusions	Hb BoS (g/dL) mean ± SD (median; min–max)	Hb EoS (g/dL) mean ± SD (median; min–max)	ΔHb (g/dL) mean ± SD (median; min–max)	% responder (ΔHb >1 g/dL)
76–85 years	1210.4 ± 308.4 (1205.6; 1205.6–1724.0)	763.2 ± 297.7 (500; 500–1500)	(1–3)	10.42 ± 0.85 (10.3; 8.8–11.8)	11.31 ± 1.17 (11.9; 9.5–14.3)	0.54 ± 1.49 (0.9; 0.0–3.2)	8/17 (41%)
>85 years	1022.5 ± 263.7 (1046.4; 500.0–1493.6)	770.8 ± 249.1 (500; 500–1000)	(1–2)	11.00 ± 1.52 (10.7; 8.8–13.5)	11.75 ± 0.86 (11.9; 10.2–13)	0.69 ± 1.10 (0.9; 0.0–2.6)	10/21 (48%)
All	1105.6 ± 299.2 (1085.6; 478.2–1724.0)	784.4 ± 271.7 (500; 500–1500)	(1–3)	10.74 ± 1.30 (10.5; 8.8–13.5)	11.68 (11.35; 8.8–14.3)	0.62 ± 1.58 (0.9; 0.0–3.2)	18/38 (47%)

BoS: beginning of study; EoS: end of study.

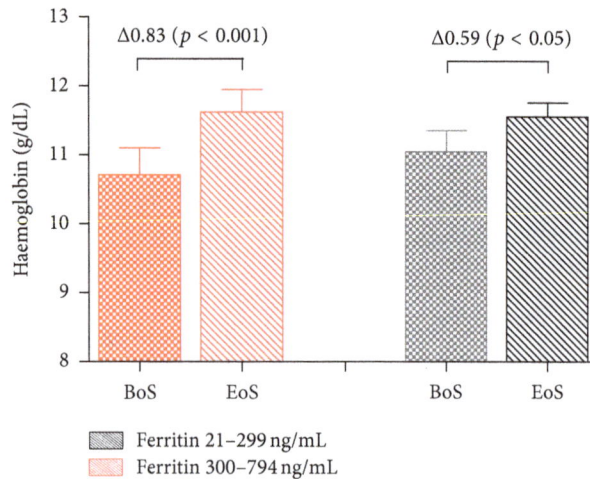

FIGURE 1

TABLE 4: Novel iron dosing strategy based on body weight and Hb levels as proposed by Evstatiev et al. [34].

Haemoglobin g/L	Body weight <70 kg	Body weight ≥70 kg
≥100	1000 mg	1500 mg
70–100	1500 mg	2000 mg
<70	2000 mg	2500 mg

were transient increases of liver enzymes (APT and/or ALT) of greater than twice the upper normal level ($n = 5$, 13.2%), which completely resolved within a few days. Transient increases of liver enzymes are scarce but have also been reported in the FERGIcor [34] and PROCEED [35] trials. Skin and subcutaneous tissue disorders, such as rash, hand and/or feet oedema, and pruritus, which were considered study drug-related were reported in 3 patients (7.8%). Leukocyte counts and CRP levels were stable until hospital discharge in both age groups. There was no report of anaphylaxis, anaphylactoid reaction, or death or of any other SAE, during the twelve-month data extraction period.

3.2. Efficacy. The number of responders, defined by increase in Hb of ≥1.0 g/dL from baseline, was 18 out of 38 (47%). Mean Hb increased from 9.1 ± 1.30 g/dL (95% CI = 8.86; 9.26) at baseline to 9.5±1.34 g/dL (95% CI = 9.25; 9.72) at 2 weeks after initial dose of FCM and continued to increase throughout the observation period, reaching 10.3±1.63 g/dL (95% CI = 10.06; 10.58) at hospital discharge.

There was no significant difference between the two age groups (age 76–85 versus > 85 years) regarding percentage of responders or change in mean Hb levels (Table 3). There was also no significant difference between the two ferritin groups, defined as ≤300 versus >301 ng/mL, as regards magnitude of Hb response to i.v. iron (Figure 1).

4. Discussion

Studies show that morbidity and mortality can be reduced by treating ID in a wide range of conditions, including chronic heart failure [36, 37], chronic kidney disease [38, 39], cancer therapy [40, 41], inflammatory bowel disease [34, 42], and rheumatoid arthritis [38, 39]. Preoperative iron administration results in faster normalisation of Hb levels and lower incidences of postoperative blood transfusion, postoperative morbidities, and infection [19, 43–45].

IDA is common in geriatric patients, and even mild anaemia is associated with poorer outcomes, extended hospitalisation, and increased mortality. Geriatric patients should therefore be routinely assessed for anaemia and causes individually identified to allow prompt initiation of therapy. However, specific guidelines for the management of anaemia in the elderly are lacking.

While particularly in outpatients oral iron preparations are commonly preferred, intravenous ferric carboxymaltose (FCM, Ferinject) provides a new, convenient option for rapid iron substitution, especially in cases where oral substitution is ineffective or not tolerated. FCM allows single-dose i.v. application of 1000 mg iron in only 15 minutes. A recent meta-analysis of published clinical studies concluded that i.v. administration of FCM is safe and effective in the various populations studied [29]. Similar data have also been published for other iron formulations such as LMW ID [46], ferumoxytol [47], and isomaltose 1000 (only available in Europe) [35].

Our retrospective chart data analysis aimed to assess the safety of intravenous FCM in anaemic geriatric patients aged 75 years and over and to evaluate the efficacy of FCM in correcting iron deficiency and Hb levels in this patient population.

Based on the Ganzoni formula, subjects were undertreated, receiving only two-thirds of the Ganzoni-calculated dose for iron store replenishment. This comes as no surprise. The complexity of the Ganzoni formula makes it impractical for everyday use. Consequently, iron requirements are often freely estimated, with physicians instinctively erring on the side of caution (or nonuse of i.v. iron) due to conceived risks of i.v. iron, especially in elderly patients. Reduced haemoglobin levels are still widely (erroneously) assumed to be an acceptable consequence of aging (see above); therefore target Hb levels are frequently lower in geriatric than in nongeriatric patients. A novel and simple dosing method based on body weight in kg and baseline Hb was recently shown by Evstatiev et al. [34] to be safe and effective in patients with inflammatory bowel disease. The calculation table used in this study (Table 4) can be used as a practical dosage guide.

Despite being undertreated, 47% of subjects were treatment responders, achieving a clinically relevant increase in Hb level of ≥1.0 g/dL after receiving iron as FCM. Clinically relevant increases (from 10.74 g/dL at baseline to 11.68 g/dL at discharge) were observed in the majority of patients, attributable to the administration of i.v. iron as FCM. These findings compare favourably with data published recently by Dossabhoy et al. [28].

The current study also examines the effectiveness of i.v. iron in the context of "*an increase in ferritin level accompanied by a decrease in TSAT that is suggested to lead to inflammation-mediated reticuloendothelial blockade*" [38]. Data from the 2007 Drive Study, a well-designed, open-label, randomised, controlled, multicentre trial in dialysis patients, clearly demonstrated that ferritin values did not predict responsiveness to intravenous iron and that i.v. iron supplementation (here, ferric gluconate at doses of up to 200 mg) was successful even at ferritin levels of 500–1200 ng/mL [38]. These findings were echoed by our results. Other studies have also shown ferritin to be unpredictive of iron responsiveness when ferritin is <500 ng/mL. Therefore, ferritin cannot be recommended as a guiding parameter for therapy except when being low (<300 ng/mL), in which case it is highly predictive of iron deficiency [48, 49].

Our study has three main limitations. Firstly, due to its retrospective design, only laboratory parameters collected as clinical routine were assessable. Due to prohibitive costs, concentrations of hepcidin, a liver-made peptide which is thought to regulate iron metabolism, were not routinely measured; thus, any correlation between hepcidin concentration, degree of functional iron deficiency, and response to i.v. iron could not be addressed. Secondly, after exclusion of patient data with confounding conditions and after screening for advanced age, IDA, and a hospital stay of at least two weeks, the number of data sets analysed, at 38, was relatively small. Thirdly, the study focused on hospitalised geriatric patients rather than outpatients. Results may therefore lack consistency and may be unrepresentative for elderly patients as a whole. The results should therefore be interpreted with caution.

5. Conclusions

The importance of IDA in the general population is increasingly recognised. Guidelines for the detection, evaluation, and management of IDA recommend i.v. supplementation as the preferred route in a variety of medical and surgical situations. However, safety and efficacy data for i.v. iron in elderly and very elderly populations have been lacking. The data presented here suggest that i.v. iron supplementation, even in cumulative doses of up to 1500 mg in one to three infusions, is safe and effective in this population.

Disclaimer

The sponsor's role was limited to financial support only. The founding sponsor had no role in the design of the study; in the collection, analyses, or interpretation of data; in the writing of the paper; or in the decision to publish the results.

Conflict of Interests

Tabea Geisel, Julia Martin, and Bettina Schulze have no conflict of interests. Garth Virgin is an employee of Vifor Pharma Deutschland GmbH. Roland Schaefer has acted as a Consultant for Vifor Pharma Deutschland GmbH. Matthias Bach has received speaker honoraria for Vifor Pharma Deutschland GmbH. Juergen Stein has received speaker honoraria and research grants from Vifor Pharma Deutschland GmbH and is a member of the company's advisory board.

Authors' Contribution

All authors contributed to the concept and design of the work and to the acquisition and interpretation of data. Juergen Stein and Matthias Bach drafted the paper. All authors provided important intellectual input and revisions to the paper and approved the final version for publication.

Acknowledgments

This work was funded by Vifor Pharma Deutschland GmbH. The authors would like to thank Janet Collins (ICCC Rhein-Main) for proofreading and language and writing support.

References

[1] J. M. Guralnik, R. S. Eisenstaedt, L. Ferrucci, H. G. Klein, and R. C. Woodman, "Prevalence of anemia in persons 65 years and older in the United States: evidence for a high rate of unexplained anemia," *Blood*, vol. 104, no. 8, pp. 2263–2268, 2004.

[2] M. Tettamanti, U. Lucca, F. Gandini et al., "Prevalence, incidence and types of mild anemia in the elderly: the 'Health and Anemia'population-based study," *Haematologica*, vol. 95, no. 11, pp. 1849–1856, 2010.

[3] T. Geisel, J. Martin, B. Schulze et al., "An etiologic profile of anemia in 405 geriatric patients," *Anemia*, vol. 2014, Article ID 932486, 7 pages, 2014.

[4] I. Petrosyan, G. Blaison, E. Andrès, and L. Federici, "Anaemia in the elderly: an aetiologic profile of a prospective cohort of 95 hospitalised patients," *European Journal of Internal Medicine*, vol. 23, no. 6, pp. 524–528, 2012.

[5] L. Ferrucci, R. D. Semba, J. M. Guralnik et al., "Proinflammatory state, hepcidin, and anemia in older persons," *Blood*, vol. 115, no. 18, pp. 3810–3816, 2010.

[6] L. Balducci, "An overlooked problem: anemia in the elderly patient with cancer," *The Journal of Supportive Oncology*, vol. 5, no. 3, pp. 115–116, 2007.

[7] E. A. Price, R. Mehra, T. H. Holmes, and S. L. Schrier, "Anemia in older persons: etiology and evaluation," *Blood Cells, Molecules, & Diseases*, vol. 46, no. 2, pp. 159–165, 2011.

[8] A. R. Nissenson, L. T. Goodnough, and R. W. Dubois, "Anemia: not just an innocent bystander?" *Archives of Internal Medicine*, vol. 163, no. 12, pp. 1400–1404, 2003.

[9] S. D. Denny, M. N. Kuchibhatla, and H. J. Cohen, "Impact of anemia on mortality, cognition, and function in community-dwelling elderly," *The American Journal of Medicine*, vol. 119, no. 4, pp. 327–334, 2006.

[10] B. W. J. H. Penninx, M. Pahor, R. C. Woodman, and J. M. Guralnik, "Anemia in old age is associated with increased mortality and hospitalization," *Journals of Gerontology. Series A Biological Sciences and Medical Sciences*, vol. 61, no. 5, pp. 474–479, 2006.

[11] M. Andro, P. Le Squere, S. Estivin, and A. Gentric, "Anaemia and cognitive performances in the elderly: a systematic review,"

European Journal of Neurology, vol. 20, no. 9, pp. 1234–1240, 2013.

[12] M. Thein, W. B. Ershler, A. S. Artz et al., "Diminished quality of life and physical function in community-dwelling elderly with anemia," *Medicine*, vol. 88, no. 2, pp. 107–114, 2009.

[13] B. W. J. H. Penninx, M. Pahor, M. Cesari et al., "Anemia is associated with disability and decreased physical performance and muscle strength in the elderly," *Journal of the American Geriatrics Society*, vol. 52, no. 5, pp. 719–724, 2004.

[14] B. W. J. H. Penninx, J. M. Guralnik, G. Onder, L. Ferrucci, R. B. Wallace, and M. Pahor, "Anemia and decline in physical performance among older persons," *The American Journal of Medicine*, vol. 115, no. 2, pp. 104–110, 2003.

[15] E. Riva, M. Tettamanti, P. Mosconi et al., "Association of mild anemia with hospitalization and mortality in the elderly: the Health and Anemia population-based study," *Haematologica*, vol. 94, no. 1, pp. 22–28, 2009.

[16] N. A. Zakai, R. Katz, C. Hirsch et al., "A prospective study of anemia status, hemoglobin concentration, and mortality in an elderly cohort: the Cardiovascular Health Study," *Archives of Internal Medicine*, vol. 165, no. 19, pp. 2214–2220, 2005.

[17] U. Lucca, M. Tettamanti, P. Mosconi et al., "Association of mild anemia with cognitive, functional, mood and quality of life outcomes in the elderly: the 'Health and Anemia' study," *PLoS ONE*, vol. 3, no. 4, Article ID e1920, 2008.

[18] R. Woodman, L. Ferrucci, and J. Guralnik, "Anemia in older adults," *Current Opinion in Hematology*, vol. 12, no. 2, pp. 123–128, 2005.

[19] P. Beris, M. Muñoz, J. A. García-Erce, D. Thomas, A. Maniatis, and P. van der Linden, "Perioperative anaemia management: consensus statement on the role of intravenous iron," *British Journal of Anaesthesia*, vol. 100, no. 5, pp. 599–604, 2008.

[20] L. T. Goodnough and S. L. Schrier, "Evaluation and management of anemia in the elderly," *The American Journal of Hematology*, vol. 89, no. 1, pp. 88–96, 2014.

[21] S. F. Clark, "Iron deficiency anemia," *Nutrition in Clinical Practice*, vol. 23, no. 2, pp. 128–141, 2008.

[22] J. Stein, F. Hartmann, and A. U. Dignass, "Diagnosis and management of iron deficiency anemia in patients with IBD," *Nature Reviews Gastroenterology & Hepatology*, vol. 7, no. 11, pp. 599–610, 2010.

[23] M. H. Bross, K. Soch, and T. Smith-Knuppel, "Anemia in older persons," *The American Family Physician*, vol. 82, no. 5, pp. 480–487, 2010.

[24] S. B. Silverstein and G. M. Rodgers, "Parenteral iron therapy options," *American Journal of Hematology*, vol. 76, no. 1, pp. 74–78, 2004.

[25] A. Shander, L. T. Goodnough, M. Javidroozi et al., "Iron deficiency anemia-bridging the knowledge and practice gap," *Transfusion Medicine Reviews*, vol. 28, no. 3, pp. 156–166, 2014.

[26] M. Auerbach, L. T. Goodnough, and A. Shander, "Iron: the new advances in therapy," *Best Practice & Research: Clinical Anaesthesiology*, vol. 27, no. 1, pp. 131–140, 2013.

[27] M. Auerbach and H. Ballard, "Clinical use of intravenous iron: administration, efficacy, and safety," *Hematology/the Education Program of the American Society of Hematology. American Society of Hematology. Education Program*, vol. 2010, pp. 338–347, 2010.

[28] N. R. Dossabhoy, S. Turley, R. Gascoyne, M. Tapolyai, and K. Sulaiman, "Safety of total dose iron dextran infusion in geriatric patients with chronic kidney disease and iron deficiency anemia," *Renal Failure*, vol. 36, no. 7, pp. 1033–1037, 2014.

[29] R. A. Moore, H. Gaskell, P. Rose, and J. Allan, "Meta-analysis of efficacy and safety of intravenous ferric carboxymaltose (Ferinject) from clinical trial reports and published trial data," *BMC Blood Disorders*, vol. 11, article 4, 2011.

[30] G. Röhrig, T. Steinmetz, J. Stein et al., "Efficacy and tolerability of ferric carboxymaltose in geriatric patients with anemia. Data from three non-interventional studies," *MMW Fortschritte der Medizin*, vol. 156, pp. 48–53, 2014.

[31] World Health Organization, "Nutritional anemia: report of a WHO Scientific Group," Technical Report Series 405, 1968.

[32] S. van Santen, E. C. van Dongen-Lases, F. de Vegt et al., "Hepcidin and hemoglobin content parameters in the diagnosis of iron deficiency in rheumatoid arthritis patients with anemia," *Arthritis and Rheumatism*, vol. 63, no. 12, pp. 3672–3680, 2011.

[33] A. M. Ganzoni, "Intravenous iron-dextran: therapeutic and experimental possibilities," *Schweizerische Medizinische Wochenschrift*, vol. 100, no. 7, pp. 301–303, 1970.

[34] R. Evstatiev, P. Marteau, T. Iqbal et al., "FERGIcor, a randomized controlled trial on ferric carboxymaltose for iron deficiency anemia in inflammatory bowel disease," *Gastroenterology*, vol. 141, no. 3, pp. 846.e2–853.e2, 2011.

[35] W. Reinisch, M. Staun, R. K. Tandon et al., "A randomized, open-label, non-inferiority study of intravenous iron isomaltoside 1,000 (Monofer) compared with oral iron for treatment of anemia in IBD (PROCEED)," *The American Journal of Gastroenterology*, vol. 108, no. 12, pp. 1877–1888, 2013.

[36] E. A. Jankowska, S. von Haehling, S. D. Anker, I. C. MacDougall, and P. Ponikowski, "Iron deficiency and heart failure: diagnostic dilemmas and therapeutic perspectives," *European Heart Journal*, vol. 34, no. 11, pp. 816–826, 2013.

[37] M. Kapoor, M. D. Schleinitz, A. Gemignani, and W.-C. Wu, "Outcomes of patients with chronic heart failure and iron deficiency treated with intravenous iron: a meta-analysis," *Cardiovascular & Hematological Disorders—Drug Targets*, vol. 13, no. 1, pp. 35–44, 2013.

[38] D. W. Coyne, T. Kapoian, W. Suki et al., "Ferric gluconate is highly efficacious in anemic hemodialysis patients with high serum ferritin and low transferrin saturation: results of the Dialysis Patients' Response to IV Iron with Elevated Ferritin (DRIVE) study," *Journal of the American Society of Nephrology*, vol. 18, no. 3, pp. 975–984, 2007.

[39] G. Wong, K. Howard, E. Hodson, M. Irving, and J. C. Craig, "An economic evaluation of intravenous versus oral iron supplementation in people on haemodialysis," *Nephrology Dialysis Transplantation*, vol. 28, no. 2, pp. 413–420, 2013.

[40] H. T. Steinmetz, "The role of intravenous iron in the treatment of anemia in cancer patients," *Therapeutic Advances in Hematology*, vol. 3, no. 3, pp. 177–191, 2012.

[41] M. Auerbach and H. Ballard, "Intravenous iron in oncology," *Journal of the National Comprehensive Cancer Network*, vol. 6, no. 6, pp. 585–592, 2008.

[42] O. Schröder, O. Mickisch, U. Seidler et al., "Intravenous iron sucrose versus oral iron supplementation for the treatment of iron deficiency anemia in patients with inflammatory bowel disease—a randomized, controlled, open-label, multicenter study," *The American Journal of Gastroenterology*, vol. 100, no. 11, pp. 2503–2509, 2005.

[43] J. A. García-Erce, J. Cuenca, F. Martínez, R. Cardona, L. Pérez-Serrano, and M. Muñoz, "Perioperative intravenous iron preserves iron stores and may hasten the recovery from postoperative anaemia after knee replacement surgery," *Transfusion Medicine*, vol. 16, no. 5, pp. 335–341, 2006.

[44] J. Cuenca, J. A. García-Erce, and M. Muñoz, "Efficacy of intravenous iron sucrose administration for correcting preoperative anemia in patients scheduled for major orthopedic surgery," *Anesthesiology*, vol. 109, no. 1, pp. 151–152, 2008.

[45] M. Muñoz, S. Gómez-Ramírez, E. Martín-Montañez, J. Pavía, J. Cuenca, and J. A. García-Erce, "Perioperative intravenous iron: an upfront therapy for treating anaemia and reducing transfusion requirements," *Nutrición Hospitalaria*, vol. 27, no. 6, pp. 1817–1836, 2012.

[46] M. Auerbach, J. A. Pappadakis, H. Bahrain, S. A. Auerbach, H. Ballard, and N. V. Dahl, "Safety and efficacy of rapidly administered (one hour) one gram of low molecular weight iron dextran (INFeD) for the treatment of iron deficient anemia," *The American Journal of Hematology*, vol. 86, no. 10, pp. 860–862, 2011.

[47] M. Auerbach, W. Strauss, S. Auerbach, S. Rineer, and H. Bahrain, "Safety and efficacy of total dose infusion of 1,020 mg of ferumoxytol administered over 15 min," *American Journal of Hematology*, vol. 88, no. 11, pp. 944–947, 2013.

[48] C.-L. Chuang, R.-S. Liu, Y.-H. Wei, T.-P. Huang, and D.-C. Tarng, "Early prediction of response to intravenous iron supplementation by reticulocyte haemoglobin content and high-fluorescence reticulocyte count in haemodialysis patients," *Nephrology Dialysis Transplantation*, vol. 18, no. 2, pp. 370–377, 2003.

[49] N. Tessitore, G. P. Solero, G. Lippi et al., "The role of iron status markers in predicting response to intravenous iron in haemodialysis patients on maintenance erythropoietin," *Nephrology Dialysis Transplantation*, vol. 16, no. 7, pp. 1416–1423, 2001.

23

Prevalence of Anemia and Its Associated Factors among Pregnant Women Attending Antenatal Care in Health Institutions of Arba Minch Town, Gamo Gofa Zone, Ethiopia: A Cross-Sectional Study

Alemayehu Bekele,[1] Marelign Tilahun,[2] and Aleme Mekuria[1]

[1]*Department of Public Health Nursing, Arba Minch College of Health Sciences, P.O. Box 155, Arba Minch, Ethiopia*
[2]*Department of Public Health, College of Health Sciences, Debre Tabor University, P.O. Box 272, Debre Tabor, Ethiopia*

Correspondence should be addressed to Aleme Mekuria; alemmekurishet@gmail.com

Academic Editor: Eitan Fibach

Background. Anemia during pregnancy is a major cause of morbidity and mortality of pregnant women in developing countries and has both maternal and fetal consequences. Despite its known serious effect on health, there is very little research based evidence on this vital public health problem in Gamo Gofa zone in general and in Arba Minch town of Southern Ethiopia in particular. Therefore, this study aims to assess the prevalence and factors associated with anemia among pregnant women attending antenatal care in health institutions of Arba Minch town, Gamo Gofa zone, Southern Ethiopia. *Method.* Institution-based, cross-sectional study was conducted from February 16 to April 8, 2015, among 332 pregnant women who attended antenatal care at government health institutions of Arba Minch town. Interviewer-administered questionnaire supplemented by laboratory tests was used to obtain the data. Bivariate and multivariate logistic regressions were used to identify predictors of anemia. *Result.* The prevalence of anemia among antenatal care attendant pregnant women of Arba Minch town was 32.8%. Low average monthly income of the family (AOR = 4.0; 95% CI: 5.62–11.01), having birth interval less than two years (AOR = 3.1; 95% CI: 6.01, 10.23), iron supplementation (AOR = 2.31; 95% CI: 7.21, 9.31), and family size >2 (AOR = 2.8; 95% CI: 1.17, 6.81) were found to be independent predictors of anemia in pregnancy. *Conclusion.* Anemia is found to be a moderate public health problem in the study area. Low average monthly income, birth interval less than two years, iron supplementation, and large family size were found to be risk factors for anemia in pregnancy. Awareness creation towards birth spacing, nutritional counselling on consumption of iron-rich foods, and iron supplementation are recommended to prevent anemia among pregnant women with special emphasis on those having low income and large family size.

1. Background

Anemia is defined as a decrease in the concentration of circulating red blood cells or in the haemoglobin concentration and a concomitant impaired capacity to transport oxygen. It has multiple precipitating factors that can occur in isolation but more frequently cooccur. These factors may be genetic, such as haemoglobinopathies; infectious diseases, such as malaria, intestinal helminths, and chronic infection or nutritional deficiency, which includes iron deficiency as well as deficiencies of other vitamins and minerals, such as folate, vitamins A and B12, and copper [1].

Anemia is a global public health problem affecting both developing and developed countries with major consequences on human health as well as social and economic development. It occurs at all stages of the life cycle but is more prevalent in pregnant women and young children [2]. Although the prevalence of anemia is estimated at 9% in countries with high development, in countries with low development the prevalence is 43%. Children and women of reproductive age are most at risk, with global anemia prevalence estimates of 47% in children younger than 5 years, 42% in pregnant women, and 30% in nonpregnant women aged 15–49 years and with Africa and Asia accounting for more than 85% of the absolute anemia burden in high risk groups [3].

Anemia during pregnancy is a major cause of morbidity and mortality of pregnant women in developing countries and has both maternal and fetal consequences. Anemia during pregnancy is considered severe when haemoglobin concentration is less than 7.0 g/dL, moderate when haemoglobin falls between 7.0 and 9.9 g/dL, and mild when haemoglobin concentration is from 10.0 to 11 g/dL [1, 3–5].

Low maternal haemoglobin levels are associated with increased risk of preterm delivery, Low Birth Weight (LBW) babies, APGAR score <5 at 1 min, and intrauterine growth retardation (IUGR). Haemoglobin adjusted for altitude and smoking status in Ethiopia shows that 22% of pregnant women in Ethiopia are anemic and the prevalence varies by residence and educational and wealth status of women. The Health Sector Development Plan IV (HSDP IV) in Ethiopia targets reducing the national level of anemia to 12% [3, 6].

Nutritional, genetic, and infectious diseases are contributing factors for anemia. However, iron deficiency is the cause of 75% of anemia cases. The understanding of how these factors vary by geography, level of development, and other social and economic factors will make it easier to design interventions that are more effective and integrative in addressing multiple contributing factors at the same time [1, 7].

In Ethiopia, even though the HSDP IV target is to reduce anemia prevalence nationally to 12 percent, still anemia is severe problem and affecting 22% of pregnant mothers [6, 8]. Given the multifactorial nature of this disease, correcting anemia often requires an integrated approach. In order to effectively combat anemia, the contributing factors must be identified and addressed. The availability of local prevalence statistics has a major role in the management and control of anemia in pregnancy. Besides the limited studies done in Ethiopia, the prevalence of anemia in pregnant women in our study area is not well known so far. Therefore, this study aims at assessing the prevalence of anemia and its associated factors among pregnant women attending ANC in health institutions of Arba Minch town, Gamo Gofa zone, Southern Ethiopia.

2. Methods

2.1. Study Area. The study was conducted at Arba Minch General Hospital, Arba Minch, and Secha Health Centers in Arba Minch town, Ethiopia. All the three health institutions are located in Arba Minch town which is the capital of Gamo Gofa zone. The catchment area of the two health centres is Arba Minch town and that of the hospital is Gamo Gofa zone. The altitude of the area is 1285 m (4216 ft) above sea level. The total population of the town is about 103,965 people; by using conversion factor for 2014/15 of SNNPR pregnant women in the town it is expected to be 3296 [9]. The three health institutions are the only institutions which provide ANC service for pregnant women in Arba Minch town. The ANC service is provided by midwives who had got special training on focused antenatal care model.

2.2. Study Design. Institution-based, cross-sectional study design was employed.

2.3. Study Participants. The study participants for this study were pregnant women who were attending antenatal care at the selected health institutions during the study period.

2.4. Inclusion Criteria. Pregnant women who reside in Arba Minch for more than six months and who came for ANC during the study period were included in the study.

2.5. Exclusion Criteria. Pregnant women who were seriously ill during the survey were excluded.

2.6. Sample Size and Sampling Procedure. A sample size of 332 was calculated using single proportion formula assuming 16.6% proportion of anemia in pregnancy (from previous study in Ethiopia [10]) at a 95% confidence limit, 80% power, and 4% margin of error and adding 10 % as contingency for nonresponse.

We have reviewed the last year records of monthly flow of pregnant women for ANC utilization in the three health institutions (340 attendees from Arba Minch General Hospital, 220 from Arba Minch Health Center, and 200 attendees from Secha Health Center). The calculated sample size (332) was proportionally allocated to these three health institutions based on the above records: 149 pregnant women for Arba Minch General Hospital, 96 for Arba Minch Health Centre, and 87 for Secha Health Center. Then, after systematic random sampling technique was employed, for instance, in the case of Arba Minch Hospital, the total monthly number of mothers who attended ANC (340) was divided into the current allocated sample size (149) to get the interval that is two, and then lottery method was used to get the random start. Therefore, randomly selected starting point was number two. The interview was started from the second mother, and then every two mothers were interviewed till the allocated sample was achieved. The same method was applied across the rest centres (Figure 1).

2.7. Data Collection. A structured pretested interviewer-administered questionnaire was used to obtain sociodemographic information and present and past obstetric history in pregnant women. To obtain dietary habit, standard food frequency questionnaire adjusted for local food item was adapted and used to assess the usual intake of various food groups for the past one month with their respective consumption frequency [10]. The questionnaire was developed in English and then translated into Amharic language for simplicity then back-translated to English language for its consistency by two different language expert individuals who speak both English and Amharic fluently. Pretesting of the questionnaire was done on 5% of the sample size among ANC attendees who were not included in the study; that was a week before commencement of the actual data collection. To ensure reliable data collection and attain standardization and maximize interviewer reliability, midwives who speak both Amharic and the local language (Gamogna) were recruited and given training on data collection procedure.

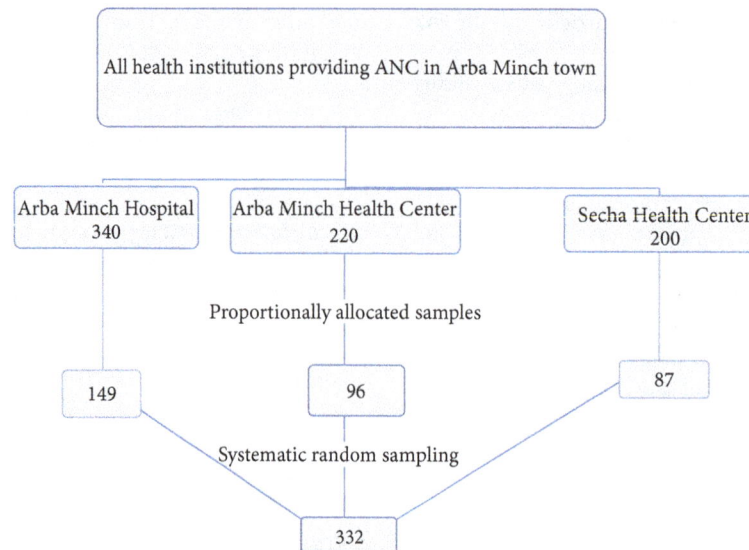

FIGURE 1: Schematic presentation of sampling procedure in public health institutions of Arba Minch town, 2014 ($n = 332$).

Exit interview was done. The data collectors were regularly supervised for proper data collection; all the questionnaires were checked for completeness and consistency in daily basis.

2.8. Specimen Collection and Processing. The specimen collection process in the three health institutions was carried out by two trained laboratory technologists. Each step of specimen collection, processing, and analysis was supervised by experienced and trained laboratory technologist supervisors. The blood for hematocrit/packed cell volume (PCV) measurement was done based on the Standard Operational Procedures (SOPs).

A venous blood sample was taken from the study participants; using heparinized hematocrit tube, three-fourths of the tube was filled and labeled with identification number. The capillary tube after being sealed at one end was centrifuged in the microhematocrit centrifuge at 10,000 g for 5 minutes. Then, the result was read using hematocrit reader.

Stool samples were collected by using a clean and labeled container from the study participants. A portion of the stool was processed with direct microscopic technique to detect intestinal parasites immediately. For detection of helminths, eggs, larvae, and cysts of protozoan parasites, the samples were examined microscopically first with 10x and then with 40x objective. The remaining part of the sample was emulsified in a 10% formalin solution.

Stool examinations were done using formal ether concentration technique, which is considered the most sensitive for most intestinal helminthes. The same method was carried out across all centres.

The hematocrit values in our study area were adjusted in line with the WHO graded adjustment for altitudes; since the altitude of our study area is 4216 feet above sea level, the normal increase for hematocrit values related to long-term

exposure is 1%. Therefore, the value is adjusted with the given range [11].

2.9. Operational Definitions and Definition of Terms

Anemia in Pregnancy. It is when the hematocrit value for a pregnant woman is less than 33% irrespective of her gestational age [11].

Public Health Importance of Anemia. It is a mild public health problem, when prevalence of anemia is <20%; a moderate public health problem, when the prevalence of anemia is between 20 and 40%; a severe public health problem, when the prevalence of anemia is >40% [11].

Mild Anemia. Hematocrit value is ≥30% and <33%.

Moderate Anemia. Hematocrit value is ≥21% and <30%.

Severe Anemia. Hematocrit value is from <21%.

Eating Habits. Different eating habits include eating animal foods, green leafy vegetables, taking fruit after meal, and drinking tea/coffee; this is measured by using food frequency questioner [10].

Permanent Resident. Pregnant women lived at least six months in the study area.

Monthly Income of the Family. Monthly income of the family is <1000 Ethiopian Birr (low), 1000–2575 Ethiopian Birr (medium), and >2575 Ethiopian Birr (high).

2.10. Data Analysis. Data was entered to Epi Info version 3.5.3 software and then exported to SPSS version 20 statistical packages for analysis. Descriptive statistics were done and summarized by frequencies and proportion for categorical predictors. The presence of association was assessed using bivariate analysis and associations with a p value <0.05 considered as statistically significant. Multivariate logistic regression was used to control confounding effects and the strength of association was estimated in odds ratio and its 95% confidence interval.

2.11. Ethical Consideration. Ethical approval was obtained from Joint MPH program, Arba Minch University, and Addis Continental Institute of Public Health Institutional Ethical Review Committee. Official letter to the hospital and health centres was obtained from College of Medicine and Health Sciences, Arba Minch University. To ensure confidentiality, it was anonymous type whereby names of the study subjects were not written on the questionnaire. Written consent from the study participants was obtained after they were briefed about the research intent and asked for their willingness to participate in the study. Their right of denial to participate in the study was also assured.

3. Result

3.1. Sociodemographic Characteristics of Study Subjects. A total of 332 representative ANC attendees participated in the study yielding the response rate of 100%.

The median age of the participants was 25 ± 4.28. Majority, 256 (77.1%), of the participants were within the age range of 20–29. Three hundred and twenty-five (97.9%) of the attendees were married but only four (1.2%) were single. With regard to religion, 174 (52.4%) were Protestants followed by Orthodox Christians, 147 (44.3%). Pertaining to educational status, 103 (31%) of the participants achieved secondary school and above. However, 62 (18.7%) had no formal education. The mean family size in this study group is 3.51 ± 1.66. One hundred and eighteen (35.5%) and 80 (24.1%) of the attendees had a family size of less than or equal to two and greater than or equal to five, respectively (Table 1).

3.2. Obstetrics and Medical History. Two hundred and seven (62.3%) of the ANC attendees had previous history of pregnancy. From those who had previous history of pregnancy, 51 (24.6%) and 63 (32.8%) had history of miscarriage or wilful abortion and at least history of one child, respectively. One hundred and twenty-five (69.1%) had their last births in health facilities. Fifteen (4.5%) of the ANC attendees had history of bleeding on the current pregnancy. One hundred and seventy-six (89.3%) had history of ANC follow-up in the previous pregnancy. From those who had history of birth, 28 (13.5%) and 179 (86.5%) had birth interval of less than two years and more than two years between the last and the current pregnancy, respectively.

More than half of the ANC attendees, 202 (60.8%), had history contraceptive use. More than quarter, 103 (31%), of the participants had history of malaria attack in the last one year. About 123 (38.0%) were using iron during the current pregnancy. Concerning gestational age, 48 (14.5%), 178 (53.6%), and 106 (31.9%) were in first, second, and third trimester of pregnancy, respectively (Table 2).

TABLE 1: Sociodemographic characteristics of ANC attendees in government health institutions of Arba Minch town, February to April 2015 ($n = 332$).

Variables	Number	%
Age		
15–19	32	9.6
20–29	256	77.1
30 and above	44	13.3
Marital status		
Single	4	1.2
Married	325	97.9
Divorced	3	0.9
Religion		
Orthodox	147	44.3
Protestant	174	52.4
Muslim	11	3.3
Educational status		
No formal education	62	18.7
Primary	88	26.5
Secondary	79	23.8
Above secondary	103	31
Family size		
≤2	118	35.5
3-4	134	40.4
≥5	80	24.1
Ethnicity		
Gamo	215	64.8
Wolayita	31	9.3
Amhara	35	10.5
Gofa	18	5.4
Others[*]	33	10

[*]Gurage, Oromo, Tigray, Konso, Burji, Derashe, Ari, Gidicho, Zayise, Oyida, Amaro, and Sidama.

Prevalence of Anemia. About one-third, 109 (32.8%), of the 332 ANC attendees were anemic (hematocrit < 33%). From those who were anemic, the majority, 57 (52.3%), were mild (hematocrit value ≥ 30% and <33%) and 4 (3.7%) were severely anemic (hematocrit value < 21%). Eleven (3%) of the pregnant women were found to be HIV positive. *Giardia lamblia*, 30 (9%); *Entamoeba histolytica*, 5 (1.5%); hookworm, 2 (0.6%), were among intestinal parasites detected in the pregnant women (Table 3).

Factors Associated with Anemia among Pregnant Women. Factors associated with anemia in pregnancy were assessed. During the bivariate analysis, educational status, family size, iron supplementation on current pregnancy, and monthly income had statistically significant association with anemia in pregnancy (Tables 4–6).

In multivariate logistic regression, monthly income of the family (AOR = 4.0; 95% CI: 5.62–11.01), family size (AOR = 2.8; 95% CI: 1.17–6.8), birth interval (AOR = 3.1; 95% CI: 6.01, 10.23), iron tablet supplementation (AOR = 2.31; 95% CI: 7.21, 9.31), and eating food made from "*Enset*" and its

TABLE 2: Obstetrics related characteristics among ANC attendees in health institutions of Arba Minch town, February to April 2015 ($n = 332$).

Variables	Number	%
History of previous pregnancy		
Yes	207	62.3
No	125	37.7
History of abortion		
Yes	51	24.6
No	156	75.4
Number of children		
1	63	32.8
2-3	102	53.1
≥4	27	14.1
Birth interval between the last and current		
Primigravida	125	37.7
<2 years	28	13.5
>2 years	179	86.5
Parity		
Nullipara (0)	125	37.6
Primipara (1)	28	8.4
Multipara (2–4)	159	47.9
Grand multipara (≥5)	30	9.0
Gestational age		
1st trimester	48	14.5
2nd trimester	178	53.6
3rd trimester	103	31.9
Place of delivery of previous pregnancy		
Home	64	30.9
Health facility	143	69.1
ANC follow-up in previous pregnancy		
Yes	176	89.3
No	21	10.7
Bleeding on current pregnancy		
Yes	15	4.5
No	317	95.5
Contraceptive use		
Yes	202	60.8
No	130	39.2
Malaria in the last one year		
Yes	103	31
No	229	69
Iron supplementation on current pregnancy		
Yes	123	37
No	209	63

TABLE 3: Laboratory findings of ANC attendees in government health institutions of Arba Minch town, February to April 2015 ($n = 332$).

Variable	Number	%
HIV serostatus		
Negative	321	96.7
Positive	11	3.3
Stool examination		
Giardia lamblia	30	9
Hookworm	2	0.6
Ascaris lumbricoides	1	0.3
Entamoeba histolytica	5	1.5
Taenia species	2	0.6
No parasite	291	87.7

TABLE 4: Sociodemographic factors associated with anemia in pregnancy among ANC attendees in government health institutions of Arba Minch town from February to April 2015 ($n = 332$).

Variables	Anemia Yes	Anemia No	COR (95% CI)
Occupation			
House wife	56 (33.5%)	111 (66.5%)	1.00
Civil servant	13 (20.3)	51 (79.7%)	0.5 (0.25–1.01)
Merchant	18 (37.5%)	30 (62.5%)	1.2 (0.61–2.32)
Day labourer	12 (60%)	8 (40%)	**2.9 (1.15–7.69)**
Others	10 (30.3%)	23 (69.7%)	0.9 (0.38–1.94)
Monthly income			
<1000 ETB	61 (41.2%)	87 (58.8)	**3 (7.41–10.67)**
1000–2575 ETB	38 (36.2%)	67 (63.8%)	0.81 (0.48–1.35)
>2575 ETB	10 (12.7%)	69 (87.3%)	**1**
Educational status			
Illiterate	29 (46.8%)	33 (53.2%)	1.00
Primary	29 (33%)	59 (67%)	0.44 (0.18–1.05)
Secondary	26 (32.9%)	53 (67.1%)	0.66 (0.31–1.39)
Above secondary	25 (24.3%)	78 (75.7%)	**0.36 (0.18–0.71)**
Marital status			
Married	105 (32.3%)	220 (67.7%)	1.00
Others	4 (57.1%)	3 (42.9%)	2.8 (0.61–12.71)
Family size			
≤2	35 (29.7%)	83 (70.3%)	1.00
3-4	40 (29.9%)	94 (70.1%)	1.5 (0.69–3.18)
≥5	34 (42.5%)	46 (57.5%)	**2.1 (6.42–10.83)**

products (AOR = 5.11; 95% CI: 16.18, 21.35) were found to be independent predictors of anemia in pregnancy (Table 7).

4. Discussion

The current study assessed the prevalence of anemia and its associated risk factors among pregnant women attending ANC in government institutions of Arba Minch town, Gamo Gofa zone, Southern Ethiopia. The overall prevalence of anemia among pregnant women attending ANC in the current study was found to be 32.8% which is lower than a study conducted in India (87–100%), Boditi (61.6%), and Gode town, Eastern Ethiopia (56.8%) [12–15]. This discrepancy could be resulting from geographical variation of factors across different areas and due to time gap between the current study and the 2011 Ethiopian Demographic and Health Survey.

TABLE 5: Obstetrics factors associated with anemia in pregnancy among ANC attendees in government health institutions of Arba Minch town from February to April 2015 (n = 332).

Variables	Anemia		COR (95% CI)
	Yes	No	
Trimester			
First	12 (25%)	36 (75%)	1.00
Second	65 (36.5%)	113 (63.5%)	1.7 (0.84–3.55)
Third	32 (30.2%)	74 (69.8%)	1.3 (0.59–2.81)
History of malaria attack (last 1 year)			
No	78 (34.1%)	151 (65.9%)	1.00
Yes	31 (30.1%)	72 (69.9%)	0.83 (0.51–1.37)
Intestinal parasite on current pregnancy			
No	97 (33.3%)	194 (66.7%)	1.00
Yes	12 (29.3%)	29 (70.7%)	0.83 (0.41–1.69)
HIV serostatus			
Negative	106 (33%)	215 (67%)	1.00
Positive	3 (27.3%)	8 (72.7%)	0.76 (0.19–2.93)
Iron supplementation on current pregnancy			
No	73 (34.9%)	136 (65.1%)	**1.9 (6.4–9.10)**
Yes	36 (29.3%)	87 (70.7%)	1
Birth interval			
≤2 years	15 (53.6%)	13 (46.4%)	**2.3 (4.41–7.23)**
>2 years	52 (29.1%)	127 (70.9%)	1

TABLE 6: Dietary habits associated with anemia in pregnancy among ANC attendees in government health institutions of Arba Minch town from February to April 2015 (n = 332).

Variables	Anemia		COR (95% CI)
	Yes	No	
Eating food made from "*Enset*" and its products			
Twice/month	10 (43.5%)	13 (56.5%)	1.00
1-2 per week	25 (35.7%)	45 (64.3%)	0.72 (0.27–1.88)
3-4 per week	15 (17.9%)	69 (82.1%)	**0.28 (0.10–0.76)**
Once/day	38 (36.5%)	66 (63.5%)	0.75 (0.30–1.87)
>1 per day	21 (41.2%)	30 (58.8%)	**0.91 (0.34–2.46)**
Eating food made from cereals, grains			
2 times/wk	7 (43.8%)	9 (56.2%)	1.00
3-4/wk	7 (33.3%)	14 (66.7%)	0.64 (0.17–2.45)
Once/day	22 (18.3%)	98 (81.7%)	0.28 (0.09–0.86)
>1/day	73 (32.8%)	102 (67.2%)	0.92 (0.33–2.58)
Drinking tea or coffee			
2/month or less	6 (2.4%)	19 (76%)	1.00
1–4/wk	6 (20%)	24 (80%)	0.79 (0.22–2.85)
1/day	33 (25%)	99 (75%)	1.1 (0.38–2.86)
>1/day	64 (44.1%)	81 (55.9%)	2.5 (0.94–6.63)
Eating fruit			
≤2 wk	20 (45.5%)	24 (54.5%)	1.00
3-4/wk	25 (30.5%)	57 (69.5%)	0.53 (0.25–1.12)
1/day	38 (28.1%)	97 (71.9%)	0.47 (0.23–0.95)
>1/day	25 (35.7%)	45 (64.3%)	0.67 (0.31–1.44)
Eating beef, goat, chicken, or other kinds of organ meat			
Never	15 (23.1%)	50 (76.9%)	1.00
1-2/month	55 (37.4%)	92 (62.6%)	1.9 (1.02–3.88)
1-2/week	30 (34.9%)	56 (65.1%)	1.8 (0.86–3.69)
≥3/wk	9 (26.5%)	25 (73.5%)	1.2 (0.46–3.12)

TABLE 7: Multivariate logistic regression analysis results showing factors associated with anemia in pregnancy among ANC attendees in government health institutions of Arba Minch town from February to April 2015 (n = 332).

Variables	Anemia		COR (95% CI)	AOR (95% CI)
	Yes	No		
Monthly income				
<1000 Birr	61 (41.2%)	87 (58.8)	**3 (7.41–10.67)**	**4.0 (5.62–11.01)**
1000–2575 Birr	38 (36.2%)	67 (63.8%)	0.81 (0.48–1.35)	0.9 (0.54–1.75)
>2575 Birr	10 (12.7%)	69 (87.3%)	1	1
Family size				
≤2	35 (29.7%)	83 (70.3%)	1.00	1.00
3-4	40 (29.9%)	94 (70.1%)	1.01 (0.59–1.73)	1.5 (0.69–3.18)
≥5	34 (42.5%)	46 (57.5%)	**2.1 (6.42–10.83)**	**2.8 (1.17–6.80)**
Iron supplementation on current pregnancy				
No	73 (34.9%)	136 (65.1%)	1.9 (6.4–9.10)	**2.31 (7.21, 9.31)**
Yes	36 (29.3%)	87 (70.7%)	1	1
Birth interval				
≤2 years	15 (53.6%)	13 (46.4%)	**2.3 (4.41–7.23)**	**3.1 (6.01, 10.23)**
>2 years	52 (29.1%)	127 (70.9%)	0.81 (0.49–1.32)	1
Eating food made from "*Enset*" and its products				
Twice/month	10 (43.5%)	13 (56.5%)	1.00	**1.00**
1-2 per week	25 (35.7%)	45 (64.3%)	0.72 (0.27–1.88)	**0.22 (0.07–0.73)**
3-4 per week	15 (17.9%)	69 (82.1%)	**0.28 (0.10–0.76)**	**0.12 (0.03–0.39)**
Once/day	38 (36.5%)	66 (63.5%)	0.75 (0.30–1.87)	0.36 (0.12–1.11)
>1 per day	21 (41.2%)	30 (58.8%)	**0.91 (0.34–2.46)**	**0.17 (0.05–0.62)**

However, the prevalence of anemia in the current study was found to be higher as compared to the study conducted in Addis Ababa (21.3%) and Gondar Northwest Ethiopia (16.6%) [10, 14, 16]. In addition, the current prevalence of anemia is also higher than the national anemia prevalence (22%) [6]. This might be attributed to the fact that the majority of the participants in the current study consume plant based foods as a staple food which is rich in nonheme iron with bioavailability of not more than 10%. The high consumption of tea and coffee in the study area might reduce the bioavailability of the nonheme iron from plant based staple foods.

In the current study among the pregnant women, mild anemia was found to be common and followed by moderate anemia. Consistent result was reported from studies conducted in some African countries and elsewhere in the world [12–15, 17–21].

Monthly income was significantly associated with anemia in pregnancy. Pregnant women who had low monthly family income (less than 2575 Ethiopian Birr) were four times more likely to be anemic as compared to those with high monthly family income (greater than 2575 Ethiopian Birr). This is in agreement with some studies [10, 14]. This could be explained by the reality that more than 57% of the total expenditure among Ethiopians is spent on food [15, 22]. Hence, pregnant women with low income groups could not get adequate nutrition so that they were at risk of anemia.

Pregnant women having birth interval less than two years were at higher risk of becoming anemic as compared to those with birth interval more than two years. This finding

is consistent with a study conducted in Saudi Arabia [23]. This might be related with decreased iron store of women due to occurrence of pregnancy in quick succession between subsequent pregnancies.

Pregnant women who have had no iron supplementation on the current pregnancy were in about two times higher risk of developing anemia as compared to those who have had iron supplementation. This finding is consistent with the findings from Gode town (Eastern Ethiopia) and Vietnam [15, 24], which indicated that lack of iron supplementation was among the most significant risk factors for developing anemia during pregnancy. This is likely due to the fact that the requirement for iron increases for pregnant women as compared to nonpregnant women; this is associated with the reality that blood volume increases by 50% during pregnancy and the requirement of iron to growing fetus and placenta. Therefore, supplementation of iron during pregnancy is crucial to fulfil this need.

In this study, family size was also significantly associated with anemia; pregnant women with family size greater than 5 were at higher risk of developing anemia than those with family size less than five. This finding is comparable with a study conducted in Shala woreda (West Arsi) in which the prevalence of anemia was higher among women with family size >5 as compared to their counterparts [25]. The direct relationship of family size with anemia in this study could be associated with food insecurity for large family size.

Study Limitations. This study is limited by its cross-sectional nature, whereby it may not explain the temporal relationship between the outcome variable and some explanatory variables; this limits interpretation of the estimated associations. Recall bias might be introduced on food frequency. Thus, the findings of this study should be interpreted within these limitations.

5. Conclusion

The overall prevalence of anemia among women attending ANC in government health institutions of Arba Minch town was 32.8%. Anemia is a moderate public health problem in Arba Minch, which is by far higher than the national prevalence, 22%. Monthly income, family size, birth interval, and iron supplementation were significantly associated with anemia. We recommend awareness creation on birth spacing and nutritional counselling on consumption of iron-rich foods and iron supplementation to prevent anemia among pregnant women with special emphasis on those from low income group and large family size.

Conflict of Interests

The authors declare that they have no conflict of interests.

Authors' Contribution

Alemayehu Bekele designed, conducted, and analyzed the data as part of his thesis work. Aleme Mekuria assisted in the design of the study and conducted critical review. Marelign Tilahun assisted in and supervised the design of the study. All the authors read and approved the paper.

Acknowledgments

The authors are very thankful to Joint MPH Program, Arba Minch University, and Addis Continental Institute of Public Health for enabling them to go through this research undertaking process. They would like also to extend their heartfelt thanks and appreciation to Arba Minch College of Health Sciences for the financial support. Last but not least, their special thanks go to the study participants for their willingness to share their experience and giving time for the interview.

References

[1] E. McLean, M. Cogswell, I. Egli, D. Wojdyla, and B. De Benoist, "Worldwide prevalence of anaemia, WHO Vitamin and Mineral Nutrition Information System, 1993-2005," *Public Health Nutrition*, vol. 12, no. 4, pp. 444–454, 2009.

[2] WHO/CDC, *Worldwide Prevalence of Anemia 1993–2005 WHO Global Database on Anemia*, WHO Press, Geneva, Switzerland, 2008.

[3] Y. Balarajan, U. Ramakrishnan, E. Özaltin, A. H. Shankar, and S. V. Subramanian, "Anaemia in low-income and middle-income countries," *The Lancet*, vol. 378, no. 9809, pp. 2123–2135, 2011.

[4] WHO, *Micronutrients Indicators Haemoglobin Concentrations for the Diagnosis of Anemia and Assessment of Severity*, Vitamin and Mineral Nutrition Information System, 2011.

[5] A. Meseret, B. Enawgaw, A. Gelaw, T. Kena, M. Seid, and Y. Olkeba, "Prevalence of anemiaand associated risk factors among pregnant women attending antenatal care in Azezo Health Center, Gondar town, Northwest Ethiopia," *Journal of Interdisciplinary Histopathology*, vol. 1, no. 3, pp. 137–144, 2013.

[6] CSA, *Ethiopia Demographic and Health Survey: Preliminary Report*, CSA, Addis Ababa, Ethiopia, 2011.

[7] F. W. Lone, R. N. Qureshi, and F. Emanuel, "Maternal anaemia and its impact on perinatal outcome," *Tropical Medicine & International Health*, vol. 9, no. 4, pp. 486–490, 2004.

[8] J. Jennings and M. B. Hirbaye, *Review of Incorporation of Essential Nutrition Actions into Public Health Programs in Ethiopia*, section 1–25, The Food and Nutrition Technical Assistance Project (FANTA), Equinet, 2008.

[9] Central Statitical Authority of Ethiopia (CSA), *Population and Housing Census of Ethiopia: Ethiopia Statistical Abstract*, CSA, Addis Ababa, Ethiopia, 2007.

[10] R. S. Gibson, *Principles of Nutritional Assessment*, Oxford University Press, New York, NY, USA, 2nd edition, 2005.

[11] WHO, *Iron Defficiency Anemia, Assessment, Prevention, and control: A Guide for Program Managers*, World Health Organization, Geneva, Switzerland, 2001.

[12] M. Melku, Z. Addis, M. Alem, and B. Enawgaw, "Prevalence and predictors of maternal anemia during pregnancy in Gondar, Northwest Ethiopia: an institutional based cross-sectional study," *Anemia*, vol. 2014, Article ID 108593, 9 pages, 2014.

[13] P. O. Lokare, V. D. Karanjekar, P. L. Gattani, and A. P. Kulkarni, "A study of prevalence of anemiaand sociodemographic factors associated with anemia among pregnant women in Aurangabad city, India," *Annals of Nigerian Medicine*, vol. 6, no. 1, pp. 30–34, 2012.

[14] B. Vemulapalli and K. K. Rao, "Prevalence of anemiaamong pregnant women of rural community in Vizianagram, North coastal Andhra Pradesh, India," *Asian Journal of Medical Science*, vol. 5, no. 2, pp. 21–25, 2014.

[15] K. A. Alene and A. M. Dohe, "Prevalence of anemia and associated factors among pregnant women in an urban area of Eastern Ethiopia," *Anemia*, vol. 2014, Article ID 561567, 7 pages, 2014.

[16] D. Lelissa, M. Yilma, W. Shewalem et al., "Prevalence of anemia among women receiving antenatal care at Boditii Health Center, Southern Ethiopia," *Clinical Medicine Research*, vol. 4, no. 3, pp. 79–86, 2015.

[17] A. Hailu Jufar and T. Zewde, "Prevalence of anemia among pregnant women attending antenatal care at Tikur Anbessa Specialized Hospital, Addis Ababa, Ethiopia," *Journal of Hematology & Thromboembolic Diseases*, vol. 2, no. 1, article 125, 2013.

[18] C. C. Dim and H. E. Onah, "The prevalence of anemia among pregnant women at booking in Enugu, South Eastern Nigeria," *Medscape General Medicine*, vol. 9, no. 3, article 11, 2007.

[19] A. Olubukola, A. Odunayo, and O. Adesina, "Anemia in pregnancy at two levels of health care in Ibadan, south west Nigeria," *Annals of African Medicine*, vol. 10, no. 4, pp. 272–277, 2011.

[20] E. O. Uche-Nwachi, A. Odekunle, S. Jacinto et al., "Anaemia in pregnancy: associations with parity, abortions and child spacing in primary healthcare clinic attendees in Trinidad and Tobago," *African Health Sciences*, vol. 10, no. 1, pp. 66–70, 2010.

[21] K. S. Okunade and M. A. Adegbesan-Omilabu, "Anemia among pregnant women at the booking clinic of a teaching hospital in South-Westeren Nigeria," *International Journal of Medicine and Biomedical Research*, vol. 3, no. 2, pp. 114–120, 2014.

[22] CSA, *Ethiopia Demographic and Health Survey*, CSA, Addis Ababa, Ethiopia, 2011.

[23] A. M. Abdelhafez and S. S. El-Soadaa, "Prevalence and risk factors of anemia among a sample of pregnant females attending primary health care centers in Makkah, Saudi Arabia," *Pakistan Journal of Nutrition*, vol. 11, no. 12, pp. 1113–1120, 2012.

[24] R. Aikawa, N. C. Khan, S. Sasaki, and C. W. Binns, "Risk factors for iron-deficiency anaemia among pregnant women living in rural Vietnam," *Public Health Nutrition*, vol. 9, no. 4, pp. 443–448, 2006.

[25] N. Obse, A. Mossie, and T. Gobena, "Magnitude of anemia and associated risk factors among pregnant women attending antenatal care in Shalla Woreda, West Arsi Zone, Oromia Region, Ethiopia," *Ethiopian Journal of Health Sciences*, vol. 23, no. 2, pp. 165–173, 2013.

24

Hyperglycaemic Environment: Contribution to the Anaemia Associated with Diabetes Mellitus in Rats Experimentally Induced with Alloxan

Oseni Bashiru Shola and Fakoya Olatunde Olugbenga

Department of Biomedical Sciences, Faculty of Basic Medical Sciences, College of Health Sciences,
Ladoke Akintola University of Technology, Ogbomosho 210214, Oyo State, Nigeria

Correspondence should be addressed to Fakoya Olatunde Olugbenga; dantuned85@yahoo.com

Academic Editor: Aurelio Maggio

Background. Diabetes mellitus characterized by hyperglycaemia presents with various complications amongst which anaemia is common particularly in those with overt nephropathy or renal impairment. The present study has examined the contribution of the hyperglycaemic environment in diabetic rats to the anaemia associated with diabetes mellitus. Method. Sixty male albino rats weighing 175–250 g were selected for this study and divided equally into control and test groups. Hyperglycaemia was induced with 170 kgbwt^{-1} alloxan intraperitoneally in the test group while control group received sterile normal saline. Blood samples obtained from the control and test rats were assayed for packed cell volume (PCV), haemoglobin (Hb), red blood cell count (RBC), reticulocyte count, glucose, plasma haemoglobin, potassium, and bilirubin. *Result.* Significant reduction ($P < 0.01$) in PCV (24.40 ± 3.87 versus 40.45 ± 3.93) and haemoglobin (7.81 ± 1.45 versus 13.39 ± 0.40) with significant increase ($P < 0.01$) in reticulocyte count (12.4 ± 1.87 versus 3.69 ± 0.47), plasma haemoglobin (67.50 ± 10.85 versus 34.20 ± 3.83), and potassium (7.04 ± 0.75 versus 4.52 ± 0.63) was obtained in the test while plasma bilirubin showed nonsignificant increase (0.41 ± 0.04 versus 0.24 ± 0.06). *Conclusion.* The increased plasma haemoglobin and potassium levels indicate an intravascular haemolytic event while the nonsignificant increased bilirubin showed extravascular haemolysis. These play contributory roles in the anaemia associated with diabetes mellitus.

1. Introduction

Diabetes mellitus is a disorder of impaired carbohydrate metabolism resulting from a relative or an absolute deficiency of the hormone insulin. It is documented to have a global prevalence, ranking among the top causes of death in the Western world [1].

Without preference to classification, diabetes mellitus generally presents with hyperglycaemia. Hyperglycaemia is referred to as blood sugar greater than the upper reference limit for age, sex, and environmental and physiological condition [2]. In hyperglycaemic state, glucose supplies to metabolizing cells are usually impaired but not to the red blood cell. The glucose transporter on the red cell membrane, *glucose-permease*, is non-insulin-dependent; hence an excessively high concentration of red cell intracellular glucose in hyperglycaemic state is imminent [3].

Studies have shown that accumulation of intracellular glucose may increase peroxidation of red cell membrane predisposing to cell membrane defects [4]. This may influence deformability [5] as observed in the red cells of patients with diabetic retinopathy [6, 7] and also contribute to reduced blood flow in the capillaries and microcirculation as hypothesized by other research workers [8–10]. It has also been reported that effective erythropoietin synthesis may be impaired following pathologic conditions of the kidneys, contributing to the anaemia observed in diabetes mellitus [11]. These factors and several others play a role in the anaemia associated with diabetes; the effect of the hyperglycaemic environment on the red cell survival is therefore investigated by this study.

2. Materials and Methods

The experimental study was conducted at the Mercyland Campus of Ladoke Akintola University of Technology (LAUTECH), Osogbo. Sixty (60) white male albino rats weighing 175–250 g were acclimated for 14 days to the animal house of the Mercyland Campus of Ladoke Akintola University, Osogbo. The selected animals were housed in wire mesh, well aerated cages at normal atmospheric temperature (25 ± 5°C) and normal 12-hour light/dark cycle. They had free access to water and supplied daily with standard diet of known composition *ad libitum*. All animal procedures were in accordance with the standard recommendations for care and use of laboratory animals [12].

2.1. Chemicals, Reagent, and Equipment. Alloxan monohydrate was purchased from Sigma-Aldrich Chemicals Co. (St. Louis, MO, USA), protected from direct light exposure, and stored at 2–4°C. All other chemicals including stains (Leishman) were of analytical grade and obtained from licensed laboratory reagent suppliers. Machines and equipment used were properly calibrated and quality-controlled before respective analyses.

2.2. Induction of Diabetes. Rats were weighed and blood samples collected from the tail vein for baseline plasma glucose (glucose oxidase method) estimation using Randox glucose kit (Randox Laboratories Ltd., BT29 QY, United Kingdom). Subsequently, the animals were divided equally into two (2) groups.

Group 1 (control group) were injected with freshly prepared sterile saline. Group 2 (test group) received 170 kgbwt^{-1} alloxan preparation (2,4,5,6-tetraoxypyrimidine; 2,4,5,6-pyrimidinetetrone). All injections were done through single intraperitoneal administration using a total volume of 0.5 mL after estimating the effective dose and administered volume with respect to their weights [13].

2.3. Experimental Design. On days 3, 6, and 9 after injection, rats were reweighed and glucose estimation was done in all the two (2) groups described above. On day 10, twenty-four (24) rats had very high plasma glucose level greater than 250 mg/dL and were included for group 2 while four (4) lower responsive rats were excluded. Animals were sacrificed by exposure to chloroform within a closed system and blood samples were collected for the various investigations into appropriate specimen bottles. The following investigations were carried out in the course of the study: haematocrit (HCT), haemoglobin (Hb), and red blood cell count (RBC), extracted from a complete blood count analysis using SYSMEX Automated Hematology Analyzer (KX-21N, Sysmex Corporation, Chuo-ku, Kobe 651-0073, Japan); peripheral blood for reticulocyte count incubated with new methylene blue at 37°C, smeared, and estimated manually; serum total

TABLE 1: The effect of alloxan on plasma glucose level.

Control (n = 30) Saline injection		Test (n = 28) Alloxan injection	
Days	Average plasma glucose (mg/dL)	Days	Average plasma glucose (mg/dL)
0	79	0	79
3	82	3	102
6	80	6	207
9	80	9	267
12	79	12	308

bilirubin estimated using Randox kit (Randox Laboratories Ltd., BT29 QY, United Kingdom); calorimetric method on BSA 3000 Semiautometed Biochemistry Analyser (SFRI San, Lieu dit Berganton, 33127 Saint Jean d'Illlac, France); and Plasma haemoglobin according to Dacie and Lewis [14]. Plasma potassium was estimated using ISE 6000 electrolyte analyzer (SFRI San, Lieu dit Berganton, 33127 Saint Jean d'Illlac, France).

2.4. Statistical Analysis. Data obtained were analyzed using statistical package for social sciences version 15 (SPSS Inc., Chicago, IL) for windows and expressed as mean ± 1standard deviation. Test of significance comparing control and test was done using Student's t-test and defined as $P < 0.01$.

3. Results

A total of fifty-four (54) rats, 30 controls and 24 (80%) alloxan induced hyperglycaemic tests rats, were used for this study. Two (6.6%) of the test rats were lost to death on days 2 and 3 after induction. In Table 1 we summarize the effect of alloxan administration on plasma glucose level. On day 9 after induction, significant hyperglycaemia (≥250 mg/dL) was observed in 24 (80%) rats. Four (13.3%) test rats showed no significant increase in plasma glucose after alloxan induction; there was no significant difference between the baseline glucose and glucose concentration after alloxan induction in these rats. Average plasma glucose level on day 9 after induction was significantly higher ($P < 0.01$) than the control (267 mg/dL versus 80 mg/dL). Since significant hyperglycaemia was not established in four (13.3%) of the rats, they were excluded from further studies. Data comparing the average mean values and standard deviations between parameters of the test and control group were summarized in Tables 2 and 3. In Table 2, we compare the results of plasma haemoglobin, plasma potassium, and total bilirubin concentration between the two groups. There was a significant increase ($P < 0.01$) in plasma haemoglobin and potassium concentration in hyperglycaemic rats; total bilirubin, however, was not significantly increased between the two groups although average mean was increased in the test group. Table 3 showed the relationship between the haematocrit, haemoglobin, total red blood cell count, and reticulocyte count in the two groups. We observed a statistically significant reduction ($P < 0.01$) in haematocrit, haemoglobin, and red blood cell count among

TABLE 2: Table of significance comparing test and control plasma haemoglobin, potassium, and bilirubin concentration.

Subject	Plasma Hb (mg/L)	Plasma K$^+$ (mmol/L)	Plasma total bilirubin (mg/dL)
Test mean ($n = 24$)	67.50 ± 10.85	7.04 ± 0.75	0.41 ± 0.04
Control mean ($n = 30$)	34.20 ± 3.83	4.52 ± 0.63	0.24 ± 0.06
t-test	26.4	11.52	0.28
P value	<0.01	<0.01	>0.01

TABLE 3: The test of significance of hyperglycaemia on PCV, Hb, RBC, and reticulocyte count.

Subject	PCV (%)	Hb (g/dL)	RBC ($\times 10^{12}$/L)	Retics. count (%)
Test mean ($n = 24$)	24.40 ± 3.87	7.81 ± 1.45	3.47 ± 0.29	12.4 ± 1.87
Control mean ($n = 30$)	40.45 ± 3.93	13.39 ± 0.40	7.16 ± 0.25	3.69 ± 0.47
t-test	-13.04	-16.61	-42.77	-20.19
P value	<0.01	<0.01	<0.01	<0.01

the hyperglycaemic rats; reticulocyte count was statistically higher in this group also. The red cell parameters (HCT, Hb, and RBC) were higher and stable in the control sets and reticulocyte count remained within normal limits.

4. Discussion

Induction of diabetes experimentally by alloxan (2,4,5,6-tetraoxypyrimidine; 2,4,5,6-pyrimidineterione) remains one of the most effective methods of establishing experimental diabetes. It is a well-known diabetogenic agent and has been widely reported to generate stable hyperglycaemia for prolong period [15]. In our study as summarized in Table 1, there was progressive induction of hyperglycaemia following alloxan administration and a stable hyperglycaemic state in 24(80%) of the alloxan induced rats. This is in consonance with several research studies that induced hyperglycaemia using alloxan [13, 16]. Misra and Aiman [17] in their study observed alloxan induced diabetes in 60% of rats using the same dosage as in our study; however they reported a dose-dependent mortality in 40% of the rats in this group. They hypothesized that susceptibility to diabetogenic and toxic effects of alloxan differs among animals of the same species. Alloxan has a narrow diabetogenic range of 160-180 kgbwt^{-1} [13]; induction therefore with a lower dose may autorevert the hyperglycaemic state following a regeneration of the pancreatic beta cells [18] while a higher dose may be cytotoxic, damaging not only the pancreatic cells but other important organs [19].

Hyperglycaemia was established on the sixth day of our study. This showed that the onset of alloxan action may be delayed [18]. Optimization of the diabetogenic agent is dependent on the dose range, route of administration, rate of injection, and age and species of experimental animal used [13, 17–20]. A study on the pharmacokinetic and pharmacodynamic profile of alloxan hypothesized unpredictable diabetes inducing alloxan effect except when administered by rapid intravenous injection [18]. Hyperglycaemic response and stability were monitored in the animals throughout the experimental process to rule out autoreversion (Table 1). Significant increase in plasma potassium and haemoglobin in the test group as depicted in Table 2 suggests episodes of intravascular red cell destruction (haemolysis within the peripheral circulation). This may be attributable to fragmentation of the red blood cells in the peripheral circulation as a result of the glucose *permease* enabled accumulated red cell intracellular glucose and generation of reactive substances, distorting the well programmed structural and functional character of the cell [3]. In addition, some red cells withstanding breakage in the circulation getting to the spleen lose deformability and are phagocytosed by the reticuloendothelial macrophages, releasing bilirubin [21]. We posit that this incidence must have informed the nonsignificant increase in total bilirubin seen in this study.

The red blood cells are clinically important haematologic cells and uniquely identified as one of the early cells affected in diabetes [22], before development of other diabetic complications. Carroll and colleagues recorded that the red cells play important role in the onset and development of several diabetic complications [23]. The mechanism underlying red cell destruction in hyperglycaemia is complex. Normal erythrocytes are biconcave shaped cells, measuring about 8 μm in diameter, with an average volume of 90fL and surface area of 140 μm^2. According to Mohandas and Gallagher, red blood cell has a membrane which is highly elastic, rapidly responds to applied fluid stress, and is stronger than steel in terms of structural resistance [24]. Despite this unique feature, a slight alteration in structural composition, small increased surface area, haemoglobin hyperviscosity, and autooxidation, amongst others, poses a challenge to the oxygen transporting cell and results in cell lysis [25, 26]. In the process of performing oxygen transport function, RBCs are exposed to high level of endogenous and exogenous oxidative metabolites [27]. These accumulating reactive substances potentiate complex oxidative processes with severe damaging consequence on the cell membrane, structure, and function. However, to optimize their exclusive role as well as to survive the rigors of circulation, the highly specialized blood cells have evolved an extensive array of enzymatic and nonenzymatic antioxidants systems, including membrane oxidoreductases, cellular antioxidants such as catalase and superoxide dismutase (SOD), and enzymes that continuously produce reducing agents through the glutathione (GSH) system [28]. In hyperglycaemic state, generation of reactive oxidative substances is markedly increased creating a redox imbalance within the red cell environment and limiting the cell antioxidative potential [22, 29]. Tiwari and Ndisang reported that glucose mediated increase in reactive oxygen species is one of the biochemical changes associated with type 1 diabetes (enhanced hyperglycaemia-mediated oxidative stress) [30]; other biochemical reactions associated with hyperglycaemia are diacylglycerol production and subsequent activation of the protein kinase C pathway, flux through the polyol metabolic pathway, secretion of cytokines, and modification of proteins and lipids that becomes nonenzymatically glycated forming Schiff bases and amadori products with resultant, irreversible generation and accumulation of glycated end products [31–35]. The red cells demonstrating an unregulated access to glucose uptake are in this state exposed to high glucose concentration both intracellularly and within the vascular environment [35]; this increases glucose oxidation and accumulates glucose metabolites, including NADPH which promotes susceptibility to lipid peroxidation, membrane damage, and intravascular cell death [4]. One of the greatest challenges to the well-equipped red cell antioxidant system as documented by Mohanty and colleagues is the increased autoxidation of haemoglobin (Hb) bound to the membrane in hyperglycaemic state which is relatively inaccessible to the antioxidant system [36]. Besides haemoglobin, ROS also critically affects other proteins in the red cell since they are easy target of ROS, majorly the spectrin, ankyrin, actin, and protein 4.1 [37]. Oxidation of biomolecules at amino acid active sites can also trigger rapid deactivation of enzyme and shut down the antioxidant system [22]. RBCs thus become highly susceptible to oxidative damage from accumulated reactive substance generation. A number of *in vitro/in vivo* studies have shown that several RBCs parameters are negatively affected by increased oxidative stress as observed in diabetes [38–41]. One of these is an assessment of heme degradation products (HDP) to determine the red cell oxidative status which was increased in older RBC as they tend to senescence [36]; this was also observed in RBC of diabetics [42] suggesting reduced membrane deformability [23]. In addition, oxidative stress also inhibits Ca-ATPase, responsible for regulating the intracellular concentration of calcium [43, 44]. With increased intracellular calcium, the Gardos channel is activated causing leakage of intracellular potassium; this alters cation homeostasis resulting in cell shrinking and lysis [45] as described in our study. Besides the red cell are the vascular endothelial cells with high amount of glucose transporter and also an unrestricted access to glucose in-flow [35]. Vascular complications in diabetes are associated with formation of cross-links between key molecules in the basement membrane of ECM and eruption of basement membrane lesions; this results in thickening of the blood vessels subjecting the already weakened red blood cells to fragmentation and contributing to premature destruction of the red cell in circulation [46]. Hence, red cell fragmentation and intravascular haemolysis are common events associated with damaged blood vessels, especially within the microvascular environment (microangiopathy).

Despite the undoubted fact that hyperglycaemia battles all the tissues in the body, it is established that diabetic complications are observed in a subset of cell types; capillary endothelial cells in the retina, mesangial cells in the renal glomerulus, and neurons and Schwann cells in peripheral nerves. Brownlee explained that, in hyperglycaemic state, most cells reduce transport of glucose inside the cell so that their internal glucose concentration stays constant. However, the cells damaged by hyperglycemia, including the red blood cells, are those that cannot do this efficiently because glucose transport rate does not decline rapidly, leading to high glucose inside the cell [35]. In view of this we propose that oxidative stress distorted biochemical processes and impaired deformability and cell membrane weakness, fragmentation, and intravascular and extravascular destructions; as observed in our study are the features characterizing the onset of anaemia associated with type 1 diabetes.

Anaemia stimulated hypoxia has been shown to increase hypoxia-inducible factor 1 which promotes synthesis of erythropoietin, inducing reticulocytosis [47]. The bone marrow responsiveness to the haemolysis through significant reticulocytosis indicates that alloxan toxicity has no destructive effect on the bone marrow at dosage used. It is further established that anaemia observed in earlier diabetes is contributed to by intravascular and extravascular haemolysis while anaemia of chronic long standing diabetics is caused by renal pathology [48].

In conclusion, we infer from our study that red cell destruction due to hyperglycaemic environment is predominantly intravascular with minor contribution from the extravascular environment and the presenting anaemia is a responsive type differing from the nonresponsive chronic anaemia associated with diabetic nephropathy documented by other workers.

Conflict of Interests

The authors declare that there is no conflict of interests regarding the publication of this paper.

Acknowledgment

The authors are grateful to the technical staff of Mercyland, Animal House, Osogbo, for helping out with care of animals and scientists of LAUTECH Teaching Hospital.

References

[1] A. C. Guyton and J. E. Hall, *A TextBook of Medical Physiology*, W.B. Saunders Company, Philadelphia, Pa, USA, 12th edition, 2012.

[2] O. J. Ochei and A. A. Kolhatkar, *Medical Laboratory Science Theory and Practice*, Tata McGraw-Hill, New Delhi, India, 1st edition, 2001.

[3] R. K. Murray, D. K. Granner, P. A. Mayes, and V. W. Rodwell, *Harper's Iluustrated Biochemistry*, McGraw-Hill, New Delhi, India, 26th edition, 2003.

[4] S. K. Jain, "Hyperglycemia can cause membrane lipid peroxidation and osmotic fragility in human red blood cells," *The Journal of Biological Chemistry*, vol. 264, no. 35, pp. 21340–21345, 1989.

[5] C. D. Brown, H. S. Ghali, Z. Zhao, L. L. Thomas, and E. A. Friedman, "Association of reduced red blood cell deformability and diabetic nephropathy," *Kidney International*, vol. 67, no. 1, pp. 295–300, 2005.

[6] R. Agrawal, R. Bhatnagar, T. Smart et al., "Assessment of red blood cell deformability by optical tweezers in diabetic retinopathy," *Investigative Ophthalmology & Visual Science*, vol. 56, no. 7, p. 5183, 2015.

[7] T. Rimmer, J. Fleming, and E. M. Kohner, "Hypoxic viscosity and diabetic retinopathy," *British Journal of Ophthalmology*, vol. 74, no. 7, pp. 400–404, 1990.

[8] Y. I. Cho, M. P. Mooney, and D. J. Cho, "Hemorheological disorders in diabetes mellitus," *Journal of Diabetes Science and Technology*, vol. 2, no. 6, pp. 1130–1138, 2008.

[9] S. Shin, Y. Ku, M.-S. Park, J.-H. Jang, and J.-S. Suh, "Rapid cell-deformability sensing system based on slit-flow laser diffractometry with decreasing pressure differential," *Biosensors and Bioelectronics*, vol. 20, no. 7, pp. 1291–1297, 2005.

[10] S. Chien, "Red cell deformability and its relevance to blood flow," *Annual Review of Physiology*, vol. 49, pp. 177–192, 1987.

[11] C. Hasslacher, "Anaemia in patients with diabetic nephropathy—prevalence, causes and clinical consequences," *European Cardiology Review*, vol. 3, no. 1, pp. 80–82, 2007.

[12] Committee for the Update of the Care and Use of Laboratory Animals, *Guide for the Care and Use of Laboratory Animals*, Committee for the Update of the Care and Use of Laboratory Animals, Washington, DC, USA, 2001, http://grants.nih.gov/grants/olaw/guide-for-the-care-and-use-of-laboratory-animals.pdf.

[13] D. C. Ashok, N. P. Shrimant, M. G. Pradeep, and U. A. Akalpita, "Optimization of Alloxan dose is essential to induce stable diabetes for prolonged period," *Asian Journal of Biochemistry*, vol. 2, no. 6, pp. 402–408, 2007.

[14] J. Babara and B. Imelda, "Basic haematological techniques," in *Practical Hematology*, S. M. Lewis, B. J. Bain, and I. Bates, Eds., pp. 139–140, Edinburgh ChurchHill LivingStone, Edinburgh, UK, 2004.

[15] R. Ankur and A. Shahjad, "Alloxan induced diabetes: mechanisms and effects," *International Journal of Research in Pharmaceutical and Biomedical Sciences*, vol. 3, pp. 819–823, 2012.

[16] T. Szkudelski, "The mechanism of alloxan and streptozotocin action in B cells of the rat pancreas," *Physiological Research*, vol. 50, no. 6, pp. 537–546, 2001.

[17] M. Misra and U. Aiman, "Alloxan: an unpredictable drug for diabetes induction," *Indian Journal of Pharmacology*, vol. 44, no. 4, pp. 538–539, 2012.

[18] D. K. Jain and R. K. Arya, "Anomalies in alloxan-induced diabetic model: it is better to standardize it first," *Indian Journal of Pharmacology*, vol. 43, article 91, 2011.

[19] I. J. Pincus, J. J. Hurwitz, and M. E. Scott, "Effect of rate of injection of alloxan on development of diabetes in," *Proceedings of the Society for Experimental Biology and Medicine.*, vol. 86, no. 3, pp. 553–554, 1954.

[20] C. C. Rerup, "Drugs producing diabetes through damage of the insulin secreting cells," *Pharmacological Reviews*, vol. 22, no. 4, pp. 485–518, 1970.

[21] A. W. Harman and L. J. Fischer, "Alloxan toxicity in isolated rat hepatocytes and protection by sugars," *Biochemical Pharmacology*, vol. 31, no. 23, pp. 3731–3736, 1982.

[22] K. B. Pandey and S. I. Rizvi, "Biomarkers of oxidative stress in red blood cells," *Biomedical Papers of the Medical Faculty of the University Palacký, Olomouc, Czech Republic*, vol. 155, no. 2, pp. 131–136, 2011.

[23] J. Carroll, M. Raththagala, W. Subasinghe et al., "An altered oxidant defense system in red blood cells affects their ability to release nitric oxide-stimulating ATP," *Molecular BioSystems*, vol. 2, no. 6, pp. 305–311, 2006.

[24] N. Mohandas and P. G. Gallagher, "Red cell membrane: past, present, and future," *Blood*, vol. 112, no. 10, pp. 3939–3948, 2008.

[25] E. Evans, N. Mohandas, and A. Leung, "Static and dynamic rigidities of normal and sickle erythrocytes. Major influence of cell hemoglobin concentration," *The Journal of Clinical Investigation*, vol. 73, no. 2, pp. 477–488, 1984.

[26] G. S. Redding, D. M. Record, and B. U. Raess, "Calcium-stressed erythrocyte membrane structure and function for assessing glipizide effects on transglutaminase activation," *Proceedings of the Society for Experimental Biology and Medicine*, vol. 196, no. 1, pp. 76–82, 1991.

[27] J. P. Fruehauf and F. L. Meyskens Jr., "Reactive oxygen species: a breath of life or death?" *Clinical Cancer Research*, vol. 13, no. 3, pp. 789–794, 2007.

[28] M. F. McMullin, "The molecular basis of disorders of red cell enzymes," *Journal of Clinical Pathology*, vol. 52, no. 4, pp. 241–244, 1999.

[29] M. Maurizio, A. Luciano, and M. Walter, "The microenvironment can shift erythrocytes from a friendly to a harmful behavior: pathogenetic implications for vascular diseases," *Cardiores*, vol. 75, no. 1, pp. 21–28, 2007.

[30] S. Tiwari and J. F. Ndisang, "The heme oxygenase system and type-1 diabetes," *Current Pharmaceutical Design*, vol. 20, no. 9, pp. 1328–1337, 2014.

[31] P. Xia, T. Inoguchi, T. S. Kern, R. L. Engerman, P. J. Oates, and G. L. King, "Characterization of the mechanism for the chronic activation of diacylglycerol-protein kinase C pathway in diabetes and hypergalactosemia," *Diabetes*, vol. 43, no. 9, pp. 1122–1129, 1994.

[32] E. P. Feener, P. Xia, T. Inoguchi, T. Shiba, M. Kunisaki, and G. L. King, "Role of protein kinase C in glucose- and angiotensin II-induced plasminogen activator inhibitor expression," *Contributions to Nephrology*, vol. 118, pp. 180–187, 1996.

[33] A. Y. W. Lee and S. S. M. Chung, "Contributions of polyol pathway to oxidative stress in diabetic cataract," *The FASEB Journal*, vol. 13, no. 1, pp. 23–30, 1999.

[34] A. Goldin, J. A. Beckman, A. M. Schmidt, and M. A. Creager, "Advanced glycation end products: sparking the development of diabetic vascular injury," *Circulation*, vol. 114, no. 6, pp. 597–605, 2006.

[35] M. Brownlee, "The pathobiology of diabetic complications: a unifying mechanism," *Diabetes*, vol. 54, no. 6, pp. 1615–1625, 2005.

[36] J. G. Mohanty, E. Nagababu, and J. M. Rifkind, "Red blood cell oxidative stress impairs oxygen delivery and induces red blood cell aging," *Frontiers in Physiology*, vol. 5, article 84, 2014.

[37] M. Bryszewska, I. B. Zavodnik, A. Niekurzak, and K. Szosland, "Oxidative processes in red blood cells from normal and diabetic individuals," *Biochemistry and Molecular Biology International*, vol. 37, no. 2, pp. 345–354, 1995.

[38] B. Halliwell and J. M. C. Gutteridge, "Cellular responses to oxidative stress: adaptation, damage, repair, senescence and death," in *Free Radicals in Biology and Medicine*, pp. 187–267, Oxford University Press, New York, NY, USA, 4th edition, 2007.

[39] I. Maridonneau, P. Barquet, and R. P. Garay, "Na$^+$/K$^+$ transport damage induced by oxygen free radicals in human red cell membranes," *The Journal of Biological Chemistry*, vol. 258, pp. 3107–3117, 1983.

[40] K. B. Pandey and S. I. Rizvi, "Protective effect of resveratrol on markers of oxidative stress in human erythrocytes subjected to in vitro oxidative insult," *Phytotherapy Research*, vol. 24, no. 1, pp. S11–S14, 2010.

[41] K. B. Pandey and S. I. Rizvi, "Protective effect of resveratrol on formation of membrane protein carbonyls and lipid peroxidation in erythrocytes subjected to oxidative stress," *Applied Physiology, Nutrition and Metabolism*, vol. 34, no. 6, pp. 1093–1097, 2009.

[42] M. Goodarzi, A. A. Moosavi-Movahedi, M. Habibi-Rezaei et al., "Hemoglobin fructation promotes heme degradation through the generation of endogenous reactive oxygen species," *Spectrochimica Acta Part A: Molecular and Biomolecular Spectroscopy*, vol. 130, pp. 561–567, 2014.

[43] M. Samaja, A. Rubinacci, R. Motterlini, A. De Ponti, and N. Portinaro, "Red cell aging and active calcium transport," *Experimental Gerontology*, vol. 25, no. 3-4, pp. 279–286, 1990.

[44] C. R. Kiefer and L. M. Snyder, "Oxidation and erythrocyte senescence," *Current Opinion in Hematology*, vol. 7, no. 2, pp. 113–116, 2000.

[45] P. A. Ney, M. M. Christopher, and R. P. Hebbel, "Synergistic effects of oxidation and deformation on erythrocyte monovalent cation leak," *Blood*, vol. 75, no. 5, pp. 1192–1198, 1990.

[46] A. V. Hoffbrand, S. M. Lewis, and E. G. D. Tuddenham, *Postgraduate Haematology*, Arnold Medical Books, London, UK, 4th edition, 2001.

[47] N. Bersch, J. E. Groopman, and D. W. Golde, "Natural and biosynthetic insulin stimulates the growth of human erythroid progenitors in vitro," *Journal of Clinical Endocrinology and Metabolism*, vol. 55, no. 6, pp. 1209–1211, 1982.

[48] E. Ritz and V. Haxsen, "Diabetic nephropathy and anaemia," *European Journal of Clinical Investigation, Supplement*, vol. 35, no. 3, pp. 66–74, 2005.

25

Sickle-Cell Disease Healthcare Cost in Africa: Experience of the Congo

L. O. Ngolet,[1] **M. Moyen Engoba,**[2] **Innocent Kocko,**[1] **Alexis Elira Dokekias,**[1] **Jean-Vivien Mombouli,**[3] **and Georges Marius Moyen**[1]

[1]*Clinical Hematology Unit, Brazzaville Teaching Hospital, Auxence Ickonga Avenue, P.O. Box 32, Brazzaville, Congo*
[2]*Pediatric Intensive Care Unit, Brazzaville Teaching Hospital, Brazzaville, Congo*
[3]*National Laboratory of Public Health, Brazzaville Teaching Hospital, Brazzaville, Congo*

Correspondence should be addressed to L. O. Ngolet; lngolet@yahoo.fr

Academic Editor: Duran Canatan

Background. Lack of medical coverage in Africa leads to inappropriate care that has an impact on the mortality rate. In this study, we aimed to evaluate the cost of severe acute sickle-cell related complications in Brazzaville. *Methods.* A retrospective study was conducted in 2014 in the Paediatric Intensive Care Unit. It concerned 94 homozygote sickle-cell children that developed severe acute sickle-cell disease related complications (average age 69 months). For each patient, we calculated the cost of care complication. *Results.* The household income was estimated as low (<XAF 90,000/<USD 158.40) in 27.7%. The overall median cost for hospitalization for sickle-cell related acute complications was XAF 65,460/USD 115.21. Costs were fluctuating depending on the generating factors of the severe acute complications ($p = 0.041$). They were higher in case of complications generated by bacterial infections (ranging from XAF 66,765/USD 117.50 to XAF 135,271.50/USD 238.07) and lower in case of complications associated with malaria (ranging from XAF 28,305/49.82 to XAF 64,891.63/USD 114.21). The mortality rate was 17% and was associated with the cost of the case management ($p = 0.006$). *Conclusion.* The case management cost of severe acute complications of sickle-cell disease in children is high in Congo.

1. Introduction

Sickle-cell disease is the most frequent haemoglobin disorder in the world, mostly in sub-Saharan Africa where 75% of the 300,000 babies are born each year with haemoglobin disorders live [1, 2]. Homozygous form of SCD is associated with very high child mortality, but reliable data are lacking. WHO estimates that 70% of deaths are avoidable by putting in place "preventive" measures [3]. These measures encompass early diagnosis, information, education, and prophylaxis of infections [4–6]. In sub-Saharan Africa, medical coverage program like Medicaid that supports patients in the expenses generated by medical management of their disease does not exist or is very insufficient. In Congo where 1% of the population is affected by the homozygous form of the disease,

such program does not exist [7]. The nonaccessibility to care and medicines is linked in 54.61% to financial challenges [8]. This inaccessibility is higher at the tertiary level of medical facilities such as the teaching hospital where the costs of care are far higher. The consequence of this is the arrival of patients at an advanced stage of the disease. Overall, in Africa and in Congo, contrary to the Western countries, morbidity and mortality are associated with the costs of sickle-cell disease (SCD) care. Although hospitalization appears to drive the majority of SCD treatment cost [9–11], only one study published in Africa has examined the hospitalization cost of SCD [12]. That small study was conducted on adult in the Hematology Unit in Congo in 2012. None studies report the cost of care for SCD children inpatient hospitalization. The purpose of this study is to report the cost of severe acute complications of SCD related care for pediatric inpatients hospitalization in the Emergency Department of the Brazzaville Teaching Hospital in Congo.

2. Material and Methods

Brazzaville Teaching Hospital has a total of 4 pediatric departments: Intensive Care, Neonatology, Infant Care, and Toddler/Teenager care where a total of 5,657 children were admitted during the period of our study. This study was conducted from January 1 to December 31, 2014, in the Pediatric Intensive Care Unit (PICU) of Brazzaville Teaching Hospital. PICU manages all medical emergencies that involve immediate vital prognostic of children aged 1 month to 16 years old.

2.1. Data Collection and Assessment Procedures. We enrolled in the study all pediatric patients that were developing severe acute SCD related complications. SCD children with no severe SCD related complications were not included in the study. We defined as severe acute complications all life threatening sickle-cell disease related acute complications. These are

(1) acute exacerbation of anemia due to acute splenic sequestration or acute hyperhemolysis;

(2) major acute pain syndromes;

(3) acute chest syndrome;

(4) stroke;

(5) mixed severe acute crisis that combines acute exacerbation of anemia and major pain syndromes;

(6) severe infection: in the context of functional asplenia, a temperature over 38, 5°C with or without a source is an emergency and considered as severe infection.

Generated Factors. Generated factors are factors that trigger acute exacerbation anemia, pain syndromes, acute chest syndrome, stroke, and mixed crisis. These factors are infectious or physical such as environmental heat, stress, wearing heat retaining clothing, and dehydration.

Thus, 94 sickle-cell disease children presenting one severe acute complication have been included in the study.

2.2. Cost Assessment of the Case Management of Severe Acute Complications. Costs generated correspond to the fees encountered for the diagnosis and treatment of acute complications and generating factors. The global cost was calculated by adding costs of medicines, hospitalization and diagnosis tests.

Hospitalization fees depend on the length of admission of the patient. Patients are charged XAF 25,000/USD 42.64 for the total of 5 days (first five days at the hospital) and then XAF 5,000/USD 11.72 for each day from the 6th day of hospitalization. Costs of medicines and diagnostic tests have been calculated from the fares displayed by the teaching hospital. The consumables, dressing, syringes, and infusion sets as well as the hospitalization or physician visits fees before the patient's admission to the PICU, were not included.

Income of the family was interpreted based on the official lowest salary fixed by the government (XAF 90,000/USD 153.53). The income was low when it was lower than XAF 90,000/USD 153.53, middle when it was between XAF 90,000/USD 153.53 and XAF 500,000/USD 852.96, and high when it was above USD XAF 500,000/USD 852.96.

The data were computed on Microsoft Excel 2013 and processed and analyzed with the software STATA (version 12, Texas, USA). For the description of each quantitative variable, the mean/average value, median, and standard deviation were calculated. For the comparison of qualitative data, the ANOVA and Student tests were used. The tests were significantly significant when p value <0.05. The different costs have been calculated in XAF and then converted into USD using the exchange rate of USD 1 = XAF 568.19.

3. Results

3.1. Characteristics of the Population. 1278 children were admitted in PICU during our study. Among them, 136 (10.64%) had sickle-cell disease and 94 (69.11%) had developed severe acute complications. These were 48 boys (51.1%) and 46 girls (48.9%) making a sex ratio of 1.04. the patients were aged from 6 to 192 months with an average age of 69 ± 50 months. Fifty-eight patients (61.7%) were coming to the hospital from their homes whereas 24 children (25.5%) were referred by primary and secondary health facilities. Twelve children (12.8%) were from other teaching hospital departments. It had been possible to determine the income of 50 families (53.2%). Among them, 26 (52%) had low status income while 18 (36%) had middle and 6 (12%) had high one (Table 1).

3.2. Costs of Hospital Expenses. The average length of hospitalization has been 5.5 days (extremes of 1 and 16 days) generating a median cost of XAF 30,000/USD 52.79 (range XAF 25,000/USD 42.64 and XAF 80,000/USD 136.47). Sixteen children (17%) died during their hospitalization. The mortality rate was significantly higher in the age group older than 120 months with no influence of referral origin of the patient ($p = 0.004$).

The median global cost care of SCD related acute complications was XAF 65.460/USD 111.67 (range XAF 28,305/USD 49.81 and XAF 365,740/USD 643.69). Diagnostic tests, hospitalizations, and medicines represented, respectively, 16%, 38%, and 49% of the global cost (Table 2).

Bacterial infections were the most frequent acute complication associated with SCD related crisis with 50 cases (53.2%). Care of bacterial infections whatever the type of sickle-cell crisis they were triggering was the most expensive since the quotation for their care was the highest (range: XAF 62,800/USD 107.13 and XAF 135271.5/USD 230.76), followed by malaria (range: XAF 28.305/USD 48.28 and XAF 99,944/USD 170.49). Vascular complications were represented by acute chest syndrome and stroke with respective costs care of XAF 42,800/USD 73.01 and XAF 103,492/USD 176.55 ($p = 0.041$) Table 3.

TABLE 1: Characteristics of the population.

Gender	n (%)
Female	46 (48.9)
Male	48 (51.1)
Sex ratio	1.04
Age (months)	
Mean ± Ecart type	69.26 ± 50.40
Min–max	6–192
Referred by	n (%)
Teaching hospital's departments	12 (12.8)
Primary and secondary public offices	14 (14.9)
Private offices	10 (10.6)
Home	58 (61.7)
Hospitalization length (days)	n (%)
1-2	44 (46.8)
3–8	34 (36.2)
9–16	16 (17)
Income	n (%)
Low	26 (27.7)
Middle	6 (6.4)
High	18 (19.1)
Unknown	44 (46.8)
Death	n (%)
Yes	78 (83.0)
No	16 (17.0)
Age of death*	n (%)
0–24	1 (12.5)
25–60	0 (00)
61–120	6 (37.5)
>120	8 (50)

*$p = 0.004$.

4. Discussion

This first study has allowed estimating the cost of care of severe acute complications SCD related in pediatric population admitted in intensive care. The global cost borne by families is high since it is on average XAF 65,460/USD 111.67 per episode, representing 2/3 of the minimum wage salary in Congo officially set at XAF 90,000/USD 153.53. Our study has several limits. First, the analysis of these results does not take into account the fees generated by consumables (syringes, infusion sets, and dressings). They are also to be paid by the patient, as well as fees for preadmission physician visit or hospitalization in different hospitals or units that concerned 38.3% of our sample population. The second limitation is the care costs estimations. Estimated costs were calculated from the teaching hospital costing that has the lowest fees. Nevertheless, fees displayed by the teaching hospital do not allow a real cost recovery, limiting a sustainable procurement in reagents but also in medicines. Referring to a WHO study, availability of medicines is limited. Only 60% of essential medicines are available in public pharmacies [8]. These parameters, which are difficult to evaluate since many medicines and tests are bought and used out of the teaching hospital, could contribute to underestimating the real care cost of SCD related acute complications. A similar study conducted on adults in the clinical hematology department reported a comparable average global cost care: XAF 88,365/USD 155.520 [12]. Nevertheless, some reservation must be expressed in comparing these costs, since the hospitalization fees in the clinical hematology department are fixed at XAF 10,000/USD 17.05 no matter the length of hospitalization. Consequently, the fees for hospitalization represented only 8.8% of the global expense in that study compared to 38% in ours [12].

Bacterial infections are the first cause of admission of sickle-cell disease children and adults in Africa [13–16]. The cost of care for their management is higher whatever the type of associated severe acute complications (XAF 66,765/USD 113.89 to XAF 135,271/USD 230.78). This is the consequence of the high cost of antibiotics in the continent [8, 17, 18]. Despite an ambitious essential medicines policy (with antibiotics in priority position) in Congo that aims to reduce the cost of medicines, these medicines remain inaccessible for the majority of the population [8]. Additionally, only 57% of antibiotics are prescribed by their international nonpropriety name (INN) [9]. This trend seems similar in sub-Saharan Africa as a study in private pharmacies in Mali showed that only 48.2% of antibiotics were prescribed in INN [18]. Also, procurement challenges at the hospital pharmacy, limited availability of essential medicines, and presence of fake antibiotics on the market are some elements pushing for prescription and purchase of branded medicines. Besides, microbiologic proof of infections barely provided by our laboratories is responsible of an overprescription of antibiotics and then an over cost care. Lastly, the absence of standard therapeutic chart has a perceptible impact on the cost of the prescription by irrational use of antibiotics.

Malaria represented the second cause of admission of sickle-cell disease children with a total of 29.8%. Malaria is widely considered a major cause of illness and death in SCD patients [14, 19, 20]. Even though we find in our study strong association between hyperhemolysis crisis and malaria, the association of this comorbidity is controversial. Some investigators have associated it with the anemic hyperhemolysis crisis while others suggest that patients living with SCD are protected from malaria [21, 22]. Despite the fact that the National Programme on Malaria has chosen the combination of artesunate and amodiaquine as first-line treatment, quinine is still used in first intention in almost 85% of health facilities [9].

The additional costs of the prescription in our study come from the purchase of pain killers and labile blood products. Blood transfusion is a major therapeutic element in the treatment of sickle-cell disease crisis since it is performed on 47% of sickle-cell disease children [14]. The supply cost for a bag of erythrocyte concentrate is XAF 7,500/USD 12.79, whereas the effective expenses for its preparation are estimated at XAF 65,000/USD 110.88. This causes supply challenges as mentioned earlier.

TABLE 2: Acute severe sickle-cell complications global treatment cost in XAF (USD).

	Hospitalization cost	Diagnosis test cost	Medicines cost	Global cost care
Mean	33,085.1 (58.23)	12,068.18 (21.23)	53,647.67 (94.41)	93,889.21 (165.24)
Ecart type	16,535.4 (29.1)	10,493.76 (18.46)	59,461.21 (104.65)	78,622.47 (138.37)
Median	30,000 (52.79)	10,500 (18.47)	32,267.5 (56.79)	65,460 (111.67)
Min–max	25,000–80,000 (42.64–136.47)	0–48,000 (0–84.47)	3,305–272,740 (5.81–480.02)	28,305–365,740 (49.81–643.69)

$t = 2028$, $p = 0.026$.

TABLE 3: Severe acute sickle-cell complications and its generated factors treatment cost.

Diagnostic	n	%	Global management care XAF (USD)	p value
Major acute pain + bacterial infections	12	12.8	66,765 (117.50)	
Hyperhemolysis + bacterial infections	18	19.2	103,492 (182.14)	$p = 0.041$
Mixed severe acute crisis + bacterial infections	28	29.8	135,271 (238.07)	
Major acute pain + malaria	4	4.2	28,305 (49.82)	
Hyperhemolysis + malaria	16	17,1	64,891.63 (114.21)	
Mixed severe acute crisis + malaria	8	8.5	99,944 (175.90)	
Major acute pain + acute chest syndrome	2	2.1	42,800 (75.33)	
Hyperhemolysis + acute chest syndrome	2	2.1	62,800 (110.52)	
Mixed severe acute crisis + stroke	4	4.2	130,333 (229.38)	
Total	94	100		

5. Conclusion

This study has examined the cost of severe acute SCD related complications in intensive care. Severe acute SCD related complications remain worrisome not only due to their graveness, but mainly due to the expenses that families must bear for their care. This study is the first to examine the cost of all components of care for pediatrics population with SCD admitted in intensive care. It is an important input to SCD treatment strategies, health care planning, and research prioritization. This study has also shown that infections and malaria remain persistently high. Additional research is needed to better understand infectious pattern of children with SCD.

Conflict of Interests

The authors declare that there is no conflict of interests regarding the publication of this paper.

Acknowledgment

The authors are grateful to Dr. Lapnet Mustapha to his assistance in the translation.

References

[1] World Health Organisation, *Management of Birth Defects and Hemoglobin Disorders: Report of a Joint Who-March of Dimes Meeting*, World Health Organization, Geneva, Switzerland, 2006.

[2] B. Modell and M. Darlison, "Global epidemiology of haemoglobin disorders and derived service indicators," *Bulletin of the World Health Organization*, vol. 86, no. 6, pp. 480–487, 2008.

[3] D. C. Rees, T. N. Williams, and M. T. Gladwin, "Sickle-cell disease," *The Lancet*, vol. 376, no. 9757, pp. 2018–2031, 2010.

[4] T. N. William and S. K. Obaro, "Sickle cell disease and malaria morbidity: a tale with two tails," *Trends in Parasitology*, vol. 27, no. 7, pp. 315–320, 2011.

[5] A. B. John, A. Ramlal, H. Jackson, G. H. Maude, A. W. Sharma, and G. R. Serjeant, "Prevention of pneumococcal infection in children with homozygous sickle cell disease," *British Medical Journal*, vol. 288, no. 6430, pp. 1567–1570, 1984.

[6] M. H. Gaston, J. I. Verter, G. Woods et al. et al., "Prophylaxis with oral penicillin in children with sickle cell anemia," *The New England Journal of Medicine*, vol. 314, no. 25, pp. 1593–1599, 1986.

[7] A. B. Mpemba Loufoua, P. Makoumbou, J. R. Mabiala Babela et al., "Dépistage néonatal de la drépanocytose au Congo Brazzaville," *Annales de l'Université Marien Ngouabi*, vol. 11, no. 5, pp. 21–25, 2010.

[8] *Rapport: Evaluation du Secteur Pharmaceutique du Congo*, OMS, Juillet, 2006.

[9] S. Lanzkron, C. Haywood Jr., J. B. Segal, and G. J. Dover, "Hospitalization rates and costs of care of patients with sickle-cell anemia in the state of Maryland in the era of hydroxyurea," *American Journal of Hematology*, vol. 81, no. 12, pp. 927–932, 2006.

[10] H. Davis, R. M. Moore Jr., and P. J. Gergen, "Cost of hospitalizations associated with sickle cell disease in the United States," *Public Health Reports*, vol. 112, no. 1, pp. 40–43, 1997.

[11] R. D. Moor, S. Charache, M. L. Terrin et al., "The costs of children with sickle cell anemia. Preparing for managed care,"

Journal of Pediatric Hematology/Oncology, vol. 20, no. 6, pp. 528–533, 1998.

[12] L. O. Ngolet, H. Ntsiba, and A. Elira Dokekias, "Le coût de la prise en charge hospitalière des crises drépanocytaires," *Annales de l'Université Marien Ngouabi*, vol. 14, no. 5, pp. 14–19, 2013.

[13] E. Barett-Connor, "Bacterial infection and sickle cell anemia," *Medicine*, vol. 50, pp. 94–112, 1971.

[14] J. R. Mabiala-Babela, T. Nkanza-Kaluwako, P. S. Ganga-Zandzou, S. Nzingoula, and P. Senga, "Causes d'hospitalisation des enfants drépanocytaires : influence de l'âge (C.H.U. de Brazzaville, Congo)," *Bulletin de la Société de Pathologie Exotique*, vol. 98, no. 5, pp. 392–393, 2005.

[15] G. R. Serjeant, "Mortality from sickle cell disease in Africa," *British Medical Journal*, vol. 330, no. 7489, pp. 432–433, 2005.

[16] S. D. Grosse, I. Odame, H. K. Atrash, D. D. Amendah, F. B. Piel, and T. N. Williams, "Sickle cell disease in Africa. A neglected cause of early childhood mortality," *American Journal of Preventive Medicine*, vol. 41, no. 6, supplement 4, pp. S398–S405, 2011.

[17] Y. Coulibaly, A. Konate, D. Done, and F. Bougoudogo, "Étude de la prescription des antibiotiques en milieu hospitalier malien," *Revue Malienne D'infectiologie et de Microbiologie*, vol. 3, pp. 2–8, 2014.

[18] IFMT, "Antibiotiques dans les pays en développement," MS.IFMT//M05, 2004.

[19] D. Diallo and G. Tchernia, "Sickle cell disease in Africa," *Current Opinion in Hematology*, vol. 9, no. 2, pp. 111–116, 2002.

[20] A. Elira Dokekias, "Etude analytique des facteurs d'aggravation de la maladie drépanocytaire au Congo," *Médecine d'Afrique Noire Électronique*, vol. 43, no. 5, pp. 279–285, 1996.

[21] I. Diagne, G. M. Soares, A. Gueye et al., "Infections in Senegalese children and adolescent with sickle cell anemia presenting with severe anaemia in a malarious area," *Tropical Doctor*, vol. 45, no. 1, pp. 55–58, 2000.

[22] A. I. Juwah, A. Nlemadim, and W. Kaine, "Clinical presentation of severe anemia in pediatric patients with sickle cell anemia seen in Enugu, Nigeria," *American Journal of Hematology*, vol. 72, no. 3, pp. 185–191, 2003.

26

Management of Sickle Cell Disease: A Review for Physician Education in Nigeria (Sub-Saharan Africa)

Ademola Samson Adewoyin

Department of Haematology and Blood Transfusion, University of Benin Teaching Hospital, PMB 1111, Benin City, Edo State, Nigeria

Correspondence should be addressed to Ademola Samson Adewoyin; drademola@yahoo.com

Academic Editor: Maria Stella Figueiredo

Sickle cell disease (SCD) predominates in sub-Saharan Africa, East Mediterranean areas, Middle East, and India. Nigeria, being the most populous black nation in the world, bears its greatest burden in sub-Saharan Africa. The last few decades have witnessed remarkable scientific progress in the understanding of the complex pathophysiology of the disease. Improved clinical insights have heralded development and establishment of disease modifying interventions such as chronic blood transfusions, hydroxyurea therapy, and haemopoietic stem cell transplantation. Coupled with parallel improvements in general supportive, symptomatic, and preventive measures, current evidence reveals remarkable appreciation in quality of life among affected individuals in developed nations. Currently, in Nigeria and other West African states, treatment and control of SCD are largely suboptimal. Improved knowledge regarding SCD phenotypes and its comprehensive care among Nigerian physicians will enhance quality of care for affected persons. This paper therefore provides a review on the aetiopathogenesis, clinical manifestations, and management of SCD in Nigeria, with a focus on its local patterns and peculiarities. Established treatment guidelines as appropriate in the Nigerian setting are proffered, as well as recommendations for improving care of affected persons.

1. Introduction

Sickle cell disease (SCD) is one of the most common genetic diseases worldwide and its highest prevalence occurs in Middle East, Mediterranean regions, Southeast Asia, and sub-Saharan Africa especially Nigeria [1, 2].

SCD is a chronic haemolytic disorder that is marked by tendency of haemoglobin molecules within red cells to polymerise and deform the red cell into a sickle (or crescent) shape resulting in characteristic vasoocclusive events and accelerated haemolysis. It is inherited in an autosomal recessive fashion either in the homozygous state or double heterozygous state. When inherited in the homozygous state, it is termed sickle cell anaemia (SCA). Other known SCD genotypes include haemoglobin SC disease, sickle beta plus thalassaemia, and sickle beta zero thalassemia (which has similar severity with sickle cell anaemia), haemoglobin SD Punjab disease, haemoglobin SO Arab disease, and others.

In Nigeria, SCD forms a small part of the clinical practice of most general duty doctors, as there is gross absence of dedicated sickle cell centres. Thus, it may be difficult to keep abreast of current knowledge and practices in the treatment of SCD. The purpose of this paper therefore is to provide a comprehensive and concise review of SCD and its management for physician education in Nigeria. Particular attention is given to its local epidemiology, clinical phenotypes and complications, current treatment guidelines, practice challenges, and recommendations for improved care. Relevant literatures and local references including clinical studies, reviews, and texts were gathered, summarized, and presented in this paper.

2. Epidemiology

About 5–7% of the global population carries an abnormal haemoglobin gene [3, 4]. The most predominant form of haemoglobinopathy worldwide is sickle cell disease. The greatest burden of the disease lies in sub-Saharan Africa and Asia [5].

The prevalence of sickle cell trait ranges between 10 and 45% in various parts of sub-Saharan Africa [6–8]. In Nigeria, carrier prevalence is about 20 to 30% [9, 10]. SCD affects about 2 to 3% of the Nigerian population of more than 160 million [9]. Recent estimate from a large retrospective study by Nwogoh et al. in Benin City, South-South Nigeria revealed an SCD prevalence of 2.39% and a carrier rate of about 23% [11].

3. Brief History and Genetic Origin of SCD

In 1874, Dr. Horton, a Sierra Leonian medical Doctor, reportedly gave the first description of clinical symptoms and signs which is now referred to as sickle cell disease [12]. Herrick, a Chicago physician, also gave a formal description of the disease in 1910 when he observed abnormal sickle shaped red cells in the blood of a dental student from West Indies who had anaemia [13]. In 1927, Hahn and Gillespie observed that sickling of red cells was associated with conditions of low oxygen tension. In 1949, Linus Pauling and colleagues demonstrated that haemoglobin in these patients was different from normal subjects using protein electrophoresis [14]. However, Venon Ingram and J. A. Hunt in 1956 sequenced the sickle haemoglobin molecule and showed that the abnormality was due to valine substitution for glutamate on the 6th position of the sickle beta-haemoglobin gene. Marotta and coworkers in 1977 showed that the corresponding change in codon 6 of the beta-globin gene was GAG to GTG [14]. Since then, further insights have been gained into understanding the origin, complex pathophysiology, and treatment of the disease through molecular biology techniques.

Africa and Asia are considered as the birthplace of the sickle cell mutation. Sickle cell disease is believed to be a consequence of natural mutation of the beta-globin gene (HBB) affecting the gametes and transferred to subsequent generations. Using restriction fragment length polymorphism analysis, four main African haplotypes and one Asian haplotype of the beta-globin chain genes have been characterized and are believed to originate differently in these regions. The main African haplotypes include Senegal, Benin, Bantu (central-African republic), and Cameroon haplotype [15–18]. The Bantu haplotype is associated with the most severe disease phenotype while the Asian (also called Arab-Indian) haplotype is associated with a mild phenotype [19].

SCD is found in other parts of the world including USA and Europe due to migration and interracial marriages [5, 20]. The high prevalence of SCD in sub-Saharan Africa has been attributed to survival advantage conferred by the sickle cell trait against *Plasmodium falciparum*. Resistance of individuals with sickle cell trait to *Plasmodium falciparum* creates a selective pressure that has maintained the sickle cell gene within human populations in malaria endemic regions like sub-Saharan Africa. This phenomenon is termed balanced polymorphism [21, 22].

4. Aetiopathogenesis of Sickle Cell Disease

SCD is a qualitative haemoglobinopathy resulting from a structural change in the sequence of amino acids on the beta globin chain of the haemoglobin molecule due to a point mutation. The sickling mutation causes a single base change from adenine to thymine on the 17th nucleotide of the beta globin chain gene (HBB). This invariably translates into substitution of valine for glutamate on the 6th amino acid of the beta globin chain. The abnormal biochemistry of this mutant haemoglobin induces polymerization of Hb S molecules within the red cells, so called sickling. On the sickle haemoglobin, the glutamate protein molecule, which is hydrophilic, polar, and negatively charged, is replaced by a less polar, hydrophobic, neutral amino acid, valine. Under deoxy conditions, the abnormal valine residue causes intraerythrocytic hydrophobic interaction of sickle haemoglobin tetramers, leading to their precipitation and polymer formation, so called gelation [23]. Eventually, all cytosolic haemoglobin molecules precipitate into seven (one inner and six outer) double strands with cross-links which are called tactoids. Upon reoxygenation, unsickling occurs and the red cell assumes its normal shape. However, repeated sickling and unsickling of the red cell damages the red cell membrane, due to herniation of sickle haemoglobin polymers through the cytoskeleton, thus rendering the red cell permanently sickled. These appear as irreversibly sickled cells (ISCs) on peripheral blood cytology.

The kinetics of red cell sickling is highly heterogenous. Several variables are known to affect the rate and degree of sickling of the red cells. Intracellular dehydration of sickle red cells increases mean cell haemoglobin concentration (MCHC) [14]. Higher MCHC favours sickling. As such, very high Hb S level of about 80 to 90% seen in the homozygous disease is associated with a worse disease while the presence of alpha thalassemia (one or two gene deletions) ameliorates the disease. Another variable is the presence of other interacting nonsickle haemoglobin. Of note is fetal haemoglobin (Hb F). Higher proportion of Hb F is associated with mild disease. When present, high levels of Hb F are uniformly dispersed within the red cell and it retards the sickling process. Thus, coinheritance of sickle haemoglobin with hereditary persistence of fetal haemoglobin (HPFH) is associated with mild disease [24]. Similarly, this advantage is positively utilized through clinical use of fetal haemoglobin inducing drug such as hydroxyurea. Vascular beds that have intrinsically sluggish venous outflow such as bone marrow, spleen, or inflamed tissues are at higher risk of infarctive events due to prolonged microvascular transit time [25]. Whenever and wherever microvascular transit time becomes longer than sickling delay time, sickling and vascular occlusion become imminent. Intracellular pH is another important variable. With acidosis, the haemoglobin molecules give off their oxygen more readily and sickling occurs more readily.

Repeated sickling of the red cell induces cellular injury which has been shown to activate membrane ion channels such as the Gardos pathway (calcium gated potassium channels) and KCL cotransporter [25]. There are influx of calcium ions and efflux of potassium and water, hence intracellular dehydration. High intracellular calcium levels provoke activity of proteolytic enzymes such as phospholipases and proteases causing the digestion of membrane phospholipids and proteins, respectively. Subsequently, there is perturbation of the membrane lipids with exteriorization of lipids such as phosphatidyl serine and ethanolamine which are normally located in the inner leaflets of the membrane lipid bilayer [26].

The diverse clinical heterogeneity of SCD is related to two main pathogenetic processes: chronic haemolysis and high viscosity/vascular occlusion. Infarctive events in SCD result from erythrostasis caused by rigid sickled cells in various vascular beds especially organs with sluggish blood flow such as the spleen and the bone marrow. Capillaries are about 2-3 microns in diameter. Sickle cells due to loss of flexibility are unable to transit the microvasculature, hence vessel occlusion. Aside from these mechanistic processes, sickle cells are also shown to exhibit increased adhesiveness to vascular endothelium, leucocytes, platelets, and themselves [27–29]. Sickle reticulocytes are even more adhesive to the endothelium than sickle discocytes [30]. Molecular interactions between the red cells and the vascular endothelium include CD36 and thrombospondin, VLA4 and VCAM-1, respectively [30, 31]. Fibronectin and von Willebrand factor are also involved in these interactions. Currently, it is known that increased adhesiveness of different cellular surfaces with formation of heterocellular aggregates is believed to propagate the phenomenon of vascular occlusion, especially in the postcapillary venules [26]. Also note that destruction of red cell membrane causes exposure of membrane proteins, thereby inciting autoantibody formation. These antibodies such as IgG anti-band 3 antibodies are believed to promote erythrophagocytosis [25].

Episodic microvascular occlusion in sickle cell disease even in steady state results in ischaemic-reperfusion injury which sets the stage for an increased inflammatory tone, thus significant elevations in total leucocyte counts, platelet counts, and positive serum acute phase reactants. Even in steady state, SCD is a chronic inflammatory condition; the attendant inflammation induced oxidative stress further contributes to progressive tissue damage [32, 33]. The leucocytes in SCD also express higher levels of L-selectins and also have stimulated adhesiveness. Increased adhesiveness coupled with phosphatidyl serine exposure on the red cell surface makes SCD a procoagulant and a hypercoagulable state [34].

Erythrocyte lifespan in SCD averages about 16–20 days in contrast to about 100–120 days in normal state [35, 36]. Haemolysis in sickle cell disease is both extravascular and intravascular. Abnormal shape of the ISCs creates an abnormal rheology, associated with heightened clearance by the reticuloendothelial system. Because of their increased fragility and reduced deformability, some red cells undergo intravascular haemolysis. High plasma haemoglobin level is associated with low haptoglobin levels and high levels of lactate dehydrogenase (LDH), arginase-1, and AST [37]. Plasma haemoglobin is an avid scavenger of nitric oxide (NO). High plasma haemoglobin levels resulting from chronic haemolysis reduce NO bioavailability. Normally, NO relaxes the endothelium and maintains vascular tone (vasodilator) [37]. Low circulating levels of NO propagate vasospasm which is observed even in large vessels in SCD. Contributing to this is dysfunction of endothelial nitric oxide synthetase [37]. This is the underlying basis of vasculopathic complications such as

cerebrovascular diseases, priapism, pulmonary hypertension, and chronic leg ulcers. Arginase 1 is normally involved in formation of urea in protein excretion. Accelerated haemolysis of red cells leads to higher levels of arginase 1. As such, more ornithine is produced, further depleting plasma arginine levels. Excess ornithine is channeled to alternate pathways which produce excess prolenes and polyamines. These byproducts promote endothelial smooth muscle proliferations, further narrowing the vascular chamber [38]. Chronic haemolysis results in excess breakdown of haemoglobin molecules and high levels of bilirubin, which is associated with formation of bilirubin pigment stones in the gall bladder (cholelithiasis).

Some authorities have attempted to categorize SCD patients into two clinical subphenotypes based on the overriding pathogenic process [25, 39]. Clinically, there is some degree of overlap between the two groups. Some patients experience more of viscosity/vasoocclusive complications and tend to have higher baseline haematocrit levels. Others experience more of vasculopathic complications due to more intense haemolysis associated with a lower baseline haematocrit [14, 39].

5. Clinical Phenotypes and Complications in Sickle Cell Disease

There is marked intraindividual and interindividual variability in SCD. Clinical heterogeneity of the disease has been explained by both genetic and environmental factors. Known genetic factors contributing to variations in clinical severity of the disease include the pattern of sickle cell inheritance, nature of b-globin haplotype, Hb F level, and FCP loci [15]. Other modulators of the disease include presence of alpha thalassemia and other probable genetic influences as well as environmental factors such as access to optimal health care, ambient living conditions, and availability of finance [15].

Physical Effects of Sickle Cell Disease. Body habitus in SCD ranges from a normal build to a tall, lanky physique depending on the clinical severity. Other physical changes include prognathism, arachnodactyly, and increased AP chest diameter (barrel chest) [40, 41]. In childhood, sickle cell patients may be shorter or smaller than normal. Puberty is often delayed but considerable growth takes place in late adolescence such that adults with sickle cell anaemia are at least as tall as normal [14]. However, adults that have suffered vertebral infarction and collapse may be shorter than normal. Many of these physical changes are due to the chronic hypoxaemia associated with severe anaemia. Severe haemolysis in infancy causes marrow hyperplasia of the skull and facial bones, resulting in frontal bossing, prognathism, or malocclusion [42]. The abnormal facies results from extension of the marrow into the cortical bone causing widening of the diploe spaces and thinning of the bone cortex. The chronic haemolytic process is associated with pallor, jaundice, splenomegaly in early childhood.

5.1. Acute Sickle Syndromes/Complications

5.1.1. Bone Pain Crisis (BPC). BPC is the most consistent and characteristic feature of SCD [43]. The pain results from activation of nociceptive afferent nerve endings in the ischemic bones. Commonly affected bones include the long bones such as femur and humerus, vertebrae, pelvis, ribs, and sternum [24]. Multiple sites may be involved. An early manifestation of bone infarction is the hand and foot syndrome. This is characterized by dactylitis involving the small bones of the hand or foot, marked by diffuse swelling over the involved area. It often resolves spontaneously within one to two weeks and is rare after 2-3 years of life. Frequency of bone pain crisis is higher in patients with homozygous sickle cell disease, low Hb F, and higher baseline haemoglobin. It is said to be more common in young adults but its frequency tends to wane at older ages. Pain episodes vary in intensity and tend to resolve within a few days. In about 57% of cases, no precipitating factor is identified [44]. However, known precipitants include exposure to cold, dehydration, intercurrent infections such as malaria, physical exertion, tobacco smoke, alcohol use, hard drugs, high altitude, hypoxic conditions, physical pain, pregnancy, hot weather, emotional stress, or onset of menses [32, 45]. Suggested treatment guideline for uncomplicated BPC is presented as follows.

Treatment Guidelines for Bone Pain Crisis

(i) Principles of treatment include adequate analgesia, hydration, warmth, prophylactic or therapeutic antibiotics if pyrexial after necessary culture samples are taken, as well as oxygenation if hypoxic (Sp O_2 < 90%) [45–48].

(ii) Oral hydration must be adequate with at least 1.5 L/m^2 of water based fluid per day in children and 60–70 mL/kg in adults. If parenteral, not more than 1.5 times maintenance is given in order to prevent volume overload considering baseline anaemia in most patients [49, 50].

(iii) Patients and parents should be encouraged to keep a stock of simple analgesics at home in event of a painful episode. However, mild to moderate pain that does not succumb to home-based oral analgesia and hydration within 2 days requires hospitalization.

(iv) Analgesia should be commenced within 15 to 30 minutes of presentation in the emergency room or day hospital. Effective analgesia should be achieved within 1 hour. There should be an ongoing assessment of analgesic efficacy every 30 minutes until pain is controlled, thereafter every 2 hours [49, 50].

(v) Treatment should be individualized. The choice of analgesia depends on the severity of the pain and the patient's prior analgesic needs/history.

(vi) Nonopioids such as simple paracetamol and NSAIDS (nonsteroidal anti-inflammatory drugs) may be used in mild VOC. Weak opioids such as tramadol and DF118 (dihydrocodeine) are used for moderate pain while severe pain requires stronger opioids/narcotics such as morphine [45, 46].

(vii) Adjuvants for pain control help in achieving better analgesia. They may include mild sedatives such as promethazine or diazepam. Combination of paracetamol or NSAIDS with opiates gives better analgesia because of their synergistic actions. Oversedation should be avoided. Laxatives should be prescribed for prevention and treatment of constipation, a side effect of opioid use.

(viii) More than five to seven days of sequential NSAID use should be avoided to reduce the risk of peptic ulceration and GIT haemorrhage. Also, NSAIDS are potentially nephrotoxic and are better avoided in established renal disease.

(ix) Severe VOC requires parenteral opioid analgesia and hydration in a hospital setting. The dose of the analgesia should be titrated with the severity of the pain until adequate control is achieved in a fixed dose schedule (FDS), interspersed with short-acting agents for breakthrough pains.

(x) Prophylactic incentive spirometry is recommended for prevention of acute chest syndrome especially in BPC involving the chest wall. In the absence of a spirometer, 10 deep breaths every 2 hours while awake between 8 a.m. and 10 p.m. are an alternative.

(xi) If pain persists, patient controlled analgesia (PCA) should be considered where available. PCA is sparsely available in Nigeria, except in very few private facilities. PCA reduces the risk of pain undertreatment.

(xii) Short-acting opioids in clinical use include tramadol, morphine, hydrocodeine, hydromorphine, fentanyl, oxymorphine, and oxycodeine. Longer acting opioids include methadone and slow release preparations of tramadol, morphine, and oxycodeine. Access to a wide range of opioids may not always be readily available in Nigeria; however, the available ones should be used.

(xiii) In difficult cases, where pain is unremitting after 48 hours of well conducted analgesia, exchange blood transfusion (EBT) may be offered [51].

(xiv) Hospitalization for severe BPC occurring on 3 or more occasions per year is an indication for initiation of hydroxyurea therapy or chronic transfusion therapy in patients that are intolerant of hydroxyurea.

(xv) Pain in SCD is majorly nociceptive in origin. However, it may also have a neuropathic component marked by tingling/burning sensation or numbness. In such cases, drugs such as pregabalin or carbamazepine will be useful [46].

(xvi) Pain control in SCD is essentially pharmacologic. However, nonpharmacologic measures such as physical therapy with heat or ice packs, relaxation, distraction, music, menthol rub, meditation, and transcutaneous electrical nerve stimulation (TENS) are also helpful [46].

Treatment of acute sickle cell pain in a dedicated day hospital is associated with better outcome due to prompt triage and familiarity with analgesic needs of individual patients, hence reduced risk of pain undertreatment. Invariably, there is reduction in overall patient admission rates and better outcomes compared to emergency room settings [52–54]. However, most institutions in Nigeria lack daycare settings for management of sickle cell crisis.

Furthermore, it is important to note that BPC may be complicated by a concurrent hyperhaemolytic crisis with resultant acute severe anaemia or may even progress to acute chest syndrome or multiorgan failure syndrome (MOFS). MOFS is defined as sudden onset, severe organ dysfunction simultaneously involving at least two major organ systems (such as the liver, lung, and kidney) in the setting of an acute sickle cell crisis. MOFS is partly explained by significant vasoocclusive events in vital organs with major functional compromise and organ failure [55]. This life-threatening complication requires immediate intensive care and a multispecialist attention including the intensivists, nephrologist, hepatologist, respiratory physicians, and others.

5.1.2. Acute Abdominal Pain.

Acute abdominal pain in SCD may be due to sequestration crisis, vasoocclusion of mesenteric vessels, gall bladder/biliary tract disorders, or other non-SCD specific causes. In a Nigerian study by Akingbola et al., the aetiology of acute abdominal pain in a population of adult Nigerian SCD patients presenting in a tertiary facility were found to include SCD related complications such as abdominal VOC and acute cholecystitis, as well as other infective causes such as cystitis, gastroenteritis, appendicitis, and bowel obstruction [56]. About 38% of the cases were due to abdominal infarction/crisis [56]. In Ile-Ife, Akinola et al. observed abdominal pain due to VOC in 26% of sickle cell anaemia patients [57]. Microvascular occlusion may involve the mesenteric bed causing ischaemic abdominal pain. Abdominal pain of presumed vasoocclusive origin is termed abdominal crisis. Girdle syndrome, otherwise called mesenteric syndrome, is a rare complication owing to extensive collateral blood supplies to the mesentery and bowel wall [58]. Girdle syndrome or mesenteric syndrome is said to be present when there is an established paralytic ileus, which may be associated with vomiting, silent distended abdomen, dilated bowel loops, and air-fluid levels on abdominal radiography. Typically, a patient with girdle syndrome presents with generalized abdominal pain and rarely in shock if there is massive bowel gangrene (third space losses). Other abdominal findings may include localized or rebound tenderness, board-like rigidity, and lack of movement on respiration. Abdominal radiography and ultrasound scan are helpful as well as investigations to rule out differentials such as pancreatitis, acute appendicitis, cholecystitis, biliary colic, splenic abscess, ischaemic colitis, and other forms of acute abdomen. Intravenous hydration, analgesia, and antibiotics are indicated. For an established ileus, NPO (nothing by mouth) should be commenced, as well as nasogastric aspiration, if there is vomiting. Urgent surgical opinion should be sought. Exchange blood transfusion may be necessary in

mesenteric (girdle) syndrome. Biliary/gall bladder anomalies commonly observed in SCD include cholelithiasis and biliary sludge [59]. Recent studies among Nigerian patients observed an age-related prevalence of about 5 to 10% for cholelithiasis [60, 61].

5.1.3. Visceral Sequestration Crisis.

Infants and children less than 7 years are at greatest risk of sequestration crisis especially splenic sequestration. Children above this age group and adults are at less risk of splenic sequestration because the spleen tends to become fibrotic with repeated infarctions and cannot enlarge [24]. However, in haemoglobin SC disease, older children and adults can experience sequestration crisis. If not corrected rapidly, acute sequestration results in hypovolaemia, severe anaemia, and possibly death. A typical patient is irritable with rapidly enlarging spleen or liver and pain in the upper abdomen. Features of acute anaemia include worsening pallor, generalized weakness, and tachycardia. Early presentation in the hospital and close monitoring are important. Blood transfusion is necessary if haemoglobin level falls 2 g/dL below steady state haemoglobin levels or evidence of cardiac decompensation. A major sequestration crisis is defined by haemoglobin level below 6 g/dL. There is risk for recurrence; therefore parents and caregivers must be taught how to examine the child's spleen regularly and report any abnormal finding to the physician immediately. Splenectomy is recommended after the second episode in children above two years of age. For children below 2 years of age, chronic blood transfusion should be offered [62]. Majority of SCD sequestration crisis involves the spleen. Though less common, the liver and lymph nodes may also be sites of sequestration in SCD.

5.1.4. Aplastic Crisis.

Aplastic crisis usually occurs in those less than 16 years of age. It is commonly caused by parvovirus B19 infection which causes transient selective suppression of erythroid progenitors. In Nigeria, prevalence of parvovirus B19 infection is shown to be similar among sickle cell patients and the general population [63]. In normal subjects, parvovirus B19 infection is asymptomatic. However, in patients with chronic haemolytic anaemia such as SCD, parvoviral infection is potentially devastating. Reticulocytopenia often lasts about 7 to 10 days, followed by spontaneous remission with reticulocytosis. Aplastic crisis may follow a recent upper respiratory tract infection and the patient may have flu-like symptoms such as headache, mild fever, and lethargy. Other findings include pallor and worsening anaemia. The condition is self-limiting. Treatment is to give red cell transfusion support until erythroid activity resumes.

5.1.5. Worsening (Acute) Anaemia in SCD.

Baseline haemoglobin level in sickle cell disease ranges between 6 and 9 g/dL [64]. A study among adult SCD patients in Lagos by Akinbami et al. shows mean steady state haemoglobin levels of 7.92 ± 1.49 g/dL [65]. Average haemoglobin concentration of an SCD patient over a minimum of 4 weeks is considered steady state (or stable) haemoglobin level in the absence of any form of crisis in the preceding three months. Anaemia in

SCD is usually well compensated. Occasionally, some patients have high steady state haematocrit level above 10 g/dL and they tend to present with more vasoocclusive complications. This has been termed high haematocrit syndrome [26]. Therapeutic phlebotomy when haemoglobin level is higher than 12 g/dL may benefit such patients [59]. However, in most other patients, significant decline of more than 2 g/dL below steady state level has functional consequences. Untreated severe anaemia is symptomatic and may precipitate heart failure. Causes of worsening anaemia in sickle cell disease may include hyperhaemolysis from any cause, aplastic crisis, megaloblastic crisis, iron deficiency, haemorrhage, renal failure, sequestration crisis, and extreme bone marrow necrosis. Treatment requires both definitive and supportive care. If patient shows signs of cardiac decompensation, blood transfusion should be given. The cause of worsening anaemia should be sought and treated accordingly.

5.1.6. Cerebrovascular Disease (CVD).

5.1.6. Cerebrovascular Disease (CVD). CVD is a significant cause of morbidity and mortality in sickle cell disease [56]. CVD or stroke refers to a sudden onset focal or global neurologic deficit of vascular origin lasting more than 24 hours. It may be ischaemic or haemorrhagic. TIA or stroke occurs in 25% of patients with sickle cell disease. Overt stroke occurs in 10 to 15% of homozygous patients under the age of 10 years [66–68]. The prevalence of overt stroke among SCA children in Port Harcourt, Nigeria, is reported as 4.3% [69]. In Abuja, Nigeria, Oniyangi et al. reported a stroke prevalence of 5.2% among SCD children seen in a tertiary center [70]. The risk of CVD is higher in those with low baseline haemoglobin, low fetal haemoglobin, high white blood cell count, and high systolic blood pressure. CVD is rare in infants. Incidence of CVD is higher in Hb SS disease compared with SC disease, S/b+thalassemia, and S/b zero thalassemia [36, 59].

Infarctive CVD is commonest and occurs in patients aged less than 20 years and older than 30 years (peak incidence: 10–15 years) [71]. Infarction is often associated with stenosis or occlusion of affected vessels most commonly the distal internal carotid, proximal middle cerebral, and anterior cerebral arteries. The patient may present with antecedent history of TIA or seizures, which eventually progresses to an overt stroke, characterized by hemiparesis, speech, or visual impairment, or even coma if immediate therapy is not instituted. Suggested guideline on acute and long-term treatment of an ischaemic stroke in SCD is provided as follows.

Treatment Guidelines for Sickle Cell Ischaemic Stroke

  (i) After initial evaluation of patient's airway, breathing, and circulation (ABC of resuscitation), further stabilization should be pursued through prevention and control of hypoxaemia, hypotension, hyperthermia, and glycaemic imbalance, which would worsen the cerebral insult.

 (ii) Presence of seizures should be controlled with appropriate anticonvulsants. Prophylactic antiseizure therapy is not necessary.

(iii) Urgent noncontrast CT/MRI is required to distinguish haemorrhage and infarction. This important distinction has to be made early, as this will impact subsequent therapeutic decisions.

(iv) In the early stage of brain ischaemia (<3 hours), cranial CT may be negative or show only subtle inconclusive signs. Magnetic resonance imaging (MRI) provides better details but should be deferred until treatment has been initiated.

 (v) Early institution of exchange transfusion is crucial to improving treatment outcome. EBT should be targeted at reducing sickle Hb level below 30%. Simple transfusions may be offered in the interim while EBT is being planned. Simple transfusions at 10–15 mL per kg red cells reduce sickle haemoglobin levels to about 60%.

(vi) Adequate hydration not more than 1.5 times the maintenance should be instituted with isotonic fluids preferably 0.9% normal saline.

(vii) In untransfused SCD patients, stroke recurrence rate is 67%, with 70% of recurrent strokes occurring in the first 3 years after the initial stroke [72]. As such, EBT should be followed up with hypertransfusion therapy to maintain sickle Hb level below 30% at a haemoglobin concentration of about 10 to 11 g/dL.

(viii) Chronic blood transfusion (CBT) has been shown to be beneficial in primary and secondary prevention of CVD [70, 73–75]. However, clear definitions on when and how CBT should be stopped is yet to be made. Often times, transfusions continue till late adolescence or early adulthood.

(ix) Hydroxyurea therapy reduces cerebral blood flow. Though less effective, hydroxyurea may be considered an alternative to chronic transfusion therapy, where transfusion is not feasible [67, 68].

 (x) Thrombolysis with recombinant tissue plasminogen activator (rTPA) within the first 3 hours of ischaemic CVD in adult patients should be considered after careful patient evaluation [76]. TPA is not recommended in children. However, the current prospect of TPA use among Nigerian patients is remote due to challenges of its availability, cost, delayed diagnosis, and clinical experience with its use.

(xi) Antiplatelet agent, aspirin 325 mg, is recommended if TPA is not used and should be avoided for the first 24 hours if TPA is used [77].

(xii) Adult SCD patients should be evaluated and treated for modifiable risk factors such as dyslipidaemia.

(xiii) Acute stroke should be treated in a dedicated stroke unit with input of both neurologist and haematologist.

Haemorrhagic stroke tends to occur between 20 and 29 years of age and is associated with low steady state haemoglobin levels and high steady state leucocyte counts [71]. Hemorrhage often results from rupture of vessels within the circle of Willis. Clinical presentation is similar to ischaemic CVD. However, patients with haemorrhagic CVDs are more likely to present with coma. In haemorrhagic CVD, patient may present with severe headache, vomiting, and other features suggesting raised intracranial pressure. Haemorrhagic CVD is rare but more fatal. Cerebral oedema is worse in haemorrhagic stroke. Prompt confirmation of diagnosis through imaging studies is required. Treatment of cerebral oedema with hypertonic solution such as mannitol is desirable. Antiplatelet and anticoagulants are contraindicated in haemorrhagic stroke. Though its exact role in haemorrhagic CVD is not clear, EBT is recommended especially for patients billed to undergo magnetic resonance angiography [76]. Surgical interventions by vascular surgeons may include ligation of accessible aneurysms and surgical vascular bypass procedure for moyamoya syndrome. Nimodipine, a calcium channel blocker, improves outcome in adults with subarachnoid haemorrhage by counteracting delayed arterial vasospasm [76, 78].

Risk evaluation for an overt ischaemic stroke and the need for early preventive intervention are performed by assessment of cerebral blood flow velocity using transcranial Doppler (TCD) ultrasound. Cerebral blood flow in excess of 2 meters per second portends a high risk for CVD. Typically, TCD ultrasound assessment is commenced by age of 2 years. TCD between 1.7 and 2 should be reassessed in 3-4 months. If stable, assessment should be annual until 16 years of age [59]. Cerebral blood flow in excess of 2 meters/second is an indication for commencement of hypertransfusion therapy and this is shown to reduce stroke occurrence by about 90% [66]. MRI scan every 5 years may also be used in periodic evaluation of the brain for silent infarctions where resources are available [79].

Subclinical cerebral infarcts (SCI) in sickle cell disease patients occur in 27% and 37% of patients before their 6th and 14th birthdays, respectively [80]. Silent stroke is defined by an abnormal MRI in the absence of history and physical signs of an overt CVD. Risk factors for SCI include male gender, low steady state haemoglobin levels, higher baseline systolic blood pressure, and previous seizures [80]. Subclinical strokes are associated with neuropsychiatric dysfunction in apparently healthy SCD patients [79, 81] and are a risk factor for overt stroke [82]. In confirmed silent brain infarctions with neurocognitive delay and behavioural disturbances, chronic transfusion therapy is indicated.

5.1.7. Acute Chest Syndrome (ACS). ACS is a leading cause of mortality in sickle cell disease even among Nigerian patients, accounting for about 25% of all deaths [83–85]. Risk factors for acute chest syndrome includes older age, low fetal haemoglobin level, high haematocrit level, homozygous SS disease, chest VOC, smoking, general anaesthesia and surgery, asthma, and possibly opioid use [86]. ACS is defined by new pulmonary infiltrates (on chest radiography) in at least one complete lung segment, fever, and at least one respiratory symptom (pleuritic chest pain, cough, dyspnoea, and tachypnoea) [86]. ACS may follow a painful crisis especially in adults. ACS may also complicate the immediate

postoperative state. As such, there is need to maintain proper protocols for preventing or treating ACS during BPC and after surgery.

The underlying pathophysiology of ACS includes vaso-occlusion of pulmonary vessels and microbial involvement. Implicated microbes include bacteria such as Pneumococcus, *Haemophilus influenza*, respiratory viruses, and atypical organisms such as *Mycoplasma*, Chlamydia, or *Legionella*. Respiratory viruses are more likely in children while bacterial causes are more frequent in adults [24]. Furthermore, hypoxia induced by ACS can trigger widespread sickling and vasoocclusion, with possibility of multiorgan failure and death. Fat laden pulmonary macrophages in the airways are observed in about half of the cases, suggesting possible contributions from bone marrow fat embolisation [83]. Bone pain crisis involving the chest cage can also trigger ACS as a result of pain induced hypoventilation, which encourages sickling in the pulmonary bed and microbial growth. Similarly, over-sedation with opioids may predispose to ACS.

During BPC or in the immediate postoperative period, care should be taken to prevent ACS. In such patients, prophylactic incentive spirometry is helpful [87]. In the absence of a spirometer, 10 deep breaths every 2 hours of the day is an alternative. Treatment of an established ACS also includes incentive spirometry/chest physiotherapy, parenteral broad-spectrum antibiotics, effective pain relief, and supplemental oxygen therapy (2–4 liters per minute). Opioid is the mainstay of pain control in SCD. Its liberal use is encouraged in order to prevent pain undertreatment, prolonged treatment, and hypoventilation. However, care should be taken to avoid oversedation. Recommended antibiotic combinations include quinolones, 2nd or 3rd generation cephalosporin alongside macrolides (for atypical bacteria). Antibiotic choice should be further directed by local susceptibility profile if available.

Bronchodilator therapy is also required as most patients may have a bronchoreactive component. EBT is indicated in worsening lung consolidation or persistent hypoxia, any neurological deficit (confusion, motor deficit, epilepsy), intractable pain or opioid intolerance, haemodynamic instability, nosocomial infections, acute worsening of anaemia or cardiovascular insufficiency, and acute enlargement of spleen or liver [59]. Mechanical ventilation is required in rapidly progressive cases. Inhaled nitric oxide and steroid may be helpful in life-threatening cases. Evidence suggests that recurrent episodes of ACS can be prevented by hydroxyurea [88]. Also chronic transfusion therapy is beneficial in secondary prevention of ACS and is indicated in patients with two or more episodes annually, who are unresponsive to hydroxyurea [89].

5.1.8. Priapism. Priapism is another acute complication of sickle cell disease. It is defined as persistent, purposeless, painful penile erection that is unassociated with sexual pleasure. Generally, reports of lifetime prevalence of priapism in sickle cell disease range from 2 to 35% [90]. Its prevalence is found to be as high as 44.9% among Nigerian male SCD patients [91]. Peak incidence occurs in 2nd and 3rd decade (median age: 18.5 years) [24, 91]. SCD priapism is a "low-flow" type. The penile ischaemia results from outflow obstruction (poor venous drainage) caused by sickled cells. Usually, it affects the corpora cavernosa alone while the spongiosum is spared. A typical genital examination reveals a hard penis with soft glans; tricorporeal involvement is rare. The priapism may also be defined as stuttering, minor, or major (prolonged) depending on the duration of the attack and its frequency. Stuttering priapism typically last about 30 minutes to 2 hours, tends to become recurrent (occurs several times a week), and may herald episodes of prolonged priapism. Minor attacks occur infrequently or isolated. Major or severe attacks last longer than 3 to 4 hours and should be treated as a urological emergency. Severe (major) and recurrent priapism (penile ischaemia) is associated with irreversible organ damage, fibrosis, and impotence.

The goal of treatment is to preserve erectile function and prevent recurrences. As such, there is need for early presentation in the hospital if home remedies are unsuccessful within 2 hours of onset. At the onset, patients should be counseled to drink extra fluid, use home-based simple or compound analgesia, and attempt to void. Other self-help strategies such as warm baths and gentle exercises like jogging may be helpful. Oral dose of pseudoephedrine or terbutaline may be given. If the priapism persists more than 2 hours, hospital care is required. This includes intravenous hydration and opioid analgesia. If the priapism persists more than 3 hours, aspiration and irrigation of the corpora with dilute phenylephrine, epinephrine, or etilefrine is indicated. Frequently, aspiration of blood from the cavernosal bodies is performed with a 23-gauge sterile needle, followed by irrigation with a 1 : 1,000,000 dilution of epinephrine in saline, after adequate counseling, conscious sedation, and local anaesthesia [92]. If detumescence is achieved lasting more than one hour, patient may be discharged home on oral analgesic, pseudoephedrine, and clinic follow-up. Penile aspiration and irrigation may be repeated up to 3 or 4 episodes if detumescence is not achieved early.

Simple early self-intracavernosal injection (SICI) of etilefrine and other adrenergic agonists such as metaraminol may achieve detumescence within one hour of onset, hence removing the need for hospital-based surgical aspiration and irrigation [93–95]. Sympathomimetics (adrenergic agonists) may be associated with untoward effects such as blood pressure changes and are yet to be licensed for SICI. EBT is indicated in recalcitrant cases. Surgical shunt procedures such as proximal shunt of quackel or distal shunt of winter may be tried, if conservative measures remain unsuccessful. However, surgical penile shunts may also be unsuccessful and may induce impotence [96]. Often, priapism will resolve with one or a combination of medical interventions.

In preventing priapism, male sickle cell patients ought to be adequately informed and counseled about priapism from adolescence. Patients with frequent episodes (≥2 per month, ≥4 per year) should receive priapism prophylaxis with oral pseudoephedrine 30 mg daily if they are less than 10 years of age and 60 mg per day if they are older than 10 years. Etilefrine and diethylstilbestrol (DES) may be used prophylactically although evidence for its usefulness is limited [97, 98]. DES use has been limited by its feminizing effects, though a short course of 5 mg daily may be used to abort a stuttering episode [99]. Similarly use of injectable leuprolide, a GnRH antagonist, which works through endogenous suppression of androgen production, is associated with longstanding hypogonadism and rebound priapism after discontinuation [97]. Use of hydroxyurea may also be beneficial [97]. There is recent evidence that use of phosphodiesterase (PDE) 5 inhibitor such as sildenafil is useful in preventing recurrent episodes of priapism [100–102]. Though not always successful, penile prosthesis may be remedial in those with established erectile difficulties persisting more than 12 months [103].

5.1.9. Ocular Disease. Central retinal artery occlusion by sickled red cell sludge is an ocular emergency. It manifests as sudden change in vision. It is treated like stroke. Treatment requires EBT, hyperoxygenation, and reduction of intraocular pressure with carbonic anhydrase inhibitors [24]. Prognosis is however poor.

5.1.10. Osteomyelitis. Osteomyelitis is one of the commonest skeletal complications of SCD [104, 105]. About 29% of Nigerian SCD patients experience this complication in their lifetime [106]. It often originates from bacteremia, as also observed in septic arthritis. Diagnosis may be quite difficult due to its similar presentation to acute bone infarction. Diagnosis requires a high index of suspicion. Serial blood cultures, as well as culture of local bone aspirates, may be required [59]. The commonest cause of osteomyelitis in SCD population is *salmonella* spp, followed by *staphylococcus* species [24, 107, 108]. Treatment requires involvement of the orthopedic surgeon and clinical microbiologist. Broad spectrum antibiotic based on the common local isolates and their susceptibility profile should be commenced after culture samples have been taken.

5.2. Chronic Morbidities in Sickle Cell Disease

5.2.1. Delayed Growth and Development. Children with sickle cell disease have normal body weight at birth. However, by one year of life, there might be obvious weight lag when compared with normal infants. This weight deficit persists till adulthood and typically imparts a thin (asthenic) build [14]. Obesity may be seen in some cases [24]. Pubertal growth spurt may be delayed 1-2 years compared to their peers. Growth deficits in children with SCD may be due to multiple factors including severe anaemia, long-term effects of repeated vasoocclusion, endocrine failure, low dietary intake, and low socioeconomic status [109]. However, delay in skeletal maturation allows for bone growth such that final adult height is reached. Menarche may also be delayed for 1-2 years in females [24].

5.2.2. Chronic Pain Syndromes. There are two forms of chronic pain in SCD: chronic pain due to obvious tissue damage such as AVN or leg ulcers, and intractable chronic pain with no obvious cause. Suboptimal treatment of recurrent severe acute painful crisis may progress to an intractable chronic pain syndrome. There is need for prompt and adequate treatment of acute pain episodes. Opioids coupled with nonopioids and adjuvant remain the mainstay of analgesia in SCD [45].

5.2.3. Immunological and Infectious Complication. SCD patients have a subnormal immunity, which partly accounts for their increased susceptibility to infections [32]. Immunologic dysfunction in SCD is attributable to autosplenectomy with the resultant defective cellular and humoral immunity [110]. About 30% loss of splenic function occurs by first year of life and 90% by sixth year of life [111]. Normal splenic synthesis of immunoglobulins, properdin, and tuftsin is impaired, leading to increased susceptibility to infections. They are particularly susceptible to encapsulated organisms such as pneumococcus especially in children aged less than 5 years, hence the rationale behind pneumococcal vaccination and penicillin prophylaxis from four months of life till age five in western societies. Previous infections with *pneumococcus* confer lifelong prophylaxis. Studies reveal that, without preventive actions, invasive pneumococcal infection is 30 to 600 times more likely to occur in SCD children compared to normal persons [112]. *Haemophilus influenza* is the next most common organism and affects children older than 5 years. In Africa, *Salmonella, Klebsiella, Escherichia coli,* and *staphylococcus* seem to be more common than *pneumococcus* [113, 114]. As such, routine prophylaxis against *pneumococcus* is not an established practice in Nigeria [115]. However, there is recent compelling evidence from other parts of Africa that *pneumococcus* contributes significantly to infections in SCD [116–118]. Since infection has been documented as the commonest cause of death among SCD patients in Nigeria, the role of pneumococcus in SCD related infections and mortalities needs to be clarified through further research. There is a need for vaccination and chemoprophylaxis against common infections [83]. Current national immunization schedule in Nigeria routinely includes vaccinations against polio, tuberculosis, Diphtheria, tetanus, pertussis, hepatitis B, *Haemophilus influenza* infections, measles, and Yellow fever. Before one year of life, the infant should have completed the vaccination schedule and is entitled to subsequent booster doses [119]. However, for persons affected with sickle cell disease, additional compulsory vaccinations should be administered to cover for *Streptococcus pneumonia, Influenza virus,* and *Neisseria meningococcus, human papillomavirus (HPV).* Children less than two years of age should have four doses of the 7 valent pneumococcal vaccine between 2 and 15 months of life. The 23 valent pneumococcal vaccine should be administered at age of 2 years and older and should be repeated every 3 to 5 years till 10 years of age and every 5 years for those older than 10 years. Influenza vaccines should be administered during cold seasons beginning at 6 months of life. HIB vaccine should be commenced at 2 months of life. Meningococcal vaccination is recommended for patient at 5 years and older and is repeated every two years. HPV vaccine is administered to females under 26 years.

Also contributing to increased risk of infection in sickle cell disease is repeated tissue infarctions, which are potential foci for pathogens. Similarly, iron overload in patients that have had several transfusions favors growth of iron dependent bacteria such as *Yersinia enterocolitica.* Furthermore, micronutrient deficiency especially zinc deficiency is associated with lymphopenia and decreased immunity [120]. About 60–70% of SCD patients are zinc deficient. In Nigeria, a case-control study showed the serum zinc level to be significantly lower among SCD children compared with healthy controls [121]. Other studies have also shown significant deficiencies of other micronutrients such as magnesium and selenium [122, 123].

5.2.4. Sickle Cell Chronic Lung Disease. Sickle cell chronic lung disease (SCCLD) is an age related morbidity. It affects at least a third of adult SCD patients [59]. Patterns of the lung involvement among Nigerian patients include restrictive lung disease, obstructive lung disease, chronic hypoxaemia, and pulmonary hypertension (PHT) [59, 124–126]. A Study in Nigeria reported a prevalence of 18.9% for SCCLD among adult SCD patients [127]. Chronic complications occur more frequently in those with history of acute chest syndrome. In about 20% of patients, echocardiography shows elevated pulmonary artery systolic blood pressure >35 mmHg. Incidence of PHT is higher in patients with high haemolytic rates and high LDH. PHT is associated with 10-fold increase in the relative risk of death and it confers poor prognosis [128]. Primary PHT is not the only cause of elevated TRV (tricuspid regurgitation jet velocity) in SCD patients. Patients with elevated TRV have increased risk of mortality in the next 3 years [59]. Treatment includes hydroxyurea therapy, chronic transfusion, vasodilator use, anticoagulation, and oxygen therapy.

5.2.5. Hepatobiliary Complications. Chronic liver damage in sickle cell disease is caused by intrahepatic trapping of sickle cells, transfusion transmitted hepatotropic infections, and transfusion siderosis [59, 129]. Evidence suggests that post-transfusion hepatitis and other transfusion transmissible infections are still a significant problem in Nigeria [130, 131]. In Ibadan, Nigeria, Fashola and Otegbayo observed a post-transfusion viral hepatitis prevalence rate of 12.5% in 2002 [130]. In rare instances, vasoocclusion in the liver with cholestasis may precipitate acute liver failure. Pigment gallstones are found in about two-thirds of sickle cell patients, especially those with sickle cell anaemia [129]. Symptomatic gallstones require cholecystectomy. Cholecystitis is treated with antibiotics. Treatment of asymptomatic cholelithiasis may require watchful waiting. Gall stones associated with common bile duct stones require endoscopic retrograde cholangiopancreatography (ERCP). The risk of hepatic damage is reduced by ensuring viral safety of all transfused blood components and prompt institution of iron chelation therapy if iron overload is present. In hepatic failure, liver transplantation is a veritable option.

5.2.6. Other Abdominal Complications. Incidence of peptic ulcer disease (PUD) is higher in SCD patients. PUD occurs in about 35% of SCD patients with epigastric pain [58]. In Ile-Ife, Nigeria, Akinola et al. observed PUD among 28% and 50% of Hb SS and Hb SC disease patients presenting with abdominal pains, respectively. Interestingly, duodenal ulcers are not associated with high acid outputs; rather, ulcers are secondary to decreased mucosal resistance, possibly due to bowel ischaemia and NSAID abuse.

5.2.7. Renal Complications. The hypoxic, acidotic, and hypertonic state of the renal medulla favors vasoocclusion and destruction of the vasa recta. By the first year of life, SCD infants may develop hyposthenuria manifesting as nocturia or enuresis [24]. Local studies have shown that the prevalence of nocturnal enuresis is higher among children with homozygous sickle cell disease [132]. This further makes them susceptible to dehydration, especially in hot climate. In addition, distal type IV tubulopathy in SCD promotes acidosis, further predisposing to vasoocclusive events. Papillary necrosis (usually of the left kidney) presents with haematuria. Other possible causes of haematuria include infections, stones, and tumor. Recommended guidelines for treatment and prevention of sickle cell nephropathy (SCN) are presented as follows.

Recommended Guidelines for Management of Sickle Cell Nephropathy

(i) SCN is an age-related morbidity. Among Nigerian patients, its prevalence and severity increases with advancing age, longer survival, and homozygous SS disease [133, 134].

(ii) Relevant clinical history and examination findings such as facial puffiness, loin pain, painless haematuria, leg and abdominal swelling, frothy urine, worsening anaemia, and hypertension, which may suggest renal disease, should be elicited at regular intervals during visits.

(iii) At least once annually during maintenance visits, SCD patients should be assessed for their renal status. Recommended laboratory assays include urinalysis (on every visit), serum electrolytes, urea and creatinine (semiannually), creatinine clearance/estimated glomerular filtration rate (eGFR), and tests for microalbuminuria (albumin creatinine ratio, ACR; urinary protein to creatinine ratio, uPCR). A normal creatinine level does not exclude renal disease in SCD due to supranormal kidneys precipitated by hyperfiltration and increased secretion of creatinine and uric acid. Emphasis and therapeutic decisions should be placed on significant adverse changes in the renal markers rather than single absolute values.

(iv) Consultations and comanagement with experienced nephrologist is recommended in the following setting: patients with uPCR >50 mg/mmol (442 mg/g), persistent microscopic haematuria, declining renal function (>10% fall in eGFR per annum), or eGFR

$<60 \, \text{mL/min/1.73 m}^2$. Further evaluations including renal biopsy are necessitated in settings of sudden onset heavy proteinuria with or without nephrotic syndrome [135, 136].

(v) Treatment of haematuria includes bed rest, hydration, and blood transfusion if indicated in events of a significant blood loss. Most times, haematuria is caused by papillary necrosis. However, the possibility of a renal medullary cell carcinoma must be excluded in these patients.

(vi) Progression of SCN to ESRD is often heralded by worsening proteinuria, anaemia, and hypertension. This may be delayed with adequate control of hypertension and proteinuria. Introduction of angiotensin converting enzyme inhibitors (ACEIs) or angiotensin receptor blockers (ARBs) reduces proteinuria [136]. For blood pressure control, diuretics are better avoided.

(vii) Similarly, early commencement of hydroxyurea helps to delay progression to ESRD except hydroxyurea is contraindicated for other reasons.

(viii) NSAIDS for pain control are better avoided in patients with established SCN, in order to prevent worse organ damage. NSAIDS cause significant decline in renal blood flow and glomerular filtration.

(ix) Urinary tract infection in these patients should be treated aggressively. Patients with ESRD should be on regular EBT especially if renal transplant is being planned. End stage renal disease is managed with repeated dialysis, erythropoietin therapy, and/or renal transplant.

5.2.8. Ocular Disease. Incidence of ocular disease is higher in Hb SC disease, Hb SB+thal compared to Hb SS [59, 137]. Repeated vasoocclusion in the vascular beds of the eye especially the retina causes progressive ophthalmopathy, which manifests as comma-shaped conjunctival vessels, iris atrophy, retinal pigmentary changes, and retinal hemorrhages. Neovascularization leads to sea-fanning, so called proliferative retinopathy. Eventually, vitreous haemorrhage and retinal detachment may occur. For prevention, annual eye examination is recommended for all SCD patients from the 2nd decade of life [59]. Treatment options for proliferative retinopathy include laser photocoagulation and vitrectomy.

5.2.9. Sickle Cell Leg Ulcer. Leg ulcers are frequent in adults SCD patients especially males with SS phenotype and patients with low steady state haemoglobin levels [138, 139]. In a report from Benin City, Nigeria, Bazuaye et al. observed a prevalence rate of 9.6 and 22.4% for current ulcers and previous ulcers, respectively [139]. Ulcers commonly arise near the medial or lateral malleolus and may be single or multiple. The aetiology is often multifactorial and they include vasoocclusion of skin microvasculature, made worse by trauma, infection, warm climate, and iron overload [24]. Commonly isolated microbes include *pseudomonas aeruginosa*, *staphylococcus aureus*, and *streptococcus* species. Chronic SCD ulcers are painful and resistant to healing. Treatment of these ulcers requires multidisciplinary approach involving the haematologist, plastic surgeon, specialist nurses, and orthopaedic surgeon [24]. Generally, treatment includes pain relief (including local pain control before wound dressing), elevation of the leg, debridement (to remove necrotic tissue), elastic dressing/support bandage, and zinc sulphate therapy (600 mg/day). Some patients may benefit from chronic blood transfusion and skin grafting.

5.2.10. Musculoskeletal Complications.
Known musculoskeletal complications in SCD include medullary hyperplasia, dystrophic intramedullary calcification, H-vertebra, osteolysis, osteopenia, septic arthritis, dactylitis, ulcers, pathologic fracture, and osteomyelitis. H-vertebra or Cod-fish vertebra is due to infarction of the vertebral body, giving a fish-mouth appearance on radiography. In a study by Balogun et al., musculoskeletal complications occurred in 31.4% of adult Nigerian SCD patients [140]. Avascular osteonecrosis of the femoral and humeral head is particularly associated with reduced quality of life. AVN develops in about 50% of patients who survive to above 35 years of age and about 60% of patients who survive to 60 years of age [141]. Another recent study revealed that AVN occurred in about 13 per 1000 Nigerian SCD patients [142]. Exact mechanism for development of AVN is yet to be clearly described. Even patients with high fetal haemoglobin levels may not be totally protected from developing AVN. However, high steady state platelet count has been correlated with AVN in Nigerian SCD patients [142]. Other clinical and laboratory correlations of AVN include high haematocrit, coexistence of alpha thalassemia, and frequent VOC [143–145].

In older patients, humeral head necrosis is more common than femoral head necrosis, although femoral head necrosis is associated with more devastating pain due to weight bearing [146]. Treatment of musculoskeletal complications of SCD requires comanagement with an orthopedic surgeon with special interest in SCD. Persisting pain in a joint or at least a stage 3 arthropathy is indication for referral to an orthopedic specialist [146]. X-ray features of AVN may not be obvious until repair processes have changed the density of the bone. MRI is the investigation of choice in SCD patients with persisting hip or shoulder pain. Every patient with confirmed AVN should be staged with MRI. Initial conservative treatment should include counseling/patient education, analgesia, partial weight bearing on crutches, and physiotherapy. Option of joint replacement/arthroplasty is available for patients with severe joint destruction.

5.2.11. Cardiovascular System Changes.
Sickle cell disease is associated with cardiac abnormalities including dilated cardiomyopathy, ventricular hypertrophy, cardiac iron overload, dysrhythmias, pulmonary hypertension, myocardial infarction, and sudden death [147, 148]. Chronic anaemia in SCD potentiates ventricular hypertrophy and dilatation which may progress to left ventricular diastolic dysfunction and exercise intolerance [147]. Pulmonary arterial hypertension is defined by end systolic pressure in the right ventricle greater than 25 mmHg (normal is less than 15 mmHg). In a cohort of Nigerian SCD patients, 2 (3.6%) out of 56 met the criteria for pulmonary hypertension [125]. Tricuspid regurgitation jet velocity of >2.5 m/sec is associated with a high risk of pulmonary hypertension and is an independent risk factor for death [128].

5.2.12. Transfusion Related Morbidities.
Blood transfusion is a key therapeutic modality in SCD. In a cohort of Nigerian SCD children, the prevalence of blood transfusion is as high as 57% [149]. Benefits of transfusion in sickle cell disease include correction of the baseline anaemia, dilution of sickle haemoglobin levels, and suppression of endogenous sickle red cell production, as well as reduction in chronic haemolysis and circulating sickle cell levels [150–152]. Transfusion modalities in SCD include simple transfusions, exchange blood transfusion, or chronic blood transfusion (hypertransfusion). Simple transfusion refers to top up correction of anaemia. Indications for chronic blood transfusion include prevention of first stroke, prevention of repeat stroke, TCD USS >2 m/sec, delayed growth and development in children, frequent ACS, severe disease, severe SCD lacking HLA match, sickle chronic lung disease, pregnant women with bad obstetric history and frequent bone pains, and sickle cell leg ulcers [150, 151]. Indications for exchange blood transfusion include moderate to severe ACS, refractory painful VOC, stroke, central retinal artery thrombosis, and acute refractory priapism [36]. The choice of blood component for transfusion in SCD should be a sickle negative, recently donated (less than 7 days old), leucodepleted, and phenotypically matched for at least Rh and Kell antigens, racial and minority matched red cell concentrate. Cytomegalovirus (CMV) negative component should be used for transfusion in all CMV negative children, as they may be candidates for bone marrow transplantation. Target haemoglobin level should not exceed 10-11 g/dL in SCD as there are concerns for hyperviscosity and vasoocclusion [26, 153].

Transfusion of blood and blood components is not without risks. In particular, delayed haemolytic transfusion reaction and alloimmunisation are among the immunologic complications of blood transfusion associated with sickle cell disease. Due to their tendency for repeated transfusion from chronic prophylactic transfusion or otherwise, the risk of iron overload in body tissues with irreversible organ damages ensues, hence the need for close monitoring and prompt iron chelation when indicated. Reports on alloimmunisation rate among Nigerian SCD patients are lacking and may be related to the lack of routine alloantibody screening and extended red cell phenotyping in most blood banks in Nigeria.

Among nonimmunologic complications of transfusion therapy in SCD in Nigeria, transmission of viruses and iron overload is of note [89, 131]. Recent evidence suggests that transmission of viruses is still a major challenge to transfusion safety in Nigeria [131]. This calls for a better national transfusion service. SCD patients, particularly those on hypertransfusion therapy, are at particular risk for iron overload, with resultant damage to vital organs [89]. Iron status should be monitored in SCD patients, particularly those who have received a cumulative transfusion dose of more than 20 to 30 units. Chelation therapy should be instituted promptly if serum ferritin levels exceed 1000 ug/L [154].

5.2.13. Psychosocial Issues/Psychiatric Complications. Psychosocial complications of SCD include poor self-image, negative thoughts and feelings about the condition, stigmatization, depression, cognitive impairments, fears, anxieties, hatred for parents and others, dropping out of school, and tendency for substance abuse [24, 155]. These complications are associated with the chronic nature, recurrent pain, reduced health related quality of life, and unpredictable course of the disease. Some degree of psychologic trauma is also rendered to parents and health caregivers. A recent report by Anie et al. revealed that about half of Nigerian SCD patients had depressive feelings [156]. Adequate psychological support should be provided for patients by physicians, other health care staff, parents, and support groups. Those requiring more definite intervention should be comanaged with clinical psychologists and psychiatrists.

A study in Jamaica revealed that 29% of SS patients had a psychiatric disorder, compared to 25% in the control population [157]. Association of psychiatric morbidity included leaving school early, difficulties in social adjustment, impaired cognition, and previous psychiatric difficulties [157]. Asthenic body builds and abnormal facies may be associated with poor self-image. Such patients should be identified early and treated. Other complications such as undereducation and underemployment may require the services of medical social worker and occupational therapy unit.

6. Special Care Situations

6.1. Sickle Cell Disease and Pregnancy. Typically, pregnancy in female SCD patients is attended by anaemia which may be worsened by pregnancy related plasma volume expansion and folate deficiency. VOC is more common in 3rd trimester [158]. Increased incidence of preeclampsia, maternal mortality, and perinatal complications such as abortions, stillbirths, low birth weight, and neonatal deaths are associated with SCD pregnancy [158–160]. As such, pregnant SCD patients require special care by specialists including experienced obstetrician, haematologist, midwives, and anaesthesiologist. Preferably, oral contraception should be recommended for sexually active SCD females and pregnancy should be planned. Folate supplementation should be ensured. A local study has shown that preconceptual care and early antenatal booking produce better outcome and less obstetric complications in SCD pregnancies [161]. Hypertransfusion is indicated in cases of bad obstetric history and severe sickle cell disease in pregnancy. SCD and pregnancy are procoagulant states. Coupled with obstetric surgeries, the risk of VTE is significantly increased and appropriate anticoagulation may also be necessary in their care-plan [45].

6.2. Perioperative Care in Sickle Cell Disease. Perioperative complications of surgery in SCD patients include hypoxia, dehydration, bone pain crisis, significant anaemia, and acute chest syndrome [162]. Anaesthesia may be associated with hypoxia and dehydration [163]. Good anaesthetic expertise and experience is indicated when undertaking surgical procedure in SCD patients [163]. Early surgical complications such as pain and haemorrhage should be well controlled. Optimal analgesia and tact surgical skills are indicated. Other strategies to improve perioperative outcomes in SCD include conservative preoperative blood transfusion therapy, epidural analgesia, and adequate postoperative pain control with opiate and nonopiate analgesia [164, 165]. Aggressive or exchange transfusion therapy has not been associated with better surgical outcomes [162, 164].

6.3. Sickle Cell Disease and Radiology. Infusion of radiologic contrast media may precipitate VOC. Hypertonic nature of contrast media triggers marked intracellular dehydration and marked increment in red cell MCHC, thus precipitating sickling. This complication may be averted by preprocedure red cell exchange to achieve target sickle haemoglobin level of 50%. Traditional iodinated contrast media (due to its high osmolality) are relatively contraindicated in SCD. Isotonic contrasts are safer to use in SCD [166].

7. Laboratory Diagnosis of Sickle Cell Disease

The science behind laboratory diagnosis of sickle cell disorder entails phenotypic testing for the presence the sickle haemoglobin and genetic analysis. Physicochemical properties of the sickle haemoglobin such as decreased solubility and sickling under deoxy conditions, its pattern of mobility in an electric field, and rate of elution from solution unto adsorbents are applied in its laboratory detection. Phenotypic tests may be used as screening tests or diagnostic tests. Screening tests chosen for the purpose of mass screening should be highly sensitive and cheap to run. Examples of screening tests include sickling test, solubility test, and alkaline haemoglobin electrophoresis. On the other hand, high specific, diagnostic tests include isoelectric focusing, citrate agar electrophoresis, and high performance liquid chromatography [167, 168]. Quantification of haemoglobin variants and globin chain studies are used in evaluation of compound heterozygous disease states such as sickle thalassemia syndrome [167, 169]. Hb A2 levels in excess of 3.5% are suggestive of haemoglobin S-beta thalassemia [168]. Other ancillary laboratory investigations useful in detection and monitoring of the disease include FBC, reticulocyte count, and peripheral blood film. Reticulocyte count usually range from 5 to 15% in sickle cell disease. On peripheral blood film examination, findings may include irreversible sickled red cells, polychromasia, occasional nucleated red cells, and schistocytes, as well as Howell-Jolly bodies [24, 111]. Target cells are seen in sickle haemoglobinopathies. In sickle cell thalassemia syndromes, target cells are seen alongside microcytes and moderate-severe hypochromia. Red cell indices may suggest macrocytosis due to increased reticulocytosis or compliance with hydroxyurea therapy. However, oval macrocytosis with hypersegmented neutrophils may suggest folic acid deficiency. Biochemical changes include high LDH, low haptoglobin, high total and indirect bilirubin, and high AST [35]. Genetic studies such as PCR are used for prenatal and pre-implantation diagnosis [170].

8. Prognosis and Life Expectancy

Severe SCD is associated with poor outcomes, if no intervention is rendered. Known modulators of clinical severity include fetal haemoglobin levels, beta globin haplotype, amd coinheritance of alpha-thalassemia, as well as geographical and other unknown genetic factors [15, 16]. In a study by Emmanuelchide et al., a higher leucocyte count was associated with more SCD complications in a Nigerian SCD population [171]. Another recent Nigerian study in a cohort of 115 children with SCD showed the presence of dactylitis at first presentation and higher total WBC, neutrophil count, platelet count, and serum bilirubin levels to be significantly higher among those with severe disease, while a higher fetal haemoglobin level was associated with a milder disease [172]. Other notable poor prognostic factors include low haemoglobin F production, Hb less than 7 g/dL, Hb greater than 7 g/dL, high VOC rate, pulmonary HTN, and nocturnal hypoxaemia (more strokes) [59].

From a large cooperative study in USA in 1994, the median survival for SCA was reported as 42 and 48 years in men and women, respectively. For haemoglobin SC disease, it was reported as 60 years and 68 years for men and women, respectively [84]. In USA, 95% of children with SCD survive till adulthood [173]. In Jamaica, survival estimates for persons with SCA were reported as 53 years and 58.5 years for men and women, respectively [174].

Life expectancy in SCD is substantially reduced especially in those with severe disease. In a 10-year retrospective study reported in 2009 from Ilorin, Nigeria, by Chijioke and Kolo, the mean age of sickle cell anaemia patients was found to be 23 years compared to 40 years in the control population, suggesting reduced life expectancy [175]. Findings from that study also revealed that age correlated negatively with survival [175]. As recently reported by Ogun et al., the leading causes of mortality in Nigerian SCD patients include infections, acute chest syndrome, anaemia, acute sequestration crisis, and stroke. According to the study, the mean age at death was 21.3 years. Though some patients now attain fifth decade, most mortality occurs in their second and third decades of life [83].

9. Sickle Cell Disease Control and Current Challenges in Nigeria

Control of SCD begins with public education and definite strategies to prevent further transmission of the trait. Carrier detection and genetic counseling have been proven to be successful in curbing the spread of other haemoglobinopathies like thalassaemia [176]. Carrier detection should be offered at designated centres after proper genetic counselling through antenatal and newborn screening, couple/premarital screening, and other forms of population screening. Genetic counselling by trained personnel helps individuals at risk to take informed decisions about their reproductive life choices. The option of prenatal diagnosis and selective abortion in Nigeria is controversial and relatively unavailable. Local studies show that a significant proportion of Nigerians are averse to selective abortion, even if legally permitted [177–179]. Early detection and diagnosis of sickle cell disease is crucial to reducing mortality and mortality associated with sickle cell disease, as affected persons are offered early supportive and preventive treatments. Despite the huge burden of SCD, currently, there is lack of national or regional SCD newborn screening programme in Nigeria, as at the time of this publication. Specialized centers dedicated to care of SCD patients with requisite multidisciplinary teams and other facilities are grossly absent. Ideally, SCD infants diagnosed prenatally or through newborn screening should be routed to comprehensive SCD centers for optimal treatment [180]. Conversely, Nigerian SCD is still associated with delayed diagnosis [181].

Continuous training of healthcare professionals involved in care of SCD patients is also desirable. Further efforts should be directed at education of the patients and their parents or caregivers. The health caregivers should also constantly undergo professional refresher and update courses in order to optimize their knowledge and skills in care of SCD. Recent surveys still suggest a dearth of public health knowledge on sickle cell disease in Nigeria [182]. Despite Nigeria being the most populous black nation on earth with the highest burden of sickle cell disease, till now, there are no coordinated nationwide efforts aimed at controlling the disease. Current evidence suggests that the care available for patients with SCD in Nigeria is still suboptimal [183]. Secondary control measures such as chronic transfusion therapy and use of hydroxyurea are faced with peculiar challenges in developing nations such as Nigeria [89]. Such challenges include unavailability of blood and blood components, the need for patients and relatives to regularly source for blood and blood donors, cost of iron chelation, risk of transfusion transmissible infections, and overall cost of chronic blood transfusion [73, 89]. A recent study estimated the mean annual cost of hypertransfusion in Ibadan among paediatric SCD patient to be 3,276 US Dollars (SD = 1,168) [73]. Also, treatment of iron overload with metal chelators, which is a potentially inevitable complication of chronic transfusion, increases cost.

Furthermore, HSCT, which is the only potentially curative disease modifying intervention in sickle cell disease, is currently available in Nigeria and has been reported [171]. However, its practice is bewildered by ample challenges including poor government commitment, weak political will, poor infrastructure, unaffordability by the average eligible Nigerian SCD patient, lack of local bone marrow registries, absence of specialized molecular diagnostic laboratories, and epileptic electric power supply [184, 185].

10. Comprehensive Care in Sickle Cell Disease and Recommendations in Nigeria

Comprehensive care incorporates provision of holistic health-care services including state-of-the-art diagnosis, standard therapies, preventive care, rehabilitative therapy, and other ancillary services, by a team of specialists in a given location, with maximum accessibility for all patients. Comprehensive sickle cell centers are grossly lacking in Nigeria. Holistic care has been shown to provide better outcomes in sickle cell disease evidenced by significant reduction in mortality, hospitalizations, and blood transfusion rates among Nigerian patients [186]. As well, WHO recommends that in areas where hemoglobin disorders are common, special dedicated centers with a high degree of autonomy are required in appropriate numbers and locations, with a high degree of autonomy [187]. Treatment of SCD requires a multispecialist team including professionals such as hematologist, pediatrician, orthopedic surgeons, plastic surgeons, ophthalmologists, nephrologist, specialist nurses, clinical psychologists, and social workers.

Provision of comprehensive health centers is crucial to improving SCD disease outcomes in Nigeria. At such facilities, treatment should be tailored to individual patient's needs. At diagnosis, proper education regarding the nature of the disease, possible complications, and its prevention and treatment should be offered to the patient and parents. Regular health maintenance visits should be scheduled and patients should be counseled on the need for adherence [188]. Compliance on the part of the patient depends on having adequate information on the disease and confidence in the health professionals. Similarly, timely and regular medical education should be provided to health care professionals involved in management of SCD in order to improve their expertise and skills. Also, establishment of support groups among patients is encouraged.

Comprehensive care centers must possess facilities for outpatient care, day-case admissions (day hospital services), and hospitalizations on a 24-hour basis [52]. Patients should have direct access (including phone contact) to such centers and their physicians. For acute complications and emergencies, a quick triage is carried out and prompt therapy is instituted. Standard protocols should be provided for management of specific complications, as well as general health maintenance. Scheduled review and strict adherence to protocols are advised.

Patients and parents should be counseled on avoidance of known precipitants of sickle cell crisis. Keeping a diary of pain episodes is helpful in identifying and avoiding triggers for pain crisis. Infections especially malaria have been reported as a major precipitant of sickle cell crisis among Nigerian patients. As such, vector control and chemoprophylaxis for malaria is recommended in all patients [189]. All forms of undue physical exertion or exhaustion should be discouraged. Mothers should be regularly reminded about routine national vaccination schedule as well as vaccination against organisms to which SCD children and adults are particularly susceptible, especially encapsulated organisms.

Adequate and regular hydration is important. At least 60–70 mL/kg of oral fluids or at least $1.5 L/m^2$ every 24 hours is recommended [45, 187]. Hydration helps with haemodilution, which reduces the propensity for sickling and vasoocclusion. Regular hydration also prevents dehydration which they are prone to due to impaired concentrating ability of the kidneys. Exercise caution with fluid administration especially in those with renal disease or severe anaemia. Excessive fluids may precipitate pulmonary oedema and death.

Moreover, physicians should administer, monitor, and encourage patient's compliance with routine medications at follow-up visits. Routine medications include prophylactic antimalarial [190] and folic acid. Others may include antioxidants, aspirin, and prophylactic antibiotic (oral penicillin from 2-3 months of life until at least age 5 in areas where pneumococcal infection is prevalent). Malaria has been described as one of the major precipitants of VOC for patients in Malaria endemic regions including Nigeria, hence the rationale behind continuous life-long chemoprophylaxis [190–192]. However, according to a local study, no significant benefit or advantage was associated with routine chemoprophylaxis for malaria in SCD patients as both patients and controls had equal rates of asymptomatic parasitaemia and similar frequency of malarial attacks [193]. In Nigeria, the actual benefits of malaria chemoprophylaxis in SCD need to be clarified through further research.

Early institution of broad spectrum antibiotics is recommended in febrile SCD patients [187]. Antibiotic use should be guided by local bacteriological profile and should be commenced after necessary bacterial cultures are taken. A switch to appropriate antibiotic is based on sensitivity pattern of the offending isolate especially if the fever is persistent (unresponsive to the former antibiotic).

11. Disease Modifying Therapies

11.1. Hydroxyurea Therapy. Currently, hydroxyurea (HU) is the only approved disease modifying drug in SCD used for selected patients above 24 months of age [194]. HU is a cytotoxic agent that has been mainly used in treatment of CML and other myeloproliferative disorders. Its usefulness in SCD is related to its ability to induce increased levels of fetal haemoglobin production in sickle cells thus mitigating tendencies for red cell sickling. The exact mechanism is not fully understood, but, as a ribonucleotide reductase inhibitor, it prevents formation of deoxyribonucleotides, causing S-phase arrest of all replicating cells, thereby inducing stress erythropoiesis, which favors increased production of fetal haemoglobin [24]. HU is also known to increase steady state haemoglobin levels and reduce leucocyte and platelet counts. Also, as a rheological agent, HU improves cell hydration, limits interaction of the sickle cells with the vascular endothelium, and acts as a nitric oxide donor [195]. HU is of benefit to patients with moderate to severe sickle cell disease. Indications for HU therapy include recurrent VOC (3 or more severe episodes requiring admission in the last 12 months), recurrent ACS (2 or more episodes in a lifetime), severe symptomatic anaemia, and recurrent priapism, alternative to transfusion to prevent new or recurrent stroke especially where transfusion is not feasible [194]. Usually, HU therapy is commenced at 10–15 mg/kg once daily. Baseline investigations prior to commencement of hydroxyurea should include FBC, reticulocyte count, %Hb F, electrolyte urea and creatinine level, liver function test, uric acid, and LDH levels. Full blood counts are monitored weekly for the first 4 weeks, fortnightly for the next 8 weeks, and thereafter monthly if the counts remain stable [14, 194]. Its dose is increased by 2.5 to 5 mg/kg/day every 12 weeks (range of 4 weeks to 6 months) if absolute neutrophil count (ANC) >2000, Haemoglobin concentration >4.5 g/dL, and platelet count >80,000/μL [14, 195]. As marrow suppression occurs, HU is withheld to allow for marrow recovery and then restarted at a dose of 2.5 mg/kg less than dose causing myelosuppression. This is known as the maximum tolerable dose [88, 195]. However, the ceiling dose for HU therapy is 35 mg/kg [151]. Minimum time interval for evaluation of therapeutic efficacy is 6 to 9 months [165]. Hb F levels should be monitored. HbF level in excess of 20% significantly ameliorates the disease. Complications of HU include myelotoxicity, mouth ulceration, macrocytosis and megaloblastoid changes, nausea, skin toxicity rashes, and hyperpigmentation [88, 194].

11.2. Haemopoietic Stem Cell Transplantation (HSCT). Suggested eligibility criteria for HSCT in SCD include the following [196, 197]: (A) age <17 years; (B) at least one of the following complications: brain infarct/ischaemia (MRI), secondary cognitive impairment with cerebral vasculopathy, severe and recurrent ACS, ≥3 VOC per annum requiring hospitalization (>3 Hospitalisations for severe VOC in consecutive 3 to 4 years), moderate glomerular dysfunction, multiple epiphyseal aseptic necrosis, and grade I/II sickle chronic lung disease; (C) availability of HLA matched sibling donor. Exclusion criteria include donor with major haemoglobinopathy and one or more of the following: Karnofsky performance <70%, Portal fibrosis (moderate or severe), renal failure (GFR <30%), major intellectual impairment, stage III or IV chronic sickle lung disease, cardiomyopathy, or HIV infection. Older adults are considered less favorable candidates for HSCT due to the higher risk for severe organ toxicities and greater susceptibility to severe graft versus host disease [198]. HSCT should be performed in centers experienced in transplant for sickle cell disease.

11.3. Future Therapies. Aside from Hydroxyurea, other promising drugs that have been shown to modulate Hb F production but are still under investigation/trials include decitabine, 5-azacytidine, and short chain fatty acids such as butyrates [199, 200]. Other novel therapies are also being investigated. Their therapeutic efficacy is designed based on their targets against specific pathophysiological processes in SCD such as the abnormal membrane cation transport systems, increased/stimulated red cell-endothelial adhesiveness, endothelial activation and vasospasm, cellular dehydration, prooxidant state, and hypercoagulability in SCD. Gardos

channel blockers such as clotrimazole and its analog, Senicapoc (ICA 17043), have been shown to reduce red cell dehydration and abate haemolytic rate and are well tolerated in SCD patients [201, 202]. Administration of magnesium salts is also observed to reduce red cell dehydration by inhibiting the KCL cotransporter. It is reported that infusion of magnesium sulfate reduced the length of hospital stay in patients with VOC [203]. However, this is not yet an established practice. Similarly, antiadhesive agents such as anti-P-selectin and heparin, as well as agents such as warfarin and aspirin for normalization of hypercoagulable state and Flocor for reduction of whole blood viscosity, and specific monoclonal antibodies for inhibition of red cell-endothelial adhesion are also being considered [199]. Inhalational nitric oxide and its precursor, L-arginine, are shown to be beneficial in acute vasoocclusive crisis and other ischaemic complications by increasing NO bioavailability [200, 203].

Theoretically, gene therapy offers a great hope of cure. However, effective vector for safe transfer and stable, erythroid specific expression of normal beta globin gene are still under investigation [204, 205].

12. Conclusion

Sickle cell disease is a major public health disease worldwide. There is still a high burden of the disease in Nigeria. There is still a significantly high rate of SCD complications and mortality among Nigerian patients. Current evidence suggests that available care is suboptimal. Largely speaking, prevention, control, and treatment of SCD in Nigeria are still in infancy. Yester efforts albeit present measures appear meager in the face of the enormous disease burden. There is need for a better coordinated effort towards control of SCD by the government at all levels and other concerned stakeholders. Appropriate interventional programmes backed by an effective national policy should be instituted. In addition, physicians involved in the care of SCD patients should be conversant with current knowledge and standard practices in the treatment of sickle cell disease in order to improve treatment outcomes.

Conflict of Interests

The author declares that there is no conflict of interests regarding the publication of this paper.

References

[1] B. Modell, Ed., *Guidelines for the Control of Haemoglobin Disorders*, WHO, Sardinia, Italy, 1989.

[2] G. R. Serjeant, "Sickle-cell disease," *The Lancet*, vol. 350, no. 9079, pp. 725–730, 1997.

[3] B. Modell and M. Darlison, "Global epidemiology of haemoglobin disorders and derived service indicators," *Bulletin of the World Health Organization*, vol. 86, no. 6, pp. 480–487, 2008.

[4] World Health Organisation 2008, "Management of haemoglobin disorders," in *Proceedings of the Report of Joint WHO-TIF Meeting*, Nicosia, Cyprus, November 2007.

[5] F. B. Piel, A. P. Patil, R. E. Howes et al., "Global epidemiology of Sickle haemoglobin in neonates: a contemporary geostatistical model-based map and population estimates," *The Lancet*, vol. 381, no. 9861, pp. 142–151, 2013.

[6] WHO Regional office for Africa, Sickle cell disease prevention and control, 2013, http://www.afro.who.int/en/nigeria/nigeria-publications/1775-sickle cell disease.html.

[7] G. R. Serjeant and B. E. Serjeant, "The epidemiology of sickle cell disorder: a challenge for Africa," *Archives of Ibadan Medicine*, vol. 2, no. 2, pp. 46–52, 2001.

[8] A. L. Okwi, W. Byarugaba, C. M. Ndugwa, A. Parkes, M. Ocaido, and J. K. Tumwine, "An up-date on the prevalence of sickle cell trait in Eastern and Western Uganda," *BMC Blood Disorders*, vol. 10, article 5, 2010.

[9] A. F. Fleming, J. Storey, L. Molineaux, E. A. Iroko, and E. D. Attai, "Abnormal haemoglobins in the Sudan savanna of Nigeria. I. Prevalence of haemoglobins and relationships between sickle cell trait, malaria and survival," *Annals of Tropical Medicine and Parasitology*, vol. 73, no. 2, pp. 161–172, 1979.

[10] P. N. Uzoegwu and A. E. Onwurah, "Prevalence of haemoglobinopathy and malaria diseases in the population of old Aguata Division, Anambra State, Nigeria," *Biokemistri*, vol. 15, no. 2, pp. 57–66, 2003.

[11] B. Nwogoh, A. S. Adewoyin, O. E. Iheanacho, and G. N. Bazuaye, "Prevalence of haemoglobin variants in Benin City, Nigeria," *Annals of Biomedical Sciences*, vol. 11, no. 2, pp. 60–64, 2012.

[12] J. A. B. Horton, *The Diseases of Tropical Climates and Their Treatment*, Churchill, London, UK, 1874.

[13] J. B. Herrick, "Peculiar elongated and sickle-shaped red blood corpuscles in a case of severe anemia," *Archives of Internal Medicine*, vol. 6, no. 5, pp. 517–521, 1910.

[14] E. Beutler, "Disorders of haemoglobin structure: sickle cell anaemia and related abnormalities," in *Williams Haematology*, M. A. Lichtman and W. J. Williams, Eds., vol. 47, pp. 667–700, McGraw-Hill, New York, NY, USA, 2006.

[15] G. R. Serjeant, "The natural history of sickle cell disease," *Cold Spring Harbor Perspectives in Medicine*, vol. 3, no. 10, Article ID a011783, 2013.

[16] J. Pagnier, J. G. Mears, O. Dunda-Belkhodja et al., "Evidence for the multicentric origin of the sickle cell hemoglobin gene in Africa," *Proceedings of the National Academy of Sciences of the United States of America*, vol. 81, no. 6 I, pp. 1771–1773, 1984.

[17] A. E. Kulozik, J. S. Wainscoat, G. R. Serjeant et al., "Geographical survey of β(S)-globin gene haplotypes: evidence for an independent Asian origin of the sickle-cell mutation," *American Journal of Human Genetics*, vol. 39, no. 2, pp. 239–244, 1986.

[18] C. Lapoumeroulie, O. Dunda, R. Ducrocq et al., "A novel sickle gene of yet another origin in Africa: the Cameroon type," *Human Genetics*, vol. 89, no. 3, pp. 333–337, 1992.

[19] M. H. Steinberg, "Predicting clinical severity in sickle cell anaemia," *British Journal of Haematology*, vol. 129, no. 4, pp. 465–481, 2005.

[20] B. Modell, M. Darlison, H. Birgens et al., "Epidemiology of haemoglobin disorders in Europe: an overview," *Scandinavian Journal of Clinical and Laboratory Investigation*, vol. 67, no. 1, pp. 39–69, 2007.

[21] D. Desai and H. Dhanani, "Sickle cell disease: history and origin," *The Internet Journal of Hematology*, vol. 1, no. 2, 2003.

[22] A. C. Allison, "Protection afforded by sickle-cell trait against subtertian malareal infection," *British Medical Journal*, vol. 1, no. 4857, pp. 290–294, 1954.

[23] C. Madigan and P. Malik, "Pathophysiology and therapy for haemoglobinopathies; Part I: sickle cell disease," *Expert Reviews in Molecular Medicine*, vol. 8, no. 9, pp. 1–23, 2006.

[24] A. Lal and E. P. Vinchinsky, "Sickle cell disease," in *Postgraduate Haematology*, A. V. Hoffbrand, D. Catovsky, E. G. D. Tuddenham, and A. R. Green, Eds., vol. 7, pp. 109–125, Blackwell Publishing, 6th edition, 2011.

[25] M.-H. Odièvre, E. Verger, A. C. Silva-Pinto, and J. Elion, "Pathophysiological insights in sickle cell disease," *Indian Journal of Medical Research*, vol. 134, no. 10, pp. 532–537, 2011.

[26] W. F. Rosse, M. Narla, L. D. Petz, and M. H. Steinberg, "New views of sickle cell disease pathophysiology and treatment," *Haematatogy*, vol. 2000, no. 1, pp. 2–17, 2000.

[27] M. H. Steinberg, "Management of sickle cell disease," *The New England Journal of Medicine*, vol. 340, no. 13, pp. 1021–1030, 1999.

[28] P. S. Frenette, "Sickle cell vasoocclusion: heterotypic, multicellular aggregations driven by leukocyte adhesion," *Microcirculation*, vol. 11, no. 2, pp. 167–177, 2004.

[29] J. E. Brittain and L. V. Parise, "The $\alpha 4 \beta 1$ integrin in sickle cell disease," *Transfusion Clinique et Biologique*, vol. 15, no. 1-2, pp. 19–22, 2008.

[30] J. E. Brittain, J. Han, K. I. Ataga, E. P. Orringer, and L. V. Parise, "Mechanism of CD47-induced $\alpha 4 \beta 1$ integrin activation and adhesion in sickle reticulocytes," *The Journal of Biological Chemistry*, vol. 279, no. 41, pp. 42393–42402, 2004.

[31] J. E. Elion, M. Brun, M. H. Odièvre, C. L. Lapouméroulie, and R. Krishnamoorthy, "Vaso-occlusion in sickle cell anemia: role of interactions between blood cells and endothelium," *Hematology Journal*, vol. 5, no. 3, pp. S195–S198, 2004.

[32] S. G. Ahmed, "The role of infection in the pathogenesis of vaso-occlusive crisis in patients with sickle cell disease," *Mediterranean Journal of Hematology and Infectious Diseases*, vol. 3, no. 1, Article ID e2011028, 2011.

[33] F. Fasola, K. Adedapo, J. Anetor, and M. Kuti, "Total antioxidants status and some hematological values in sickle cell disease patients in steady state," *Journal of the National Medical Association*, vol. 99, no. 8, pp. 891–894, 2007.

[34] M. Westerman, A. Pizzey, J. Hirschman et al., "Microvesicles in haemoglobinopathies offer insights into mechanisms of hypercoagulability, haemolysis and the effects of therapy," *British Journal of Haematology*, vol. 142, no. 1, pp. 126–135, 2008.

[35] S. D. Roseff, "Sickle cell disease: a review," *Immunohematology*, vol. 25, no. 2, pp. 67–74, 2009.

[36] M. M. Hsieh, J. F. Tisdale, and G. P. Rodgers, "Haemolytic anaemia: thalassemias and sickle cell disorders," in *The Bethesda Handbook of Clinical Haematology*, G. P. Rodgers and N. S. Young, Eds., vol. 4, pp. 37–56, Lippincott Williams & Wilkins, Philadelphia, Pa, USA, 3rd edition, 2013.

[37] P. S. Frenette and G. F. Atweh, "Sickle cell disease: old discoveries, new concepts, and future promise," *The Journal of Clinical Investigation*, vol. 117, no. 4, pp. 850–858, 2007.

[38] R. P. Hebbel, R. Osarogiagbon, and D. Kaul, "The endothelial biology of sickle cell disease: inflammation and a chronic vasculopathy," *Microcirculation*, vol. 11, no. 2, pp. 129–151, 2004.

[39] G. J. Kato, M. T. Gladwin, and M. H. Steinberg, "Deconstructing sickle cell disease: reappraisal of the role of hemolysis in the development of clinical subphenotypes," *Blood Reviews*, vol. 21, no. 1, pp. 37–47, 2007.

[40] T. M. Walker, D. T. Dunn, and G. R. Serjeant, "The metacarpal index in homozygous sickle-cell disease," *British Journal of Radiology*, vol. 61, no. 724, pp. 280–281, 1988.

[41] N. C. G. Stevens, R. J. Hayes, and G. R. Serjeant, "Body shape in young children with homozygous sickle cell disease," *Pediatrics*, vol. 71, no. 4, pp. 610–614, 1983.

[42] F. A. Oredugba and K. O. Savage, "Anthropometric finding in Nigerian children with sickle cell disease," *Pediatric Dentistry*, vol. 24, no. 4, pp. 321–325, 2002.

[43] O. S. Platt, B. D. Thorington, D. J. Brambilla et al., "Pain in sickle cell disease: rates and risk factors," *The New England Journal of Medicine*, vol. 325, no. 1, pp. 11–16, 1991.

[44] V. Vijay, J. D. Cavenagh, and P. Yate, "The anaesthetist's role in acute sickle cell crisis," *British Journal of Anaesthesia*, vol. 80, no. 6, pp. 820–828, 1998.

[45] S. Delicou and K. Maragkos, "Pain management in patients with Sickle cell disease—a review," *European Medical Journal*, vol. 1, pp. 30–36, 2013.

[46] S. K. Ballas, "Current issues in sickle cell pain and its management," *ASH Education Book*, vol. 2007, no. 1, pp. 97–105, 2007.

[47] S. H. Yale, N. Nagib, and T. Guthrie, "Approach to the vaso-occlusive crisis in adults with sickle cell disease," *American Family Physician*, vol. 61, no. 5, pp. 1349–1356, 2000.

[48] I. Okpala and A. Tawil, "Management of pain in sickle-cell disease," *Journal of the Royal Society of Medicine*, vol. 95, no. 9, pp. 456–458, 2002.

[49] L. R. Solomon, "Pain management in adults with sickle cell disease in a medical center emergency department," *Journal of the National Medical Association*, vol. 102, no. 11, pp. 1025–1032, 2010.

[50] D. C. Rees, A. D. Olujohungbe, N. E. Parker, A. D. Stephens, P. Telfer, and J. Wright, "Guidelines for the management of the acute painful crisis in sickle cell disease," *British Journal of Haematology*, vol. 120, no. 5, pp. 744–752, 2003.

[51] S. C. Davies and M. Brozovic, "The presentation, management and prophylaxis of sickle cell disease," *Blood Reviews*, vol. 3, no. 1, pp. 29–44, 1989.

[52] A. H. Adewoye, V. Nolan, L. McMahon, Q. Ma, and M. H. Steinberg, "Effectiveness of a dedicated day hospital for management of acute sickle cell pain," *Haematologica*, vol. 92, no. 6, article 854, 2007.

[53] L. J. Benjamin, G. I. Swinson, and R. L. Nagel, "Sickle cell anemia day hospital: an approach for the management of uncomplicated painful crises," *Blood*, vol. 95, no. 4, pp. 1130–1137, 2000.

[54] M. A. Ware, I. Hambleton, I. Ochaya, and G. Serjeant, "Day-care management of sickle cell painful crisis in Jamaica: a model applicable elsewhere?" *British Journal of Haematology*, vol. 104, no. 1, pp. 93–96, 1999.

[55] K. L. Hassell, J. R. Eckman, and P. A. Lane, "Acute multiorgan failure syndrome: a potentially catastrophic complication of severe sickle cell pain episodes," *The American Journal of Medicine*, vol. 96, no. 2, pp. 155–162, 1994.

[56] T. S. Akingbola, B. Kolude, E. C. Aneni et al., "Abdominal pain in adult sickle cell disease patients: a Nigerian experience," *Annals of Ibadan Postgraduate Medicine*, vol. 9, no. 2, pp. 100–104, 2011.

[57] N. O. Akinola, R. A. Bolarinwa, and A. F. Faponle, "The import of abdominal pain in adults with sickle cell disorder," *West African Journal of Medicine*, vol. 28, no. 2, pp. 83–86, 2009.

[58] E. C. Ebert, M. Nagar, and K. D. Hagspiel, "Gastrointestinal and hepatic complications of sickle cell disease," *Clinical Gastroenterology and Hepatology*, vol. 8, no. 6, pp. 483–489, 2010.

[59] F. Galacteros and M. de Montalembert, "Sickle cell disease: a short guide to management," in *ESH Handbook on Disorders of Erythropoiesis, Erythrocytes and Iron Metabolism*, C. Beaumont, P. Beris, Y. Beuzard, and C. Brugnara, Eds., vol. 13, pp. 276–309, 2009.

[60] M. E. Odunvbun and A. A. Adeyekun, "Ultrasonic assessment of the prevalence of gall stones in sickle cell disease children seen at the University of Benin Teaching Hospital, Benin City, Nigeria," *Nigerian Journal of Paediatrics*, vol. 41, no. 4, pp. 370–374, 2014.

[61] C. A. Agholor, A. O. Akhigbe, and O. M. Atalabi, "The prevalence of cholelithiasis in Nigerians with sickle cell disease as diagnosed by ultrasound," *British Journal of Medicine and Medical Research*, vol. 4, no. 15, pp. 2866–2873, 2014.

[62] National Heart and Lung and Blood Institute, *The Management of Sickle Cell Disease*, NIH Publication 02-2117, National Institutes of Health, 2002.

[63] M. C. Iheanacho, A. S. Akanmu, and B. Nwogoh, "Seroprevalence of human parvovirus B19 antibody in paediatric sickle cell disease patients seen at the Lagos University Teaching Hospital," *Annals of Biomedical Sciences*, vol. 13, no. 1, pp. 123–129, 2014.

[64] "Genetic disorders of haemoglobin," in *Essential Haematology*, A. V. Hoffbrand, P. A. H. Moss, and J. E. Pettit, Eds., vol. 6, pp. 72–93, Blackwell Publishing, Southampton, UK, 5th edition, 2006.

[65] A. Akinbami, A. Dosunmu, A. Adediran et al., "Steady state hemoglobin concentration and packed cell volume in homozygous sickle cell disease patients in Lagos, Nigeria," *Caspian Journal of Internal Medicine*, vol. 3, no. 2, pp. 405–409, 2012.

[66] R. J. Adams, V. C. Mckie, L. H. Su et al., "Prevention of a first stroke by transfusions in children with sickle cell anemia and abnormal results on transcranial Doppler ultrasonography," *The New England Journal of Medicine*, vol. 339, pp. 5–11, 1998.

[67] O. S. Platt, "Preventing stroke in sickle cell anemia," *The New England Journal of Medicine*, vol. 353, no. 26, pp. 2743–2745, 2005.

[68] R. E. Ware, S. A. Zimmerman, and W. H. Schultz, "Hydroxyurea as an alternative to blood transfusions for the prevention of recurrent stroke in children with sickle cell disease," *Blood*, vol. 94, no. 9, pp. 3022–3026, 1999.

[69] I. O. George and A. I. Frank-Biggs, "Stroke in Nigerian children with sickle cell anaemia," *Journal of Public Health and Epidemiology*, vol. 3, no. 9, pp. 407–409, 2011.

[70] O. Oniyangi, P. Ahmed, O. T. Otuneye et al., "Strokes in children with sickle cell disease at the National Hospital, Abuja, Nigeria," *Nigerian Journal of Paediatrics*, vol. 40, no. 2, pp. 158–164, 2013.

[71] A. Ferster, P. Tahriri, C. Vermylen et al., "Five years of experience with hydroxyurea in children and young adults with sickle cell disease," *Blood*, vol. 97, no. 11, pp. 3628–3632, 2001.

[72] D. Powars, B. Wilson, C. Imbus, C. Pegelow, and J. Allen, "The natural history of stroke in sickle cell disease," *The American Journal of Medicine*, vol. 65, no. 3, pp. 461–471, 1978.

[73] I. A. Lagunju, B. J. Brown, and O. O. Sodeinde, "Chronic blood transfusion for primary and secondary stroke prevention in Nigerian children with sickle cell disease: a 5-year appraisal," *Pediatric Blood and Cancer*, vol. 60, no. 12, pp. 1940–1945, 2013.

[74] S. T. Miller, E. Wright, M. Abboud et al., "Impact of chronic transfusion on incidence of pain and acute chest syndrome during the Stroke Prevention Trial (STOP) in sickle-cell anemia," *The Journal of Pediatrics*, vol. 139, no. 6, pp. 785–789, 2001.

[75] T. L. McCavit, L. Xuan, S. Zhang, G. Flores, and C. T. Quinn, "National trends in incidence rates of hospitalization for stroke in children with sickle cell disease," *Pediatric Blood & Cancer*, vol. 60, no. 5, pp. 823–827, 2013.

[76] J. J. Strouse, S. Lanzkron, and V. Urrutia, "The epidemiology, evaluation and treatment of stroke in adults with sickle cell disease," *Expert Review of Hematology*, vol. 4, no. 6, pp. 597–606, 2011.

[77] W. C. Wang, "The pathophysiology, prevention, and treatment of stroke in sickle cell disease," *Current Opinion in Hematology*, vol. 14, no. 3, pp. 191–197, 2007.

[78] M. R. Mayberg, H. H. Batjer, R. Dacey et al., "Guidelines for the management of aneurysmal subarachnoid hemorrhage," *Stroke*, vol. 25, no. 11, pp. 231–232, 1994.

[79] O. S. Platt, "Prevention and management of stroke in sickle cell anemia," *Hematology*, pp. 54–57, 2006.

[80] M. R. DeBaun, F. D. Armstrong, R. C. McKinstry, R. E. Ware, E. Vichinsky, and F. J. Kirkham, "Silent cerebral infarcts: a review on a prevalent and progressive cause of neurologic injury in sickle cell anemia," *Blood*, vol. 119, no. 20, pp. 4587–4596, 2012.

[81] M. R. DeBaun, J. Schatz, M. J. Siegel et al., "Cognitive screening examinations for silent cerebral infarcts in sickle cell disease," *Neurology*, vol. 50, no. 6, pp. 1678–1682, 1998.

[82] S. T. Miller, E. A. Macklin, C. H. Pegelow et al., "Silent infarction as a risk factor for overt stroke in children with sickle cell anemia: a report from the cooperative study of sickle cell disease," *Journal of Pediatrics*, vol. 139, no. 3, pp. 385–390, 2001.

[83] G. O. Ogun, H. Ebili, and T. R. Kotila, "Autopsy findings and pattern of mortality in Nigerian sickle cell disease patients," *The Pan African Medical Journal*, vol. 18, article 30, 2014.

[84] O. S. Platt, D. J. Brambilla, W. F. Rosse et al., "Mortality in sickle cell disease. Life expectancy and risk factors for early death," *The New England Journal of Medicine*, vol. 330, no. 23, pp. 1639–1644, 1994.

[85] A. Gray, E. N. Anionwu, S. C. Davies, and M. Brozovic, "Patterns of mortality in sickle cell disease in the United Kingdom," *Journal of Clinical Pathology*, vol. 44, no. 6, pp. 459–463, 1991.

[86] R. N. Paul, O. L. Castro, A. Aggarwal, and P. A. Oneal, "Acute chest syndrome: sickle cell disease," *European Journal of Haematology*, vol. 87, no. 3, pp. 191–207, 2011.

[87] P. S. Bellet, K. A. Kalinyak, R. Shukla, M. J. Gelfand, and D. L. Rucknagel, "Incentive spirometry to prevent acute pulmonary complications in sickle cell diseases," *The New England Journal of Medicine*, vol. 333, no. 11, pp. 699–703, 1995.

[88] S. Charache, M. L. Terrin, R. D. Moore et al., "Effect of hydroxyurea on the frequency of painful crises in Sickle cell anemia," *The New England Journal of Medicine*, vol. 332, no. 20, pp. 1317–1322, 1995.

[89] A. S. Adewoyin and J. C. Obieche, "Hypertransfusion therapy in sickle cell disease in Nigeria," *Advances in Hematology*, vol. 2014, Article ID 923593, 8 pages, 2014.

[90] G. M. Crane and N. E. Bennett, "Priapism in sickle cell anemia: emerging mechanistic understanding and better preventative strategies," *Anemia*, vol. 2011, Article ID 297364, 6 pages, 2011.

[91] B. Nwogoh, A. Adewoyin, G. N. Bazuaye, and I. A. Nwannadi, "Prevalence of priapism among male sickle cell disease patients at the University of Benin Teaching Hospital, Benin City," *Nigerian Medical Practitioner*, vol. 65, no. 1-2, pp. 3–7, 2014.

[92] E. M. Isoa, "Current trends in the management of sickle cell disease: an overview," *Benin Journal of Postgraduate Medicine*, vol. 11, no. 1, pp. 50–64, 2009.

[93] R. Virag, D. Bachir, K. Lee, and F. Galacteros, "Preventive treatment of priapism in sickle cell disease with oral and self-administered intracavernous injection of etilefrine," *Urology*, vol. 47, no. 5, pp. 777–781, 1996.

[94] M. McDonald and R. A. Santucci, "Successful management of stuttering priapism using home self-injections of the alpha-agonist metaraminol," *International Braz J Urol*, vol. 30, no. 2, pp. 121–122, 2004.

[95] C. Teloken, E. P. Ribeiro, M. Chammas Jr., P. E. Teloken, and C. A. V. Souto, "Intracavernosal etilefrine self-injection therapy for recurrent priapism: one decade of follow-up," *Urology*, vol. 65, no. 5, p. 1002, 2005.

[96] J. Cherian, A. R. Rao, A. Thwaini, F. Kapasi, I. S. Shergill, and R. Samman, "Medical and surgical management of priapism," *Postgraduate Medical Journal*, vol. 82, no. 964, pp. 89–94, 2006.

[97] G. J. Kato, "Priapism in sickle-cell disease: a hematologist's perspective," *The Journal of Sexual Medicine*, vol. 9, no. 1, pp. 70–78, 2012.

[98] A. D. Gbadoé, Y. Atakouma, K. Kusiaku, and J. K. Assimadi, "Management of sickle cell priapism with etilefrine," *Archives of Disease in Childhood*, vol. 85, no. 1, pp. 52–53, 2001.

[99] G. R. Serjeant, K. De Ceulaer, and G. H. Maude, "Stilboestrol and stuttering priapism in homozygous sickle-cell disease," *The Lancet*, vol. 2, no. 8467, pp. 1274–1276, 1985.

[100] A. L. Burnett, U. A. Anele, I. N. Trueheart, J. J. Strouss, and J. F. Casella, "Randomised Clinical Trial of sildenafil for preventing recurrent ischaemic priapism in Sickle cell disease," *American Journal of Medicine*, vol. 127, no. 7, pp. 664–668, 2014.

[101] A. Lane and R. Deveras, "Potential risks of chronic sildenafil use for priapism in sickle cell disease," *The Journal of Sexual Medicine*, vol. 8, no. 11, pp. 3193–3195, 2011.

[102] P. M. Pierorazio, T. J. Bivalacqua, and A. L. Burnett, "Daily phosphodiesterase type 5 inhibitor therapy as rescue for recurrent ischemic priapism after failed androgen ablation," *Journal of Andrology*, vol. 32, no. 4, pp. 371–374, 2011.

[103] L. Douglas, H. Fletcher, and G. R. Serjeant, "Penile prostheses in the management of impotence in sickle cell disease," *British Journal of Urology*, vol. 65, no. 5, pp. 533–535, 1990.

[104] A. Mallouh and Y. Talab, "Bone and joint infection in patients with sickle cell disease," *Journal of Pediatric Orthopaedics*, vol. 5, no. 2, pp. 158–162, 1985.

[105] A. Almeida and I. Roberts, "Bone involvement in sickle cell disease," *British Journal of Haematology*, vol. 129, no. 4, pp. 482–490, 2005.

[106] W. W. Ebong, "Acute osteomyelitis in Nigerians with sickle cell disease," *Annals of the Rheumatic Diseases*, vol. 45, no. 11, pp. 911–915, 1986.

[107] M. Sadat-Ali, "The status of acute osteomyelitis in sickle cell disease. A 15 year review," *International Surgery*, vol. 83, no. 1, pp. 84–87, 1998.

[108] M. W. Burnett, J. W. Bass, and B. A. Cook, "Etiology of osteomyelitis complicating sickle cell disease," *Pediatrics*, vol. 101, no. 2, pp. 296–297, 1998.

[109] E. M. Barden, D. A. Kawchak, K. Ohene-Frempong, V. A. Stallings, and B. S. Zemel, "Body composition in children with sickle cell disease," *The American Journal of Clinical Nutrition*, vol. 76, no. 1, pp. 218–225, 2002.

[110] C. Booth, B. Inusa, and S. K. Obaro, "Infection in sickle cell disease: a review," *International Journal of Infectious Diseases*, vol. 14, no. 1, pp. e2–e12, 2010.

[111] F. Rahim, "The sickle cell disease," Haematology Updates, 2010.

[112] N. B. Halasa, S. M. Shankar, T. R. Talbot et al., "Incidence of invasive pneumococcal disease among individuals with sickle cell disease before and after the introduction of the pneumococcal conjugate vaccine," *Clinical Infectious Diseases*, vol. 44, no. 11, pp. 1428–1433, 2007.

[113] O. Akinyanju and A. O. Johnson, "Acute illness in Nigerian children with sickle cell anaemia," *Annals of Tropical Paediatrics*, vol. 7, no. 3, pp. 181–186, 1987.

[114] H. O. Okuonghae, M. U. Nwankwo, and E. C. Offor, "Pattern of bacteraemia in febrile children with sickle cell anaemia," *Annals of Tropical Paediatrics*, vol. 13, no. 1, pp. 55–64, 1993.

[115] S. Obaro, "Pneumococcal infections and sickle cell disease in Africa: does absence of evidence imply evidence of absence?" *Archives of Disease in Childhood*, vol. 94, no. 9, pp. 713–716, 2009.

[116] J. A. Berkley, B. S. Lowe, I. Mwangi et al., "Bacteremia among children admitted to a rural hospital in Kenya," *The New England Journal of Medicine*, vol. 352, no. 1, pp. 39–47, 2005.

[117] A. Roca, B. Sigaúque, L. Quintó et al., "Invasive pneumococcal disease in children >5 years of age in rural Mozambique," *Tropical Medicine and International Health*, vol. 11, no. 9, pp. 1422–1431, 2006.

[118] T. N. Williams, S. Uyoga, A. Macharia et al., "Bacteraemia in Kenyan children with sickle-cell anaemia: a retrospective cohort and case-control study," *The Lancet*, vol. 374, no. 9698, pp. 1364–1370, 2009.

[119] National Immunization Policy Nigeria, "National primary health care development agency 2013," 2014.

[120] P. J. Fraker, L. E. King, T. Laakko, and T. L. Vollmer, "The dynamic link between the integrity of the immune system and zinc status," *Journal of Nutrition*, vol. 130, supplement 5, pp. S1399–S1406, 2000.

[121] E. O. Temiye, E. S. Duke, M. A. Owolabi, and J. K. Renner, "Relationship between painful crisis and serum zinc level in children with sickle cell anaemia," *Anemia*, vol. 2011, Article ID 698586, 7 pages, 2011.

[122] B. O. Idonije, O. I. Iribhogbe, and G. R. A. Okogun, "Serum trace element levels in sickle cell disease patients in an urban city in Nigeria," *Nature and Science*, vol. 9, no. 3, pp. 67–71, 2011.

[123] O. G. Arinola, J. A. Olaniyi, and M. O. Akiibinu, "Evaluation of antioxidant levels and trace element status in Nigerian sickle cell disease patients with Plasmodium parasitaemia," *Pakistan Journal of Nutrition*, vol. 7, no. 6, pp. 766–769, 2008.

[124] E. S. Klings, D. F. Wyszynski, V. G. Nolan, and M. H. Steinberg, "Abnormal pulmonary function in adults with sickle cell anemia," *American Journal of Respiratory and Critical Care Medicine*, vol. 173, no. 11, pp. 1264–1269, 2006.

[125] A. O. Dosunmu, T. M. Balogun, O. O. Adeyeye et al., "Prevalence of pulmonary hypertension in sickle cell anaemia patients of a tertiary hospital in Nigeria," *Nigerian Medical Journal*, vol. 55, no. 2, pp. 161–165, 2014.

[126] A. O. Dosunmu, R. A. Akinola, J. A. Onakoya et al., "Pattern of chronic lung lesions in adults with sickle cell disease in Lagos, Nigeria," *Caspian Journal of Internal Medicine*, vol. 4, no. 4, pp. 754–758, 2013.

[127] A. E. Fawibe, "Sickle cell chronic pulmonary disease among Africans: the need for increased recognition and treatment," *African Journal of Respiratory Medicine*, pp. 13–16, 2008.

[128] M. T. Gladwin, V. Sachdev, M. L. Jison et al., "Pulmonary hypertension as a risk factor for death in patients with sickle cell disease," *The New England Journal of Medicine*, vol. 350, no. 9, pp. 886–895, 2004.

[129] H. Issa and A. H. Al-Salem, "Hepatobiliary manifestations of sickle cell anemia," *Gastroenterology Research*, vol. 3, no. 1, pp. 1–8, 2010.

[130] F. A. Fashola and I. A. Otegbayo, "Post transfusion viral hepatitis in sickle cell anaemia: retrospective—prospective analysis," *Nigerian Journal of Clinical Practice*, vol. 5, no. 1, pp. 16–19, 2002.

[131] E. U. Ejeliogu, S. N. Okolo, S. D. Pam, E. S. Okpe, C. C. John, and M. O. Ochoga, "Is human immunodeficiency virus still transmissible through blood transfusion in children with sickle cell anaemia in Jos, Nigeria?" *The British Journal of Medicine and Medical Research*, vol. 4, no. 21, pp. 3912–3923, 2014.

[132] G. O. Ogunrinde, R. O. Zubair, S. M. Mado, S. Musa, and L. W. Umar, "Prevalence of nocturnal enuresis in children with homozygous sickle cell disease in zaria," *Nigerian Journal of Paediatrics*, vol. 34, pp. 31–35, 2007.

[133] A. Abdu, M. Emokpae, P. Uadia, and A. Kuliya-Gwarzo, "Proteinuria among adult sickle cell anemia patients in Nigeria," *Annals of African Medicine*, vol. 10, no. 1, pp. 34–37, 2011.

[134] J. C. Aneke, A. O. Adegoke, A. A. Oyekunle et al., "Degrees of kidney disease in Nigerian adults with sickle-cell disease," *Medical Principles and Practice*, vol. 23, no. 3, pp. 271–274, 2014.

[135] C. C. Sharpe and S. L. Thein, "How I treat renal complications in sickle cell disease," *Blood*, vol. 123, no. 24, pp. 3720–3726, 2014.

[136] K. I. Ataga and E. P. Orringer, "Renal abnormalities in sickle cell disease," *American Journal of Hematology*, vol. 63, pp. 205–211, 2000.

[137] P. I. Condon and G. R. Serjeant, "Ocular findings in homozygous sickle cell anemia in Jamaica," *The American Journal of Ophthalmology*, vol. 73, no. 4, pp. 533–543, 1972.

[138] M. Koshy, R. Entsuah, A. Koranda et al., "Leg ulcers in patients with sickle cell disease," *Blood*, vol. 74, no. 4, pp. 1403–1408, 1989.

[139] G. N. Bazuaye, A. I. Nwannadi, and E. E. Olayemi, "Leg Ulcers in Adult sickle cell disease patients in Benin City, Nigeria," *Gomal Journal of Medical Sciences*, vol. 8, no. 2, pp. 190–194, 2010.

[140] R. A. Balogun, D. C. Obalum, S. O. Giwa, T. O. Adekoya-Cole, C. N. Ogo, and G. O. Enweluzo, "Spectrum of musculo-skeletal disorders in sickle cell disease in Lagos, Nigeria," *Journal of Orthopaedic Surgery and Research*, vol. 5, article 2, 2010.

[141] P. Hernigou, A. Habibi, D. Bachir, and F. Galacteros, "The natural history of asymptomatic osteonecrosis of the femoral head in adults with sickle cell disease," *Journal of Bone and Joint Surgery—Series A*, vol. 88, no. 12, pp. 2565–2572, 2006.

[142] A. J. Madu, A. K. Madu, G. K. Umar, K. Ibekwe, A. Duru, and A. O. Ugwu, "Avascular necrosis in sickle cell (homozygous S) patients: predictive clinical and laboratory indices," *Nigerian Journal of Clinical Practice*, vol. 17, no. 1, pp. 86–89, 2014.

[143] H. Hawker, H. Neilson, R. J. Hayes, and G. R. Serjeant, "Haematological factors associated with avascular necrosis of the femoral head in homozygous sickle cell disease," *British Journal of Haematology*, vol. 50, no. 1, pp. 29–34, 1982.

[144] M. Mukisi-Mukaza, A. Elbaz, Y. Samuel-Leborgne et al., "Prevalence, clinical features, and risk factors of osteonecrosis of the femoral head among adults with sickle cell disease," *Orthopedics*, vol. 23, no. 4, pp. 357–363, 2000.

[145] A. D. Adekile, R. Gupta, F. Yacoub, T. Sinan, M. Al-Bloushi, and M. Z. Haider, "Avascular necrosis of the hip in children with sickle cell disease and high Hb F: magnetic resonance imaging findings and influence of α-thalassemia trait," *Acta Haematologica*, vol. 105, no. 1, pp. 27–31, 2001.

[146] "Sickle cell disease in childhood. Standards and guidelines for clinical care," UK Forum on Haemoglobin Disorders, 2010.

[147] M. T. Gladwin and V. Sachdev, "Cardiovascular abnormalities in sickle cell disease," *Journal of the American College of Cardiology*, vol. 59, no. 13, pp. 1123–1133, 2012.

[148] N. I. Oguanobi, E. C. Ejim, B. C. Anisiuba et al., "Clinical and electrocardiographic evaluation of sickle-cell anaemia patients with pulmonary hypertension," *ISRN Hematology*, vol. 2012, Article ID 768718, 6 pages, 2012.

[149] B. Otaigbe, "Prevalence of blood transfusion in sickle cell anaemia patients in South-South Nigeria: a two-year experience," *International Journal of Biological and Medical Research*, vol. 1, no. 1, pp. 13–18, 2013.

[150] H. H. Al-Saeed and A. H. Al-Salem, "Principles of blood transfusion in sickle cell anemia," *Saudi Medical Journal*, vol. 23, no. 12, pp. 1443–1448, 2002.

[151] Z. Y. Aliyu, A. R. Tumblin, and G. J. Kato, "Current therapy of sickle cell disease," *Haematologica*, vol. 91, no. 1, pp. 7–11, 2006.

[152] N. Win, "Blood transfusion therapy for Haemoglobinopathies," in *Practical Management of Haemoglobinopathies*, I. E. Okpala, Ed., pp. 99–106, Blackwell Publishing, 2004.

[153] C. D. Josephson, L. L. Su, K. L. Hillyer, and C. D. Hillyer, "Transfusion in the patient with sickle cell disease: a critical review of the literature and transfusion guidelines," *Transfusion Medicine Reviews*, vol. 21, no. 2, pp. 118–133, 2007.

[154] E. P. Vinchinsky, "Transfusion therapy in sickle cell disease," 2014, http://sickle.bwh.harvard.edu/transfusion.html.

[155] J. L. Levenson, "Psychiatric issues in adults with sickle cell disease," *Primary Psychiatry*, vol. 15, no. 5, pp. 45–49, 2008.

[156] K. A. Anie, F. E. Egunjobi, and O. O. Akinyanju, "Psychosocial impact of sickle cell disorder: perspectives from a Nigerian setting," *Globalization and Health*, vol. 6, article 2, 2010.

[157] C. Hilton, M. Osborn, S. Knight, A. Singhal, and G. Serjeant, "Psychiatric complications of homozygous sickle cell disease among young adults in the Jamaican cohort study," *The British Journal of Psychiatry*, vol. 170, pp. 69–76, 1997.

[158] V. J. Rappaport, M. Velazquez, and K. Williams, "Hemoglobinopathies in pregnancy," *Obstetrics and Gynecology Clinics of North America*, vol. 31, no. 2, pp. 287–317, 2004.

[159] R. P. Naik and S. Lanzkron, "Baby on board: what you need to know about pregnancy in the hemoglobinopathies," *Hematology*, vol. 2012, pp. 208–214, 2012.

[160] B. B. Afolabi, N. C. Iwuala, I. C. Iwuala, and O. K. Ogedengbe, "Morbidity and mortality in sickle cell pregnancies in Lagos, Nigeria: a case control study," *Journal of Obstetrics & Gynaecology*, vol. 29, no. 2, pp. 104–106, 2009.

[161] A. Omole-Ohonsi, O. A. Ashimi, and T. A. Aiyedun, "Preconception care and sickle cell anemia in pregnancy," *Journal of Basic and Clinical Reproductive Sciences*, vol. 1, no. 1, pp. 12–18, 2012.

[162] Z. M. Al-Samak, M. M. Al-Falaki, and A. A. Pasha, "Assessment of perioperative transfusion therapy and complications in sickle cell disease patients undergoing surgery," *Middle East Journal of Anesthesiology*, vol. 19, no. 5, pp. 983–995, 2008.

[163] W. A. Marchant and I. Walker, "Anaesthetic management of the child with sickle cell disease," *Paediatric Anaesthesia*, vol. 13, no. 6, pp. 473–489, 2003.

[164] E. P. Vichinsky, C. M. Haberkern, L. Neumayr et al., "A comparison of conservative and aggressive transfusion regimens in the perioperative management of sickle cell disease," *The New England Journal of Medicine*, vol. 333, no. 4, pp. 206–213, 1995.

[165] H. M. Dix, "New advances in the treatment of sickle cell disease: focus on perioperative significance," *Journal of the American Association of Nurse Anesthetists*, vol. 69, no. 4, pp. 281–286, 2001.

[166] P. Losco, G. Nash, P. Stone, and J. Ventre, "Comparison of the effects of radiographic contrast media on dehydration and filterability of red blood cells from donors homozygous for hemoglobin A or hemoglobin S," *American Journal of Hematology*, vol. 68, no. 3, pp. 149–158, 2001.

[167] T. R. Kotila, "Guidelines for the diagnosis of the haemoglobinopathies in Nigeria," *Annals of Ibadan Postgraduate Medicine*, vol. 8, no. 1, pp. 25–29, 2011.

[168] Y. Daniel, "Haemoglobinopathy diagnostic tests: blood counts, sickle solubility test, haemoglobin electrophoresis and high-performance liquid chromatography," in *Practical Management of Haemoglobinopathies*, I. E. Okpala, Ed., pp. 10–19, Blackwell Publishing, 2004.

[169] B. J. Bain, "Haemoglobinopathy diagnosis: algorithms, lessons and pitfalls," *Blood Reviews*, vol. 25, no. 5, pp. 205–213, 2011.

[170] G. M. Clarke and T. N. Higgins, "Laboratory investigation of hemoglobinopathies and thalassemias: review and update," *Clinical Chemistry*, vol. 46, no. 8, part 2, pp. 1284–1290, 2000.

[171] O. Emmanuelchide, O. Charle, and O. Uchenna, "Hematological parameters in association with outcomes in sickle cell anemia patients," *Indian Journal of Medical Sciences*, vol. 65, no. 9, pp. 393–398, 2011.

[172] S. A. Adegoke and B. P. Kuti, "Evaluation of clinical severity of sickle cell anaemia in Nigerian children," *Journal of Applied Hematology*, vol. 4, no. 2, pp. 58–64, 2013.

[173] C. T. Quinn, Z. R. Rogers, and G. R. Buchanan, "Survival of children with sickle cell disease," *Blood*, vol. 103, no. 11, pp. 4023–4027, 2004.

[174] K. J. J. Wierenga, I. R. Hambleton, and N. A. Lewis, "Survival estimates for patients with homozygous sickle-cell disease in Jamaica: a clinic-based population study," *The Lancet*, vol. 357, no. 9257, pp. 680–683, 2001.

[175] A. Chijioke and P. M. Kolo, "The longevity and clinical pattern of adult sickle cell anaemia in Ilorin," *European Journal of Scientific Research*, vol. 32, no. 4, pp. 528–532, 2009.

[176] M. Angastiniotis, S. Kyriakidou, and M. Hadjiminas, "How thalassaemia was controlled in Cyprus," *World Health Forum*, vol. 7, no. 3, pp. 291–297, 1986.

[177] M. A. Durosinmi, A. I. Odebiyi, I. A. Adediran, N. O. Akinola, D. E. Adegorioye, and M. A. Okunade, "Acceptability of prenatal diagnosis of sickle cell anaemia (SCA) by female patients and parents of SCA patients in Nigeria," *Social Science and Medicine*, vol. 41, no. 3, pp. 433–436, 1995.

[178] A. S. Adeyemi and D. A. Adekanle, "Knowledge and attitude of female health workers towards prenatal diagnosis of sickle cell disease," *Nigerian Journal of Medicine*, vol. 16, no. 3, pp. 268–270, 2007.

[179] M. B. Kagu, U. A. Abjah, and S. G. Ahmed, "Awareness and acceptability of prenatal diagnosis of sickle cell anaemia among health professionals and students in North Eastern Nigeria," *Nigerian Journal of Medicine*, vol. 13, no. 1, pp. 48–51, 2004.

[180] World Health Organisation, *Guidelines for the Control of Haemoglobin Disorders*, WHO, Sardinia, Italy, 1994.

[181] S. O. Akodu, I. N. Diaku-Akinwumi, and O. F. Njokanma, "Age at diagnosis of sickle cell anaemia in lagos, Nigeria," *Mediterranean Journal of Hematology and Infectious Diseases*, vol. 5, no. 1, Article ID e2013001, 2013.

[182] F. A. Olatona, K. A. Odeyemi, A. T. Onajole, and M. C. Asuzu, "Effects of health education on knowledge and attitude of youth corps members to sickle cell disease and its screening in Lagos State," *Journal of Community Medicine & Health Education*, vol. 2, article 163, 2012.

[183] N. Galadanci, B. J. Wudil, T. M. Balogun et al., "Current sickle cell disease management practices in Nigeria," *International Health*, vol. 6, no. 1, pp. 23–28, 2014.

[184] A. A. Oyekunle, "Haemopoietic stem cell transplantation: prospects and challenges in Nigeria," *Annals of Ibadan Postgraduate Medicine*, vol. 4, no. 1, pp. 17–27, 2006.

[185] N. Bazuaye, B. Nwogoh, D. Ikponmwen et al., "First successful allogeneic hematopoietic stem cell transplantation for a sickle cell disease patient in a low resource country (Nigeria): a case report," *Annals of Transplantation*, vol. 19, no. 1, pp. 210–213, 2014.

[186] O. O. Akinyanju, A. I. Otaigbe, and M. O. O. Ibidapo, "Outcome of holistic care in Nigerian patients with sickle cell anaemia," *Clinical and Laboratory Haematology*, vol. 27, no. 3, pp. 195–199, 2005.

[187] I. E. Okpala, "Sickle cell crisis," in *Practical Management of Haemoglobinopathies*, I. E. Okpala, Ed., pp. 63–71, Blackwell Publishing, 2004.

[188] I. Okpala, V. Thomas, N. Westerdale et al., "The comprehensive care of sickle cell disease," *European Journal of Haematology*, vol. 68, no. 3, pp. 157–162, 2002.

[189] J. Makani, S. F. Ofori-Acquah, O. Nnodu, A. Wonkam, and K. Ohene-Frempong, "Sickle cell disease: new opportunities and challenges in Africa," *The Scientific World Journal*, vol. 2013, Article ID 193252, 16 pages, 2013.

[190] O. Oniyangi and A. A. A. Omari, "Malaria chemoprophylaxis in sickle cell disease," *The Cochrane Library*, vol. 1, pp. 1–18, 2009.

[191] E. O. Ibe, A. C. J. Ezeoke, I. Emeodi et al., "Electrolyte profile and prevalent causes of sickle cell crisis in Enugu, Nigeria," *African Journal of Biochemistry Research*, vol. 3, no. 11, pp. 370–374, 2009.

[192] R. A. Bolarinwa, N. O. Akinola, O. A. Aboderin, and M. A. Durosinmi, "The role of malaria in vaso-occlusive crisis of adult patients with sickle cell disease," *Journal of Medicine and Medical Sciences*, vol. 1, pp. 407–411, 2010.

[193] R. Kotila, A. Okesola, and O. Makanjuola, "Asymptomatic malaria parasitaemia in sickle-cell disease patients: how effective is chemoprophylaxis?" *Journal of Vector Borne Diseases*, vol. 44, no. 1, pp. 52–55, 2007.

[194] R. E. Ware, "How I use hydroxyurea to treat young patients with sickle cell anemia," *Blood*, vol. 115, no. 26, pp. 5300–5311, 2010.

[195] S. C. Davies and A. Gilmore, "The role of hydroxyurea in the management of sickle cell disease," *Blood Reviews*, vol. 17, no. 2, pp. 99–109, 2003.

[196] S. C. Davies and I. A. G. Roberts, "Bone marrow transplant for sickle cell disease—an update," *Archives of Disease in Childhood*, vol. 75, no. 1, pp. 3–6, 1996.

[197] I. Roberts, "Current status of allogeneic transplantation for haemoglobinopathies," *British Journal of Haematology*, vol. 98, no. 1, pp. 1–7, 1997.

[198] S. Shenoy, "Hematopoietic stem cell transplantation for sickle cell disease: current practice and emerging trends," *Hematology*, vol. 2011, pp. 273–279, 2011.

[199] L. De Franceschi, "Pathophysiology of sickle cell disease and new drugs for the treatment," *Mediterranean Journal of Hematology and Infectious Diseases*, vol. 1, no. 1, 2009.

[200] L. De Franceschi and R. Corrocher, "Established and experimental treatments for sickle cell disease," *Haematologica*, vol. 89, no. 3, pp. 348–356, 2004.

[201] K. I. Ataga and J. Stocker, "Senicapoc (ICA17043): a potential therapy for the prevention and treatment of hemolysis-associated complications in sickle cell anemia," *Expert Opinion on Investigational Drugs*, vol. 18, no. 2, pp. 231–239, 2009.

[202] K. I. Ataga, W. R. Smith, L. M. De Castro et al., "Efficacy and safety of the Gardos channel blocker, senicapoc (ICA-17043), in patients with sickle cell anemia," *Blood*, vol. 111, no. 8, pp. 3991–3997, 2008.

[203] I. E. Okpala, "New therapies for sickle cell disease," *Hematology/Oncology Clinics of North America*, vol. 19, no. 5, pp. 975–987, 2005.

[204] M. J. Stuart and R. L. Nagel, "Sickle-cell disease," *The Lancet*, vol. 364, no. 9442, pp. 1343–1360, 2004.

[205] M. C. Walters, "Stem cell therapy for sickle cell disease: transplantation and gene therapy," *Hematology*, vol. 2005, no. 1, pp. 66–73, 2005.

Correlation between Plasma Interleukin-3, the α/β Globin Ratio, and Globin mRNA Stability

S. Rouhi Dehnabeh,[1] R. Mahdian,[2] S. Ajdary,[3] E. Mostafavi,[4] and S. Khatami[1]

[1] Biochemistry Department, Pasteur Institute of Iran, Pasteur Street, No. 69, Tehran 1316943551, Iran
[2] Molecular Medicine Department, Pasteur Institute of Iran, Pasteur Street, No. 69, Tehran 1316943551, Iran
[3] Immunology Department, Pasteur Institute of Iran, Pasteur Street, No. 69, Tehran 1316943551, Iran
[4] Department of Epidemiology, Pasteur Institute of Iran, Pasteur Street, No. 69, Tehran 1316943551, Iran

Correspondence should be addressed to S. Khatami; khatamibiochem@yahoo.com

Academic Editor: Aurelio Maggio

Background. Globin chain synthesis (GCS) analysis is used in the diagnosis of thalassemia. However, the wide reference range limits its use as a decisive diagnostic tool. It has been shown that α and β *globin mRNA* increase through stimulation of cells by interleukin-3 (IL-3). Therefore, this study investigates the relationship between plasma IL-3 and the β/α *globin* ratio. *Methods.* Blood samples were collected from 32 healthy participants on two occasions one month apart. GCS analysis, real-time PCR, and ELISA tests were conducted to determine the β/α *globin* ratio, *globin mRNA* expression and stability rate, and IL-3 levels. *Results.* On the basis of IL-3 levels, the participants were divided in two groups. One group included participants who showed a significant increase in IL-3 as indicated by a significant rise in mean values of α, β, and γ *globin mRNA*, α and β *globin*, RBC, and hemoglobin. The other group included participants who showed no difference in IL-3 levels with no significant variations in the above-mentioned parameters. *Conclusion.* The results of this study indicate that IL-3 has an equivalent positive effect on α and β *globin* chain synthesis. Therefore, IL-3 levels do not explain the wide reference range of the α/β *globin* ratio.

1. Introduction

Thalassemia is one of the most common genetic diseases in Iran. In an attempt to limit the emergence of new cases of major β-thalassemia, health authorities are developing a national program to accurately diagnose different types of thalassemia. With more than 200 genetic mutations, thalassemia has different clinical manifestations ranging from no symptoms to severe disease. Currently, despite the fact that *DNA* analysis provides useful information on thalassemia, it cannot be used alone as a decisive diagnostic tool. This is because the disease involves unknown deletions and mutations, mutations in gene regulation sites, and mutations in genes generating trans-elements for globin gene expression (nonglobin gene related thalassemia). In some cases, globin chain synthesis is required for diagnosis because it enables monitoring of gene expression at different levels, including transcription (*mRNA* production), generation of stable

mRNA, and translation on ribosomes [1]. In the globin chain synthesis carried out to determine the α/β *globin* ratio, all intermediate stages of globin generation (from no generation of *mRNA* or unstable *mRNA* to no translation on ribosomes) are controlled. Therefore, the results of this test indicate the final efficiency of globin genes and are very valuable for diagnosis. However, the wide reference range [2, 3], a consequence of the greater influence of biological changes compared with methodological changes [2, 4], limits the use of this method as a decisive and final diagnostic tool. To address this, it is necessary to study the effects of biological substances on globin chain synthesis test results.

Previous research has shown that interleukin-3 (IL-3) can alter globin chain synthesis, which in turn affects translation levels. In this way, IL-3 generates hemoglobin F through its stimulating effect on α *globin* and γ *globin* chain synthesis [5].

(γ)	Seq $5' \rightarrow 3'$	Tm	GC%	L	L
F	CAAGGTGAATGTGGAAGATGCTG	60.5	48	23	115 bp
R	GATGGCAGAGGCAGAGGACAG	60.9	62	21	
(β)	Seq $5' \rightarrow 3'$	Tm	GC%	L	L
F	CGTGGATGAAGTTGGTGGTGAG	61.3	55	22	112 bp
R	GCCCATAACAGCATCAGGAGTG	60.5	55	22	
(α)	Seq $5' \rightarrow 3'$	Tm	GC%	L	L
F	GCACAAGCTTCGGGTGGAC	60.2	63	19	157 bp
R	GGTATTTGGAGGTCAGCACGGT	61.1	55	22	

IL-3 is lymphocytes, epithelial cells, and astrocytes secreted cytokine. The IL-3 molecule has a glycoprotein structure and is generated as a result of antigenic or mitogenic stimulation. It affects the reproduction and differentiation of blood cells and other cells through special receptors [6]. IL-3 can promote erythropoiesis by activating the Ras pathway, resulting in apoptosis control and a Jak2/stat5 cascade, and by stimulating DNA synthesis [7].

The hemoglobin molecule has a complex structure, and the components contributing to the molecular structure are coordinated through complex mechanisms. However, coordinated generation of the chains contributing to the structure of hemoglobin depends on other factors, including blood iron level, ferritin concentration, transferrin receptors, cytokine concentration, and heme concentration [8]. In addition, the generation of protein subunits contributing to the hemoglobin structure is coordinated so the generation rate of α chains almost approaches that of non-α chains. This process prevents cell damage from increases in levels of one type of chain but is disrupted in thalassemia.

The present study aims to investigate the specific effect of IL-3 on α globin mRNA and β globin mRNA stability, α globin and β globin production, and the range of the α/β globin ratio, assuming that antigenic and mitogenic stimulation results in different concentrations of IL-3 in the blood at different times (affecting the stability of the exclusive mRNA globin as well as the generation of α and β chains).

2. Material and Methods

Blood samples were collected from 32 healthy participants, on two occasions one month apart. The participants were divided in two groups based on IL-3 levels. Group 1 included participants who showed a significant increase in IL-3 levels over the month, and Group 2 included participants who showed no change or decrease in IL-3 levels.

Inclusion criteria based on blood sample analysis were as follows: MCV > 80 fL, MCH > 27 pg, normal levels of total iron, TIBC, and ferritin, and normal hemoglobin electrophoresis. All participants provided written, informed consent prior to taking part in the study.

Complete blood count (CBC) tests were carried out using a Sysmex KX-1000 apparatus and hemoglobin electrophoresis was performed on acetate cellulose. Total iron concentration and TIBC and ferritin levels were measured using

the colorimetric method (Darman Kav Co. kit) and the ELISA method (Padtan-Teb Company kit), respectively.

At the start of the study and after one month, globin chain synthesis, real-time PCR, and ELISA tests were conducted to determine the α/β globin ratio (globin chain generation), globin mRNA expression and stability rate, and the level of IL-3, respectively.

The Weatherall and Clegg method [9] was used for globin chain synthesis to determine the α/β globin ratio. Globin chain analyses were done using Mono-S ion exchange columns and a high-performance liquid chromatography (HPLC) device [2].

The IL-3 concentration was measured using the ELISA method (R&D Company kit Lot. no. 765250.1).

Real-time PCR was used to investigate the expression and stability of α globin mRNA, β globin mRNA, and γ globin mRNA, [10–12]. First, the mRNA was purified and cDNA was produced, and real-time PCR was performed. Standard graphs were constructed using a serial dilution of cDNA samples from healthy people to determine the efficiency of PCR for each gene, including the α globin, β globin, and γ globin genes, and the GAPDH reference gene.

Tri Reagent (Sigma, DB) was used to purify mRNA, which was kept in water containing diethyl pyrocarbonate (DEPC). To verify the quality of the mRNA, the optical absorption was measured at 260 and 280 nm wavelengths using a Nanodrop spectrometer (Implen, Munich, Germany). The mean optical absorption of the purified samples was 2.02. A Qiagen kit (cat. number 205311) was used to make cDNA. The real-time PCR test was performed using an ABI 7300 Sequence Detection System (Applied Biosystems, Foster City, CA, USA). The oligonucleotide primers for α, β, and γ globin genes and the GAPDH reference gene were designed with Primer Express software Ver. 3 (Applied Biosystems, Foster City, CA). The specificity of the primer sequences was confirmed on a search of the NCBI/BLAST database. The characteristics of the primers are shown in Table 1.

Following the determination of the best concentration of cDNA, to avoid the generation of dimer primers, a real-time PCR test was conducted on special plates to ensure the optimal reaction and concentration of primers. For each reaction, a solution with a volume of 25 mL was prepared. The contents of the solution were as follows: Power SYBR Green Master Mix (Applied Biosystems, UK), 12.5 mL; α, β, and γ primers, 3 pmol; GAPDH primer, 5 pmol; water, 6.5–7 mL;

TABLE 2: Determination of the real-time PCR efficiencies.

	Concen.	Log	Mean Ct	Ct1	Ct2	Ct3	Slope	Effic. %
α	50	1.69897	16.32	16.32	16.31	16.33	−3.30089	
	25	1.39794	17.22	17.21	17.23	17.22		101
	12.5	1.09691	18.17667	18.22	18.15	18.16		
	6.25	0.79588	19.31333	19.27	19.31	19.36		
β	50	1.69897	16.48667	16.46	16.47	16.53	−3.24109	
	25	1.39794	17.29	17.28	17.3	17.29		103
	12.5	1.09691	18.27667	18.32	18.17	18.34		
	6.25	0.79588	19.41	19.45	19.36	19.42		
γ	100	2	24.76667	24.54	24.92	24.84	−3.61426	
	50	1.69897	25.85	25.82	25.95	25.78		
	25	1.39794	26.91	26.94	26.88	26.91		89
	12.5	1.09691	28.04333	28.05	28.05	28.03		
	6.25	0.79588	29.11	29.02	29.14	29.17		
GAPDH	100	2	31.395	31.3		31.49	−3.65744	
	50	1.69897	32.11	32.06		32.16		88
	25	1.39794	33.775	33.52	34.03			
	12.5	1.09691	34.51		34.85	34.17		

and cDNA, 25 ng. The test was conducted for all four genes in two simultaneous series and the mean Ct was computed for each gene.

The following schedule was used for the real-time PCR test.

The first cycle was carried out at 95°C for 10 min, to achieve primary separation of the expression pattern cDNA. Next, two thermal schedules were repeated for 40 cycles: 95°C for 15 s and 60°C for 1 min.

For every complete reproduction stage, a separation step was carried out to analyze the melting curve: 95°C for 15 s, 60°C for 30 s, and 90°C for 15 s.

To determine the efficiency of reproduction [11, 12] of α, β, and γ globin genes and the GAPDH reference gene, a serial dilution of the cDNA sample from one of the study participants was prepared and a real-time PCR test was carried out separately, using different primers and different concentrations. Finally, a standard graph was drawn for each of the four gene sections. The efficiency of PCR for all four genes was calculated through the determination of the standard graph slope and was derived from the following equation:

$$\text{Efficiency} = \left[10^{(-1/\text{Slope})}\right] - 1. \tag{1}$$

When the efficiency was sufficient to allow the use of the $2^{-\Delta\Delta Ct}$ method (Table 2 and Figure 1), the real-time PCR test was performed on α, β, and γ globin genes in the samples from the participants and the GAPDH reference gene. When reproduction was complete, a graph was drawn for each PCR reaction, based on the Ct (Figures 2 and 3). A ΔCt index was calculated for standard and study samples by deducing the mean Ct of the target genes and of the reference

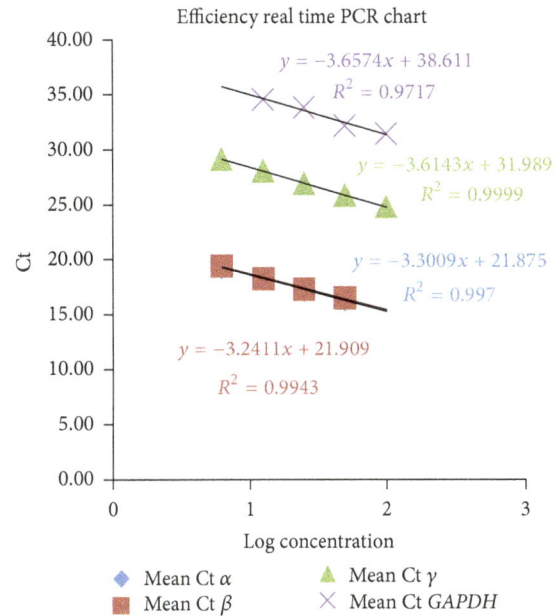

FIGURE 1: The standard curves of the real-time PCR assay.

gene, resulting in the ΔΔCt factor, which is derived from the following equation:

$$\Delta\Delta Ct$$
$$= \left[\text{mCt } \alpha \, (\text{test Sample}) - \text{mCT } GAPDH \, (\text{test Sample})\right]$$
$$- \left[\text{mCT } \alpha \, (\text{normal Sample})\right.$$
$$\left. -\text{mCT } GAPDH \, (\text{normal Sample})\right]. \tag{2}$$

Delta Rn versus cycle

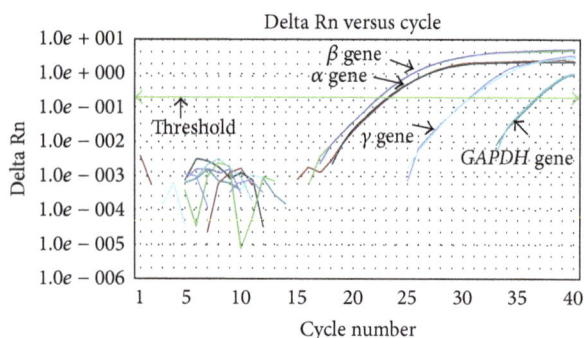

FIGURE 2: Delta Rn versus cycle for different genes.

Dissociation curve

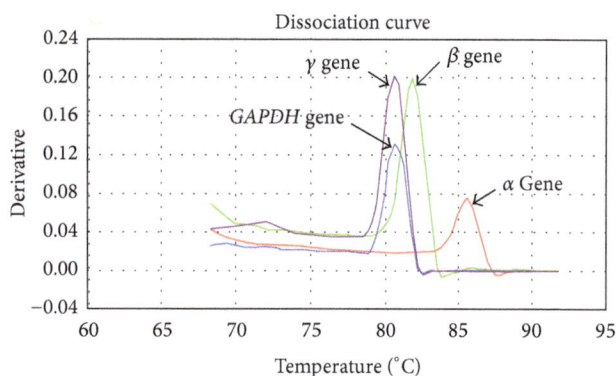

FIGURE 3: Dissociation curve for different genes.

Finally, the expression rate of the α, β, and γ globin was determined using the $2^{-\Delta\Delta Ct}$ formula.

Based on the research objectives and assumptions, the results were analyzed, compiled, and interpreted using SPSS ver. 16 (SPSS, Chicago, IL, USA).

3. Results

On the basis of IL-3 levels, the participants were divided in two groups. One group included 15 participants who showed a significant increase in IL-3 after one month and the other group included 17 participants who showed no difference or decrease in IL-3 levels.

Table 3 shows the mean ± standard deviation of the results and demonstrates that all participants had normal MCV and MCH values and no evidence of iron deficiency.

The Kolmogorov-Smirnov test was used to test the dispersion of the studied variables, and the mean values of the following variables were statistically analyzed and compared: α globin mRNA, β globin mRNA, γ globin mRNA, α globin, β globin, γ globin, α/β globin ratio, RBC, hemoglobin, IL-3, ferritin, and the reticulocyte count. Table 4 presents a summary of the results. The variables followed a normal distribution. Therefore, a paired t-test was used to compare the variables between groups. In Group 1 (participants with increased IL-3), the mean values of α globin mRNA, β globin mRNA, γ globin mRNA, α globin, β globin, RBC, hemoglobin, and IL-3 all increased over the month of

TABLE 3: Hematological and biochemical data.

Variables	Group 1 Mean ± 2 SD	Group 2 Mean ± 2 SD
WBC ($\times 10^3$/L)	6.7 ± 2.0	6.5 ± 2.2
RBC ($\times 10^{12}$/L)	4.89 ± 0.80	4.84 ± 0.80
Hb (g/dL)	14.0 ± 2.0	13.8 ± 2.6
Hct (%)	41.7 ± 5.4	41.3 ± 6.8
MCV (fL)	85.4 ± 5.2	85.5 ± 5.0
MCH (pg)	28.7 ± 1.8	28.5 ± 1.4
MCHC (g/dL)	33.6 ± 1.2	33.0 ± 2.4
RDW	12.0 ± 0.7	12.4 ± 1.8
Reticulocytes (%)	0.9 ± 0.8	0.8 ± 0.6
Hb A (%)	97.1 ± 0.6	97.2 ± 0.5
Hb A$_2$ (%)	2.3 ± 0.6	2.4 ± 0.4
Hb F (%)	0.5 ± 0.4	0.4 ± 0.3
Total iron (ug/d)	86 ± 33	99 ± 57
TIBC (ug/dL)	339 ± 88	328 ± 138
Ferritin (ng/dL)	46 ± 102	56 ± 132
Number of total cases	15	17

the study. The increase was significant for α globin mRNA, β globin mRNA, and γ globin mRNA at a significance level of 90% and for hemoglobin, RBC, and IL-3 at a significance level of 95%. In Group 2, the mean concentration of IL-3 showed a decrease after one month, which was significant at a level of 95%. Among the parameters studied using the paired t-test, none showed a significant difference between the two test steps with a resampling interval of one month. In the present study of healthy participants, the α/β globin ratio range was 0.74–1.31, which agrees well with the findings of recent studies [2, 3].

4. Discussion

Many studies have demonstrated that transcriptional control mechanisms regulate gene expression, and recently, research has confirmed the importance of posttranscriptional mechanisms in the regulation of eukaryotic gene expression [1]. Increased mRNA reading by ribosomes [13], increased protection against proteins produced from degradation mechanisms [14], and increased stability of mRNA are possible mechanisms underlying changes in translation levels. Previous research has shown that, in addition to increases in transferrin (CD71) receptors, α globin mRNA and β globin mRNA increase through stimulation of cells by IL-3. This increase is attributed to the stabilization of α globin mRNA and β globin mRNA molecules [5].

The decrease in ferritin levels in the group 1 with increased IL-3 in the present study could be attributed to increased CD71 receptors as well as increased IL-3 (CDw123) receptors. The decreased ferritin levels could be attributed to the requirement for iron to produce heme molecules. The presence of CD71 receptors and CDw123 receptors on reticulocytes has been confirmed [5]. It has also been shown that

TABLE 4: Summary of the results.

Parameter	Step 1 of sampling in Group 1 ($n = 15$) Mean (SD)	Step 2 of sampling in Group 1 ($n = 15$) Mean (SD)	Step 1 of sampling in Group 2 ($n = 17$) Mean (SD)	Step 2 of sampling in Group 2 ($n = 17$) Mean (SD)
α globin mRNA	1.00 (0.0)	3.99 (5.10)	1.00 (0.0)	1.24 (1.16)
β globin mRNA	1.00 (0.0)	3.73 (5.14)	1.00 (0.0)	1.23 (0.97)
γ globin mRNA	1.00 (0.0)	2.79 (3.08)	1.00 (0.0)	1.12 (0.84)
α globin	100.00 (0.0)	129.87 (17.63)	100.00 (0.0)	100.11 (41.45)
β globin	100.00 (0.0)	134.93 (72.46)	100.00 (0.0)	102.29 (46.56)
γ globin	100.00 (0.0)	105.07 (28.49)	100.00 (0.0)	98 (41.65)
α/β globin ratio	1.083 (0.118)	1.058 (0.129)	0.99 (0.14)	0.96 (0.13)
RBC	4.69 (0.44)	4.89 (0.36)	4.83 (0.46)	4.83 (0.42)
Hemoglobin	13.58 (1.05)	14.01 (0.96)	13.95 (1.40)	13.78 (1.34)
IL-3	25.67 (28.76)	67.07 (75.60)	46.64 (50.95)	29.35 (23.28)
Ferritin	52.87 (59.81)	44.80 (51.51)	57.00 (56.34)	56.12 (66.37)
Concentrated reticulocyte	2.13 (0.80)	2.18 (0.75)	1.87 (0.52)	1.78 (0.52)

the number of CD71 receptors increases as IL-3 concentration increases [5]. This may occur because an increase in *globin mRNA* will result in an increase in translation levels. Further, since the generation of hemoglobin molecules requires a heme component, the number of CD71 receptors will increase to enable the generation of heme molecules.

The complex process of hemoglobin generation is dependent on many factors, including the blood iron level, ferritin concentration, transferrin receptors, cytokine (IL-3 and IL-9) concentrations, heme concentration, the hematopoietic GTPase RhoH required for adjusting the signal effects of IL-3 [15], and the presence or absence of CD133 on the surface of erythroid cells. These factors cause adult cells to react to IL-3 to more strongly activate erythropoiesis [16]. It is difficult to explain why the reference range of the α/β globin ratio is so wide and future comprehensive research is required to answer this question. Recent studies have shown that the expression of IL-3 receptors, as well as signal transducers and activators of transcription (STAT) activity, is adjusted under the influence of GTPase RhoH, which in turn results in the adjustment of IL-3 signals [15].

The results of this study on the α/β globin ratio imply that because IL-3 has an equivalent positive effect on the generation of α globin and β globin, it is not likely to be the biological factor underlying the wide range of α/β globin ratios in globin chain synthesis tests.

Consent

Signed informed consent was obtained from the participants in the study.

Conflict of Interests

The authors declare that there is no conflict of interests regarding the publication of this paper.

Acknowledgments

The authors are grateful to colleagues in the Biochemistry Department, Molecular Medicine Department, and Immunology Department of the Pasteur Institute of Iran for their cooperation in the project. They would also like to offer special thanks to participants for their collaboration in this project.

References

[1] D. A. Day and M. F. Tuite, "Post-transcriptional gene regulatory mechanisms in eukaryotes: an overview," *Journal of Endocrinology*, vol. 157, no. 3, pp. 361–371, 1998.

[2] S. Khatami, S. R. Dehboneh, S. Sadeghi et al., "Globin chain synthesis is a useful complementary tool in the differential diagnosis of thalassemias," *Hemoglobin*, vol. 31, no. 3, pp. 333–341, 2007.

[3] A. Villegas, J. Sanchez, F. Gonzalez et al., "Red blood cell phenotypes in α thalassemias in the Spanish population," *Hematologica*, vol. 83, no. 2, pp. 99–103, 1998.

[4] P. C. Giordano, P. van Delft, D. Batelaan, C. L. Harteveld, and L. F. Bernini, "Haemoglobinopathy analyses in the netherlands: a report of an in vitro globin chain biosynthesis survey using a rapid, modified method," *Clinical and Laboratory Haematology*, vol. 21, no. 4, pp. 247–255, 1999.

[5] D. Reinhardt, R. Ridder, W. Kugler, and A. Pekrun, "Post-transcriptional effects of interleukin-3, interferon-γ, erythropoietin and butyrate on in vitro hemoglobin chain synthesis in congenital hemolytic anemia," *Haematologica*, vol. 86, no. 8, pp. 791–800, 2001.

[6] http://www.rightdiagnosis.com/medical/interleukin_3.htm.

[7] http://www.biocarta.com/genes/CytokinesChemokines.asp.

[8] A. D. Sheftel, A. B. Mason, and P. Ponka, "The long history of iron in the Universe and in health and disease," *Biochimica et Biophysica Acta*, vol. 1820, no. 3, pp. 161–187, 2012.

[9] D. J. Weatherall and J. B. Clegg, *The Thalassemia Syndromes*, Blackwell Scientific Publications, Oxford, UK, 3rd edition, 1981.

[10] C. Chaisue, S. Kitcharoen, P. Wilairat, A. Jetsrisuparb, G. Fucha-roen, and S. Fucharoen, "α/β-Globin mRNA ratio determina-tion by multiplex quantitative real-time reverse transcription-polymerase chain reaction as an indicator of globin gene function," *Clinical Biochemistry*, vol. 40, no. 18, pp. 1373–1377, 2007.

[11] K. J. Livak and T. D. Schmittgen, "Analysis of relative gene expression data using real-time quantitative PCR and the $2^{-\Delta\Delta CT}$ method," *Methods*, vol. 25, no. 4, pp. 402–408, 2001.

[12] J. L. Vaerman, P. Saussoy, and I. Ingargiola, "Evaluation of real-time PCR data," *Journal of Biological Regulators & Homeostatic Agents*, vol. 18, no. 2, pp. 212–214, 2004.

[13] J. Ross, "Messenger RNA turnover in cell-free extracts from higher eukaryotes," *Methods in Molecular Biology*, vol. 118, pp. 459–476, 1999.

[14] A. Krowczynska and G. Brawerman, "Structural features in the $3'$-terminal region of polyribosome-bound rabbit globin messenger RNAs," *Journal of Biological Chemistry*, vol. 261, no. 1, pp. 397–402, 1986.

[15] M. S. Gündogdu, H. Liu, D. Metzdorf et al., "The haematopoi-etic GTPase RhoH modulates IL3 signalling through regulation of STAT activity and IL3 receptor expression," *Molecular Can-cer*, vol. 9, article 225, 2010.

[16] R. M. Böhmer, "Erythropoiesis from adult but not fetal blood-derived CD133+ stem cells depends strongly on interleukin-3," *Growth Factors*, vol. 22, no. 1, pp. 45–50, 2004.

28

Antianemic Treatment of Cancer Patients in German Routine Practice: Data from a Prospective Cohort Study—The Tumor Anemia Registry

Tilman Steinmetz,[1] Jan Schröder,[2] Margarete Plath,[3] Hartmut Link,[4] Michèle Vogt,[5] Melanie Frank,[5] and Norbert Marschner[6]

[1]Outpatient Clinic for Hematology and Oncology, Sachsenring 69, 50677 Cologne, Germany

[2]Outpatient Clinic for Oncology, Kettwiger Strasse 62, 45468 Mülheim an der Ruhr, Germany

[3]Outpatient Clinic for Oncology, Prinzregentenstrasse 1, 86150 Augsburg, Germany

[4]Department for Internal Medicine I, Westpfalz-Klinikum, Hellmut-Hartert-Strasse 1, 67655 Kaiserslautern, Germany

[5]iOMEDICO, Hanferstrasse 28, 79108 Freiburg, Germany

[6]Outpatient Clinic for Interdisciplinary Oncology and Hematology, Wirthstrasse 11c, 79110 Freiburg, Germany

Correspondence should be addressed to Tilman Steinmetz; steinmetz@oncokoeln.de

Academic Editor: Bruno Annibale

The aim of this prospective cohort study was to assess current antianemic treatment of cancer patients in German routine practice, including diagnostics, treatments, and quality of life (QoL). 88 study sites recruited 1018 patients at the start of antianemic treatment with hemoglobin (Hb) levels <11 g/dL (females) or <12 g/dL (males). Patients were followed up for 12 weeks. 63% of the patients had inoperable solid tumors, 22% operable solid tumors, and 15% hematological malignancies. Over 85% received chemotherapy. Median age was 67 years; 48% were male. Red blood cell transfusions (RBCTx) were given to 59% of all patients and to 55% of the patients with Hb ≥8 g/dL on day 1 of the observation period (day 1 treatment). Erythropoiesis-stimulating agents (ESAs) were the second most frequently applied day 1 treatment (20%), followed by intravenous (IV) iron (15%) and ESA + IV iron (6%). Only about a third of patients were tested for blood serum iron parameters at the start of treatment. Overall, more than half of the patients had long-term responses to antianemic therapy. Our data suggest that in routine practice diagnostics for treatable causes of anemia are underused. A high proportion of cancer patients receive RBCTx. It should be discussed whether thorough diagnostics and earlier intervention could decrease the need for RBCTx. This trial is registered with NCT01795690.

1. Introduction

Anemia is defined as a hemoglobin (Hb) level of <12 g/dL for nonpregnant women and <13 g/dL for men, according to the World Health Organization [1]. It is a common complication of multifactorial etiology among patients with malignant diseases. The European Cancer Anemia Survey (ECAS) reported an overall anemia incidence (Hb <12 g/dL) of more than 50% during the 6-month survey period for patients with solid or hematological tumors who received their first anticancer treatment. Anemia incidence was almost 65% in patients receiving chemotherapy [2]. Low Hb levels are associated with poor physical performance status [2–5] and decreased quality of life (QoL) [3, 6–9], indicating a need for early antianemic treatment.

Treatment strategies include red blood cell transfusions (RBCTx), erythropoiesis-stimulating agents (ESAs), and iron supplementation either alone or in combination with ESAs. Treatment decision-making should be based on the best benefit-to-risk ratio for each patient and depends on patients' Hb level, the presence of symptoms, and the underlying cause for anemia as evaluated by blood parameters such as ferritin, transferrin saturation (TSAT), folate, and vitamin B12 [10–12]. While the National Comprehensive Cancer Network

(NCCN) has published a comprehensive guideline on anemia management, current guidelines in Europe focus on the application of ESAs and/or transfusions. The administration of intravenous (IV) iron is the treatment of choice for cancer patients with anemia due to absolute iron deficiency (AID). It has been shown to improve efficacy and is thus recommended in combination with ESAs for patients with functional iron deficiency (FID) [10–12]. If iron deficiency is excluded, the European Organization for Research and Treatment of Cancer (EORTC) recommends ESAs to treat symptomatic anemia with Hb levels ≥9 g/dL and to assess whether transfusions are required in case of Hb levels <9 g/dL [10]. The NCCN advises thorough diagnostics for possible causes of anemia and subsequent treatment of these. If no treatable cause can be identified, transfusions are recommended depending on the presence of symptoms and comorbidities. ESAs are suggested for anemic patients undergoing palliative cancer treatment but not for patients receiving chemotherapy with curative intent [12]. The German guideline on the use of transfusions considers them an option depending on severity and symptoms of anemia, especially when rapid, short-term improvement of Hb levels <8 g/dL is required [13].

Prospective, observational studies can be used to assess the current state of care. In 2001/2002, the ECAS assessed prevalence, incidence, and treatment of anemia in more than 15,000 cancer patients in Europe. Over all patients, ESA therapy was the most frequently used antianemic treatment, while transfusions were most commonly applied in anemic patients with Hb levels ≤9.9 g/dL receiving chemotherapy [2]. In 2004/2005, the German Cancer Anemia Registry (CAR) was a survey on the planned anemia management of almost 2,000 cancer patients in German routine care. Overall, the three predefined treatment strategies "to correct underlying disorder causative of anemia" (e.g., iron or vitamin deficiency or bone marrow infiltration), "to use transfusions as first-line treatment," and "to use ESA as first-line treatment" were selected equally frequently, while diagnostic measures were used in two-thirds of patients only [3].

Here, we present data on the current anemia management in cancer patients from the Clinical Tumor Anemia Registry (TAR) conducted in 2012/2013. This paper addresses the treatment reality of patients with cancer and/or therapy related anemia, the use of diagnostic measures, and effectiveness of treatment based on changes in Hb values and QoL within three months after the start of antianemic treatment.

2. Patients and Methods

2.1. Study Design.
The TAR was an open, prospective, multicenter, longitudinal, observational study investigating the treatment reality of patients with cancer-induced anemia in Germany. It was conducted according to the Declaration of Helsinki, reviewed by an ethics committee, and registered in the ClinicalTrials.gov registry (NCT01795690).

2.2. Patients.
Eligible patients were ≥18 years old, with diagnosed cancer, irrespective of tumor type, and about to start antianemic therapy with baseline Hb levels <11 g/dL (females) or <12 g/dL (males). Antianemic treatment was started no longer than 7 days prior to signing written informed consent. Additional inclusion criteria comprised an Eastern Cooperative Oncology Group performance status of 0–3 and life expectancy of >16 weeks. Patients with myelodysplastic syndrome or an experimental antianemic therapy as part of a clinical trial were excluded. Study sites were encouraged to enroll patients consecutively to ensure unselected recruitment. Patients were treated according to physicians' choice based on patients' individual needs.

2.3. Data Collection.
At the time of enrolment, data on patients' sociodemographics, tumor entity, type of antineoplastic treatment, concomitant diseases, previous antianemic treatments, and current laboratory parameters were documented. Comorbidity was assessed using the Charlson Comorbidity Index [16]. During the 12-week observational period, antianemic treatment and laboratory parameters were documented. Data were collected from patients' medical files and transferred to a secure web-based electronic case report form (eCRF) by physicians or trained study nurses. Implemented automatic completeness and plausibility checks, and if necessary direct contact with the study site, were done for quality assurance. To determine QoL, patients completed the Functional Assessment of Cancer Therapy Anemia (FACT-An) questionnaire at enrolment and 6 and 12 weeks later. The initial questionnaire was filled at the study site; the remaining two were mailed to the patients, filled at home, and returned by mail in prepaid envelopes. All patients who returned the baseline questionnaire were included in the analysis of patient-reported outcomes.

2.4. Patient Cohort and Statistical Analysis.
Of all patients recruited, those with documented baseline Hb (measured no longer than 7 days before the start of antianemic treatment) were eligible for the final analysis. Patients who received one of the four standard antianemic treatments (RBCTx, ESA, IV iron, or ESA + IV iron) on day 1 of the observation period (day 1 treatment) were included in the present analysis. Patients were categorized by (1) their type of disease (solid operable tumor/potentially curative, solid inoperable tumor/palliative intention, and hematological tumor) and by (2) their day 1 treatment. The frequency of diagnostic measurements at the start of treatment was calculated. For this purpose, the number of patients for whom specified blood parameters were measured at least once within 4 weeks until 2 weeks after the beginning of antianemic treatment was determined. To analyze the effectiveness of treatments, the proportion of "responders" and ΔHb(final) and ΔHb(max) were determined. ΔHb(final) was defined as the difference between the baseline Hb and the last Hb documented within the observation period, but at least 4 weeks after the start of treatment. ΔHb(max) was defined as the difference between the baseline Hb and the highest Hb documented. "Responders" were all patients with final Hb of >11 g/dL or with ΔHb(final) of ≥1.5 g/dL, with the final Hb being the last documented Hb within the observation period, but at least 4 weeks after the start of antianemic treatment.

The FACT-An total score and the anemia-specific sub-scale score were determined according to the questionnaire's manual. Missing data within a questionnaire were handled according to the questionnaire's manual [17]. Median scores were calculated for each time point and patient sample. No imputations for missing questionnaires were performed. Improvements of seven points on the FACT-An total scale and four points on the anemia subscale were considered clinically meaningful [14, 15]. The statistical analysis was performed using STATISTICA (StatSoft, Inc.) version 10.0, R version 2.15.1, and IBM SPSS Statistics version 19.0.

3. Results and Discussion

3.1. Patients' Characteristics and Day 1 Treatment. Between March 2012 and September 2013, 216 office-based medical oncologists from 88 study sites recruited 1018 patients. Of these patients, 984 were eligible for analysis. 22 patients were excluded because treatment sample sizes were too small for meaningful analysis. They received nonstandard day 1 treatments (8 oral iron, 5 ESA + RBCTx, 4 oral iron + RBCTx, 2 oral iron + IV iron + RBCTx, 2 IV iron + RBCTx, and 1 oral iron + IV iron), and to this end 962 patients were included in the present study (Figure 1).

Table 1 displays the baseline sociodemographic and clinical characteristics. Overall, 85% of the patients ($n = 813$) had solid tumors, predominantly breast, colorectal, and non-small cell lung cancer (NSCLC), whereas the remaining patients (15%, $n = 149$) were affected by hematological malignancies. 75% of the solid tumors were inoperable (palliative patients, $n = 606$). Mean baseline Hb was 8.9 g/dL.

The majority of patients (88%, $n = 850$) received chemotherapy, of which about half were platinum based (Table 1). Figure 2 presents the frequency of the most common day 1 treatments according to type of disease ($n = 962$). Overall, 59% ($n = 571$) of the patients received RBCTx, 20% ($n = 196$) underwent ESA therapy, and 15% ($n = 142$) were treated with IV iron. A combination of ESAs and IV iron was the treatment of choice for the minority of patients (6%, $n = 53$) (Table 1). Thus, approximately 40% of the patients received antianemic therapy with ESA, IV iron, or ESA + IV iron.

Patients with inoperable solid tumors and patients with hematological malignancies were treated more often with RBCTx (60% and 64%, resp.) than patients with operable solid tumors (55%). ESA therapy was used less frequently in patients with inoperable solid tumors than in patients with operable solid tumors and hematological malignancies (18% versus 25%). Of all patients with solid tumors receiving ESAs, patients with breast cancer constitute approximately one-third. 20–30% of the patients with solid tumors and treated with IV iron had colorectal cancer (Table 1).

Approximately 20% of the patients had received previous antianemic therapies within 4 weeks before day 1 of the observation period, mostly RBCTx (data on file).

Our data show that in 2012/2013 transfusions accounted for almost 60% of day 1 antianemic treatments in German routine practice, while ESA (alone or with IV iron) was used in 26% and IV iron alone in 15% of patients. In 2004/2005, the

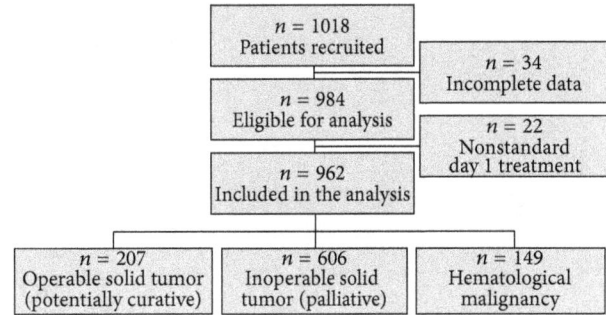

FIGURE 1: Patient recruitment, patient cohort, and type of disease.

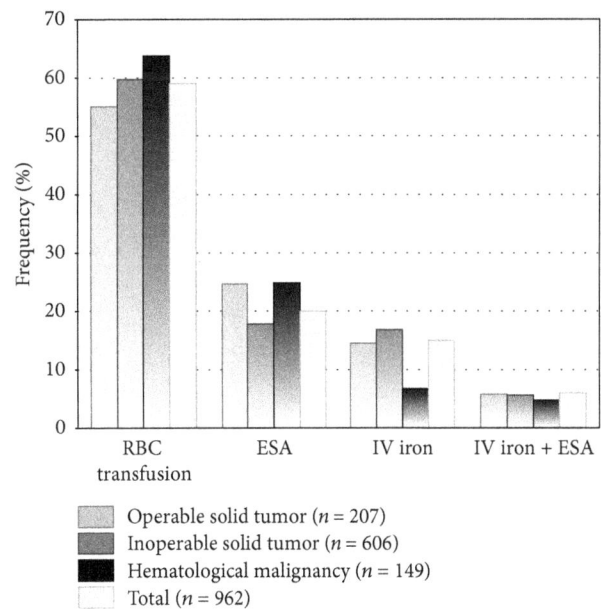

FIGURE 2: Frequency of antianemic day 1 treatments by type of disease.

German CAR study reported that transfusions were planned as "first-line" antianemic therapy for almost 35% of anemic cancer patients, whereas ESAs were chosen for 39% and strategies "correcting the underlying disorder" for 26% of patients [3]. Mean Hb for requiring treatment was 9.4 g/dL in CAR, while mean Hb at the start of treatment was 8.9 g/dL in TAR. Mean Hb triggering transfusion was 8.7 g/dL in CAR, while mean Hb at the start of transfusion as day 1 treatment was 8.6 g/dL in TAR. Mean Hb when ESAs, IV iron, and ESA + IV iron were chosen was 9.7 g/dL in CAR and between 9 and 10 g/dL in TAR (data on file).

In 2001/2002, the ECAS reported that approximately 38% of those patients receiving any antianemic therapy were treated with transfusions (alone or in combination with iron) at any time during the observational period, while approximately 45% received ESAs (alone or in combination with iron and/or transfusion) [2].

It has to be noted that CAR also included patients with Hb levels <12 g/dL (females) or <13 g/dL (males), who are less likely to receive transfusions. On the other hand, 33% of patients in CAR had a lymphoproliferative malignancy

TABLE 1: Characteristics of patients receiving antianemic treatments in German routine practice.

Day 1 treatment	Operable solid tumor (n = 207)				Inoperable solid tumor (n = 606)				Hematological malignancy (n = 149)				Total
	Transfusion	ESA	IV iron	ESA + IV iron	Transfusion	ESA	IV iron	ESA + IV iron	Transfusion	ESA	IV iron	ESA + IV iron	
Number of patients [n]	114	51	30	12	362	108	102	34	95	37	10	7	962
Sex													
Male [%]	36.8	27.5	40.0	50.0	50.0	43.5	52.9	58.8	57.9	51.4	80.0	57.1	48.0
Age at start of therapy													
Mean ± StD	66.0 ± 12.8	64.2 ± 12.5	66.2 ± 9.5	66.4 ± 8.8	66.6 ± 10.6	64.4 ± 9.7	66.8 ± 10.6	69.1 ± 9.2	69.2 ± 11.5	64.8 ± 17.0	67.7 ± 14.3	67.4 ± 10.4	66.5 ± 11.3
CCI[a] [0–36]													
Mean ± StD	0.6 ± 1.6	0.5 ± 0.9	0.5 ± 0.9	0.8 ± 1.1	0.8 ± 1.3	0.6 ± 1.2	0.6 ± 1.1	0.6 ± 1.0	0.5 ± 0.9	0.8 ± 1.3	0.3 ± 0.7	1.4 ± 2.9	0.7 ± 1.2
Karnofsky Index [0–100]													
Mean ± StD	81.6 ± 11.5	82.2 ± 9.2	87.7 ± 8.2	86.7 ± 4.9	78.7 ± 12.8	82.5 ± 8.8	78.8 ± 12.0	80.6 ± 10.7	82.6 ± 12.5	82.2 ± 10.0	77.0 ± 14.9	88.6 ± 6.9	80.7 ± 118
Most frequent solid cancers [%]													
Breast	16.7	41.2	16.7	8.3	14.1	25.0	11.8	14.7	—	—	—	—	14.7
Colorectal	15.8	13.7	30.0	33.3	9.1	5.6	20.6	2.9	—	—	—	—	10.3
Lung (NSCLC)	10.5	11.8	3.3	16.7	10.8	15.7	3.9	5.9	—	—	—	—	8.6
Tumor therapy [%]													
No therapy	6.1	—	3.3	—	2.5	0.9	2.0	—	6.3	5.4	20.0	—	3.1
Chemotherapy	92.1	98.0	93.3	100.0	88.1	95.4	86.3	94.1	76.8	81.1	40.0	85.7	88.4
Other	1.8	2.0	3.4	—	90.6	96.3	88.3	5.9	16.9	13.5	40.0	14.3	91.5
Baseline Hb [g/dL]													
Median	8.7	9.3	9.6	9.6	8.6	9.5	9.6	9.4	8.5	9.2	9.6	10.8	8.9

[a]Charlson Comorbidity Index.

compared to 15% in TAR, with these patients being more likely to receive transfusions in both data sets. The ECAS recruited all patients, independently of anemia, and also anemic patients that did not require treatment. Mean Hb at the start of treatment was higher in ECAS (9.7 g/dL) than in TAR (8.9 g/dL). Patients undergoing chemotherapy and whose Hb was <9 g/dL at the start of antianemic treatment were treated most frequently with transfusions (53%). In contrast, 71% of TAR patients receiving transfusions had Hb of <9 g/dL.

In summary, our data indicate that the use of transfusions as antianemic treatment might have increased in the last decade, while the use of ESA has decreased. Due to the limitations of historic controls, it cannot be excluded that the differences seen in the frequencies of treatments in ECAS, CAR, and TAR are at least partially caused by differences in the design of these studies (inclusion criteria) resulting in different patients recruited (e.g., with lower Hb in TAR) and thus receiving different treatments (e.g., more transfusions in TAR).

3.2. RBC Transfusions in Patients with Hb Levels ≥8 g/dL.
In general, patients receiving RBCTx as day 1 treatment showed lower baseline Hb values than patients receiving other antianemic therapies (Table 1).

Overall, 85% (n = 813) of all patients had baseline Hb levels ≥8 g/dL. Of these patients, 55% (n = 443) received RBCTx. This also means that, of all patients receiving transfusions (n = 571), almost 80% (n = 443) had baseline Hb values ≥8 g/dL. Study sites reported the presence of anemic symptoms for 88% of patients with Hb levels ≥8 g/dL. In total, 71% (n = 406) of the patients who received transfusions (n = 571) had Hb values <9.0 g/dL at the start of treatment (data on file).

The high rates of RBCTx, especially in patients with Hb ≥8 g/dL in TAR, are concerning, considering the various risks, such as transfusion-transmitted infections, transfusion-related circulatory overload, iron overload, anaphylactic reactions, and thromboembolism [8, 12, 18]. While RBCTx are the only option when immediate correction of anemic symptoms is required, there is ongoing debate about the Hb that should trigger transfusions, which is reflected in several changes in guidelines over time [18–20]. According to the EORTC guideline on the use of ESAs, patients should be evaluated for the need of transfusions if their Hb level is <9 g/dL [21]. Guidelines of the German Medical Association indicate the use of transfusions for patients with symptomatic anemia whose Hb level is <8 g/dL and/or for patients with symptomatic cardiovascular disease and the additional presence of physiologic transfusion triggers, such as tachycardia or hypotension, along with an Hb level between 8 and 10 g/dL [13]. The high rate of transfusions in patients with Hb levels ≥8 g/dL in TAR may only partly be explained by the presence of physiologic transfusion triggers, data on which were not collected within this study. There may be other rationales for applying transfusions more often than other treatments in patients with Hb levels ≥8 g/dL and in the study cohort as a whole.

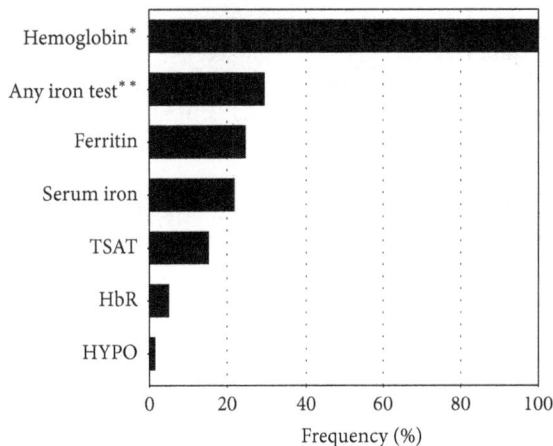

FIGURE 3: Frequency of patients tested for iron parameters at the start of antianemic treatment. *Inclusion criterion; **Patients tested for any of the listed iron parameters: ferritin, serum iron, TSAT (transferrin saturation), HbR (hemoglobin content of reticulocytes), or HYPO (hypochromic erythrocytes).

3.3. Testing for Specific Blood Serum Parameters.
About a quarter of TAR patients received ESAs as day 1 treatment, either alone or in combination with IV iron. Although a direct comparison is prevented by the reasons mentioned above, findings of the CAR and the ECAS reported a higher use of ESAs in Germany and Europe in 2001–2005 (CAR: planned ESA treatment rate of almost 40%; ECAS: approximately 45% of the patients were treated with epoetin, either alone or in combination with iron and/or transfusion) [2, 3]. Since then, safety concerns have led to revisions of existing practice guidelines [10, 12]. A summary of meta-analyses on ESA use in cancer patients from 2011 came to the conclusion that, overall, ESAs reduced the risk for RBCTx and increased the risk for thrombovascular events and mortality, while the effect of ESAs on mortality in patients receiving chemotherapy was unclear [22]. A Cochrane meta-analysis found no evidence for increased mortality in patients with target Hb <12 g/dL, undergoing chemotherapy [23]. Thus, in clinical practice, the benefits and risks of ESAs and transfusions should be carefully considered and decisions should be made based on each patient's situation and preferences.

In this context, it is of great concern that only approximately one-third (30%) of all patients in TAR were tested for iron parameters at the start of antianemic treatment, most frequently by measuring ferritin, serum iron, or TSAT within 4 weeks before the start of therapy. Testing for Hb content of reticulocytes and hypochromic erythrocytes occurred even less frequently (Figure 3). Iron parameters were measured more often in patients with colorectal cancer than in patients affected by other malignancies (43% versus 28%, data on file).

Evaluation of nutritional deficiencies other than iron was rarely done; <1% of patients were analyzed for deficits in vitamin B12 and folic acid, respectively (data on file).

While it is possible that a proportion of patients had been tested prior to the four weeks before inclusion into TAR, this is unlikely to account for almost 70% of patients without documented diagnostics. Only 20% of patients had received antianemic treatment in the four weeks prior to inclusion. Data from the CAR reported that 44% of patients had been tested for ferritin and 33% for TSAT, although the time frame was not restricted and could have been more than four weeks before treatment [3].

While the NCCN recommends thorough diagnostics for possible treatable causes of anemia, including AID and FID, and specifies the parameters to be tested, no guideline on the diagnostics and treatment of cancer-related anemia has been published in Europe to date. In the TAR study, testing for iron parameters was performed more often in patients with colorectal cancer than in patients affected by other malignancies, accompanied by a higher frequency of IV iron therapy in this patient subgroup. This indicates that physicians currently use diagnostics for specific subsets of patients rather than as a routine requirement prior to any antianemic therapy.

IV iron has been shown to improve the efficacy of ESAs in patients with FID and is thus recommended for this patient subgroup [10, 12]. In addition, IV or oral iron is the treatment of choice in patients with AID [12]. In the TANDEM study, a diagnostic algorithm to select patients to antianemic treatment was suggested [24] based on the diagnostic plot by C. Thomas and L. Thomas [25] and identified about 25% of patients with iron deficiency in a cohort primarily designated for ESA treatment.

3.4. Effectiveness. Overall, antianemic treatment was successful in approximately half of all patients ("responders," Table 2). Data on effectiveness are limited by the observational study design. There is considerable heterogeneity between the patients and thus effectiveness of treatments and QoL should not be compared between the different types of therapies. Causal relations cannot be drawn. Patient characteristics and inclusion criteria, such as baseline Hb levels <11 g/dL (females) or <12 g/dL (males), have to be considered when comparing data with other published studies.

Patients receiving transfusions had median final Hb between 1.2 and 1.6 g/dL above baseline, depending on the type of disease (ΔHb(final), Table 2). The maximum median increase after the start of treatment was between 2.6 and 2.9 g/dL (ΔHb(max), Table 2). Patients receiving ESAs showed median final Hb between 1.9 and 2.1 g/dL above baseline (ΔHb(final), Table 2). The maximum median increase was between 2.6 and 2.7 g/dL after the start of treatment (ΔHb(max), Table 2). Patients with inoperable solid tumors treated solely with IV iron, who in general had higher baseline Hb values (median 9.6 g/dL, Table 1), showed median final Hb of 1.1 g/dL above baseline. Due to the small number of patients, effectiveness parameters for other subgroups should be interpreted with caution.

The majority of patients receiving no RBCTx as antianemic therapy required no additional transfusions during the observation period (Table 2). According to the criteria defined in this study, all treatments were on average effective within the patient populations investigated. More than half of all patients showed a long-term rise in Hb levels. The main

purpose of antianemic treatment is not only to correct Hb levels, but also to improve QoL [3].

3.5. Quality of Life. While QoL is being measured more frequently in clinical trials, data on QoL in unselected, real-life patients are still rare. The FACT-An questionnaire is a validated tool to assess QoL in anemic cancer patients and to discriminate patients by their Hb levels and physical performance status [26]. In total, 78%, 70%, and 60% of the patients returned QoL questionnaires at baseline, after 6 weeks, and after 12 weeks, respectively. Median baseline FACT-An total scores (maximum 188 points) indicating overall QoL were between 104.1 and 115.9 points for all patients, with patients receiving transfusions having the lowest score (Figure 4(a)). Median baseline anemia-specific subscale scores (maximum 80 points) were <45 for all patients (transfusion: 41.6, ESA: 44.0, IV iron: 43.5, and ESA + IV iron: 41.0; Figure 4(b)). The median anemia-specific subscale scores showed improvement in all treatment groups. Clinically meaningful changes (≥4 points) were observed after 12 weeks for patients receiving ESA (44.0 to 48.2 points), IV iron (43.5 to 51.3 points), or ESA + IV iron (41.0 to 50.0 points). For patients receiving ESAs, clinically meaningful changes were already observed after 6 weeks (44.0 to 48.2 points). Overall QoL, as measured by the FACT-An total scores, also showed a median improvement after 12 weeks for patients receiving IV iron or ESA + IV iron. The difference reached the level of clinical relevance (≥7 points) for patients receiving ESA + IV iron (106.5 to 117.5 points); however, due to the small number of patients, this result should be interpreted with caution.

On average, a clinically meaningful improvement in the anemia-specific subscale scores was observed for TAR patients undergoing therapies other than RBCTx. However, this has to be interpreted with caution and might not be caused by the treatment applied, since patients receiving transfusions had lower Hb values at the start of treatment among other differences, which may also affect QoL. Improvement in QoL during antianemic treatment was also recently reported for patients receiving darbepoetin in German routine practice [7].

4. Conclusion

The aim of the TAR study was to assess the current treatment of anemia in cancer patients in German routine practice. Our data show that the majority of patients receive RBCTx, while ESAs, IV iron, or a combination of both is applied less frequently. Diagnostic testing for iron or other nutritional deficiencies is not routinely performed before treatment. All antianemic treatments were effective within the patient populations examined. Therefore, our data suggest that diagnostics for possible causes and causal therapies of anemia are underused in German routine practice. The large proportion of patients treated with transfusions, especially with Hb values ≥8 g/dL, highlights the need for systematic studies on the benefits of diagnostic-led treatment decision-making and for a European guideline on anemia management. It urgently needs to be discussed whether thorough diagnostics and

TABLE 2: Effectiveness of antianemic treatments in German routine practice.

Day 1 treatment	Operable solid tumor (n = 207)				Inoperable solid tumor (n = 606)				Hematological malignancy (n = 149)			
	Transfusion	ESA	IV iron	ESA + IV iron	Transfusion	ESA	IV iron	ESA + IV iron	Transfusion	ESA	IV iron	ESA + IV iron
ΔHb(max)[b] [g/dL]												
n[a]	78	41	18	11	257	79	71	27	67	34	7	5
Median	2.9	2.7	2.0	2.6	2.7	2.6	2.0	2.3	2.6	2.6	2.0	2.9
Mean ± StD	3.1 ± 1.5	3.0 ± 1.4	2.3 ± 1.2	2.8 ± 1.3	2.8 ± 1.8	2.8 ± 1.5	2.0 ± 1.6	2.5 ± 1.3	2.6 ± 1.5	2.5 ± 1.9	2.6 ± 1.5	2.8 ± 1.5
ΔHb(final)[c] [g/dL]												
n[a]	63	40	16	11	223	77	67	26	62	32	7	5
Median	1.6	2.0	1.6	1.7	1.5	1.9	1.1	1.8	1.2	2.1	2.0	2.3
Mean ± StD	2.0 ± 1.8	2.1 ± 1.2	1.7 ± 1.5	2.1 ± 1.3	1.6 ± 1.5	2.1 ± 1.7	1.3 ± 1.5	1.9 ± 1.5	1.6 ± 1.8	1.9 ± 2.0	2.4 ± 1.6	2.2 ± 1.9
Responders[d]												
n[a]	63	40	16	11	223	77	67	26	62	32	7	5
%	50.8	72.5	62.5	63.6	41.3	55.8	43.3	57.7	35.5	59.4	57.1	80.0
Transfusions												
n[a]	114	51	30	12	362	108	102	34	95	37	10	7
Weeks 1–4 [%]	100.0	25.5	13.3	8.3	100.0	26.9	16.7	17.6	100.0	29.7	10.0	—
Weeks 5–8 [%]	24.6	5.9	6.7	—	31.5	14.8	9.8	2.9	44.2	10.8	10.0	14.3
Weeks 9–12 [%]	17.5	3.9	3.3	—	26.2	8.3	7.8	5.9	33.7	21.6	20.0	—

[a] Number of patients for whom variable is documented or could be calculated.

[b] The maximal difference between the baseline Hb and the highest Hb documented.

[c] The difference between the baseline Hb and the last Hb documented within the 12-week observation period, but at least 4 weeks after the start of treatment.

[d] A responder is defined as a patient with final Hb > 11 g/dL or with ΔHb(final) of ≥ 1.5 g/dL, with final Hb being the last documented Hb within the observation period, but at least 4 weeks after the start of antianemic treatment.

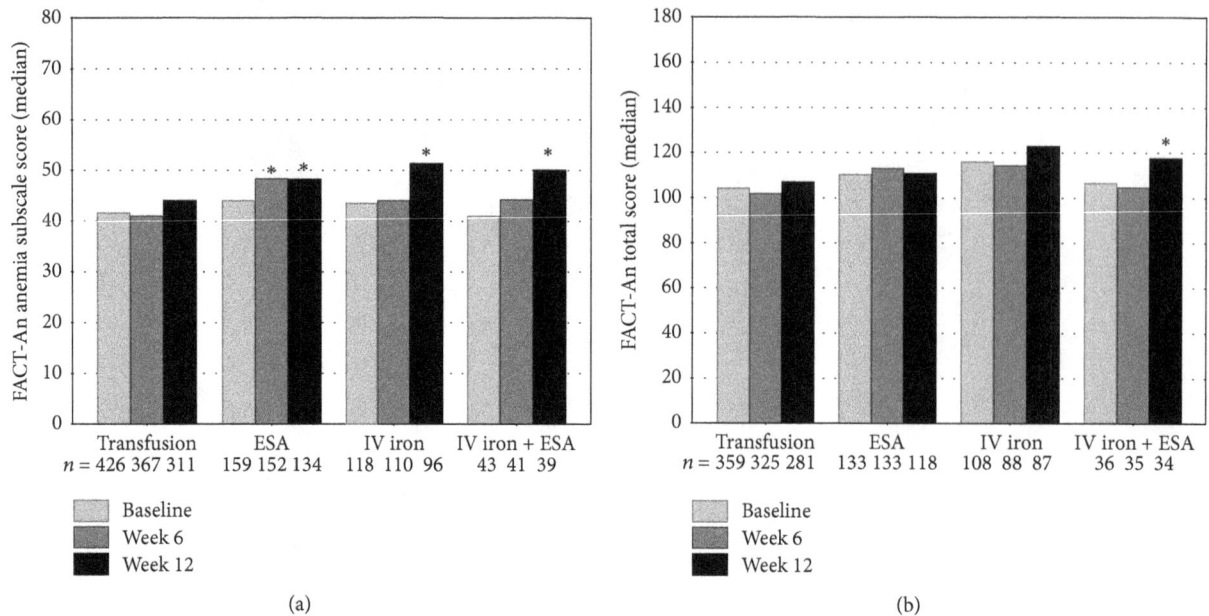

(a)

(b)

FIGURE 4: Quality of life (QoL) of patients assessed by the FACT-An questionnaire at baseline and after 6 and 12 weeks of the observation period. (a) Anemia-specific subscale score range [0–80]; *a difference of 4 points is considered clinically relevant [14, 15]; (b) FACT-An total score range [0–188]; *a difference of 7 points is considered clinically relevant [14, 15]; higher scores indicate a better QoL; numbers indicate the number of questionnaires returned.

earlier intervention can decrease the need for transfusions, at least in subsets of patients.

Conflict of Interests

The authors declare that there is no conflict of interests regarding the publication of this paper.

Acknowledgments

The authors thank all patients, physicians, and study teams participating in the TAR study. They also thank Vifor Pharma Deutschland GmbH for the supporting research grant. Moreover, they thank Holger Hartmann and Jörg Spirik (iOMEDICO) and Olof Harlin and Garth Virgin (Vifor Pharma) for support and comments during the design and setup of the project; Martina Jänicke, Anja Kaiser-Osterhues, Lisa Spring, and Susanne Tech (iOMEDICO) for support with the writing of the paper; and Beate Stremmel and Garth Virgin (Vifor Pharma) for critical comments on the paper. The study was conducted in collaboration with the Arbeitsgemeinschaft Supportive Maßnahmen in der Onkologie, Rehabilitation und Sozialmedizin (ASORS).

References

[1] WHO, "Haemoglobin concentrations for the diagnosis of anaemia and assessment of severity," Vitamin and Mineral Nutrition Information System, Geneva, Switzerland, World Health Organization (WHO/NMH/NHD/MNM/11.1), 2011, http://www.who.int/vmnis/indicators/haemoglobin.pdf.

[2] H. Ludwig, S. Van Belle, P. Barrett-Lee et al., "The European Cancer Anaemia Survey (ECAS): a large, multinational, prospective survey defining the prevalence, incidence, and treatment of anaemia in cancer patients," European Journal of Cancer, vol. 40, no. 15, pp. 2293–2306, 2004.

[3] T. Steinmetz, U. Totzke, M. Schweigert et al., "A prospective observational study of anaemia management in cancer patients—results from the German Cancer Anaemia Registry," European Journal of Cancer Care, vol. 20, no. 4, pp. 493–502, 2011.

[4] G. Birgegård, P. Gascón, and H. Ludwig, "Evaluation of anaemia in patients with multiple myeloma and lymphoma: findings of the European CANCER ANAEMIA SURVEY," European Journal of Haematology, vol. 77, no. 5, pp. 378–386, 2006.

[5] P. J. Barrett-Lee, H. Ludwig, G. Birgegård et al., "Independent risk factors for anemia in cancer patients receiving chemotherapy: results from the European Cancer Anaemia Survey," Oncology, vol. 70, no. 1, pp. 34–48, 2006.

[6] J. Bohlius, T. Tonia, E. Nüesch et al., "Effects of erythropoiesis-stimulating agents on fatigue- and anaemia-related symptoms in cancer patients: systematic review and meta-analyses of published and unpublished data," British Journal of Cancer, vol. 111, no. 1, pp. 33–45, 2014.

[7] T. Steinmetz, M. Kindler, O. Lange, U. Vehling-Kaiser, A. Kuhn, and E. Hellebrand, "A prospective cohort study on the impact of darbepoetin alfa on quality of life in daily practice following anemia treatment guideline revisions," Current Medical Research and Opinion, vol. 30, no. 9, pp. 1813–1820, 2014.

[8] J. L. Spivak, P. Gascón, and H. Ludwig, "Anemia management in oncology and hematology," Oncologist, vol. 14, supplement 1, pp. 43–56, 2009.

[9] D. Cella, M. J. Zagari, C. Vandoros, D. D. Gagnon, H.-J. Hurtz, and J. W. R. Nortier, "Epoetin alfa treatment results in clinically

significant improvements in quality of life in anemic cancer patients when referenced to the general population," *Journal of Clinical Oncology*, vol. 21, no. 2, pp. 366–373, 2003.

[10] M. S. Aapro and H. Link, "September 2007 update on EORTC guidelines and anemia management with erythropoiesis-stimulating agents," *Oncologist*, vol. 13, supplement 3, pp. 33–36, 2008.

[11] J. D. Rizzo, M. Brouwers, P. Hurley et al., "American Society of Clinical Oncology/American Society of Hematology clinical practice guideline update on the use of epoetin and darbepoetin in adult patients with cancer," *Journal of Clinical Oncology*, vol. 28, no. 33, pp. 4996–5010, 2010.

[12] NCCN, *NCCN Clinical Practice Guidelines in Oncology: Cancer- and Chemotherapy-Induced Anemia*, Version 2.2015, National Comprehensive Cancer Network, 2015, http://www.nccn.org/professionals/physician_gls/pdf/anemia.pdf.

[13] Bundesärztekammer BÄK (German Medical Association), "Cross-sectional guidelines for therapy with blood components and plasma derivatives—4th revised edition," *Transfusion Medicine and Hemotherapy*, vol. 36, pp. 345–492, 2009.

[14] K. Webster, D. Cella, and K. Yost, "The Functional Assessment of Chronic Illness Therapy (FACIT) measurement system: properties, applications, and interpretation," *Health and Quality of Life Outcomes*, vol. 1, article 79, 2003.

[15] J. Ringash, B. O'Sullivan, A. Bezjak, and D. A. Redelmeier, "Interpreting clinically significant changes in patient-reported outcomes," *Cancer*, vol. 110, no. 1, pp. 196–202, 2007.

[16] M. E. Charlson, P. Pompei, K. L. Ales, and C. R. MacKenzie, "A new method of classifying prognostic comorbidity in longitudinal studies: development and validation," *Journal of Chronic Diseases*, vol. 40, no. 5, pp. 373–383, 1987.

[17] FACIT.org, "FACT-An Scoring Guidelines," Version 4, May 2003.

[18] A. Calabrich and A. Katz, "Management of anemia in cancer patients," *Future Oncology*, vol. 7, no. 4, pp. 507–517, 2011.

[19] M. L. Thomas, "Anemia and quality of life in cancer patients: impact of transfusion and erythropoietin," *Medical Oncology*, vol. 15, supplement 1, pp. S13–S18, 1998.

[20] P. J. Barrett-Lee, N. P. Bailey, M. E. R. O'Brien, and E. Wager, "Large-scale UK audit of blood transfusion requirements and anaemia in patients receiving cytotoxic chemotherapy," *British Journal of Cancer*, vol. 82, no. 1, pp. 93–97, 2000.

[21] C. Bokemeyer, M. S. Aapro, A. Courdi et al., "EORTC guidelines for the use of erythropoietic proteins in anaemic patients with cancer: 2006 update," *European Journal of Cancer*, vol. 43, no. 2, pp. 258–270, 2007.

[22] T. Tonia and J. Bohlius, "Ten years of meta-analyses on erythropoiesis-stimulating agents in cancer patients," in *Hematopoietic Growth Factors in Oncology*, vol. 157 of *Cancer Treatment and Research*, pp. 217–238, Springer, Berlin, Germany, 2011.

[23] T. Tonia, A. Mettler, N. Robert et al., "Erythropoietin or darbepoetin for patients with cancer," *Cochrane Database of Systematic Reviews*, vol. 12, Article ID CD003407, 2012.

[24] H. T. Steinmetz, A. Tsamaloukas, S. Schmitz et al., "A new concept for the differential diagnosis and therapy of anaemia in cancer patients," *Supportive Care in Cancer*, vol. 19, no. 2, pp. 261–269, 2010.

[25] C. Thomas and L. Thomas, "Biochemical markers and hematologic indices in the diagnosis of functional iron deficiency," *Clinical Chemistry*, vol. 48, no. 7, pp. 1066–1076, 2002.

[26] S. B. Yellen, D. F. Cella, K. Webster, C. Blendowski, and E. Kaplan, "Measuring fatigue and other anemia-related symptoms with the Functional Assessment of Cancer Therapy (FACT) measurement system," *Journal of Pain and Symptom Management*, vol. 13, no. 2, pp. 63–74, 1997.

29

Prevalence and Risk Factors for Complications in Patients with Nontransfusion Dependent Alpha- and Beta-Thalassemia

**Poramed Winichakoon,[1] Adisak Tantiworawit,[1]
Thanawat Rattanathammethee,[1] Sasinee Hantrakool,[1] Chatree Chai-Adisaksopha,[1]
Ekarat Rattarittamrong,[1] Lalita Norasetthada,[1] and Pimlak Charoenkwan[2]**

[1]*Division of Hematology, Department of Internal Medicine, Faculty of Medicine, Chiang Mai University,
110 Intravaroros Road, A. Muang, Chiang Mai 50200, Thailand*
[2]*Division of Hematology and Oncology, Department of Pediatrics, Faculty of Medicine, Chiang Mai University,
110 Intravaroros Road, A. Muang, Chiang Mai 50200, Thailand*

Correspondence should be addressed to Adisak Tantiworawit; atantiwo@yahoo.com

Academic Editor: Aurelio Maggio

Background. Nontransfusion dependent thalassemia (NTDT) is a milder form of thalassemia that does not require regular transfusion. It is associated with many complications, which differ from that found in transfusion-dependent thalassemia (TDT). Currently available information is mostly derived from beta-NTDT; consequently, more data is needed to describe complications found in the alpha-NTDT form of this disease. *Methods.* We retrospectively reviewed the medical records of NTDT patients from January 2012 to December 2013. Complications related to thalassemia were reviewed and compared. *Results.* One hundred patients included 60 females with a median age of 38 years. The majority (54 patients) had alpha-thalassemia. Overall, 83 patients had one or more complications. The three most common complications were cholelithiasis (35%), abnormal liver function (29%), and extramedullary hematopoiesis (EMH) (25%). EMH, cardiomyopathy, cholelithiasis, and pulmonary hypertension were more commonly seen in beta-thalassemia. Osteoporosis was the only complication that was more common in alpha-thalassemia. The risk factors significantly related to EMH were beta-thalassemia type and hemoglobin < 8 g/dL. The risk factors related to osteoporosis were female gender and age > 40 years. Iron overload (ferritin > 800 ng/mL) was the only risk factor for abnormal liver function. *Conclusion.* The prevalence of alpha-NTDT complications was lower and different from beta-thalassemia.

1. Introduction

Thalassemia is a well-known inherited hematologic disorder caused by a decrease or an absence of globin production [1]. Patients with thalassemia suffer from chronic hemolytic anemia and its sequelae. Thalassemia originates from varying genetic abnormalities that result in different clinical presentation. Nontransfusion dependent thalassemia (NTDT) or thalassemia intermedia (TI) is a milder form of thalassemia which does not require regular blood transfusion for survival. This group of thalassemia patients was recognized earlier as a TI but no consensus on diagnostic criteria has been reached due to high clinical variations ranging from asymptomatic to multiorgan involvement [2–9]. The terminology has been changed from TI to NTDT [10]. Generally patients with NTDT can maintain hemoglobin levels at 6–10 g/dL with occasional blood transfusions that may be required with fever, infection, or pregnancy [3, 4, 7, 8, 10]. Complications of NTDT result from chronic hemolysis and tissue hypoxia, causing iron overload and problems in many organ systems [5, 6, 8, 11–20]. According to the largest observational study on thalassemia intermedia (OPTIMAL CARE study; n = 584 TI patients), the three most common complications were osteoporosis, extramedullary hematopoiesis (EMH), and hypogonadism, respectively [8].

Several complications that are associated with thalassemia intermedia are less frequently seen in thalassemia major, including EMH, leg ulcers, gallstones, and thrombophilia [8].

TABLE 1: Clinical definition required to confirm identified complications.

Complications	Definition
Extramedullary hematopoiesis (EMH)	Physical or radiologic evidence of extramedullary hematopoietic foci with or without symptoms
Pulmonary hypertension (PHT)	Systolic pulmonary artery pressure > 35 mmHg, which corresponds to a tricuspid regurgitant velocity on Doppler echocardiography of > 2.8 m/s plus exertional dyspnea without evidence of left heart disease
Thrombosis	Compression ultrasonography, contrast venography, or angiography evidence of thrombus
Cardiomyopathy	Echocardiographic, electrodiagnostic, or radiologic evidence of pathological change of myocardium such as hypertrophy, dilatation, or restriction
Cholelithiasis	Radiologic evidence of gallbladder stones
Abnormal liver function	ALT > 50 U/L
Pseudoxanthoma elasticum (PXE)	Histopathologic evidence of pathological change in elastic fibers to inelastic tissue
Leg ulcers	Ischemic or necrotic skin lesion on the lower extremity by general visual inspection
Osteoporosis (OP)	Bone densitometry T score < 2.5 SD
Abnormal plasma glucose	Fasting plasma glucose > 110 mg/dL at least one time
Hypothyroidism	TSH > 4.7 U/L and a free T4 > 0.8 ng/dL
Hypogonadism	Females: > 13 years, not yet Tanner B2 (i.e., prepubertal breast development) or > 14 years requiring estrogen replacement therapy or > 15 years with primary amenorrhea; males: > 14 years, not yet Tanner G2 (i.e., prepubertal genital development) or on androgen replacement therapy or > 17 years, not yet Tanner G4 (i.e., midpubertal genital development)
Iron overload	Maximum ferritin level >800 ng/mL with or without radiologic or histopathologic evidence

Adapted from [8].

One of the most serious complications in NTDT is pulmonary hypertension which can be found in 11–50% of patients and leads to heart failure; the most common cause of death in NTDT patients [3, 4, 6, 8, 11, 13, 14, 16].

In our region, the proportion of patients classified by thalassemia type is changing due to advances in prenatal diagnoses and early detection. Higher numbers of NTDT patients are diagnosed and more fetuses with severe thalassemia are terminated.

Many previous studies aim to establish predictive factors for thalassemia complications and report that mechanisms for complications in thalassemia are multifactorial [3, 6, 8, 12, 15, 21–27].

In our region, the prevalence of alpha-thalassemia is greater than that of beta-thalassemia which is different from the prevalence found in other regions [25, 26, 28–30]. The lack of studies and clear guidelines in this group can present a significant clinical challenge. This study aims to elucidate the prevalence of complications and identify predictive factors affecting complication of both alpha- and beta-NTDT patients.

2. Material and Method

We retrospectively reviewed medical records of NTDT patients who attended the Chiang Mai University Hospital Adult Hematology Clinic for the two-year period from January 1, 2012, to December 31, 2013.

2.1. Population. The NTDT patients, age 15 years or older, were included in the study. NTDT is defined by thalassemia disease that does not require regular transfusion for survival [10]. However, the definition of transfusion varies among studies. We used the criteria of less than an average of three transfusions per year for the purpose of the study. The patient needed to visit the clinic at least once in order to be enrolled.

The diagnosis for the type of NTDT patients was made by hemoglobin analysis using a high-performance liquid column chromatography (HPLC) method. The molecular confirmation of α^0-thalassemia (Southeast Asian or Thai deletion) and HbCS was done for cases with HbH disease and HbH with Hb Constant Spring (HbH/CS) disease. Molecular diagnosis of beta-globin mutations was done in cases with beta NTDT when the results from hemoglobin analysis by HPLC method showed abnormal hemoglobin peak other than Hb E.

2.2. Data Collection. From January 1, 2012, to December 31, 2013, medical records of NTDT patients who met the inclusion criteria were reviewed. Data collected from medical records included demographic characteristics and diagnosis obtained by hemoglobin analysis. Also, findings from physical examination, laboratory investigations, and records of complications were recorded. The definition of conditions and complications in this study are shown in Table 1 [8].

2.3. Complications. Complications of NTDT patients were retrospectively collected from the medical record.

All NTDT patients had regular evaluation and investigations for these complications: three-monthly liver function tests and serum ferritin, annual tests for endocrine function which included fasting plasma glucose, thyroid function test, and hormonal assays for hypogonadism. Hepatitis B and C virus test were also done annually. Chest radiograph and echocardiogram were obtained for suspected cases of cardiomyopathy. Spine radiograph and bone mass densitometry were conducted in suspected osteoporosis cases.

For other complications such as extramedullary hematopoiesis (EMH), pulmonary hypertension (PHT), thrombosis, cardiomyopathy, cholelithiasis, pseudoxanthoma elasticum (PXE), leg ulcers, and osteoporosis (OP), the information was obtained retrospectively from medical records. Investigations for complications listed in Table 1 were conducted for putative cases where risk factors were present.

2.4. Statistical Analysis. Data were entered into database, crossed-checked, and analyzed using SPSS statistics software. Descriptive results of categorical and continuous variables were expressed as mean (±SD) or median (range in continuous variables) depending on their distribution or as percentages of the group from which they were derived (categorical variables). The Chi-square test or Fisher exact test was used to compare categorical variables and Student's *t*-test was used to compare between continuous variables as appropriate. Variables that were significantly related to complications or with *p* values less than 0.05 in the univariate analysis were entered into the multivariate analyses. Multivariate logistic regression analysis was used to identify independent risk factors for complications. Odds ratios (OR) and 95% confidence intervals (CI) were calculated for all associations that emerged. A *p* value less than 0.05 was considered as statistically significant.

3. Results

3.1. Patient Characteristics. During the study period, 250 thalassemia patients attended our clinic. Of these, 100 NTDT patients who matched our inclusion criteria were included in this study, 60 patients (60%) were female. Table 2 summarized patient demographics, underlying diseases and conditions, and clinical characteristics. The median age was 38 years (range 19–78 years). More than half of patients (54%) were diagnosed with alpha-thalassemia. The mean ferritin level was 1,563.46 ng/mL while 76% and 44% of patients had ferritin levels more than 800 and 2,500 ng/mL, respectively. Chronic hepatitis B infection (27%) was the most common comorbid condition.

3.2. Complications and Treatment Outcomes. Figure 1 summarizes patient treatments and the outcomes. Fifty-five of 100 patients (55%) received iron chelation treatment for iron overload, and 33 of these patients (33%) underwent a splenectomy. Overall, complications occurred in 83% of the study population. The three most common complications

TABLE 2: Characteristics of the study populations.

Parameter	Frequency, number (%)
Gender	
Male	40 (40%)
Female	60 (60%)
Age	
<40 years	54 (54%)
≥40 years	46 (46%)
Region	
Northern Thailand	97 (97%)
Other	3 (3%)
Comorbidities	
Cerebrovascular disease	2 (2%)
Chronic lung disease	4 (4%)
Chronic kidney disease	11 (11%)
Cirrhosis	9 (9%)
Diabetes mellitus	11 (11%)
Dyslipidemia	2 (2%)
Endocrine disease	16 (16%)
Eye-ENT disease	4 (4%)
Gynecologic disease	4 (4%)
Heart disease	8 (8%)
Hypertension	7 (7%)
HBV infection	27 (27%)
HCV infection	12 (12%)
Malignancy	4 (4%)
Seizure	4 (4%)
Personal history	
Alcohol drinking	14 (14%)
Herb use	1 (1%)
Smoking	4 (4%)
Thalassemia type	
Alpha-thalassemia	54 (54%)
Hemoglobin H	38 (38%)
Hemoglobin H/CS	16 (16%)
Beta-thalassemia	46 (46%)
Beta-thalassemia and HbE disease	36 (36%)
Beta-thalassemia intermedia	10 (10%)
Hemoglobin	
Mean hemoglobin level	7.8 g/dL
Platelet	
Mean platelet count	330,900/mm^3
Serum ferritin, ng/mL	
Mean ferritin	1,563.46 ng/mL
Maximum ferritin > 800 ng/mL	76 (76%)

Hemoglobin H/CS: hemoglobin H with Hb constant spring.

were cholelithiasis (35%), abnormal liver function (29%), and EMH (25%). Other complications included osteoporosis (17%), abnormal plasma glucose (16%), pulmonary hypertension (14%), hypothyroidism (13%), cardiomyopathy (11%), thrombosis (4%), hypogonadism (7%), and leg ulcers (2%), respectively.

TABLE 3: Treatment, outcome, and complications in study population.

Parameter	Frequency N = 100 (%)	α-Thal (%) N = 54 (%)	β-Thal (%) N = 46 (%)
Treatment			
Antiplatelet	26%	3 (5.6)	23 (50)
Iron chelation	55%	21 (38.9)	34 (73.9)
Splenectomy	33%	8 (14.8)	25 (54.3)
Complications			
Abnormal plasma glucose	16%	9 (16.6)	7 (15.2)
Abnormal liver function	29%	15 (27.7)	14 (30.4)
Cardiomyopathy	11%	3 (5.5)	8 (17.4)
Cholelithiasis	35%	15 (27.7)	20 (43.5)
Cholecystectomy	25%	10 (18.5)	15 (32.6)
EMH	25%	3 (5.6)	22 (47.8)
Hypothyroidism	13%	6 (11.1)	7 (15.2)
Hypogonadism	7%	2 (3.7)	5 (10.9)
Leg ulcers	2%	1 (1.8)	1 (2.2)
Osteoporosis	17%	11 (20.4)	6 (13.0)
PHT	14%	3 (5.6)	11 (23.9)
PXE	None	None	None
Thrombosis	4%	2 (3.7)	2 (4.3)
Overall complications	83%	43 (79.6)	40 (87)

EMH: extramedullary hematopoiesis, PHT: pulmonary hypertension, PXE: pseudoxanthoma elasticum, α-Thal: alpha-thalassemia, and β-Thal: beta-thalassemia.

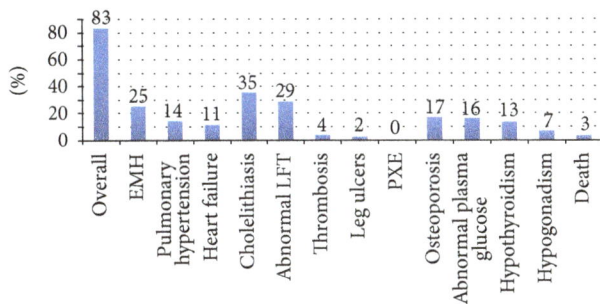

EMH: extramedullary hematopoiesis
LFT: liver function test
PXE: pseudoxanthoma elasticum

FIGURE 1: Percentage of complications and mortality in study population.

The radiologic investigations including plain film, CT scan, and MRI were used to detect EMH complications. Paravertebral soft tissue masses were found in nine patients, thalassemic bone change was found in five patients, and 11 patients had both paravertebral soft tissue and thalassemic bone change. All paravertebral soft tissue masses (20 patients) were found in the thoracic spine region. Thalassemic bone changes were found in the ribs (14 patients), femur (one patient), and spine (one patient).

3.3. Complications in Alpha and Beta-NTDT.

The differences of complications classified by type of thalassemia were summarized in Table 3. The most common complications were similar between alpha- and beta-thalassemia groups: cholelithiasis and abnormal liver function test. However, the prevalence of cardiomyopathy, cholelithiasis, and pulmonary hypertension was higher in beta-thalassemia but the differences were not statistically significant. Osteoporosis was the only complication that was more commonly seen in alpha-thalassemia.

Though not statically significant, beta-thalassemia patients tended to have higher clinical severity and required further treatment more frequently than those with alpha-thalassemia. The mean ferritin level for the beta-thalassemia group (1,971 ng/mL) was higher than the alpha-thalassemia group (1,202 ng/mL). Seventy-four percent of beta-thalassemia patients received iron chelation as compared to 39% in alpha-thalassemia patients. Splenectomy was performed in 54.3% of beta-thalassemia and only 14.8% of alpha-thalassemia patients.

3.4. Risk Factors Affecting Complications.

Results from the univariate analysis of significant risk factors for each complication were shown in Table 4. The following factors were significant in the model: extramedullary hematopoiesis, female gender ($p = 0.05$), beta-thalassemia ($p = 0.031$), hemoglobin level below 8 g/dL ($p = 0.003$), platelets above 400,000/mm^3 ($p = 0.025$), maximum ferritin more than

TABLE 4: Significant risk factors affecting complications from univariate analysis.

Complication	Significant variables	p value
Extramedullary hematopoiesis	Gender (female)	0.050
	Thalassemia type (beta)	0.031
	Hemoglobin < 8 g/dL	0.003
	Platelets > 400,000 per cumm.	0.025
	Maximum ferritin > 800 ng/mL	0.004
	Splenectomy	0.019
	Iron chelation	0.001
Pulmonary hypertension	None	—
Heart failure	Splenectomy	0.035
Cholelithiasis	None	—
Abnormal LFT (ALT >50 U/L)	Iron chelation	0.007
	Maximum ferritin > 800 ng/mL	0.041
	HCV infection*	0.143
Osteoporosis	Gender (female)	0.006
	Age > 40 years	0.003
Abnormal plasma glucose	None	—
Hypothyroidism	None	—
Hypogonadism	Splenectomy	0.016

*p value is not significant.

TABLE 5: Significant risk factors affecting complications from multivariate analysis.

Complication	Significant variables	p value	95% CI	Odd ratio
Extramedullary hematopoiesis	Thalassemia type (beta)	0.031	1.173–27.971	5.72
	Hemoglobin < 8 g/dL	0.007	1.736–31.252	7.37
Osteoporosis	Gender (female)	0.014	1.514–38.604	7.64
	Age > 40 years	0.017	1.313–16.506	4.66
Abnormal liver function	Maximum ferritin > 800 ng/mL	0.035	1.033–13.919	3.79

800 ng/mL ($p = 0.004$), iron chelation ($p = 0.001$), and splenectomy ($p = 0.019$). Splenectomy was also associated with heart failure ($p = 0.035$) and hypogonadism ($p = 0.016$). The significant risk factors affecting abnormal liver function tests were a maximum ferritin more than 800 ng/mL ($p = 0.041$) and iron chelation ($p = 0.007$). There was no statistically significant difference for the relationship between HCV infection and abnormal liver function. Female gender ($p = 0.006$) and age over 40 years ($p = 0.003$) were significant factors for osteoporosis. No significant risk factors were found in pulmonary hypertension, cholelithiasis, abnormal plasma glucose, and hypothyroidism.

From multivariate analysis, significant risk factors affecting complications in EMH were beta-thalassemia with an odds ratio 5.7 (95% CI 1.2–27.9, $p = 0.03$) and hemoglobin level below 8 g/dL with an odds ratio 7.4 (95% CI 1.7–31.3, $p = 0.007$). Significant risk factors affecting complications in osteoporosis were female gender with an odds ratio 7.4 (95% CI 1.5–38.6, $p = 0.014$) and age more than 40 years with an odds ratio 4.6 (95% CI 1.3–16.5, $p = 0.017$). Iron overload (ferritin > 800 ng/mL) was the only risk factor for abnormal liver function with an odds ratio of 3.7 (95% CI 1.0–13.9, $p = 0.035$) (Table 5).

4. Discussion

NTDT is thought to be a less severe form of thalassemia since regular transfusions are not required. However, several studies revealed that many complications occur in patients with this form of thalassemia [8, 11, 14, 19]. We compare prevalence and complications between alpha-NTDT and beta-NTDT and identify putative risk factors affecting complications in this group of patients.

Eighty-three percent of the study population (83 patients) experienced NTDT-related complications. Cholelithiasis (35%), abnormal liver function (29%), and EMH (25%) were the three most common complications found in this study. These results were similar to that found in a study of 37 NTDT patients in Lebanon [6] where common complications were cholelithiasis, pulmonary hypertension, leg ulcer, and EMH. Another study from Taher et al. [8] found that osteoporosis, EMH, hypogonadism, and cholelithiasis were the most common complications in NTDT. These findings indicate that complications from NTDT are quite different from TDT related complications which are mainly cardiomyopathy, endocrinopathy, and abnormal liver function [6].

Differences in the prevalence of complications across NTDT studies can be explained by the various complication definitions used, different in population numbers and type of NTDT (alpha or beta type). Our study had a higher portion of patients with alpha-NTDT which was different from previous studies [6, 8]. This study was done only in adult patients who tended to have more complications.

Another reason that can explain the high prevalence of EMH, cholelithiasis, and iron overload is that our study site is a referral center where most patients within the region with these complications were referred for further treatment.

The lower prevalence of thrombosis in our study may be due to a low incidence of thrombosis for the general Thai population when compared with other countries [31]. Moreover, thrombosis in thalassemia patients was largely disease related such as number of nucleated red cells, platelets $\geq 500 \times 10/mm^3$, and splenectomy. The lower number of mean platelet count and splenectomized patients from our study may also explain the lower incidence of thrombosis [8, 32]. Due to incomplete medical records, our study did not have data regarding the number of nucleated red cells and years following splenectomy which are valuable predictors of thrombosis risk.

In this study, we compared the prevalence of complications between alpha-NTDT and beta-NTDT, which contribute new information to the existing body of research focused mainly on beta-NTDT patients [4, 8, 15, 16]. In the multivariate analysis, beta-thalassemia was a significant risk factor for EMH complications (47.8% in beta-NTDT versus 5.6% in alpha-NTDT). However, this significance disappeared when further subgroup analysis into alpha and beta-NTDT populations reduced the number of patients. The alpha-NTDT group tended to have less severe clinical manifestations than the beta group such as the degree of iron overload and iron chelation therapy and splenectomy frequency.

In the OPTIMAL CARE study, splenectomy had a significant effect on almost all complications in TI patients [8] while none of complications in our study related with this condition perhaps due to the low number of splenectomized patients. The rate of splenectomy in our study was 33% compared to more than half in other studies [8].

Iron overload played a significant role in many TI related complications in previous studies and was also a risk factor for abnormal liver function tests in our study [8, 15, 24, 33, 34]. The incidence of iron overload was high in our study where 76% of patients had serum ferritin levels > 800 ng/mL. Half of these patients received iron chelation therapy while the other half could not afford iron chelation therapy. Studies indicate serum ferritin levels may underestimate liver iron burden in NTDT [8], which can explain the high prevalence of iron overload and abnormal liver function in our study. Hence, iron overload is a critical issue for NTDT patients, even ones who are not receiving regular blood transfusions.

The major limitation of this study was the retrospective data collection for some complications such as pulmonary hypertension (PHT), thrombosis, cardiomyopathy, leg ulcers, and osteoporosis (OP). The information was obtained retrospectively from medical records but not routinely accessed, which may cause an underrepresentation of these complications. The incomplete medical records could prevent us from identifying predictive risk factors. Another limitation of this study was the small number of patients comprising the alpha-NTDT and beta-NTDT subgroups.

In conclusion, despite variable clinical presentation and unclear diagnostic criteria, the prevalence of complications in NTDT was higher than and descriptively different from TDT. The prevalence of complications in alpha-NTDT was lower and descriptively different from beta-NTDT.

Conflict of Interests

The authors declare that there is no conflict of interests regarding the publication of this paper.

Authors' Contribution

Poramed Winichakoon was responsible for collecting the data, analyzing the data, interpreting the data, and writing the paper in part; Adisak Tantiworawit was responsible for conceiving and designing the study, obtaining funding and/or ethics approval, analyzing the data, interpreting the data, and writing the paper in whole; Thanawat Rattanathammethee, Ekarat Rattarittamrong, Lalita Norasetthada, Chatree Chai-Adisaksopha, Sasinee Hantrakool, and Pimlak Charoenkwan were responsible for revising the paper.

Acknowledgments

The authors thank Elizabeth Matovinovic (Faculty of Medicine, Research Administration, Chiang Mai University) for revising the paper. This work was supported by a grant from Chiang Mai University research fund.

References

[1] P. J. Giardina, "Thalassemia syndromes," in *Hematology: Basic Principles and Practice*, R. Hoffman, E. J. Benz, and S. S. Shattil, Eds., Elsevier Churchill Livingstone, Philadelphia, Pa, USA, 5th edition, 2008.

[2] C. Camaschella and M. D. Cappellini, "Thalassemia intermedia," *Haematologica*, vol. 80, no. 1, pp. 58–68, 1995.

[3] M. D. Cappellini, K. M. Musallam, and A. T. Taher, "Insight onto the pathophysiology and clinical complications of thalassemia intermedia," *Hemoglobin*, vol. 33, supplement 1, pp. S145–S159, 2009.

[4] F. El Rassi, M. D. Cappellini, A. Inati, and A. Taher, "Beta-thalassemia intermedia: an overview," *Pediatric Annals*, vol. 37, no. 5, pp. 322–328, 2008.

[5] K. M. Musallam, A. T. Taher, and E. A. Rachmilewitz, "β-thalassemia intermedia: a clinical perspective," *Cold Spring Harbor Perspectives in Medicine*, vol. 2, no. 7, Article ID a013482, 2012.

[6] A. Taher, H. Isma'eel, and M. D. Cappellini, "Thalassemia intermedia: revisited," *Blood Cells, Molecules, and Diseases*, vol. 37, no. 1, pp. 12–20, 2006.

[7] A. T. Taher, K. M. Musallam, and M. D. Cappellini, "Thalassaemia intermedia: an update," *Mediterranean Journal of Hematology and Infectious Diseases*, vol. 1, no. 1, Article ID e2009004, 2009.

[8] A. T. Taher, K. M. Musallam, M. Karimi et al., "Overview on practices in thalassemia intermedia management aiming for lowering complication rates across a region of endemicity: the OPTIMAL CARE study," *Blood*, vol. 115, no. 10, pp. 1886–1892, 2010.

[9] J. E. Maakaron, M. D. Cappellini, and A. T. Taher, "An update on thalassemia intermedia," *Journal Medical Libanais*, vol. 61, no. 3, pp. 175–182, 2013.

[10] D. J. Weatherall, "The definition and epidemiology of non-transfusion-dependent thalassemia," *Blood Reviews*, vol. 26, supplement 1, pp. S3–S6, 2012.

[11] C. Borgna-Pignatti, M. Marsella, and N. Zanforlin, "The natural history of thalassemia intermedia," *Annals of the New York Academy of Sciences*, vol. 1202, pp. 214–220, 2010.

[12] H. Isma'eel, A. H. E. Chafic, F. E. Rassi et al., "Relation between iron-overload indices, cardiac echo-Doppler, and biochemical markers in thalassemia intermedia," *American Journal of Cardiology*, vol. 102, no. 3, pp. 363–367, 2008.

[13] M. Karimi, K. M. Musallam, M. D. Cappellini et al., "Risk factors for pulmonary hypertension in patients with β thalassemia intermedia," *European Journal of Internal Medicine*, vol. 22, no. 6, pp. 607–610, 2011.

[14] B. N. Matta, K. M. Musallam, J. E. Maakaron, S. Koussa, and A. T. Taher, "A killer revealed: 10-year experience with beta-thalassemia intermedia," *Hematology*, vol. 19, no. 4, pp. 196–198, 2014.

[15] K. M. Musallam, M. D. Cappellini, and A. T. Taher, "Iron overload in β-thalassemia intermedia: an emerging concern," *Current Opinion in Hematology*, vol. 20, no. 3, pp. 187–192, 2013.

[16] A. Taher, F. El Rassi, H. Ismaeel, and A. Inati, "Complications of β-thalassemia intermedia: a 12-year Lebanese experience," *American Journal of Hematology*, vol. 83, no. 7, pp. 605–606, 2008.

[17] A. Taher, C. Hershko, and M. D. Cappellini, "Iron overload in thalassaemia intermedia: reassessment of iron chelation strategies," *British Journal of Haematology*, vol. 147, no. 5, pp. 634–640, 2009.

[18] A. T. Taher, K. M. Musallam, and A. Inati, "The hypercoagulable state in thalassemia intermedia," *Hemoglobin*, vol. 33, supplement 1, pp. S160–S169, 2009.

[19] J. E. Maakaron, "Complications and management of thalassemia intermedia," *Journal of Applied Hematology*, vol. 3, no. 4, pp. 143–146, 2012.

[20] M. D. Cappellini, K. M. Musallam, E. Poggiali, and A. T. Taher, "Hypercoagulability in non-transfusion-dependent thalassemia," *Blood Reviews*, vol. 26, no. 1, pp. S20–S23, 2012.

[21] C. Camaschella, U. Mazza, A. Roetto et al., "Genetic interactions in thalassemia intermedia: Analysis of β-mutations, α-genotype, γ-promoters, and β-LCR hypersensitive sites 2 and 4 in Italian patients," *American Journal of Hematology*, vol. 48, no. 2, pp. 82–87, 1995.

[22] C. Camaschella, G. Saglio, A. Serra et al., "Molecular characterization of thalassemia intermedia in Italy," *Birth Defects Original Article Series*, vol. 23, no. 5, pp. 111–116, 1987.

[23] F. X. Kleber, L. Niemoller, and W. Doering, "Impact of converting enzyme inhibition on progression of chronic heart failure: results of the Munich Mild Heart Failure Trial," *British Heart Journal*, vol. 67, no. 4, pp. 289–296, 1992.

[24] K. M. Musallam, M. D. Cappellini, J. C. Wood, and A. T. Taher, "Iron overload in non-transfusion-dependent thalassemia: a clinical perspective," *Blood Reviews*, vol. 26, no. 1, pp. S16–S19, 2012.

[25] L. Nuntakarn, S. Fucharoen, G. Fucharoen, K. Sanchaisuriya, A. Jetsrisuparb, and S. Wiangnon, "Molecular, hematological and clinical aspects of thalassemia major and thalassemia intermedia associated with Hb E-β-thalassemia in Northeast Thailand," *Blood Cells, Molecules, and Diseases*, vol. 42, no. 1, pp. 32–35, 2009.

[26] I. C. Verma, M. Kleanthous, R. Saxena et al., "Multicenter study of the molecular basis of thalassemia intermedia in different ethnic populations," *Hemoglobin*, vol. 31, no. 4, pp. 439–452, 2007.

[27] K. M. Musallam, A. Beydoun, R. Hourani et al., "Brain magnetic resonance angiography in splenectomized adults with β-thalassemia intermedia," *European Journal of Haematology*, vol. 87, no. 6, pp. 539–546, 2011.

[28] G. Fucharoen, H. Srivorakun, S. Singsanan, and S. Fucharoen, "Presumptive diagnosis of common haemoglobinopathies in Southeast Asia using a capillary electrophoresis system," *International Journal of Laboratory Hematology*, vol. 33, no. 4, pp. 424–433, 2011.

[29] S. Fucharoen, *Thalassemia: From Molecular Biology to Clinical Medicine*, Mahidol University, Bangkok, Thailand, 2007.

[30] S. Fucharoen and P. Winichagoon, "Haemoglobinopathies in Southeast Asia," *Indian Journal of Medical Research*, vol. 134, no. 10, pp. 498–506, 2011.

[31] P. Angchaisuksiri, V. Atichartakarn, K. Aryurachai et al., "Risk factors of venous thromboembolism in Thai patients," *International Journal of Hematology*, vol. 86, no. 5, pp. 397–402, 2007.

[32] A. T. Taher, K. M. Musallam, M. Karimi et al., "Splenectomy and thrombosis: the case of thalassemia intermedia," *Journal of Thrombosis and Haemostasis*, vol. 8, no. 10, pp. 2152–2158, 2010.

[33] E. B. Fung, P. R. Harmatz, P. D. K. Lee et al., "Increased prevalence of iron-overload associated endocrinopathy in thalassaemia versus sickle-cell disease," *British Journal of Haematology*, vol. 135, no. 4, pp. 574–582, 2006.

[34] K. M. Musallam, M. D. Cappellini, and A. T. Taher, "Evaluation of the 5mg/g liver iron concentration threshold and its association with morbidity in patients with β-thalassemia intermedia," *Blood Cells, Molecules, and Diseases*, vol. 51, no. 1, pp. 35–38, 2013.

30

Reproductive and Obstetric Factors Are Key Predictors of Maternal Anemia during Pregnancy in Ethiopia: Evidence from Demographic and Health Survey (2011)

Taddese Alemu[1] and Melaku Umeta[2]

[1]*Center of Food Science and Nutrition, College of Natural Sciences, Addis Ababa University, P.O. Box 1196, Addis Ababa, Ethiopia*
[2]*Department of Biochemistry, College of Medical Sciences, Addis Ababa University, P.O. Box 1196, Addis Ababa, Ethiopia*

Correspondence should be addressed to Taddese Alemu; tadal2005@yahoo.com

Academic Editor: Aurelio Maggio

Anemia is a major public health problem worldwide. In Ethiopia, a nationally representative and consistent evidence is lacking on the prevalence and determinants during pregnancy. We conducted an in-depth analysis of demographic and health survey for the year 2011 which is a representative data collected from all regions in Ethiopia. Considering maternal anemia as an outcome variable, predicting variables from sociodemographic, household, and reproductive/obstetric characteristics were identified for analyses. Logistic regression model was applied to identify predictors at $P < 0.05$. The prevalence of anemia among pregnant women was 23%. Maternal age, region, pregnancy trimester, number of under five children, previous history of abortion (termination of pregnancy), breastfeeding practices, and number of antenatal care visits were key independent predictors of anemia during pregnancy. In conclusion, the level of anemia during pregnancy is a moderate public health problem in Ethiopia. Yet, special preventive measures should be undertaken for pregnant women who are older in age and having too many under five children and previous history of abortion. Further evidence is expected to be generated concerning why pregnant mothers from the eastern part of the country and those with better access to radio disproportionately develop anemia more than their counterparts.

1. Introduction

Maternal death continues to be a major health and development concern globally, particularly in the developing world [1, 2]. In 2013 alone, there were an estimated 289,000 maternal deaths (210 deaths per 100,000 live births) across the globe, of which the sub-Saharan Africa region accounting for 62% (179,000) of these. During the same period, the mortality rate in developing regions (230) was 14 times higher than in developed regions (16) whilst the sub-Saharan Africa recorded the highest (510) regional MMR [2]. Astonishingly, over the 99% of these annual deaths occurring in developing countries are avoidable, as the healthcare solutions to prevent or manage complications are well known.

Regarding the major causes of maternal death, about 73% of all deaths between 2003 and 2009 were due to direct obstetric causes. Haemorrhage (27.1%), hypertensive disorders (14.0%), sepsis (10.7%), abortion (7.9%), and embolism accounted for the majority of these direct causes. On the other hand, the indirect causes contributed to over 27.5% of the maternal deaths globally and 28.6% in sub-Saharan Africa [1].

Anemia is one of the leading indirect causes of maternal mortality and it is the most common and intractable nutritional problem globally [3]. Although easily preventable and treatable, it is one of the most serious threats to the health of children and a factor in maternal mortality. In pregnant women, anemia results in an increased risk of premature delivery and low birth weight. It is also known to be an important factor in maternal death, the poor cognitive development of children, and decreased work capacity of the mother. It also decreases the health and energy of approximately 500 million women and leads to approximately 50,000 deaths in childbirth each year [4].

The World Health Organization (WHO) defines anemia as hemoglobin concentrations that are below recommended thresholds [3, 5]. The main causes of anemia are dietary iron deficiency; infectious diseases such as malaria, hookworm infections, and schistosomiasis; deficiencies of other key micronutrients including folate, vitamin B12, and vitamin A; or inherited conditions that affect red blood cells (RBCs), such as thalassaemia [6].

The prevalence of anemia during pregnancy is quite high (42%) globally and above 57.1% in Africa, signifying it as a severe public health problem in the region [3]. In Ethiopia, even if the situation seems better, the latest EDHS estimated that above 22% of women during pregnancy were found anemic [7]. On the other hand, some cross-sectional localized studies conducted at various regions of the country demonstrated that the prevalence of anemia among women of the reproductive age group in general and pregnant women in particular ranged from as low as 16.6% in the north [8] to a modest (33.2%) level in the south [9] and high up to 43.9% [10] in the eastern parts of the country.

On top of variation in the prevalence rate, the very important aspect of these local studies stipulating further investigation is the fact that none of them presented with conclusive and consistent findings on the determinants of anemia during pregnancy. A number of dissimilar and mutually exclusive determinant factors were identified in the studies. For instance, the northern study heightened hookworm infestation and HIV infection [8], whereas daily chewing of khat, restrictive dietary behavior, parity levels, and pregnancy trimesters were identified by the eastern study. Another relatively representative nationwide study [11] conducted in nine regions of the country identified other factors like chronic illnesses and deficiency of iron/folic acid as key determinants of anemia during pregnancy [11].

Generally, even if these studies have given important clues to policy makers, programmers, and other stakeholders, they mainly lack consistency and representatives to be used for national level policy making and programming by concerned bodies. Therefore, these in-depth analyses of the latest (2011) EDHS provide in-depth and explicit results on the prevalence and key proximate determinants of maternal anemia during pregnancy in Ethiopia.

2. Methods

2.1. Data Source. This study uses data from the Ethiopian Demographic and Health Survey (EDHS) conducted in 2011. The survey was conducted with nationally representative samples from all of the country's regions. The details of the sample design, including the sampling framework and sample implementation, and response rates are provided in the respective EDHS reports (http://www.measuredhs.com/).

In the DHS, there are three core questionnaires (household, women's, and male questionnaires) and nine recode files. This way of recoding is done because of two outstanding reasons: to define a standardized file that would make cross-country analysis easier and to compare data with the World Fertility Surveys (WFS) to study trends [12]. The recode files have five main and two additional digits. The first two digits of the file name correspond to the country code (e.g., ET for Ethiopia). The next two digits identify the unit of analysis (IR—women, KR—children, etc.). The fourth digit identifies the DHS phase. The fifth digit identifies the data release number and the last two digits identify whether it is a rectangular (RT) or flat (FL) file; for the hierarchical file they are left blank.

In our current analyses, we used ETIR61FL.SAV recode data files for prevalence and analyses of determinant factors. This means that we used the 2011 IR (women with completed interviews) EDHS data to describe the prevalence and determinants of anemia during pregnancy in Ethiopia.

2.2. Study Variables. The dependent variable is maternal anemia during pregnancy. According to the WHO and International Nutritional Anemia Consultative Group (INACG) [5, 13] anemia during pregnancy, after adjusting for altitude, is defined as a hemoglobin concentration of 11.0 g/dL and hemoglobin levels of 10–10.9 g/dL, 7–9.9 g/dL, and less than 7.0 g/dL were considered as mild, moderate, and severe anemia, respectively. Other cutoff points of hemoglobin concentration specific to trimesters of pregnancy are suggested by the International Nutritional Anemia Consultative Group (INACG) and others.

The selection of potential predictors of maternal anemia during pregnancy in this study is based on the literature and the availability of variables from the EDHS data sets on these potential predictors. An attempt is also made to test all potentially relevant variables existing in the EDHS data sets before concluding dropping of them; therefore, all variables which showed a statistical significance or some sort of trend during bivariate analyses are included into the analyses.

These potential predicting variables are categorized into three groups: sociodemographic characteristics, household variables, and maternal reproductive characteristics.

Sociodemographic Variables. These groups of indicators consist of both maternal and paternal (husbands') characteristics. Among the maternal characteristics, maternal age, urban/rural residence, region, educational status, and literacy level are included.

Household Variables. In this group, we included presence or absence of key household variables like electricity, radio, and television. Other variables included into this category are type of toilet facility (whether the household uses improved or nonimproved type of toilet) and sources of drinking water.

Maternal Reproductive and Obstetric Variables. Attributable to the nature of the study and availability of evidence by a wide range of literatures, a number of variables are included into this category as compared to the other two. Accordingly, pregnancy trimester, number of births in the last five years and last year, whether the current pregnancy is wanted or not, history of abortion (pregnancy termination), practice of breastfeeding, timing of first ANC visit, and number of ANC visits are all included.

TABLE 1: Sociodemographic characteristics of pregnant mothers and their association with anemia during pregnancy in Ethiopia, EDHS 2011.

Sociodemographic characteristic	Anemic (#)/(%)	Nonanemic (#)/(%)	Crude OR (95% CI)	Adjusted OR (95% CI)
(1) Age				
15–19	5 (12.5)	35 (87.5)	1	1
20–24	45 (19.1)	190 (80.9)	1.64 (0.61, 4.38)	1.57 (0.57, 4.35)
25–29	110 (23.7)	355 (76.3)	2.13 (0.82, 5.53)	2.35 (0.87, 6.35)
30–34	67 (27.1)	180 (72.9)	2.56 (0.97, 6.75)	2.65 (0.97, 7.260)
35–39	29 (20.1)	110 (79.1)	1.79 (0.65, 4.96)	2.04 (0.71, 5.85)
40–44	12 (30)	28 (70)	3.07 (0.98, 9.64)	3.43 (1.04, 11.28)[**]
45–49	2 (25)	6 (75)	1.82 (0.24, 13.70)	1.36 (0.15, 11.89)
(2) Residence				
Urban	25 (26.9)	68 (73.1)	1	1
Rural	245 (22.7)	836 (77.3)	0.77 (0.48, 1.25)	0.80 (0.43, 1.48)
(3) Region				
Tigray	16 (21.6)	58 (78.4)	1	1
Afar	7 (38.9)	11 (61.1)	2.23 (0.74, 6.71)	2.09 (0.68, 4.40)
Amhara	49 (31.2)	108 (68.8)	1.64 (0.86, 3.14)	1.62 (0.84, 3.14)
Oromia	129 (23.5)	419 (76.5)	1.11 (0.62, 1.99)	1.04 (0.57, 1.89)
Somali	29 (51.8)	27 (48.2)	3.93 (1.84, 8.39)	3.82 (1.71, 8.52)[**]
Ben.-Gumuz	5 (27.8)	13 (72.2)	1.47 (0.47, 4.61)	1.32 (0.41, 4.25)
SNNPR	30 (10.6)	252 (89.4)	0.44 (0.22, 0.85)	0.41 (0.21, 0.82)[**]
Gambella	1 (33.3)	2 (66.7)	1.79 (0.13, 23.8)	1.83 (0.11, 29.43)
Hareri	1 (33.3)	2 (66.7)	2.10 (0.14, 30.85)	2.10 (0.13, 32.89)
Addis Ababa	0 (0)	10 (100)		
Dire Dawa	3 (60)	2 (40)	4.97 (0.73, 33.64)	4.51 (0.63, 32.28)
(4) Maternal educ. status				
No education	206 (25)	617 (75)	1	1
Primary educ.	60 (18.4)	266 (81.6)	0.67 (0.48, 0.92)	0.95 (0.60, 1.51)
Sec. education	0 (0)	11 (100)	0.08 (0.002, 2.97)	0.24 (0.00, 10.82)
Higher educ.	5 (33.3)	10 (67.7)	1.31 (0.43, 4.01)	3.00 (0.66, 13.68)
(5) Maternal literacy level				
Cannot read/write	226 (23.7)	727 (76.3)	1	1
Partially read and write	25 (23.4)	82 (76.6)	0.99 (0.62, 1.59)	1.12 (0.61, 2.04)
Fully read and write	13 (13)	87 (87)	0.49 (0.27, 0.90)	0.46 (0.19, 1.11)

[**]Significant at P value < 0.05, OR: odds ratio.

2.3. *Data Analysis.* This study employed a three-stage analysis. In the first stage, univariate and bivariate analyses of the level (prevalence) of maternal anemia during pregnancy by the three categories of variables mentioned were calculated using chi-square, ANOVA, and Student's t-test.

In the later stage, binary logistic regression analyses of each variable to determine the crude odds ratio of each identified variable with maternal anemia were calculated. After making an appropriate selection of variables having a strong association with the dependent variable, we moved to the third stage of analyses of multivariate logistic regression analyses of all variables found statistically significant. SPSS version 20 software was used to run all stages of the analyses.

2.4. *Data Quality Assessment.* The data quality assessment report highlights its findings on misreporting, omission, and digit preference, which are common data quality problems observed in surveys and censuses in developing countries.

Over all, the assessment shows that the problems do not exist to the extent that might challenge the quality of the conclusions of this study.

3. Results

A total of 1,212 pregnant women were included into the initial analyses which is 10.2% of the total women of the reproductive age group from whom data was collected in the same survey. The overall prevalence of anemia in this group was found to be around 23%, varying from 12.4% milder forms to 9% and 1.6% moderate and severe forms, respectively (Figure 1 and Table 1).

In terms of maternal age, the lowest (12.5%) and the highest (30%) prevalence of anemia were seen among teenagers (15–19) and older (40–45) women, respectively. Women in the latter group had a 3.43 more added risk of developing anemia during pregnancy as compared to the reference age group

TABLE 2: Selected household characteristics of pregnant mothers and their association with anemia during pregnancy in Ethiopia, EDHS 2011.

Household characteristic	Anemic (#)/(%)	Nonanemic (#)/(%)	Crude OR (95% CI)	Adjusted OR (95% CI)
(1) Presence of electricity in the HH				
No	247 (23.7)	795 (76.3)	1	1
Yes	23 (19.7)	94 (80.3)	0.77 (0.47, 1.25)	0.73 (0.39, 1.38)
(2) Presence of radio in the HH				
No	154 (21)	578 (79)	1	1
Yes	116 (27.2)	311 (72.8)	1.39 (1.05, 1.84)	1.41 (1.01, 1.88)**
(3) Presence of television in the HH				
No	260 (23.4)	849 (76.6)	1	1
Yes	10 (20)	40 (80)	0.83 (0.41, 1.68)	0.96 (0.39, 2.37)
(4) Access to safe water source				
Safe water sources	97 (22.1)	342 (77.9)	1	1
Unsafe water sources	174 (23.6)	562 (76.4)	1.09 (0.89, 1.45)	1.09 (0.81, 1.48)
(5) Sanitation facility				
Improved sanitation	**19 (25.3)**	**561 (74.7)**	1	1
Nonimproved sanitation	**251 (22.8)**	**348 (77.2)**	0.85 (0.49, 1.45)	0.81 (0.45, 1.43)
Total	271 (23)	904 (77)		

**Significant at P value < 0.05, OR: odds ratio.

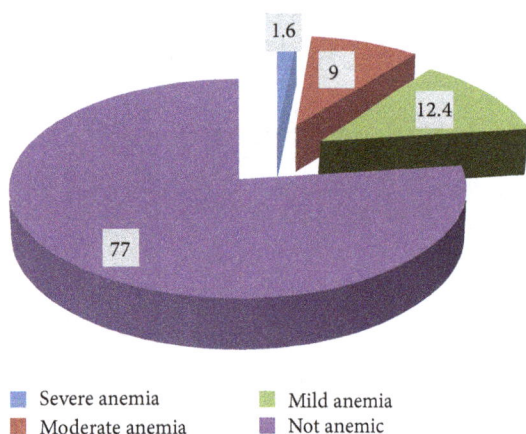

FIGURE 1: Prevalence and severity of anemia among pregnant mothers in Ethiopia, EDHS 2011.

(15–19) (AOR, 3.43; 95% CI, 1.04–11.28). Pregnant women aged (30–34) and (20–24) had the second highest (27.1%) and lowest (19.1%) prevalence of anemia, respectively ($P > 0.05$) (Table 1).

Pregnant women from urban setting had a nonsignificant but higher (26.9%) prevalence of anemia as compared to the rural counterpart (22.7%) (AOR, 0.80; 95% CI, 0.43–1.48). In the same way, the prevalence of anemia among pregnant women across different regions in the country ranged from as low as 0% in Addis Ababa followed by 10.6% and 21.6% in SNNPR and Tigray regions. It was also as high as 60%, 51.9%, and 38.9% in regions like Dire Dawa, Somali, and Afar, respectively (all of these regions are Muslim community dominated and are located in the eastern part of the country). The variation was significant for SNNPR (AOR, 0.41; 95% CI, 0.21–0.82) and Somali regions (AOR, 3.82; 95% CI, 1.71–8.52).

Considering the educational and literacy characteristics of mothers, even if a statistically significant difference was observed during the bivariate logistic regression analyses, none of these appeared in the final multivariate regression model. Yet, descriptive analysis shows that women with no formal education and those trained to tertiary level had a higher, 25% and 33.3%, prevalence of anemia during pregnancy, respectively. Literacy level showed a nonsignificant but a linear declining trend of anemia prevalence; that is, the higher the woman is literate, the lower is the risk of developing anemia during pregnancy ($P > 0.05$) (Table 1).

Table 2 shows that, among the household variables analyzed, all were found not to be associated with anemia of a pregnant women, but radio ownership. Pregnant women who reported lack of access to household variables like electricity, television, and safe water reported almost similar (23.4%–23.7%) prevalence of anemia which is lower than their counterparts. Contrarily to expectations and biological plausibility, however, pregnant women, who were supposed to have a lesser prevalence as they own/have access to radio and improved sanitation, reported a higher 27.2% (AOR, 1.41; 95% CI, 1.01–1.88) and 25.3% (AOR, 0.81; 95% CI, 0.45–1.43) prevalence of anemia than their counterparts, respectively (Table 2).

Regarding the obstetric factors analyzed, almost all of these showed a strong association (increased risk or protective benefit) with the outcome variable of interest, amongst which, pregnancy trimester, number of under five children, previous history of abortion (termination of pregnancy), practice of exclusive breastfeeding, and number of antenatal care visits showed a statistical significance association.

Pregnant women in their second and third trimesters of pregnancy had a 17-fold higher risk of developing anemia compared to those in the first and second trimesters (AOR, 17.05 and 17.71; 95% CI, 3.69–78.8 and 3.76–83.27),

TABLE 3: Selected obstetric characteristics of pregnant mothers and their association with anemia during pregnancy in Ethiopia, EDHS 2011.

Obstetric (RH) characteristics	Anemic (#)/(%)	Nonanemic (#)/(%)	Crude OR (95% CI)	Adjusted OR (95% CI)
(1) Pregnancy trimester				
First	26 (11.3)	205 (88.7)	1	1
Second	140 (27.8)	364 (72.2)	3.07 (1.95, 4.84)	17.05 (3.69, 78.8)**
Third	106 (24)	336 (76)	2.51 (1.58, 4.01)	17.71 (3.76, 83.27)**
(2) Number of under five children				
1	146 (25)	439 (75)	1	1
2	86 (18.5)	379 (81.5)	0.68 (0.50, 0.92)	0.39 (0.18, 0.84)**
3	39 (31.7)	84 (68.3)	1.40 (0.92, 2.14)	2.10 (0.52, 8.48)
(3) Ever had terminated pregnancy				
No	224 (22.6)	767 (77.4)	1	1
Yes	47 (25.5)	137 (74.5)	1.17 (0.81, 1.68)	2.63 (1.17, 5.92)**
(4) Pregnancy intention				
Wanted (then or later)	231 (22.7)	786 (77.3)	1	1
Unwanted	39 (26.5)	108 (73.5)	1.24 (0.84, 1.84)	2.39 (0.98, 5.86)
(5) Practice of breast feeding				
Ever breastfeeding	233 (23.1)	744 (76.9)	1	1
Never breastfeeding	13 (26)	37 (74)	1.15 (0.6, 2.22)	7.64 (2.28, 25.65)**
Continued breastfeeding	25 (21.9)	89 (78.1)	0.92 (0.57, 1.47)	4.05 (1.61, 10.91)**
(6) Timing of first ANC visit				
Timely (<4 months)	28 (20)	112 (80)	1	1
Delayed (4-5 months)	31 (24.8)	94 (75.2)	1.29 (0.72, 2.36)	0.85 (0.42, 1.69)
Delayed much (4–9 months)	13 (37.1)	22 (62.9)	2.26 (1.01, 5.05)	2.29 (0.82, 6.38)
(7) Number of ANC visits				
No (0) visits	130 (23.3)	429 (76.7)	1	1
Low (1-2) visits	22 (31.4)	48 (68.6)	1.53 (0.89, 2.62)	1.09 (0.50, 2.36)
Adequate (3-4) visits	34 (26.4)	95 (73.6)	1.18 (0.76, 1.83)	0.49 (0.19, 0.98)**
Frequent (4+) visits	16 (16.3)	82 (83.7)	0.64 (0.36, 1.13)	0.36 (0.08, 0.64)**
Total	271 (23)	904 (77)		

**Significant at P value < 0.05, OR: odds ratio.

respectively. In the same way, pregnant women who have two or more under five children (AOR, 0.39; 95% CI, 0.18–0.84) have previous history of pregnancy termination (AOR, 2.63; 95% CI, 1.17–5.92), who have never breastfed or continued breastfeeding to present pregnancy (AOR, 7.64 and 4.05; 95% CI, 2.28–25.65 and 1.61–10.91), and those who had adequate (3-4) and/or frequent antenatal care visits (AOR, 0.49 and 0.36; 95% CI, 0.19–0.98 and 0.08–0.64), respectively, had a statistically significant higher (increased) or lower risk of developing anemia during pregnancy (Table 3).

4. Discussion

This in-depth analysis of the latest (2011) Ethiopian demographic and health survey shows that the prevalence of anemia among pregnant women (23%) in the country is comparable to the nonpregnant women of reproductive age group (22%) and to the level of moderate public health problem. The prevalence is also lower than several other local cross-sectional studies [9, 14, 15] and previous EDHS reports [16, 17]. This shows a declining trend of anemia in the country. On the other hand, the value is far below regional

and international estimates [18–20]. This shows the results of the current study should be interpreted cautiously as the data was collected for comprehensive survey of health and demographic events and the samples included in this study might not be good representative of pregnant mothers.

On the other hand, previous similar surveys [16, 17, 21], cross-sectional studies, and other reports [9, 14, 15] in the country have revealed almost similar trend. Studies of food analysis in the country have shown that, if not for bioavailability, most staple diets are rich in iron [22, 23] which might has contributed to lesser prevalence of anemia compared to the predictions and other countries of the sub-Saharan African region where the prevalence of anemia is the highest in the world.

In this study, older women were at a higher risk of anemia compared to teenagers (AOR, 3.43; 95% CI, 1.04–11.28) and the prevalence also increased with age ($P < 0.05$). This is consistent with previous local studies [8, 14]. On the other hand, pregnant mothers from some regions in the country had relatively higher prevalence of anemia during pregnancy and others quite very low. In this regard, pregnant mothers from Somali, Dire Dawa, and Afar regions have high level and those from Addis Ababa and SNNPR as well as Tigray region had the lowest level of prevalence. Those regions with high prevalence of anemia have something in common; they are located in the eastern part of the country and are dominated by Muslim community. Another study in the area [10] has estimated a similar prevalence and identified that khat chewing and restrictive dietary behaviors are the key factors associated with the unacceptably high level of anemia among pregnant mothers [10]. On the other hand, the very low prevalence level of anemia in Addis Ababa should be interpreted very cautiously as only ten cases of pregnant women were included into the analysis. This is of course contrary to previous studies in the area [11, 24].

Contrarily to scientific plausibility [20] and other positive effects of electronic communications, pregnant mothers from households owning radio have shown a statistically inverse association with the occurrence of anemia during pregnancy. This might be attributable to the high level of adult illiteracy at rural communities whereby little comprehension of radio messages or lack of adequate and tailored information about pregnancy and pregnancy related issues in the national broadcasting services exists. Generally, as this is a new and unprecedented condition, further studies on the association between the two are demanded.

Unlike sociodemographic and household variables that exhibited little or no significant association with maternal anemia during pregnancy, most of the obstetric variables studied have either increased or reduced the risk of developing anemia during pregnancy. In this regard, pregnancy trimester, number of under five children in the household, previous history of abortion, breast feeding practices, and frequency of antenatal care visits showed a significant effect on anemia during pregnancy.

Pregnant mothers in the second or third trimester had a sevenfold raised risk of anemia during pregnancy compared to during the first trimester. This is consistent with several other local [8, 10] and international [15] similar studies. It is important, however, to interpret the results as every pregnancy has three trimesters but could only be classified once with the other variables.

Having too many under five children or too frequent birth is among the key predictors of anemia in Ethiopia identified by the current analyses. This is also consistent with the findings of other studies [14, 25–27] that limiting birth or using family planning to control and space births is a key contributing factor to the prevention of anemia during pregnancy. At the same time, women who experienced abortion or terminated pregnancy before the index pregnancy were also found to have a 2.63 times higher risk of developing anemia than those who did not (AOR, 2.63; 95% CI, 1.17–5.92). This is consistent with several other studies [28, 29].

The other important aspect of the findings is the fact that breast feeding patters of mothers contributed much to the occurrence of anemia during subsequent pregnancies. Women who have never breastfed and continued breastfeeding to the index pregnancy were almost eight and four times more likely to experience anemia during recent pregnancies compared to those who have ever breastfed (AOR, 7.64 and 4.05; 95% CI, 2.28–25.65 and 1.61, 10.91). This is not explained

by any study so far which prompts further study on these associations and requires careful interpretation, as the same holds true for the selection of samples is not directly related to the current analysis.

The other obstetric characteristic with protective finding to the occurrence of anemia during pregnancy is the frequency of antenatal care visits. Pregnant mothers who had at least 3-4 and above four visits had a 51% and 64% less chance of developing anemia during pregnancy than those who had less or none at all (AOR, 0.49; 95% CI, 0.19–0.98, and AOR, 0.36; 95% CI, 0.08–0.64), respectively. On the other hand, despite lesser (20% compared to 24.8% and 37.1%) proportion, pregnant mothers who timely (<4 months) started antenatal care visits were found to be nonanemic compared to those who started late (4-5 months) and too late (6–9 months); the occurrence was not statistically significant in the final logistic regression model (AOR, 0.85 and 2.29; 95% CI, 0.42–1.69 and 0.82–6.38). This is also consistent with several other studies conducted locally [11, 14, 30] or globally [31–33].

Limitations. The study has a limitation of selection of study participants and some potential variables. This is to say that even if the data is collected from representative population across the country, it did not take anemia and its determinants into account to determine sample sizes and the data collection tool lacked considering variables affecting anemia. Therefore, caution should be taken while interpreting some results.

5. Conclusion and Recommendation

Generally, even if the prevalence of maternal anemia during pregnancy declined over time, still it remains a moderate public health problem in Ethiopia. The occurrence of anemia is mainly guided by several sociodemographic (maternal age and region), household (access to radio), and many of the obstetric characteristics including pregnancy trimester, number of under five children in the household, previous history of abortion, breastfeeding patterns (never or continued breastfeeding), and frequency of antenatal care visits.

Therefore, policy makers and other concerned program managers should focus on the key variables in their future planning to deal with the high level of anemia in the country. They should pay attention to older age, those in the eastern region of the country, second and third pregnancy trimesters, having too many under five children, women with previous history of abortion, those with infrequent (≤2) antenatal care visiting pregnant mothers in the programming, and implementation priorities. Further studies are also recommended to be conducted on why some special group of mothers (those who have access to radio and those from the eastern parts of the country) are at special risk of developing the problem without a clear implication to the risk.

Conflict of Interests

The authors declare that they do not have competing interests.

Authors' Contribution

Taddese Alemu developed the analyses parameters, developed objectives, and secured support. He also undertook analysis of the data. Melaku Umeta made detailed analyses and was involved in the write-up and synthesis of the findings. He also reviewed and standardized the study. Both authors read and approved the final paper.

Acknowledgment

The authors acknowledge MEASURE DHS for granting access to Ethiopian DHS 2005 and 2011 data.

References

[1] L. Say, D. Chou, A. Gemmill et al., "Global causes of maternal death: a WHO systematic analysis," *The Lancet Global Health*, vol. 2, no. 6, pp. e323–e333, 2014.

[2] World Health Organization, *Trends in Maternal Mortality: 1990 to 2013*, WHO, UNICEF, UNFPA, The World Bank and the United Nations Population Division, Geneva, Switzerland, 2013.

[3] E. McLean, M. Cogswell, I. Egli, D. Wojdyla, and B. De Benoist, "Worldwide prevalence of anaemia, WHO Vitamin and Mineral Nutrition Information System, 1993–2005," *Public Health Nutrition*, vol. 12, no. 4, pp. 444–454, 2009.

[4] L. Fischer, W. Shearer, and L. Hediger, "Anemia vs iron deficiency? In a prospective study13 increased delivery," *The American Journal of Clinical Nutrition*, vol. 55, pp. 985–988, 1992.

[5] WHO, *Haemoglobin Concentrations for the Diagnosis of Anaemia and Assessment of Severity*, Vitamin and Mineral Nutrition Information System, World Health Organization, Geneva, Switzerland, 2011, http://www.who.int/vmnis/indicators/haemoglobin/en/.

[6] J. C. McCann and B. N. Ames, "An overview of evidence for a causal relation between iron deficiency during development and deficits in cognitive or behavioral function," *The American Journal of Clinical Nutrition*, vol. 85, no. 4, pp. 931–945, 2007.

[7] Central Statistical Agency and ICF International, *Ethiopia Demographic and Health Survey*, Central Statistical Agency and ICF International, Addis Ababa, Ethiopia, 2011.

[8] M. Melku, Z. Addis, M. Alem, and B. Enawgaw, "Prevalence and predictors of maternal anemia during pregnancy in Gondar, Northwest Ethiopia: an institutional based cross-sectional study," *Anemia*, vol. 2014, Article ID 108593, 9 pages, 2014.

[9] S. Gebremedhin, A. Samuel, G. Mamo, T. Moges, and T. Assefa, "Coverage, compliance and factors associated with utilization of iron supplementation during pregnancy in eight rural districts of Ethiopia: a cross-sectional study," *BMC Public Health*, vol. 14, no. 1, article 607, 2014.

[10] H. Kedir, Y. Berhane, and A. Worku, "Khat chewing and restrictive dietary behaviors are associated with anemia among pregnant women in high prevalence rural communities in eastern Ethiopia," *PLoS ONE*, vol. 8, no. 11, Article ID e78601, 2013.

[11] M. Umeta, J. Haidar, T. Demissie, G. Akalu, and G. Ayana, "Iron deficiency anaemia among women of reproductive age in nine administrative regions of Ethiopia," *Ethiopian Journal of Health Development*, vol. 22, no. 3, pp. 252–258, 2006.

[12] Guide DHS, "DHS Guide to statistics Demographic and Health Surveys Methodology," 2013.

[13] International Nutritional Anemia Consultative Group (INACG), *Adjusting Hemoglobin Values in ProgramSurveys*, International Nutritional Anemia Consultative Group (INACG), Washington, DC, USA, 2002, http://inacg.ilsi.org.

[14] S. Gebremedhin and F. Enquselassie, "Correlates of anemia among women of reproductive age in Ethiopia: evidence from Ethiopian DHS 2005," *Ethiopian Journal of Health Development*, vol. 25, no. 1, pp. 22–30, 2011.

[15] N. Obse, A. Mossie, and T. Gobena, "Magnitude of anemia and associated risk factors among pregnant women attending antenatal care in Shalla Woreda, West Arsi Zone, Oromia Region, Ethiopia," *Ethiopian Journal of Health Sciences*, vol. 23, no. 2, pp. 165–173, 2013.

[16] Central Statistical Agency and ICF International, *Ethiopia Demographic and Health Survey*, Central Statistical Agency and ICF International, Addis Ababa, Ethiopia, 2000.

[17] Central Statistical Agency Ethiopia, *Ethiopia Demographic and Health Survey*, Central Statistical Agency Ethiopia, Addis Ababa, Ethiopia, 2005.

[18] M. Atuahene, D. Mensah, M. Adjuik, and S. Obed, "Maternal anemia and its association with low birth weight: a cross-sectional study in two leading hospitals in Ghana," *International Journal of Maternal and Child Health*, vol. 3, no. 1, pp. 24–30, 2015.

[19] S. Seshadri, "Prevalence of micronutrient deficiency particularly of iron, zinc and folic acid in pregnant women in South East Asia," *British Journal of Nutrition*, vol. 85, no. 2, pp. 87–92, 2001.

[20] R. D. W. Klemm, A. E. Sommerfelt, A. Boyo et al., "Are we making progress on reducing anemia in women?" Tech. Rep., The USAID, Washington, DC, USA, 2011.

[21] I. Nfant, Y. O. C. Hild, and F. E. Iycf, "Addendum to the 2005 Ethiopia Demographic and Health Survey," 23–25, 2005.

[22] Y. Abebea, A. Bogalea, K. M. Hambidgeb, B. J. Stoeckerc, K. Baileyd, and R. S. Gibsond, "Phytate, zinc, iron and calcium content of selected raw and prepared foods consumed in rural Sidama, Southern Ethiopia, and implications for bioavailability," *Journal of Food Composition and Analysis*, vol. 20, no. 3-4, pp. 161–168, 2007.

[23] M. Umeta, C. E. West, and H. Fufa, "Content of zinc, iron, calcium and their absorption inhibitors in foods commonly consumed in Ethiopia," *Journal of Food Composition and Analysis*, vol. 18, no. 8, pp. 803–817, 2005.

[24] J. Haidar, "Prevalence of anaemia, deficiencies of iron and folic acid and their determinants in Ethiopian women," *Journal of Health, Population and Nutrition*, vol. 28, no. 4, pp. 359–368, 2010.

[25] A. Abriha, M. E. Yesuf, and M. M. Wassie, "Prevalence and associated factors of anemia among pregnant women of Mekelle town: a cross sectional study," *BMC Research Notes*, vol. 7, no. 1, article 888, 6 pages, 2014.

[26] American Society for Reproductive Medicine, *Noncontraceptive Benefits of Birth Control Pills*, American Society for Reproductive Medicine, Birmingham, Ala, USA, 2011, https://www.asrm.org/uploadedFiles/ASRM_Content/Resources/Patient_Resources/Fact_Sheets_and_Info_Booklets/Noncontraceptive%20benefits%20of%20BCP-final_1-5-12.pdf.

[27] A. M. Shojania, "Oral contraceptives: effect of folate and vitamin B12 metabolism," *Canadian Medical Association journal*, vol. 126, no. 3, pp. 244–247, 1982.

[28] E. O. Uche-Nwachi, A. Odekunle, S. Jacinto et al., "Anaemia in pregnancy: associations with parity, abortions and child spacing in primary healthcare clinic attendees in Trinidad and Tobago," *African Health Sciences*, vol. 10, no. 1, pp. 66–70, 2010.

[29] E. R. Wiebe, K. J. Trouton, and A. Eftekhari, "Anemia in early pregnancy among Canadian women presenting for abortion," *International Journal of Gynecology & Obstetrics*, vol. 94, no. 1, pp. 60–61, 2006.

[30] Y. Lakew, S. Biadgilign, and D. Haile, "Anaemia prevalence and associated factors among lactating mothers in Ethiopia: evidence from the 2005 and 2011 demographic and health surveys," *BMJ Open*, vol. 5, no. 4, Article ID e006001, 2015.

[31] I. Kisuule, D. K. Kaye, F. Najjuka et al., "Timing and reasons for coming late for the first antenatal care visit by pregnant women at Mulago hospital, Kampala Uganda," *BMC Pregnancy and Childbirth*, vol. 13, article 121, 2013.

[32] P. Christian, C. P. Stewart, S. C. Leclerq et al., "Antenatal and postnatal iron supplementation and childhood mortality in rural Nepal: a prospective follow-up in a randomized, controlled community trial," *The American Journal of Epidemiology*, vol. 170, no. 9, pp. 1127–1136, 2009.

[33] E. M. Ikeanyi and A. I. Ibrahim, "Does antenatal care attendance prevent anemia in pregnancy at term?" *Nigerian Journal of Clinical Practice*, vol. 18, no. 3, pp. 323–327, 2015.

31

Extent of Anaemia among Preschool Children in EAG States, India: A Challenge to Policy Makers

Rakesh Kumar Singh and Shraboni Patra

International Institute for Population Sciences, Mumbai 400088, India

Correspondence should be addressed to Rakesh Kumar Singh; rakeshiips5700@gmail.com

Academic Editor: Aurelio Maggio

Background. India is the highest contributor to child anemia. About 89 million children in India are anemic. The study determines the factors that contributed to child anemia and examines the role of the existing programs in reducing the prevalence of child anemia particularly in the EAG states. *Methods.* The data from the latest round of the National Family Health Survey (NFHS-3) is used. Simple bivariate and multinomial logistics regression analyses are used. *Results.* About 70% children are anemic in all the EAG states. The prevalence of severe anemia is the highest (6.7%) in Rajasthan followed by Uttar Pradesh (3.6%) and Madhya Pradesh (3.4%). Children aged 12 to 17 months are significantly seven times (RR = 7.99, $P < 0.001$) more likely to be severely anemic compared to children of 36 to 59 months. Children of severely anemic mothers are also found to be more severely anemic (RR = 15.97, $P < 0.001$) than the children of not anemic mothers. *Conclusions.* The study reveals that the existing government program fails to control anemia among preschool children in the backward states of India. Therefore, there is an urgent need for monitoring of program in regular interval, particularly for EAG states to reduce the prevalence of anemia among preschool children.

1. Introduction

Worldwide, anemia among preschool children is one of the serious public health problems. Globally 1.62 billion people are anemic, while among the preschool children the prevalence of anemia is 47.4% [1]. In India, about 89 million children are anemic [1, 2]. Thus, India is the highest contributor to child anemia among the developing countries [2, 3]. According to the latest national representative survey of India, 70% children are anemic in the age group of 6–59 months, including 3% severely anemic, 40% moderately anemic, and 26% mildly anemic (NFHS 3, 2005-06) [4]. Anemia is the most predominant factor for morbidity and child mortality [5–7], and hence, it is a critical health issue for preschool children in India [8, 9].

Anemia is considered as a proxy indicator of iron deficiency [2, 10] because it is defined as an abnormal iron biochemistry with or without anemia [11]. Iron deficiency is caused by the poor iron intake and low iron bioavailability [1, 2]. Some other factors like vitamin A, vitamin B_{12}, hookworm, and malaria infection are found associated with anemia among preschool children [2, 10]. Iron deficiency anemia affects the physical and mental development of the human body [1, 12]. For instance, many studies have shown that iron deficiency reduces the learning capacity of the children aged below five years, decreases attentiveness, and causes low intelligence [13]. Thus, anemia leads to decrease of the actual economic productivity of human resources and ultimately impacts on the development of the country [12, 14]. Few studies have shown that preschool children are more vulnerable to the risk of iron deficiency anemia [15–17]. The prevalence of iron deficiency anemia is the highest among preschool children. In this age group (6–59 months) body grows rapidly and requires high-iron-rich and nutritious food that may not be fulfilled by their normal diet. Low economic status, less education, and poor health of mothers due to meager dietary intake are the main causes of anemia [18, 19].

Numerous studies have been carried out on anemia in India since the 1980's. However, we have found very few studies on child anemia particularly focusing on children aged 6–59 months at the national [1] and regional levels [10]. Although nutritional problem is very common in all states, it is more prevalent and severe among the children below five years in the particular states, whose performances are very poor in respect of the other important demographic and socioeconomic indicators. The Government of India (GOI) has named these states as Empowered Action Groups (EAG) states, which consist of Uttarakhand, Uttar Pradesh, Madhya Pradesh, Bihar, Odisha, Jharkhand, Chhattisgarh, and Rajasthan. The EAG states comprise almost 45% of Indian population [20].

A number of studies have been conducted to show an association between the socioeconomic status (SES) and the prevalence of anemia [10]. Among the different socioeconomic factors, women's level of education and exposure to mass media are found to play a key role in determining their own and their children's health status. Moreover, preventive health care is supposed to be more effective in reducing child morbidity in those areas where accessibility of and affordability for curative health care services are much less than the other region [21]. Hence, to increase the awareness on preventive health care practices, it is always important to understand the background characteristics of women and their children. Therefore, it is obligatory to scrutinize the extent of prevalence of anemia among preschool children and its determinants in the EAG states. Although the etiology of anemia is multifactorial, there is an urgent need to determine the factors that contributed to anemia and to examine the role of the existing program in controlling child anemia especially in the less developed areas like EAG states.

2. Data and Methods

2.1. Ethics Statement. No ethics statement is needed for this work, as the study is based on an anonymous dataset which is available in the public domain and does not contain any identifiable information on the survey participants.

2.2. Sample Size. The study used National Family Health Survey (NFHS-3) data, which was conducted in 2005-06 covering 29 states in India [4]. The NFHS-3 has collected information from a nationally representative sample of 109,401 households, 124,385 women of age group 15–49 years, and 74,369 men aged 15–54 years. It provides a cross-sectional survey data on preschool children and their mother's haemoglobin status, body weight, and demographic and socioeconomic characteristics. The study has considered only the preschool children aged 6–59 months in the EAG states of India. The total sample of the preschool children is 16065 in the EAG states.

2.3. Methods

2.3.1. Variables. The study had used several variables to comprehend the differences in the prevalence of anemia among the preschool children and the interrelationships among the variables related to children and their mother's

health. The variables of the study are briefly described in the following section.

Dependent Variables. Anemia level: Preschool children with any anemia (mild, moderate, and severe) are considered for this study. The cut-off level of anemia (haemoglobin or Hb level) among the preschool children is less than 11 g/dL. Anemia variable, for preschool children of age group 6–59 months, is divided into four categories: (a) severe (<7 g/dL), (b) moderate (7.0–9.9 g/dL), (c) mild (10–10.9 g/dL), amd (d) not anemic (>11 g/dL), and is used for multinomial regression analysis.

Independent Variables. The study includes a set of independent variables to understand the extent and differentials in the level of anemia among preschool children and their mother's, and its effect on the outcomes. The independent variables are mainly socioeconomic and demographic characteristics of mothers. The socioeconomic characteristics of the children and their mothers include *age groups of the children* (6–11, 12–17, 18–23, 24–35, and 36–59 months), *age groups of mothers* (15–19, 20–29, 30–39, and 40–49 years), *place of residence* (urban, rural), *Mother's level of education* (no education, up to primary level complete, up to secondary level complete, and high school and above), *father's level of education* (no education, up to primary level complete, up to secondary level complete, and high school and above), *household structure* (nuclear family, joint family), *wealth quintile* (poorest, poorer, middle, richer, and richest), *media exposure* (no, yes), *birth order of the child* (1, 2-3, 4-5, and 6+), and *mother's anemia status* (severe, moderate, mild, and not anemic).

2.3.2. Statistical Analyses. The study used bivariate and multivariate techniques to comprehend the level of anemia among preschool children of age group 6–59 months belonging to the EAG states of India. Multivariate technique like multinomial logit regression analysis is applied to examine the effect of socioeconomic and demographic factors on the level of anemia among preschool children and their mothers.

Multinomial Logit Regression (MLR) Analysis. Multinomial regression is the most appropriate technique in a situation where the dependent variables are categorical and have more than two categories. The model allows the study to see the effect of a unit change in the predictors or independent variables on the outcome or dependent variable considering the simultaneous effects of several other variables in the form of the relative risk (RR). The multinomial regression model is a generalized form of the logistic regression model. In the present study, the multinomial regression model is used to analyze the effect of some selected socioeconomic and demographic factors on anemia among preschool children in the EAG states of India. The categories of the level of anemia among preschool children are severe (<7 g/dL), moderate (7.0–9.9 g/dL), mild (10–10.9 g/dL), and not anemic (>11 g/dL).

TABLE 1: Prevalence of anaemia among preschool children in EAG states in India, NFHS, 2005-06.

States	Anemia status by haemoglobin levels				Sample size
	Severe	Moderate	Mild	Any anaemic	
Uttarakhand	2.3	30.8	28.8	61.9	887
Rajasthan	6.7	40.8	23.2	70.6	1619
Uttar Pradesh	3.6	45.4	25.0	74.0	4788
Bihar	1.6	47.3	29.0	77.9	1995
Jharkhand	2.0	39.5	29.0	70.5	1303
Odisha	1.5	34.5	29.4	65.5	1413
Chhattisgarh	2.1	45.9	24.1	72.1	1298
Madhya Pradesh	3.4	43.6	27.0	74.0	2762
EAG states	2.9	41.0	26.9	70.8	16065

3. Results

3.1. Prevalence of Anemia among Preschool Children in the EAG States.

Table 1 illustrates that the prevalence of severe anemia among preschool children is the highest in Rajasthan (6.7%) followed by Uttar Pradesh (3.6%) and Madhya Pradesh (3.4%), and it is the lowest in Odisha (1.5%). The prevalence of moderate anemia is the highest in Bihar (47.3%) and the lowest in Uttarakhand (30.8%). The prevalence of moderate anemia is almost more than 40% in all EAG states except Odisha and Uttarakhand. About 30% preschool children are moderately anemic in Bihar, Jharkhand, and Odisha, whereas, in the rest of the states, the percentage is above 20. Among the EAG states, 3% children are found to be severely anemic, 41% are moderately anemic, and about 27% are mildly anemic.

3.2. Prevalence and Associated Factors of Anemia among Preschool Children by Their Background Characteristics.

Table 2 illustrates that the prevalence of severe anemia has been found more among 12–17 month children (5.2%) as compared to 36–59 month children (3.9%), whereas prevalence of moderate anemia has been found above 50% among 6–23 month children. Approximately, 80% preschool children have any anemia in the EAG states. The children of the mothers of age group 15 to 19 years and 40 to 49 years are found to have severe anemia (4.8% and 6.1%, resp.). Children are found to be less severely anemic (1.6%) of those women who have at least high school and above education, as compared to the children of those women who have no education (3.5%). Mother's level of education plays a significant role in determining the level of anemia among children in the EAG states. Children, belonging to the joint family, are less severely anemic than those who live in nuclear families (2.8% and 3.4%, resp.). About 12.9% preschool children have severe anemia as their mothers are found to be severely anemic. For those women who do not have anemia, their children are found to be less severely anemic (1.8%).

Table 3 provides the estimates from the multinomial regression analysis, used to find out the contributing factors to anemia among preschool children in the EAG states. It shows that children of those mothers who have severe anemia are about 16 times (RR = 15.97, $P < 0.001$) more likely to be severely anemic as compared to the children of not anemic mothers. Children belonging to the richest quintile are less likely to be severely anemic as compared to children who belong to poor or middle wealth quintile. Children are more likely to be severely anemic of those mothers who have no education (RR = 1.71, $P < 0.001$) or up to primary education, (RR = 1.61, $P < 0.001$) compared to the children of mothers with higher education. Children belonging to the nuclear family are more likely to be severely anemic than those who live in a joint family. The adolescent mother's children are two times (RR = 1.99, $P < 0.001$) more likely to be moderately anemic as compared to children of older mothers. Education, wealth quintile, and family structure are found to be significant in controlling the level (severe, moderate, and mild) of anemia.

4. Discussion

Iron deficiency anemia among preschool children is a major public health problem in Southeast Asia [10, 22]. According to the World Health Organization (WHO), anemia adds to 324,000 deaths and 12,500,000 disability adjusted life years (DALYs) in this region, which is the highest in the world [11, 13, 23]. The present study has reinforced and extended the previous findings that anemia among preschool children is an important public health problem in India. The study found anemia is clearly widespread among preschool children particularly in the EAG states. The prevalence of anemia among preschool children is about 71% in the EAG states, which is much higher than the other less developed South Asian Countries such as Vietnam [24] and Bangladesh [25]. The highest prevalence of anemia among preschool children is found in Bihar (77.9%), followed by Uttar Pradesh (74%), Madhya Pradesh (74%), Chhattisgarh (72.1%), Rajasthan (70.6%), and Jharkhand (70.5%). Contrary to this, Uttarakhand (61.9%) and Odisha (65.5%) have a lower rate of prevalence among the EAG states. Bharati et al., 2013, have shown the state-wise distribution of the prevalence of anemia among preschool children, which also authenticates the findings of the present study [1].

Among all the EAG states, the prevalence of severe anemia among preschool children is found highest in Rajasthan

TABLE 2: Percentage distribution of age 6–59 months children among EAG states by background characteristics in India, NFHS, 2005-06.

Background characteristics	Anemia status by haemoglobin levels				Sample size
	Severe	Moderate	Mild	Not anaemic	
Age groups of children (months)					
6–11	2.30	52.40	28.30	17.00	1696
12–17	5.20	57.60	22.80	14.40	1725
18–23	4.60	57.40	23.30	14.80	1841
24–35	3.90	47.20	26.20	22.60	3519
36–59	2.00	30.90	27.90	39.10	7285
Age groups of mother's (years)					
15–19	4.80	51.70	26.60	16.90	816
20–29	2.80	42.80	26.60	27.80	10678
30–39	3.30	41.30	26.10	29.40	4097
40–49	6.10	34.90	28.60	30.40	475
Place of residence					
Urban	4.10	36.70	25.60	33.60	2919
Rural	2.90	44.00	26.70	26.40	13147
Mothers level of education					
No education	3.40	45.90	26.40	24.40	9815
Up to primary level complete	3.20	41.20	27.10	28.60	2854
Up to secondary level complete	2.70	37.60	27.10	32.50	1606
High school and above	1.80	32.00	26.00	40.30	1790
Fathers level of education					
No education	3.50	47.10	26.50	22.90	5123
Up to primary level complete	2.80	43.10	26.80	27.30	2480
Up to secondary level complete	3.30	41.30	26.40	29.00	6761
High school and above	1.60	33.10	25.90	39.40	1487
Household structure					
Nuclear family	3.40	42.60	26.40	27.60	7210
Joint family	2.80	42.50	26.60	28.10	7710
Wealth quintile					
Poorest	2.80	46.90	27.70	22.50	5594
Poor	3.10	44.40	27.00	25.60	3893
Middle	3.90	41.20	25.60	29.40	2826
Rich	3.00	39.10	25.30	32.60	2188
Richest	2.80	30.90	24.50	41.80	1566
Media exposure					
No	3.10	45.40	27.20	24.30	6378
Yes	3.10	40.90	26.10	29.90	9675
Birth order of the child					
1	2.60	39.30	26.30	31.70	3942
2-3	2.90	42.60	26.70	27.90	6601
4-5	3.40	45.60	26.30	24.80	3451
6+	4.40	44.50	26.80	24.20	2072
Mothers anaemia status					
Severe	12.90	47.70	22.10	17.30	265
Moderate	5.80	52.20	23.40	18.60	2820
Mild	2.80	45.20	27.50	24.50	6607
Not anaemic	1.80	35.50	27.00	35.70	6248
Total	3.58	42.91	26.21	27.31	16065

TABLE 3: Multinomial regression analysis results on anemia status among preschool (6–59 months) children by background characteristics, EAG states in India, NFHS, 2005-06.

	Anaemia status by haemoglobin levels								
	Severe anaemia			Moderate anaemia			Mild anaemia		
	Relative risk (RR)	Confidence interval		Relative risk (RR)	Confidence interval		Relative risk (RR)	Confidence interval	
Background characteristics		Upper limit	Lower limit		Upper limit	Lower limit		Upper limit	Lower Limit
Age groups of children (months)									
6–11	2.42***	1.53	3.837	4.25***	3.607	5.008	2.45***	2.059	2.92
12–17	7.98***	5.693	11.211	5.41***	4.583	6.401	2.47***	2.061	2.97
18–23	7.33***	5.259	10.239	5.14***	4.392	6.037	2.20***	1.845	2.622
24–35	4.04***	3.092	5.298	2.77***	2.479	3.109	1.67***	1.485	1.891
36–59	1	–	–	1	–	–	1	–	–
Age groups of mothers (years)									
15–19	1.428	0.671	3.036	1.99***	1.356	2.936	1.353	0.903	2.026
20–29	0.693	0.396	1.211	1.50***	1.128	2.018	1.102	0.821	1.478
30–39	0.661	0.393	1.112	1.317*	0.998	1.738	0.982	0.743	1.297
40–49	1	–	–	1	–	–	1	–	–
Place of residence									
Urban	1.319*	0.996	1.746	0.892	0.789	1.009	1.015	0.892	1.155
Rural	1	–	–	1	–	–	1	–	–
Mothers level of education									
No education	1.708**	1.046	2.79	1.40***	1.177	1.675	1.057	0.88	1.271
Primary level complete	1.607*	0.974	2.649	1.23**	1.029	1.471	1.049	0.872	1.263
Secondary level complete	1.4	0.831	2.359	1.149	0.954	1.382	1.064	0.879	1.288
High school and above	1	–	–	1	–	–	1	–	–
Household structure									
Nuclear family	1.011	0.808	1.265	0.928	0.845	1.019	0.98**	0.811	0.988
Joint family	1	–	–	1	–	–	1	–	–
Wealth quintile									
Poorest	1.484	0.877	2.509	1.91***	1.535	2.384	1.90***	1.509	2.394
Poor	1.628*	0.994	2.666	1.64***	1.339	2.024	1.58***	1.279	1.973
Middle	1.637**	1.04	2.577	1.41***	1.17	1.719	1.34***	1.096	1.64
Rich	1.121	0.728	1.726	1.29***	1.086	1.532	1.17*	0.985	1.41
Richest	1	–	–	1	–	–	1	–	–
Media exposure									
No	0.767**	0.596	0.988	0.927	0.832	1.034	0.962	0.857	1.08
Yes	1	–	–	1	–	–	1	–	–
Birth order of the child									
1	0.927	0.472	1.819	0.882	0.663	1.173	0.904	0.668	1.223
2–3	1.14	0.647	2.009	1.012	0.789	1.297	0.98	0.753	1.275
4–5	0.97	0.652	1.442	1.06	0.882	1.273	1.001	0.823	1.217
6+	1	–	–	1	–	–	1	–	–
Mothers anaemia status									
Severe	15.97***	9.533	26.766	2.94***	2.035	4.264	1.61**	1.064	2.447
Moderate	6.271***	4.71	8.351	2.88***	2.532	3.297	1.66***	1.439	1.919
Mild	2.374***	1.821	3.095	1.78***	1.626	1.97	1.44***	1.31	1.601
Not anaemic	1	–	–	1	–	–	1	–	–

TABLE 3: Continued.

Background characteristics	Severe anaemia			Anaemia status by haemoglobin levels					
	Relative risk (RR)	Confidence interval		Moderate anaemia			Mild anaemia		
		Upper limit	Lower limit	Relative risk (RR)	Confidence interval		Relative risk (RR)	Confidence Interval	
					Upper limit	Lower limit		Upper limit	Lower Limit
States									
Uttaranchal	0.601***	0.347	1.041	0.623***	0.504	0.769	0.926	0.75	1.145
Rajasthan	1.735*	1.221	2.464	0.923	0.776	1.099	0.82**	0.684	0.995
Uttar Pradesh	1.099	0.802	1.506	1.167*	1.018	1.338	1.018	0.881	1.177
Bihar	0.543*	0.343	0.862	1.155	0.971	1.375	1.157	0.964	1.389
Jharkhand	0.322***	0.184	0.565	0.661***	0.547	0.799	0.81**	0.667	0.985
Orissa	0.319***	0.187	0.545	0.564***	0.47	0.676	0.82**	0.689	0.996
Chhattisgarh	0.573***	0.347	0.946	1.065	0.887	1.28	0.861	0.705	1.051
Madhya Pradesh	1	—	—	1	—	—	1	—	—

*** $P < 0.001$, ** $P < 0.01$, * $P < 0.05$, reference is last category of each variable and not anemic.

(6.7%). The severe anemia is a very serious problem because recovery from severe anemia is very rare, and there is a high risk of child mortality [26]. The reason of high prevalence of severe anemia in this region could be a lack of dietary energy in their diet and low protein intake by them [27]. Further, a weak economy of the state declines the availability and accessibility of nutrient rich food to the disadvantaged community [26, 27]. The study has also added that mother's anemia status also determines their children's anemia status. Children of severely anemic mothers are found more severely anemic than the children of not anemic mothers.

According to NFHS-3, the total fertility rate (TFR) in the EAG states is much higher (above three children per women in her entire reproductive lifespan) than the other states [4]. In the poor families, additional child is considered as a helping hand for domestic work and later, as the bread earner. Consequently, the higher number of children in the family increases the requirement for childcare, demand for food, and inadequate supply of nutritional diet to all the children which ultimately make the children more vulnerable to the risk of anemia [10, 28, 29]. Similar evidence emerges from the present study, which supports the fact that prevalence of severe anemia among preschool children increases with the increase of their birth order.

GOI has launched many programs to reduce the anemia level among the vulnerable populations by improving their nutritional status. One of the important programs is the National Nutritional Anemia Prophylaxis Program (NNAPP), launched in 1970 [11, 17]. In 1970, about 20% of maternal deaths occurred due to deficiency of iron and folic acid. Through this program, GOI has implemented and distributed IFA tablets to the pregnant and lactating mothers and children by the health centers [30]. Vijayaraghavan and his team had evaluated the NNAPP in 1990. It was evident that health functionaries are not properly oriented towards the program as many of them are not aware of all beneficiaries under the program. The chemical analysis of the tablets indicates that about 30% of the tablet sample was less than expected levels, and none of them had expected levels of folic acid content [31]. Therefore, the program was redesigned as the National Nutritional Anemia Control Program in 1991. The program was designed for the reduction of the incidence of the anemia among the risk population such as pregnant or lactating women, intrauterine device (IUD) consumers, and children aged 12 to 59 months. According to the program, one tablet of 20 mg iron is essential for children aged 1 to 5 years and 100 μg folic acid for 100 days in a year is required by the anemic children [11].

Initially, the program was to be implemented as part of the Reproductive and Child Health (RCH), but now it is the part of the Integrated Child Development Scheme (ICDS) under the Department of Women and Child Development. Government of India has launched ICDS to improve the nutritional status of the preschool children especially from poor or less developed areas. However, the available studies, assessing the ICDS program, have found no significant effects which can control chronic child malnutrition [32]. In 2005, the World Bank found that the services, provided by the local ICDS centers, did not focus on the youngest child (below three years) who should have benefited from the program. In addition, children from the wealthier family participated more in the evaluation compared to the children from poorer or lower caste households. Inadequate worker skills, absence of equipment, and poor monitoring diverted the program from the objective of the ICDS [33]. Some studies have suggested that the IFA tablets given to the children (below three years) were not easily acceptable and recommended the liquid IFA for young children [34]. In 2007, Government of India has modified policy and replaced tablets by liquid IFA. According to the new policy, young children (6–59 months) will get one milliliter of IFA syrup for 100 days in a year that will contain 20 mg elemental iron and 100 μg folic acid [11]. In 2011, zee research groups conducted an interview with child right officer, Chetanalaya (a Delhi based nongovernment organization), who said "The rise in anemic children in Bihar, Uttar Pradesh, and Madhya Pradesh is attributed to the poor health of pregnant and lactating mothers" [35].

5. Conclusion

The study reveals that the prevalence of anemia among preschool children is very high among each of the EAG states in India. Special program at the state level is required to control the prevalence of anemia among preschool children in the EAG states. About 45% population of India lives in the EAG states and a reduction in the prevalence of anemia among these states will inevitably decline the prevalence of anemia at the national level. Anemia remains as a serious health problem due to various causes. The present study also helps to find out the factors, such as higher education of mothers and media exposure, playing an important role in controlling the high prevalence of anemia among preschool children in the EAG states. Hence, the intervention targeting only iron and folic supplements, as we have found in the earlier studies, is not adequate to tackle this problem [36]. Now, it is a big challenge to policy makers and programmer to identify specific strategies to reduce anemia in the backward states. Therefore, there is an urgent need to use multiple interventions and new approaches addressing major preventable causes of anemia among the preschool children. Individual state government should take serious measure to improve the quality of services and to provide nutritional education to mothers to improve their children's health status. In addition, proper monitoring and evaluation of the existing programs, such as ICDS, are required to direct the programs towards their success.

Conflict of Interests

The authors declare that there is no conflict of interests regarding the publication of this paper.

Acknowledgments

The paper has been presented in the 16th Congress of International Pediatrics Nephrology Association (IPNA-2013) in August 30th-September 3rd, 2013, held in Shanghai, China.

The authors would like to thank the editor and the anonymous reviewers of this paper and the audiences of the conference for their valuable suggestions and comments, which were helpful to improve the study.

References

[1] S. Bharati, M. Pal, S. Chakrabarty, and P. Bharati, "Socioeconomic determinants of iron-deficiency anemia among children aged 6 to 59 months in India," *Asia-Pacific Journal of Public Health*, vol. 6, 2013.

[2] S. Pasricha, J. Black, S. Muthayya et al., "Determinants of anemia among young children in rural India," *Pediatrics*, vol. 126, no. 1, pp. e140–e149, 2010.

[3] B. Benoist, E. McLean, I. Egli, and M. Cogswell, *Worldwide Prevalence of Anaemia 1993-2005: WHO Global Database on Anaemia*, WHO, Geneva, Switzerland, 2008.

[4] International Institute for Population Sciences and Macro International (IIPS and Macro Int.), *National Family Health Survey (NFHS-3), 2005-06, Key Findings*, International Institute for Population Sciences, Mumbai, India, 2007.

[5] T. Walter, I. de Andraca, P. Chadud, and C. G. Perales, "Iron deficiency anemia: adverse effects on infant psychomotor development," *Pediatrics*, vol. 84, no. 1, pp. 7–17, 1989.

[6] N. Arlappa, N. Balakrishna, A. Laxmaiah, and G. N. V. Brahmam, "Prevalence of anaemia among rural pre-school children of Maharashtra, India," *Indian Journal of Community Health*, vol. 24, no. 1, pp. 4–8, 2012.

[7] W. Gao, H. Yan, S. Dang, and L. Pei, "Severity of anemia among children under 36 months old in Rural Western China," *PLoS ONE*, vol. 8, no. 4, Article ID e62883, 2013.

[8] N. B. Jain, F. Laden, U. Guller, A. Shankar, S. Kasani, and E. Garshick, "Relation between blood lead levels and childhood anemia in India," *American Journal of Epidemiology*, vol. 161, no. 10, pp. 968–973, 2005.

[9] B. J. Brabin, Z. Premji, and F. Verhoeff, "An analysis of anemia and child mortality," *Journal of Nutrition*, vol. 131, no. 2, supplement 2, pp. 636S–648S, 2001.

[10] S. Dey, S. Gosawmi, and T. Dey, "Identifying predictors of childhood anaemia in north-east India," *Journal of Health and Population Nutrition*, vol. 31, no. 4, pp. 462–470, 2013.

[11] P. V. Kotecha, "Nutritional anemia in young children with focus on Asia and India," *Indian Journal of Community Medicine*, vol. 36, no. 1, pp. 8–16, 2011.

[12] M. E. Bentley and P. L. Griffiths, "The burden of anemia among women in India," *European Journal of Clinical Nutrition*, vol. 57, no. 1, pp. 52–60, 2003.

[13] A. Zhao, Y. Zhang, Y. Peng et al., "Prevalence of anemia and its risk factors among children 6-36 months old in Burma," *The American Journal of Tropical Medicine and Hygiene*, vol. 87, no. 2, pp. 306–311, 2012.

[14] D. Kapur, K. N. Agarwal, and D. K. Agarwal, "Nutritional anemia and its control," *Indian Journal of Pediatrics*, vol. 69, no. 7, pp. 607–616, 2002.

[15] R. Katzman, A. Novack, and H. Pearson, "Nutritional anemia in an inner-city community. Relationship to age and ethnic group," *The Journal of the American Medical Association*, vol. 222, no. 6, pp. 670–673, 1972.

[16] V. S. Pablo, R. Windom, and H. A. Pearson, "Disappearance of iron deficiency anemia in a high risk infant population given supplemental iron," *The New England Journal of Medicine*, vol. 313, no. 19, pp. 1239–1240, 1985.

[17] R. E. Behrman and R. M. Kleigman, *Nelson Essentials of Pediatrics: Hematology*, WB Saunders, Philadelphia, Pa, USA, 2nd edition, 1994.

[18] F. A. Oski, "Iron deficiency in infancy and childhood," *The New England Journal of Medicine*, vol. 329, no. 3, pp. 190–193, 1993.

[19] J. D. Sargent, T. A. Stukel, M. A. Dalton, J. L. Freeman, and M. J. Brown, "Iron deficiency in Massachusetts communities: socioeconomic and demographic risk factors among children," *American Journal of Public Health*, vol. 86, no. 4, pp. 544–550, 1996.

[20] R. K. Singh, "Lifestyle behavior affecting prevalence of anemia among women in EAG states, India," *Journal of Public Health*, vol. 21, no. 3, pp. 279–288, 2013.

[21] P. Winichagoon, "Prevention and control of anemia: Thailand experiences," *Journal of Nutrition*, vol. 132, no. 4, pp. 862S–866S, 2002.

[22] E. DeMaeyer and M. Adiels-Tegman, "The prevalence of anaemia in the world," *World Health Statistics Quarterly*, vol. 38, no. 3, pp. 302–316, 1985.

[23] R. Stoltzfus, L. Mullany, and R. E. Black, "Iron deficiency anaemia," in *Comparative Quantification of Health Risks: Global and Regional Burden of Disease Attributable to Selected Major Risk Factors*, M. Ezzati, A. Lopez, A. Rodgers, and C. J. L. Murray, Eds., pp. 163–210, World Health Organization, Geneva, Switzerland, 2004.

[24] P. H. Nguyen, K. G. Nguyen, M. B. Le et al., "Risk factors for anemia in Vietnam," *Southeast Asian Journal of Tropical Medicine and Public Health*, vol. 37, no. 6, pp. 1213–1223, 2006.

[25] F. Ahmed, "Anaemia in Bangladesh: a review of prevalence and aetiology," *Public Health Nutrition*, vol. 3, no. 4, pp. 385–393, 2000.

[26] M. B. Singh, R. Fotedar, and J. Lakshminarayana, "Micronutrient deficiency status among women of desert areas of western Rajasthan, India," *Public Health Nutrition*, vol. 12, no. 5, pp. 624–629, 2009.

[27] M. B. Singh, R. Fotedar, J. Lakshminarayana, and P. K. Anand, "Studies on the nutritional status of children aged 0–5 years in a drought-affected desert area of Western Rajasthan, India," *Public Health Nutrition*, vol. 9, no. 8, pp. 961–967, 2006.

[28] T. Konstantyner, J. A. A. C. Taddei, M. N. Oliveira, D. Palma, and F. A. B. Colugnati, "Isolated and combined risks for anemia in children attending the nurseries of daycare centers," *Jornal de Pediatria*, vol. 85, no. 3, pp. 209–216, 2009.

[29] E. Tympa-Psirropoulou, C. Vagenas, O. Dafni, A. Matala, and F. Skopouli, "Environmental risk factors for iron deficiency anemia in children 12–24 months old in the area of Thessalia in Greece," *Hippokratia*, vol. 12, no. 4, pp. 240–250, 2008.

[30] U. Kapil, S. Chaturvedi, and D. Nayar, "National nutrition supplementation programmes," *Indian Pediatrics*, vol. 29, no. 12, pp. 1601–1613, 1992.

[31] K. Vijayaraghavan, G. N. V. Brahmam, K. M. Nair, D. Akbar, and N. Pralhad Rao, "Evaluation of national nutritional anemia prophylaxis programme," *The Indian Journal of Pediatrics*, vol. 57, no. 2, pp. 183–190, 1990.

[32] E. Kandpal, "An Evaluation of the Indian Child Nutrition and Development Program," Paper presented at Population Association of America, 2010.

[33] M. Gragnolati, M. Shekar, M. D. Gupta, C. Bredenkamp, and Y. K. Lee, "India's undernourished children: a call for reform and

action," in *Health, Nutrition and Population*, The World Bank, 2005.

[34] U. S. Kapil, "Technical consultation on 'Strategies for Prevention and Control of Iron-deficiency anemia amongst under three Children in India'," *Indian Pediatrics*, vol. 39, no. 7, pp. 640–647, 2002.

[35] A. Chakrabarty, "Bihar Children are Still Anemic," Zee Research Group, 2011, http://zeenews.india.com/exclusive/bihar-children-are-still-anemic_5252.html.

[36] J. A. Noronha, E. A. Khasawneh, V. Seshan, S. Ramasubramaniam, and S. Raman, "Anemia in pregnancy-consequences and challenges: a review of literature," *Journal of South Asian Federation of Obstetrics and Gynecology*, vol. 4, no. 1, pp. 64–70, 2012.

32

Trace Element Status (Iron, Zinc, Copper, Chromium, Cobalt, and Nickel) in Iron-Deficiency Anaemia of Children under 3 Years

Maria Georgieva Angelova,[1] **Tsvetelina Valentinova Petkova-Marinova,**[2]
Maksym Vladimirovich Pogorielov,[3] **Andrii Nikolaevich Loboda,**[4] **Vania Nedkova**
Nedkova-Kolarova,[2] **and Atanaska Naumova Bozhinova**[1]

[1] *Department of Chemistry and Biochemistry & Physics and Biophysics, University of Medicine-Pleven,*
  1 Kliment Ohridski Street, 5800 Pleven, Bulgaria
[2] *Department of Pediatrics, University of Medicine-Pleven, 1 Kliment Ohridski Street, 5800 Pleven, Bulgaria*
[3] *Department of Hygiene and Ecology, Sumy State University, Medical Institute, 31 Sanatornaya Street, Sumy 40007, Ukraine*
[4] *Department of Pediatrics with Medical Genetics, Sumy State University, Medical Institute, 31 Sanatornaya Street, Sumy 40007, Ukraine*

Correspondence should be addressed to Maria Georgieva Angelova; angelovamg@abv.bg

Academic Editor: Aurelio Maggio

Aim. To determine trace element status and aetiologic factors for development of trace elements deficiencies in children with iron-deficiency anaemia (IDA) aged 0 to 3 years. *Contingent and Methods*. 30 patients of the University Hospital, Pleven, Bulgaria—I group; 48 patients of the Sumy Regional Child's Clinical Hospital, Sumy, Ukraine—II group; 25 healthy controls were investigated. Serum concentrations of iron, zinc, copper, chromium, cobalt, and nickel were determined spectrophotometrically and by atomic absorption spectrophotometry. *Results*. Because the obtained serum levels of zinc, copper, and chromium were near the lower reference limits, I group was divided into IA and IB. In IA group, serum concentrations were lower than the reference values for 47%, 57%, and 73% of patients, respectively. In IB group, these were within the reference values. In II group, results for zinc, cobalt, and nickel were significantly lower ($P < 0.05$), and results for copper were significantly higher in comparison to controls higher in comparison to controls. *Conclusion*. Low serum concentrations of zinc, copper, cobalt, and nickel were mainly due to inadequate dietary intake, malabsorption, and micronutrient interactions in both studied groups. Increased serum copper in II group was probably due to metabolic changes resulting from adaptations in IDA. Data can be used for developing a diagnostic algorithm for IDA.

1. Introduction

Under conditions of iron-deficiency anaemia (IDA), a host of metabolic changes representing adaptation mechanisms for maximizing iron delivery for erythropoiesis occur [1, 2]. There are close relations between the metabolism of different trace elements including iron based on antagonistic or synergistic interactions [3, 4]. One of known links is at the level of common intestinal transporters for iron and other divalent metals. Upregulation of their expression induced by iron deficiency (ID) predisposes to metabolic imbalances and

respective changes in trace element status [1, 2]. Another known link is at the level of metal-storage proteins, metallothioneins, which bind different metals, thus acting in their storage and detoxification [5–7].

Interactions of different trace elements with iron determine the relationship between changes in trace element status in the organism and development of IDA. Increases in content of antagonistic to iron trace elements, such as cobalt, zinc, copper, chromium, and calcium, which impair iron absorption or its physiological impact, can lead to development of IDA. Deficiencies of synergistic to iron trace elements implicated in iron metabolism or processes of haematopoiesis, such as copper, chromium, nickel, sodium, and potassium, can contribute substantially to the aetiology of IDA [4].

Only 35–55% of cases of IDA in children are solely due to iron deficiency and others are associated with changes in status of multiple trace elements.

In our study, we use serum trace element concentrations as markers of trace element status in the organism.

Results published from different researchers on status of trace elements in IDA are various and often conflicting.

Most of the researchers have discovered lower serum zinc levels in subjects with IDA in comparison to nonanaemic subjects [8–11], but others have not found significant differences in serum zinc between IDA subjects and healthy controls [12–14].

In studies on copper content in serum and blood, higher [8–10, 12, 15] and lower levels [16, 17] as well as levels without significant differences [13, 14] have been discovered in subjects with ID and anaemia in comparison to nonanaemic and iron-adequate subjects. Both low and high serum copper concentrations have been observed in a subset of anaemic participants in a study of Knovich et al. [18].

Although chromium is considered synergistic to iron [4] and some researchers have found lower concentrations in blood of anaemic patients when compared to control subjects [17], it is known as an antagonistic competition between trivalent chromium and trivalent iron for binding to apotransferrin [4, 19]. On the basis of this interaction, Lukaski et al. have suggested adverse effect of high-dose and long-term chromium supplementation on iron metabolism and status in adults [20].

Cobalt and nickel are essential trace elements with significant impact on the processes of haematopoiesis—stimulation of erythropoietin production and haemoglobin synthesis [21]. Lower concentrations of nickel have been observed in blood of anaemic children as compared to healthy controls [17]. Higher concentrations of cobalt have been found in blood at low body iron stores [2].

Our literature search shows that many researchers do not explain changes in trace element status with mechanisms for transport and storage.

The aim of the study is to determine trace element status, aetiologic factors, and mechanisms for development of trace elements deficiencies in children with IDA from 0 to 3 years of age.

2. Clinical Contingent and Methods

Our investigation comprises 78 patients from 0 to 3 years of age with clinical and laboratory signs of IDA. 30 children-patients are of the University Hospital, Medical University, Pleven, Bulgaria—I group, and 48 are patients of the Sumy Regional Child's Clinical Hospital, Sumy, Ukraine—II group. Comparison group includes 25 healthy children at the same age.

Anaemia was defined according to the criteria adopted by the WHO. Haemoglobin level below 110 g/L and haematocrit

value below 0.33 l/l were used as diagnostic limits of anaemia. In I group of patients, measures of iron status, especially serum iron concentrations below 8.0 μmol/L and transferrin saturation (TS) below 16%, and low red cell indices were used to identify that anaemia was due to ID [22]. Percent TS was calculated as a ratio of serum iron and total iron-binding capacity (TIBC)—serum iron/TIBC × 100. Serum ferritin values were used as indicators for iron deficiency in II group.

All children were enrolled in the study after informed consent from their parents or guardians. Ethical approval was obtained from the Institutional research ethics committees.

A parental questionnaire was provided to collect information about feeding patterns.

Fasting venous blood samples were obtained for analysis in the morning from all children into sterile tubes untreated with heparin, EDTA, citrate, and so forth. After two hours standing and centrifugation at 3500 rpm for 10 minutes, blood serum was separated. The serum samples were put in closed plastic laboratory vessels and stored at −18°C until trace element analysis.

In I group, serum content of trace elements iron, zinc, copper, and chromium was determined spectrophotometrically: ferrozine method [23] for serum iron and total iron-binding capacity by COBAS INTEGRA 400 (Roche) analyzer, spectrophotometric methods using GIESSE diagnostics (Italy) tests for serum zinc and AUDIT diagnostics (Ireland) tests for serum copper, and spectrophotometric method [24] with our modifications for serum chromium. Serum concentrations of zinc, copper, and chromium were determined by a spectrophotometer DR2800 (Hach Lange, Germany).

The serum ferritin levels were determined by ELISA using a kit of reagents "UBI MAGIVEL FERRITIN" produced by "United Biotech Inc." (USA).

Haematological parameters, such as haemoglobin (Hb), haematocrit (Ht), red blood cell (erythrocyte) count (RBC), and the red cell indices, mean corpuscular volume (MCV), mean corpuscular haemoglobin (MCH), mean corpuscular haemoglobin concentration (MCHC), and red cell distribution width (RDW) were examined by analyzer MIKROS—18 (ABX). The reticulocyte count was determined by microscopic examination of a peripheral blood smear stained with a supravital dye.

Serum trace element concentrations and haematological parameters in I group of patients were compared to their respective reference values indicated in Table 1.

In II group, the content of trace elements iron, zinc, copper, cobalt, and nickel in blood serum and erythrocytes was determined by atomic absorption spectrophotometry (AAS) on a spectrophotometer C-115 M1 (JSC "Selmi," Ukraine) [25, 26]. All results from trace element analysis and investigated haematological parameters in II group of patients were compared to healthy controls. Content of trace elements in blood serum and erythrocytes in comparison group was determined by AAS.

Statistical data processing was performed using Excel (Microsoft Corporation, Redmond, WA), Statgraphics Plus (Manugistics, Rockville, MD), and Statistica 6.1

TABLE 1: Haematological parameters and content of trace elements in blood serum of children with IDA.

Parameter	Reference values		I group with IDA ($n = 30$)	II group with IDA ($n = 48$)	Comparison group ($n = 25$)
	Mean [27, 28]	−2 SD [27, 28]			
Haemoglobin (g/L)	120	105	90.23 ± 11.09	89.79 ± 1.23	119.15 ± 2.41
Haematocrit (L/L)	0.36	0.33	0.279 ± 0.029	0.301 ± 0.004	0.3442 ± 0.006
RBC ($\times10^{12}$ cells/L)	4.5	3.7	4.41 ± 0.65	3.58 ± 0.05	4.07 ± 0.12
Rtc (Ǧ)	10 [28]	—	—	5.5 ± 0.87	7.86 ± 0.98
MCV (fL)	78	70	64.3 ± 9.87	74.66 ± 1.08	82.52 ± 1.17
MCH (pg)	27	23	20.93 ± 4.17	24.77 ± 0.39	29.82 ± 0.56
MCHC (g/L)	330	300	322.67 ± 18.16	323.47 ± 4.34	365.17 ± 3.6
RDW (%)	1.5–15 [29]		15.58 ± 1.56	—	—
Iron (μmol/L)	8.0–24.0 [30]		4.43 ± 1.21	9.23 ± 0.86	22.92 ± 1.83
Zinc (μmol/L)	11.1–19.5 [5, 31]		11.22 ± 4.40	11.02 ± 1.79	17.96 ± 1.06
Copper (μmol/L)	11.0–24.0 [6, 32]		11.81 ± 4.39	23.80 ± 0.76	16.50 ± 0.71
Chromium (μmol/L)	0.95–9.5 [33]		0.83 ± 0.69	—	—
Cobalt (μmol/L $\times 10^{-3}$)	0.00–15.25 [34]		—	5.74 ± 0.76	9.16 ± 0.61
Nickel (μmol/L $\times 10^{-3}$)	1.70–10.22 [35]		—	8.99 ± 0.868	14.35 ± 1.09

(StatSoft, USA). All values were expressed as mean ± standard deviation (SD). Student's t-test and Wilcoxon's test were used to evaluate differences between study groups. Statistically significant differences were indicated by P values < 0.05.

3. Results

Clinical manifestations of IDA in all children were demonstrated by the presence of sideropenic and anaemic syndromes.

Anaemic syndrome is manifested by such symptoms as pallor of skin and mucous membranes, fatigue and faintness, tachycardia, and systolic murmur. In a number of patients apathy, drowsiness, or conversely, excessive irritability, and emotional lability were observed due to decreased oxygen delivery to the brain [36] and deficiency of iron which has been shown to play a key role in brain functions [22].

Manifestations of hyposiderosis were due to deficiency of iron-containing enzymes. Dryness of skin, changes in hair—fragility, and dim color were observed; signs of angular stomatitis and atrophic glossitis were also found. Most children suffered from loss of appetite. A number of patients had a syndrome of muscular hypotonia. In some of the patients with IDA increased size of the liver and spleen was observed due to extramedullary haematopoiesis (Figures 1(a) and 1(b)).

Results of investigated clinical laboratory indicators in patients with IDA, comparison group, and the respective reference values are presented in Table 1.

All haematological parameters in anaemic children exhibited changes in accordance with the presence of IDA. Mean value of serum iron in I group of patients with IDA was found to be lower than the reference values–4.43 ± 1.21 μmol/L (Table 1, Figure 2(a)), and along with the low transferrin saturation (TS)–6.23 ± 2.65%, indicated presence of ID. In II group, serum ferritin content was found to be 9.42 ± 0.75 ng/mL which is significantly lower (P < 0.001) in comparison to healthy controls −38.67 ± 4.18 ng/mL.

Mean values of serum zinc, copper, and chromium in I group were all near the lower limits of the reference ranges (Table 1, Figure 2(a)). In II group of patients with IDA, mean serum iron, zinc, cobalt, and nickel concentrations were found to be significantly lower, and mean serum copper level was found to be significantly higher in comparison to their respective controls (Table 1, Figure 2(b)) with reliability level P < 0.05.

In I group, results for serum levels of zinc, copper, and chromium (Table 1, Figure 2(a)) enable to divide examined patients into two groups for each of the investigated trace elements (Figure 3).

Patients with serum trace elements concentrations lower than the reference values—serum zinc 7.29 ± 2.54 μmol/L, copper 8.6 ± 1.46 μmol/L, and chromium 0.47 ± 0.14 μmol/L, are included in IA group. For each of the investigated trace elements, the number of patients in this group constitutes 47% ($n = 14$), 57% ($n = 17$), and 73% ($n = 22$) of total number of children with IDA in I group.

Patients with serum trace elements concentrations within the reference values—serum zinc 14.65 ± 2.21 μmol/L, copper 16.0 ± 3.2 μmol/L, and chromium 1.83 ± 0.61 μmol/L, are included in IB group. For each of the investigated trace elements, the number of patients in this group includes 53% ($n = 16$), 43% ($n = 13$), and 27% ($n = 8$) of total number of participants with IDA in I group.

There are statistically significant differences between IA and IB groups (P < 0.001).

Examination of trace element content in erythrocytes showed significantly lower values for all investigated trace elements in patients with IDA in comparison to control subjects (Table 2).

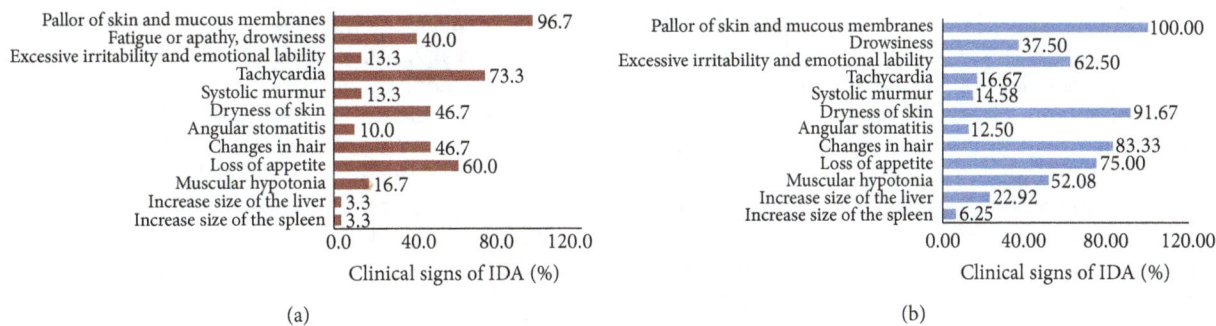

FIGURE 1: Clinical signs of IDA in I group (a) and II group (b).

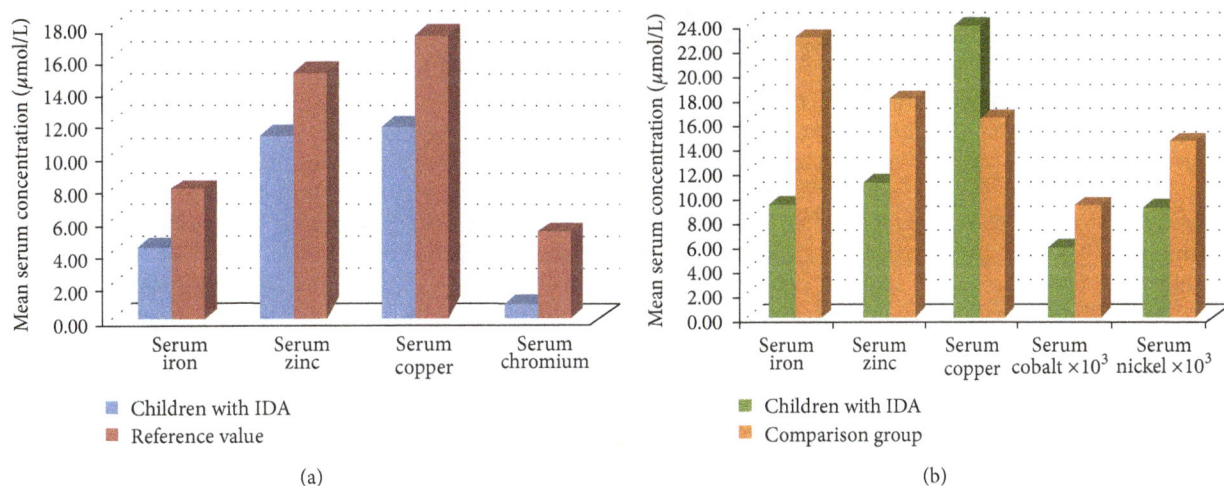

FIGURE 2: Serum concentrations of trace elements in I group (a) and II group (b) of children with IDA.

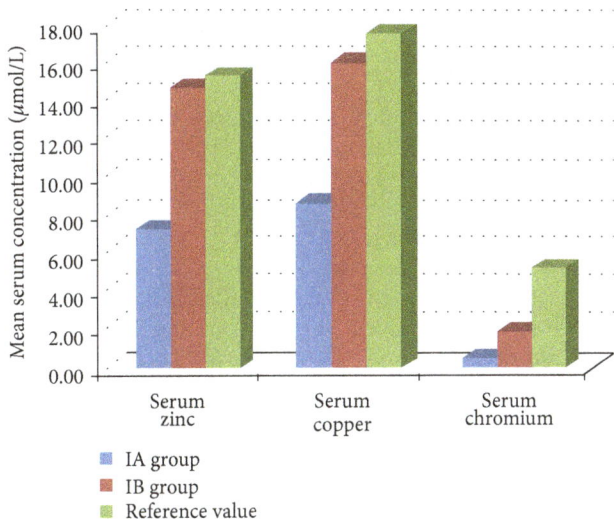

FIGURE 3: Serum concentrations of zinc, copper, and chromium among IA group and IB group of children with IDA.

4. Discussion

Under conditions of IDA, trace element status in the organism is largely influenced by metabolic interactions between

TABLE 2: Content of trace element in erythrocytes in children with IDA and healthy controls.

Trace element content (μg/mg ash)	II group with IDA ($n = 48$)	Comparison group ($n = 25$)
Iron[*]	15.58 ± 1.13	31.56 ± 1.65
Zinc[*]	0.208 ± 0.013	0.260 ± 0.012
Copper[*]	0.176 ± 0.016	0.271 ± 0.039
Cobalt[*]	0.0316 ± 0.0023	0.0411 ± 0.0034
Nickel[*]	0.0330 ± 0.0023	0.0500 ± 0.0034

[*] Reliability level $P < 0.05$.

trace elements, some of which result from adaptation mechanisms for maximizing iron delivery for erythropoiesis [1, 2, 22]. Nutrition, physiologic features in different life periods, and underlying pathological conditions also affect trace element status. It has been shown that children in infancy and early childhood are particularly susceptible to deficiencies of iron and zinc, and copper deficiency occurs mainly in infancy. This vulnerability is due to increased requirements for rapid growth which are frequently not met by the diet [6, 17, 22, 36, 37].

IDA often shows association with low serum zinc levels, as well as zinc deficiency states [8–10]. In our study, obtained values for serum zinc in patients with IDA were also lower in comparison to reference values and controls (Figures 2(b) and 3(a)). These changes in zinc status are frequently explained by coexisting deficiencies of iron and zinc due to common dietary sources of both micronutrients and decreasing their intestinal absorption by the same dietary factors [9, 11].

Lower serum levels than the reference values were also obtained for copper among most patients in I group (57%, $n = 17$).

In our research, we found a number of factors associated with low serum concentrations of zinc and copper in children with IDA.

In 20% of children with IDA from I group, there was a history of preterm birth or low birth weight which are important contributing factors for zinc and copper deficiencies because of the inadequate prenatal stores and elevated requirements for growth [6, 38].

Association between short duration of breast-feeding, exclusive cow's milk feeding and low serum levels of zinc was observed in 57.14% of patients in IA group. Association between the same dietary factors and low serum levels of copper was observed in 64.7% of patients in IA group. This relationship may probably be due to the lower zinc and copper bioavailability from cow's milk in comparison to human milk and the low copper content of cow's milk [5–7, 38, 39].

Malabsorption due to cow's milk protein-induced enteropathy may be regarded as a factor for development of micronutrient deficiencies in 10% of patients with IDA [5, 6, 18, 37].

Low serum concentrations of zinc and copper in some of the investigated children may be attributed to the inadequate consumption of foods with high bioavailability of zinc and copper—meat, poultry, and fish, which are important dietary sources of zinc and copper in children's diet [5, 15, 39, 40]. Other dietary factor is the early introduction and high intake of flour-based foods containing the inhibitors of zinc and copper absorption phytates [7, 17]. These dietary factors were observed in 78.6% of patients with low serum levels of zinc and in 76.47% of patients with low serum levels of copper from I group.

The proposed mechanisms explaining low serum zinc and copper levels in some of the investigated children are antagonistic interactions between zinc and copper within the enterocyte [7]. Impaired intestinal absorption of zinc is observed under conditions of high intake of copper attributed to competitive antagonism between both metals for absorption sites in the gastrointestinal tract [3, 5].

In relatively high dietary intake of zinc, production of metal-binding proteins metallothioneins in intestinal mucosa is induced. As metallothioneins have a greater affinity for copper than zinc, this is followed by sequestration of high proportion of dietary copper in a stable copper-metallothionein complex in intestinal mucosal cells—"mucosal block" in copper transport, reduction in copper absorption, and increased copper excretion [5, 7].

Low serum concentrations of zinc and copper, which we found in investigated children, may be considered as contributing factors for IDA due to known synergistic interactions of both trace elements with iron—participation of zinc in haemoglobin synthesis and its essentiality in erythropoiesis [7, 41], and implication of copper-containing enzymes ceruloplasmin and hephaestin, ferrochelatase and cytochrom-c oxidase in iron metabolism, formation of haemoglobin, and mechanisms of hematopoiesis [4, 6, 7, 42]. Studies in animals and humans have found that copper deficiency can lead to ID [1, 4] and IDA [6, 7, 43].

It is difficult to identify factors explaining relatively high serum levels of zinc found in some patients with IDA from IB group, as well as their relationship with development of IDA. Some studies have shown that nutritional deficiency of iron enhances the intestinal absorption of zinc suggesting the divalent metal transporter 1 (DMT1) as a common absorptive pathway for both metals and physiological basis for such an interaction [44]. Although zinc is considered antagonistic to iron [4] on the basis of absorptive competition, conflicting results have been obtained in studies evaluating effect of zinc on iron absorption, and DMT1 has been postulated as an unlikely site for competitive antagonism [7].

Discovering significantly higher serum copper in II group of patients with IDA in comparison to healthy controls and relatively high serum copper in a part of IB group may be considered as a consequence of adaptation mechanisms in ID intended to maximize iron delivery for erythropoiesis [1]. There are data for upregulating the duodenal iron transporter DMT1 which is also a physiologically relevant copper transporter and the Menkes copper ATPase (MNK protein, Atp7a) on the basolateral membrane of enterocytes under low iron conditions [1, 2, 13].

It has been shown that increased copper absorption induced by ID might contribute to IDA [12] due to known antagonistic competition between copper and iron at the level of DMT1 [4, 8]. Moreover, higher serum copper concentrations are related to high levels of serum ceruloplasmin which, because of the antagonism with zinc, lowers zinc to copper (Zn : Cu) ratio. This is known to increase hemolysis and peroxidation of erythrocytes and thereby promotes anemia [7, 43]. Therefore, higher serum levels of copper in II group of patients and relatively high although in the reference range serum levels of copper in IB group may be considered as an important contributing factor for IDA.

In addition, imbalance of erythrocyte and serum copper was observed in II group of children with IDA with significant increase of its concentration in the blood serum, but copper deficiency in red blood cells (Table 2). It is known that erythrocyte deficiency of copper impairs incorporation of iron into the haem structure [43].

The serum concentrations of chromium were found to be lower than the reference values in 73% of children with IDA in I group. Other researchers [17] have also discovered significantly lower concentrations of chromium in blood of anaemic patients when compared to control subjects. Chromium is considered synergistic to iron and its deficiency can lead to ID [4]. For the rest 27% of patients with IDA in I group, serum chromium concentrations within the reference values were found. This is explained by the fact that besides being synergistic, chromium can be antagonistic to iron due to competition for binding to apotransferrin. Significantly reduced uptake of iron by serum transferrin has been observed in the presence of chromium [4, 19]. Therefore, in these children, serum chromium levels found may be associated with negative influence of chromium on iron metabolism, thus contributing to the aetiology of IDA.

Both cobalt and nickel mean serum concentrations in our study were found to be significantly lower in children with IDA than healthy controls ($P < 0.05$). Cobalt and nickel play important roles in the processes of erythropoiesis. It has been shown that both metals stimulate erythropoietin production by activation of the transcription factor hypoxia-inducible factor 1α (HIF-1α). Cobalt influences DNA synthesis accelerating maturation of erythroid stem cells and stimulates haemoglobin synthesis [21, 45]. Nickel is considered synergistic to iron by promoting its intestinal absorption and nickel deficiency can lead to ID and anaemia [4, 17, 46]. Therefore, deficiencies of both trace elements might be a contributing factor for development of IDA in our study.

However, it is difficult to identify the contribution factors explaining these results because although serum levels of cobalt and nickel were found to be lower than the control subjects, they were within the reference values. It has been shown that the intestinal absorption of iron, cobalt, and nickel is mediated by a common transport mechanism, DMT1 [2, 47], which is known to be upregulated by ID [2, 13]. It has been found, however, that transport capacity for cobalt and nickel was lower than the iron because of a higher binding constant and lower exchange rate for both metals as compared with iron. This probably not only results in suppressed duodenal uptake of iron but also explains lower levels of cobalt and nickel which we observed in children with IDA [21].

We also found that dietary factors and malabsorption may be regarded as associated with lower serum concentrations of cobalt and nickel in our patients with IDA. Important dietary sources of cobalt are animal tissues or products, such as meat, eggs, and dairy products, which were found to be scarce in the diet of the children with IDA. High dietary intake of cow's milk, frequently observed in children of infancy and early childhood, and found as a common dietary pattern in our patients with IDA, does not obligatory provide sufficient intake of cobalt because of the known geochemical cobalt deficiency. As cow's milk has low nickel content and contains factors inhibiting nickel absorption, cow's milk-based dietary patterns observed in our study may be a possible reason for lower serum levels of nickel discovered. Intestinal malabsorption, found in certain patients with IDA, is also known as contributing to low cobalt and nickel content in the organism [48–50].

5. Conclusion

Through the present study including investigation of trace element status, we expand the aetiology of IDA. Data obtained can be used for developing a diagnostic algorithm for IDA.

Low serum trace element concentrations of zinc, copper, cobalt, and nickel, mainly due to inadequate dietary intake, malabsorption problems, and trace element interactions, were found in both studied groups (I and II groups) of children with IDA.

Profiles of trace elements iron and zinc in blood serum do not differ in the two examined groups by the means of two analytical methods applied. Increased serum concentrations of copper in II group in comparison to control subjects are probably due to metabolic changes resulting from adaptation mechanisms in IDA.

Dietary insufficiencies of micronutrients, as well as low concentrations of trace elements in blood serum, are common in children with IDA under 3 years of age. However, mechanisms for metabolic interactions between trace elements based on transport and storage molecules are not clearly investigated yet. Micronutrient deficiency in patients with IDA can lead to the formation of so-called related functional iron deficiency. In this case, it is considered that molecular mechanisms provided by trace elements responsible for iron absorption and transport and further included in haem structure are probably impaired. This could lead to low efficiency of the monotherapy by iron supplements.

High prevalence of nutrition-related disorders in trace element status under conditions of IDA indicates the need to develop and implement appropriate intervention strategies for prevention and control of micronutrient deficiencies—supplementation, fortification, and dietary diversification/modification.

Conflict of Interests

The authors declare that there is no conflict of interests regarding the publication of this paper.

Acknowledgments

This study was performed with financial support from the Medical University, Pleven, Bulgaria, and Sumy State University, Ukraine.

References

[1] P. N. Ranganathan, Y. Lu, L. Jiang, C. Kim, and J. F. Collins, "Serum ceruloplasmin protein expression and activity increases in Iron-deficient rats and is further enhanced by higher dietary copper intake," *Blood*, vol. 118, no. 11, pp. 3146–3153, 2011.

[2] E. Bárány, I. A. Bergdahl, L.-E. Bratteby et al., "Iron status influences trace element levels in human blood and serum," *Environmental Research*, vol. 98, no. 2, pp. 215–223, 2005.

[3] J. W. Choi and S. K. Kim, "Relationships of lead, copper, zinc, and cadmium levels versus hematopoiesis and Iron parameters in healthy adolescents," *Annals of Clinical and Laboratory Science*, vol. 35, no. 4, pp. 428–434, 2005.

[4] D. L. Watts, "The nutritional relationships of Iron," *Journal of Orthomolecular Medicine*, vol. 3, no. 3, pp. 110–116, 1988.

[5] World Health Organization, "Environmental health criteria 221: Zinc," Tech. Rep., World Health Organization, Geneva, Switzerland, 2001.

[6] World Health Organization, "Environmental health criteria 200: Copper," Tech. Rep., World Health Organization, Geneva, Switzerland, 1998.

[7] M. Olivares, E. Hertrampf, and R. Uauy, "Copper and zinc interactions in anemia: a public health perspective," in *Nutritional Anemia*, K. Kraemer and M. B. Zimmermann, Eds., pp. 99–109, Sight and Life Press, Basel, Switzerland, 2007.

[8] M. Wajeunnesa, N. Begum, S. Ferdousi, S. Akhter, and S. B. Quarishi, "Serum Zinc and Copper in Iron deficient adolescents," *Journal of Bangladesh Society of Physiologist*, vol. 4, no. 2, pp. 77–80, 2009.

[9] M. K. Gürgöze, A. Ölcücü, A. D. Aygün, E. Taskin, and M. Kilic, "Serum and hair levels of Zinc, Selenium, Iron, and Copper in children with Iron-deficiency anemia," *Biological Trace Element Research*, vol. 111, no. 1–3, pp. 23–29, 2006.

[10] A. Ece, B. S. Uyanik, A. Işcan, P. Ertan, and M. R. Yiğitoğlu, "Increased serum Copper and decreased serum Zinc levels in children with Iron deficiency anemia," *Biological Trace Element Research*, vol. 59, no. 1–3, pp. 31–39, 1997.

[11] C. R. Cole, F. K. Grant, E. D. Swaby-Ellis et al., "Zinc and Iron deficiency and their interrelations in low-income African American and Hispanic children in Atlanta," *American Journal of Clinical Nutrition*, vol. 91, no. 4, pp. 1027–1034, 2010.

[12] S. Turgut, A. Polat, M. Inan et al., "Interaction between anemia and blood levels of Iron, Zinc, Copper, Cadmium and Lead in children," *Indian Journal of Pediatrics*, vol. 74, no. 9, pp. 827–830, 2007.

[13] S. Turgut, S. Hacioğlu, G. Emmungil, G. Turgut, and A. Keskin, "Relations between Iron deficiency anemia and serum levels of Copper, Zinc, Cadmium and Lead," *Polish Journal of Environmental Studies*, vol. 18, no. 2, pp. 273–277, 2009.

[14] A. A. Hegazy, M. M. Zaher, M. A. Abd El-Hafez, A. A. Morsy, and R. A. Saleh, "Relation between anemia and blood levels of Lead, Copper, Zinc and Iron among children," *BMC Research Notes*, vol. 3, article 133, 2010.

[15] V. De la Cruz-Gongora, B. Gaona, S. Villalpando, T. Shamah-Levy, and R. Robledo, "Anemia and Iron, Zinc, Copper and Magnesium deficiency in Mexican adolescents: National Health and Nutrition Survey 2006," *Salud Publica Mex*, vol. 54, no. 2, pp. 135–145, 2012.

[16] S. S. Gropper, D. M. Bader-Crowe, L. S. McAnulty, B. D. White, and R. E. Keith, "Non-anemic Iron depletion, oral Iron supplementation and indices of Copper status in college-aged females," *Journal of the American College of Nutrition*, vol. 21, no. 6, pp. 545–552, 2002.

[17] F. Shah, T. G. Kazi, H. I. Afridi et al., "Evaluation of status of trace and toxic metals in biological samples (scalp hair, blood, and urine) of normal and anemic children of two age groups," *Biological Trace Element Research*, vol. 141, no. 1–3, pp. 131–149, 2011.

[18] M. A. Knovich, D. Il'yasova, A. Ivanova, and I. Molnár, "The association between serum Copper and anaemia in the adult Second National Health and Nutrition Examination Survey (NHANES II) population," *British Journal of Nutrition*, vol. 99, no. 6, pp. 1226–1229, 2008.

[19] M. Ani and A. A. Moshtaghie, "The effect of chromium on parameters related to Iron metabolism," *Biological Trace Element Research*, vol. 32, pp. 57–64, 1992.

[20] H. C. Lukaski, W. W. Bolonchuk, W. A. Siders, and D. B. Milne, "Chromium supplementation and resistance training: effects on body composition, strength, and trace element status of men," *American Journal of Clinical Nutrition*, vol. 63, no. 6, pp. 954–965, 1996.

[21] P. Maxwell and K. Salnikow, "HIF-1: an Oxygen and metal responsive transcription factor," *Cancer Biology and Therapy*, vol. 3, no. 1, pp. 29–35, 2004.

[22] World Health Organization, *Iron Deficiency Anemia: Assessment, Prevention, and Control—A Guide for Program Managers*, World Health Organization, Geneva, Switzerland, 2001.

[23] L. L. Stookey, "Ferrozine—a new spectrophotometric reagent for Iron," *Analytical Chemistry*, vol. 42, no. 7, pp. 779–781, 1970.

[24] R. Soomro, M. J. Ahmed, and N. Memon, "Simple and rapid spectrophotometric determination of trace level chromium using bis (salicylaldehyde) orthophenylenediamine in nonionic micellar media," *Turkish Journal of Chemistry*, vol. 35, no. 1, pp. 155–170, 2011.

[25] F. W. Sunderman Jr., A. Marzouk, M. C. Crisostomo, and D. R. Weatherby, "Electrothermal atomic absorption spectrophotometry of nickel in tissue homogenates," *Annals of Clinical and Laboratory Science*, vol. 15, no. 4, pp. 299–307, 1985.

[26] B. Brzozowska and T. Zawadzka, "Atomic absorption spectrophotometry method for determination of Lead, Cadmium, Zinc and Copper in various vegetable products," *Roczniki Panstwowego Zakladu Higieny*, vol. 32, no. 1, pp. 9–15, 1981.

[27] C. Brugnara, "Refernce values in infancy and childhood," in *Nathan and Oski's Hematology of Infancy and Childhood*, S. H. Orkin and D. G. Nathan, Eds., p. 1774, Elsevier Saunders, 7th edition, 2009.

[28] B. Glader, "The anemias," in *Nelson Textbook of Pediatrics*, R. M. Kliegman, R. E. Behrman, H. B. Jenson, and B. F. Stanton, Eds., p. 2003, Elsevier Saunders, Philadelphia, Pa, USA, 18th edition, 2007.

[29] N. C. Andrews, C. K. Ullrich, and M. D. Fleming, "Disorders of Iron metabolism and sideroblastic anemia," in *Nathan and Oski's Hematology of Infancy and Childhood*, S. H. Orkin and D. G. Nathan, Eds., Elsevier Saunders, 7th edition, 2009.

[30] G. Hetet, I. Devaux, N. Soufir, B. Grandchamp, and C. Beaumont, "Molecular analyses of patients with hyperferritinemia and normal serum Iron values reveal both L ferritin IRE and 3 new ferroportin (slc11A3) mutations," *Blood*, vol. 102, no. 5, pp. 1904–1910, 2003.

[31] M. A. Akl, "Spectrophotometric and AAS determinations of trace zinc(II) in natural waters and human blood after preconcentration with phenanthraquinone monophenylthiosemicarbazone," *Analytical Sciences*, vol. 17, no. 4, pp. 561–564, 2001.

[32] R. S. Gibson, *Principles of Nutritional Assessment*, Oxford University, New York, NY, USA, 2nd edition, 2005.

[33] J. B. Mason, "Chapter 237: vitamins, trace minerals, and other micronutrients," in *Cecil Medicine*, L. Goldman and D. Ausiello, Eds., Elsevier Saunders, Philadelphia, Pa, USA, 23rd edition, 2007.

[34] D. E. Leavelle, Ed., *Mayo Medical Laboratories Interpretive Handbook: Interpretive Data for Diagnostic Laboratory Tests*, The Laboratories, Rochester, Vt, USA, 2001.

[35] World Health Organization, "Environmental health criteria 108: Nickel," Tech. Rep., World Health Organization, Geneva, Switzerland, 1991.

[36] R. J. Stoltzfus, L. Mullany, and R. E. Black, "Iron deficiency anaemia," in *Comparative Quantification of Health Risks. Global and Regional Burden of Disease Attribution To Selected Major Risk Factors*, M. Ezzati, A. D. Lopez, A. Rodgers, and C. J. L. Murray, Eds., pp. 164–165, World Health Organization, Geneva, Switzerland, 2004.

[37] I. Voskaki, V. Arvanitidou, H. Athanasopoulou, A. Tzagkaraki, G. Tripsianis, and A. Giannoulia-Karantana, "Serum Copper and Zinc levels in healthy Greek children and their parents," *Biological Trace Element Research*, vol. 134, no. 2, pp. 136–145, 2010.

[38] International Zinc Nutrition Consultative Group (IZiNCG), K. H. Brown, J. A. Rivera et al., "International Zinc Nutrition Consultative Group (IZiNCG) technical document #1. Assessment of the risk of zinc deficiency in populations and options for its control," *Food and Nutrition Bulletin*, vol. 25, no. 1, supplement 2, pp. S99–S203, 2004.

[39] M. Kaji and Y. Nishi, "Growth and minerals: Zinc," *Growth, Genetics & Hormones (GGH)*, vol. 22, no. 1, pp. 1–10, 2006.

[40] A. Taylor, E. W. Redworth, and J. B. Morgan, "Influence of diet on Iron, Copper, and Zinc status in children under 24 months of age," *Biological Trace Element Research*, vol. 97, no. 3, pp. 197–214, 2004.

[41] R. S. Gibson, Y. Abebe, S. Stabler et al., "Zinc, gravida, infection, and Iron, but not vitamin B-12 or folate status, predict hemoglobin during pregnancy in Southern Ethiopia," *Journal of Nutrition*, vol. 138, no. 3, pp. 581–586, 2008.

[42] M. Olivares and R. Uauy, "Copper as an essential nutrient," *American Journal of Clinical Nutrition*, vol. 63, no. 5, pp. 791S–796S, 1996.

[43] B. A. Hayton, H. E. Broome, and R. C. Lilenbaum, "Copper deficiency-induced anemia and neutropenia secondary to intestinal malabsorption," *American Journal of Hematology*, vol. 48, no. 1, pp. 45–47, 1995.

[44] R. J. Cousins and R. J. McMahon, "Integrative aspects of Zinc transporters," *Journal of Nutrition*, vol. 130, no. 5, pp. 1384S–1387S, 2000.

[45] Y. Gluhcheva, V. Atanasov, J. Ivanova, and M. Mitewa, "Cobalt-induced changes in the spleen of mice from different stages of development," *Journal of Toxicology and Environmental Health A*, vol. 75, no. 22-23, pp. 1418–1422, 2012.

[46] M. Anke, B. Groppel, H. Kronemann, and M. Grün, "Nickel—an essential element," *IARC Scientific Publications*, no. 53, pp. 339–365, 1984.

[47] M. Muñoz, I. Villar, and J. A. García-Erce, "An update on Iron physiology," *World Journal of Gastroenterology*, vol. 15, no. 37, pp. 4617–4626, 2009.

[48] B. Glader, "Anemias of inadequate production," in *Nelson Textbook of Pediatrics*, R. M. Kliegman, R. E. Behrman, H. B. Jenson, and B. F. Stanton, Eds., p. 2013, Elsevier Saunders, Philadelphia, Pa, USA, 18th edition, 2007.

[49] "FAO/WHO expert consultation on human vitamin and mineral requirements," in *Human Vitamin and Mineral Requirements*, Food and Nutrition Division FAO, Rome, Italy, 2001.

[50] A. D. Sharma, "Low nickel diet in dermatology," *Indian Journal of Dermatology*, vol. 58, no. 3, pp. 240–247, 2013.

Permissions

The contributors of this book come from diverse backgrounds, making this book a truly international effort. This book will bring forth new frontiers with its revolutionizing research information and detailed analysis of the nascent developments around the world.

We would like to thank all the contributing authors for lending their expertise to make the book truly unique. They have played a crucial role in the development of this book. Without their invaluable contributions this book wouldn't have been possible. They have made vital efforts to compile up to date information on the varied aspects of this subject to make this book a valuable addition to the collection of many professionals and students.

This book was conceptualized with the vision of imparting up-to-date information and advanced data in this field. To ensure the same, a matchless editorial board was set up. Every individual on the board went through rigorous rounds of assessment to prove their worth. After which they invested a large part of their time researching and compiling the most relevant data for our readers.

The editorial board has been involved in producing this book since its inception. They have spent rigorous hours researching and exploring the diverse topics which have resulted in the successful publishing of this book. They have passed on their knowledge of decades through this book. To expedite this challenging task, the publisher supported the team at every step. A small team of assistant editors was also appointed to further simplify the editing procedure and attain best results for the readers.

Apart from the editorial board, the designing team has also invested a significant amount of their time in understanding the subject and creating the most relevant covers. They scrutinized every image to scout for the most suitable representation of the subject and create an appropriate cover for the book.

The publishing team has been an ardent support to the editorial, designing and production team. Their endless efforts to recruit the best for this project, has resulted in the accomplishment of this book. They are a veteran in the field of academics and their pool of knowledge is as vast as their experience in printing. Their expertise and guidance has proved useful at every step. Their uncompromising quality standards have made this book an exceptional effort. Their encouragement from time to time has been an inspiration for everyone.

The publisher and the editorial board hope that this book will prove to be a valuable piece of knowledge for researchers, students, practitioners and scholars across the globe.

List of Contributors

J. A. Wright and T. Richards
Department of Vascular Surgery, Royal Free and University College Hospitals, London, UK

M. J. Oddy
Department of Orthopaedic Surgery, University College Hospital, London, UK

Gerardo Alvarez-Uria, Praveen K. Naik, Manoranjan Midde, Pradeep S. Yalla and Raghavakalyan Pakam
Department of Infectious Diseases, Bathalapalli Rural Development Trust Hospital, Kadiri Road, Bathalapalli, Anantapur District, Andhra Pradesh 515661, India

Zeina A. Salman
Center for Hereditary Blood Diseases, Basra Maternity and Children Hospital, Basra, Iraq

Meaad K. Hassan
Center for Hereditary Blood Diseases, Basra Maternity and Children Hospital, Basra, Iraq
Department of Pediatrics, College of Medicine, University of Basra, Basra, Iraq

Mohamed ElMissiry, Mohamed Hamed Hussein, Sadaf Khalid, Cornelio Uderzo and Lawrence Faulkner
Cure2Children Foundation, Via Marconi 30, 50131 Florence, Italy

Naila Yaqub, Sarah Khan and Fatima Itrat
Children's Hospital Pakistan Institute of Medical Sciences, Islamabad, Pakistan

Abu Syed Mohammed Mujib, Abu Sayeed Mohammad Mahmud and Milton Halder
Industrial Microbiology Research Division, Bangladesh Council of Scientific and Industrial Research, Chittagong 4220, Bangladesh

Chowdhury Mohammad Monirul Hasan
Department of Biochemistry and Molecular Biology, University of Chittagong, Chittagong 4331, Bangladesh

Jéssica Barbieri
Regional University of Northwestern Rio Grande do Sul (UNIJUÍ), Ijuí, RS, Brazil

Paula Caitano Fontela
Program in Respiratory Sciences, the Federal University of Rio Grande do Sul (UFRGS), Porto Alegre, RS, Brazil

Eliane Roseli Winkelmann
Department of Life Sciences, the Regional University of Northwestern Rio Grande do Sul (UNIJUÍ), Rua do Comércio No. 3000, Bairro Universitário, 98700 000 Ijuí, RS, Brazil

Program in Integral Attention to Health (PPGAIS-UNIJUI/UNICRUZ), Ijuí, RS, Brazil

Carine Eloise Prestes Zimmermann
Program in Pharmacology of the Health Sciences Center, The Federal University of Santa Maria (UFSM), RS, Brazil
Cenecista Institute for Higher Education, Rua Dr. João Augusto Rodrigues 471, 98801 015 Santo Ângelo, RS, Brazil

Yana Picinin Sandri
Program in Integral Attention to Health (PPGAIS-UNIJUI/UNICRUZ), Ijuí, RS, Brazil
Cenecista Institute for Higher Education, Rua Dr. João Augusto Rodrigues 471, 98801 015 Santo Ângelo, RS, Brazil

Emanelle Kerber Viera Mallet
Cenecista Institute for Higher Education, Rua Dr. João Augusto Rodrigues 471, 98801 015 Santo Ângelo, RS, Brazil

Matias Nunes Frizzo
Department of Life Sciences, the Regional University of Northwestern Rio Grande do Sul (UNIJUÍ), Rua do Comércio No. 3000, Bairro Universitário, 98700 000 Ijuí, RS, Brazil
Cenecista Institute for Higher Education, Rua Dr. João Augusto Rodrigues 471, 98801 015 Santo Ângelo, RS, Brazil

Samuel Olufemi Akodu, Olisamedua Fidelis Njokanma and Omolara Adeolu Kehinde
Department of Paediatrics, Lagos State University Teaching Hospital, P.O. Box 11950, Ikeja, Lagos 100001, Nigeria

Gebremedhin Gebreegziabiher
Department of Public Health, College of Health Science, Adigrat University, P.O. Box 50, Adigrat, Ethiopia

Belachew Etana and Daniel Niggusie
School of Public Health, College of Health Science, Mekelle University, P.O. Box 1871, Mekelle, Ethiopia

Gayashan Chathuranga and Thushara Balasuriya
Medical Laboratory Sciences Unit, Department of Allied Health Sciences, Faculty of Medical Sciences, University of Sri Jayewardenepura, Gangodawila, 10250 Nugegoda, Sri Lanka

Rasika Perera
Department of Biochemistry, Faculty of Medical Sciences, University of Sri Jayewardenepura, Gangodawila, 10250 Nugegoda, Sri Lanka

Hylemariam Mihiretie
Department of Medical Laboratory Sciences, Faculty of Medical and Health Sciences,Wollega University, P.O. Box 395, Nekemte, Ethiopia
Department of Medical Laboratory Sciences, School of Allied Health Sciences, College of Health Science, Addis Ababa University, P.O. Box 1176, Addis Ababa, Ethiopia

Bineyam Taye and Aster Tsegaye
Department of Medical Laboratory Sciences, School of Allied Health Sciences, College of Health Science, Addis Ababa University, P.O. Box 1176, Addis Ababa, Ethiopia

Omar Maoujoud
Research Team of Pharmacoepidemiology & Pharmacoeconomics, Medical and Pharmacy School, Mohammed V University, Madinat Al Irfane, 10000 Rabat, Morocco
Department ofNephrology&Dialysis,MilitaryHospital Agadir, 20450 Agadir, Morocco

Samir Ahid and Yahia Cherrah
Research Team of Pharmacoepidemiology & Pharmacoeconomics, Medical and Pharmacy School, Mohammed V University, Madinat Al Irfane, 10000 Rabat, Morocco

Hocein Dkhissi
Meknes Dialysis Center (on Behalf of Moroccan Society of Nephrology), 33150 Meknes, Morocco

Zouhair Oualim
IdrissAlakbar Dialysis Center (on Behalf of the Scientific Committee, Moroccan Society of Nephrology), 12470 Rabat, Morocco

Kefyalew Addis Alene
Institute of Public Health, College of Medicine and Health Sciences, University of Gondar, P.O. Box 196, Gondar, Ethiopia

Abdulahi Mohamed Dohe
Somali Regional Health Bureau, P.O. Box 238, Jijiga, Ethiopia

Arun Kumar Aggarwal, Jaya Prasad Tripathy, Deepak Sharma and Ajith Prabhu
School of Public Health, Postgraduate Institute of Medical Education and Resear ch, Chandigarh 160012, India

Leeniyagala Gamaralalage, Thamal Darshana and Deepthi Inoka Uluwaduge
Medical Laboratory Sciences Unit, Department of Allied Health Sciences, Faculty of Medical Sciences, University of Sri Jayewardenepura, Gangodawila, Nugegoda 10250, Sri Lanka

Aysel Vehapoglu, Ayşegul Dogan Demir, Selcuk Uzuner and Mustafa Atilla Nursoy
Department of Pediatrics, School of Medicine, Bezmialem Vakif University, 34093 Istanbul, Turkey

Gamze Ozgurhan
Department of Pediatrics, Suleymaniye Obstetrics and Gynecology Hospital, 34010 Istanbul, Turkey

Serdar Turkmen
Department of Biochemistry, Istanbul Training and Research Hospital, 34098 Istanbul, Turkey

Arzu Kacan
Department of Pediatrics, Istanbul Training and Research Hospital, Istanbul, Turkey

Mulugeta Melku
Department of Hematology, School of Biomedical and Laboratory Sciences, College of Medicine and Health Sciences, University of Gondar, P.O. Box 196, 6200 Gondar, Ethiopia

Zelalem Addis
Department of Medical Microbiology, School of Biomedical and Laboratory Sciences, College of Medicine and Health Sciences, University of Gondar, 6200 Gondar, Ethiopia

Meseret Alem
Department of Immunology and Molecular Biology, School of Biomedical and Laboratory Sciences, College of Medicine and Health Sciences, University of Gondar, 6200 Gondar, Ethiopia

Bamlaku Enawgaw
Department of Hematology, School of Biomedical and Laboratory Sciences, College of Medicine and Health Sciences, University of Gondar, 6200 Gondar, Ethiopia

Peter C. Kurniali
Department of Medicine, RogerWilliams Medical Center, Providence, RI, USA
Department of Medicine, Boston University School of Medicine, Boston, MA, USA
Division of Hematology Oncology, Michigan State University and Breslin Cancer Center, 401W. Greenlawn Avenue, Lansing, MI 48910, USA

Stephanie Curry, KeithW. Brennan and Elise McCormack
Department of Medicine, RogerWilliams Medical Center, Providence, RI, USA
Department of Medicine, Boston University School of Medicine, Boston, MA, USA

Kim Velletri
Department of Medicine, RogerWilliams Medical Center, Providence, RI, USA

Mohammed Shaik and Kenneth A. Schwartz
Division of Hematology Oncology, Michigan State University and Breslin Cancer Center, 401W. Greenlawn Avenue, Lansing, MI 48910, USA

Tabea Geisel and JuliaMartin
Crohn Colitis Center Rhein-Main, 60594 Frankfurt/Main, Germany

Institute of Nutritional Science, University of Giessen, 35392 Giessen, Germany

Bettina Schulze and Matthias Bach
St. Elisabethen Krankenhaus, 60487 Frankfurt/Main, Germany

Roland Schaefer
Krankenhaus Sachsenhausen, Teaching Hospital of the J.W. von Goethe University Frankfurt/Main, 60594 Frankfurt/Main, Germany

Garth Virgin
Vifor Pharma Deutschland GmbH, 81379 Munich, Germany

Jürgen Stein
Crohn Colitis Center Rhein-Main, 60594 Frankfurt/Main, Germany
Institute of Nutritional Science, University of Giessen, 35392 Giessen, Germany
Department of Gastroenterology and Nutritional Medicine, Krankenhaus Sachsenhausen, Teaching Hospital of the J.W. von Goethe University Frankfurt/Main, 60594 Frankfurt/Main, Germany

Todd A. Koch
Luitpold Pharmaceuticals, Inc., Norristown, PA 19403, USA

Jennifer Myers
St. John's University, Jamaica, NY 11439, USA

Lawrence Tim Goodnough
Department of Pathology and Medicine (Hematology), Stanford, CA 94305, USA

Betelihem Terefe
Department of Hematology and Immunohematology, University of Gondar, Gondar, Ethiopia

Asaye Birhanu and Aster Tsegaye
School of Medical Laboratory Science, Addis Ababa University, Addis Ababa, Ethiopia

Paulos Nigussie
Ethiopian Health and Nutrition Research Institute (EHNRI), Addis Ababa, Ethiopia

Arch G. Mainous III
Department of Health Services Research,Management and Policy, University of Florida, P.O. Box 100195, Gainesville, FL 32610, USA
Department of Community Health and Family Medicine, University of Florida, P.O. Box 100237, Gainesville, FL 32610-0237, USA

Rebecca J. Tanner and Christopher A. Harle
Department of Health Services Research,Management and Policy, University of Florida, P.O. Box 100195, Gainesville, FL 32610, USA

Richard Baker
Department of Health Sciences, University of Leicester, 22-28 Princess RoadWest, Leicester LE1 6TP, UK

Navkiran K. Shokar
Department of Family and Community Medicine, Texas Tech University Health Science Center at El Paso, 9849 Kenworthy Street, El Paso, TX 79924, USA

Mary M. Hulihan
Division of Blood Disorders, CDC, National Center on Birth Defects and Developmental Disabilities, Mail-Stop E87, 1600 Clifton Road, Atlanta, GA 30333, USA

Matthias Bach and Bettina Schulze
St. Elisabethen Krankenhaus, 60487 Frankfurt/Main, Germany

Tabea Geisel and JuliaMartin
Interdisciplinary Crohn Colitis Centre Rhein-Main, 60594 Frankfurt/Main, Germany
Institute of Nutritional Science, University of Giessen, 35392 Giessen, Germany

Roland Schaefer
Krankenhaus Sachsenhausen, Teaching Hospital of the J.W. Goethe University, 60594 Frankfurt/Main, Germany

Garth Virgin
Vifor Pharma Deutschland GmbH, 81379 Munich, Germany

Juergen Stein
Interdisciplinary Crohn Colitis Centre Rhein-Main, 60594 Frankfurt/Main, Germany
Institute of Nutritional Science, University of Giessen, 35392 Giessen, Germany
Gastroenterology and Clinical Nutrition, Krankenhaus Sachsenhausen, Teaching Hospital of the J.W. Goethe University, 60594 Frankfurt/Main, Germany

Alemayehu Bekele and Aleme Mekuria
Department of Public Health Nursing, Arba Minch College of Health Sciences, P.O. Box 155, Arba Minch, Ethiopia

Marelign Tilahun
Department of Public Health, College of Health Sciences, Debre Tabor University, P.O. Box 272, Debre Tabor, Ethiopia

Oseni Bashiru Shola and Fakoya Olatunde Olugbenga
Department of Biomedical Sciences, Faculty of Basic Medical Sciences, College of Health Sciences, Ladoke Akintola University of Technology, Ogbomosho 210214, Oyo State, Nigeria

L. O. Ngolet, Innocent Kocko, Alexis Elira Dokekias and Georges Marius Moyen
Clinical HematologyUnit, Brazzaville Teaching Hospital, Auxence Ickonga Avenue, P.O. Box 32, Brazzaville, Congo

M. Moyen Engoba
Pediatric Intensive Care Unit, Brazzaville Teaching Hospital, Brazzaville, Congo

Jean-Vivien Mombouli
National Laboratory of Public Health, Brazzaville Teaching Hospital, Brazzaville, Congo

Ademola Samson Adewoyin
Department of Haematology and Blood Transfusion, University of Benin Teaching Hospital, PMB 1111, Benin City, Edo State, Nigeria

S. Rouhi Dehnabeh and S. Khatami
Biochemistry Department, Pasteur Institute of Iran, Pasteur Street, No. 69, Tehran 1316943551, Iran

R. Mahdian
Molecular Medicine Department, Pasteur Institute of Iran, Pasteur Street, No. 69, Tehran 1316943551, Iran

S. Ajdary
Immunology Department, Pasteur Institute of Iran, Pasteur Street, No. 69, Tehran 1316943551, Iran

E. Mostafavi
Department of Epidemiology, Pasteur Institute of Iran, Pasteur Street, No. 69, Tehran 1316943551, Iran

Tilman Steinmetz
Outpatient Clinic for Hematology and Oncology, Sachsenring 69, 50677 Cologne, Germany

Jan Schröder
Outpatient Clinic for Oncology, Kettwiger Strasse 62, 45468 M˙ulheim an der Ruhr, Germany

Margarete Plath
Outpatient Clinic for Oncology, Prinzregentenstrasse 1, 86150 Augsburg, Germany

Hartmut Link
Department for Internal Medicine I, Westpfalz-Klinikum, Hellmut-Hartert-Strasse 1, 67655 Kaiserslautern, Germany

Michèle Vogt and Melanie Frank
iOMEDICO, Hanferstrasse 28, 79108 Freiburg, Germany

Norbert Marschner
Outpatient Clinic for Interdisciplinary Oncology and Hematology, Wirthstrasse 11c, 79110 Freiburg, Germany

Poramed Winichakoon, Adisak Tantiworawit, Thanawat Rattanathammethee, Sasinee Hantrakool, Chatree Chai-Adisaksopha, Ekarat Rattarittamrong and Lalita Norasetthada
Division of Hematology, Department of Internal Medicine, Faculty of Medicine, Chiang Mai University, 110 Intravaroros Road, A. Muang, Chiang Mai 50200, Thailand

Pimlak Charoenkwan
Division of Hematology and Oncology, Department of Pediatrics, Faculty of Medicine, Chiang Mai University, 110 Intravaroros Road, A. Muang, Chiang Mai 50200, Thailand

Taddese Alemu
Center of Food Science and Nutrition, College of Natural Sciences, Addis Ababa University, P.O. Box 1196, Addis Ababa, Ethiopia

Melaku Umeta
Department of Biochemistry, College of Medical Sciences, Addis Ababa University, P.O. Box 1196, Addis Ababa, Ethiopia

Rakesh Kumar Singh and Shraboni Patra
International Institute for Population Sciences, Mumbai 400088, India

Maria Georgieva Angelova and Atanaska Naumova Bozhinova
Department of Chemistry and Biochemistry & Physics and Biophysics, University of Medicine-Pleven, 1 KlimentOhridski Street, 5800 Pleven, Bulgaria

Tsvetelina Valentinova Petkova-Marinova and Vania Nedkova Nedkova-Kolarova
Department of Pediatrics, University of Medicine-Pleven, 1 Kliment Ohridski Street, 5800 Pleven, Bulgaria

Maksym Vladimirovich Pogorielov
Department of Hygiene and Ecology, Sumy State University, Medical Institute, 31 Sanatornaya Street, Sumy 40007, Ukraine

Andrii Nikolaevich Loboda
Department of PediatricswithMedicalGenetics, Sumy StateUniversity,Medical Institute, 31 Sanatornaya Street, Sumy 40007,Ukraine